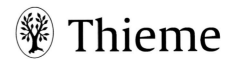

Differential Diagnosis in Ultrasound

A Teaching Atlas

Guenter Schmidt, M.D.
Director
Department of Internal Medicine
Protestant Hospital Kredenbach
Kreuztal, Germany

With contributions by

Barbara Beuscher-Willems, M.W. Max Brandt, Christian Goerg, Lucas Greiner, Christian Jakobeit, Johannes Mueller, Dieter Nuernberg

2397 illustrations

Thieme
Stuttgart · New York

Library of Congress Cataloging-in-Publication Data is available from the publisher.

This book is an authorized, revised and updated translation of the German edition published and copyrighted 2002 by Georg Thieme Verlag, Stuttgart, Germany. Title of the German edition: Sonographische Differenzialdiagnose: Lernatlas zur systematischen Bildanalyse mit über 2500 Befundbeispielen.

Translators: Dietrich Herrmann, M.D., Hameln, Germany; Terry Telger, Fort Worth, TX, USA

© 2006 Georg Thieme Verlag,
Rüdigerstrasse 14, 70469 Stuttgart, Germany
http://www.thieme.de
Thieme New York, 333 Seventh Avenue,
New York, NY 10001 USA
http://www.thieme.com

Typesetting by primustype Hurler GmbH, Notzingen
Printed in Germany by Karl Grammlich GmbH, Pliezhausen
ISBN 3-13-131891-0 (GTV)
ISBN 1-58890-179-3 (TNY)   1 2 3 4 5 6

Important note: Medicine is an ever-changing science undergoing continual development. Research and clinical experience are continually expanding our knowledge, in particular our knowledge of proper treatment and drug therapy. Insofar as this book mentions any dosage or application, readers may rest assured that the authors, editors, and publishers have made every effort to ensure that such references are in accordance with **the state of knowledge at the time of production of the book.**

Nevertheless, this does not involve, imply, or express any guarantee or responsibility on the part of the publishers in respect to any dosage instructions and forms of applications stated in the book. **Every user is requested to examine carefully** the manufacturers' leaflets accompanying each drug and to check, if necessary in consultation with a physician or specialist, whether the dosage schedules mentioned therein or the contraindications stated by the manufacturers differ from the statements made in the present book. Such examination is particularly important with drugs that are either rarely used or have been newly released on the market. Every dosage schedule or every form of application used is entirely at the user's own risk and responsibility. The authors and publishers request every user to report to the publishers any discrepancies or inaccuracies noticed. If errors in this work are found after publication, errata will be posted at www.thieme.com on the product description page.

Some of the product names, patents, and registered designs referred to in this book are in fact registered trademarks or proprietary names even though specific reference to this fact is not always made in the text. Therefore, the appearance of a name without designation as proprietary is not to be construed as a representation by the publisher that it is in the public domain.

This book, including all parts thereof, is legally protected by copyright. Any use, exploitation, or commercialization outside the narrow limits set by copyright legislation, without the publisher's consent, is illegal and liable to prosecution. This applies in particular to photostat reproduction, copying, mimeographing, preparation of microfilms, and electronic data processing and storage.

Preface

The raison d'être for a new textbook in a discipline which has been served by standard works for many years was the initial conviction of Dr. Markus Becker of the Thieme Publishing Group that a distinct need for a modern work on differential diagnosis in ultrasound existed. Realizing full well the time and effort required by such an undertaking, I was reluctant at first. But slowly and steadily the formula or blueprint to be used took shape. I was motivated in this endeavor by the joy sonography holds for me, by the still surprising diagnostic avenues it offers, and by my belief that this incredibly versatile imaging modality should be mastered by all physicians, be it in the hospital or office setting.

Today, as time is more and more of the essence in our daily work, I realize that it will be faster to order a CT scan than to spend my own time on an ultrasound study. Thus, during the early stages of this project numerous concepts were considered and discarded. How much extraneous material should be included? How could we ensure that the reader would come away with maximum knowledge gained in the least amount of time, benefiting daily practice?

The recent explosion of factual knowledge has emphasized the need for a presentation which would provide the reader with an opportunity to assimilate pertinent facts in a logical fashion. The clinical manifestations and diagnostic studies are therefore considered as a reflection of anatomy and pathophysiology. I have deliberately chosen to provide a book which is heavily illustrated since diagnostic ultrasound does not rely on text but on images. The au courant concept is hopefully apparent throughout the entire work and is exemplified by colored text boxes repeating basic tenets and deepening the reader's understanding—as one can only recognize what one knows and understand what one sees. The highlighted sonogram boxes (▣) display variant courses and atypical images or those particularly important in the differential diagnosis of a particular pathology.

As a matter of course, careful sonographic differential diagnosis of special findings has to make use of color flow and spectral Doppler imaging as well. Whenever it is deemed necessary by the clinical issue in question, the reader will find the B-mode images complemented by color flow Doppler sonograms. There is some repetition, since I see this work as providing a reference to the diagnostic study of specific diseases rather than as a book which is likely to be read from cover to cover.

As stated above, the ultimate goal has been to collate a book which is deserving of the adjective "modern." The contributing authors are acknowledged authorities in the areas in which they have written; but, more importantly, they are skilled, experienced teachers of sonography infecting others with their enthusiasm for this modality. Writing chapters is usually a thankless job, with no reward other than being recognized for one's expertise and the satisfaction of contributing to a textbook that has become, by these very efforts, a valuable resource in one's chosen field. Needless to say, I have benefited the most from all these efforts, being given undue credit for the work of so many others. I am deeply indebted to each of them for their numerous ideas in making this a textbook and guide for daily practice. They, together with all their coworkers, are to be commended for their patience in tolerating the countless delays and myriad requests from the editorial office for more, different, or revised information. Special gratitude is also due to the many practitioners of the art—and it is an art—who provided me with sonograms. It is my hope that they all will share my pride in a job well done, that their unselfish efforts will continue to sustain this textbook in the role into which it has grown, and that they will see it as a legacy worth perpetuating with future editions.

Work on the English edition began in 2003 and I owe my deep appreciation to Ms Angelika Findgott, Editor, and Ms Stefanie Langner, Production Manager, of Thieme International who have shouldered the hard work of putting together a thoroughly revised and updated edition with countless new sonograms.

Nine years have passed since I accepted the publisher's and my own self-generated challenge to develop a "new and modern" textbook of differential diagnosis in ultrasound. The favorable reception suggests that we have succeeded. As the landmark of the first English edition is completed, the frustrations and toils are erased and what remains is an immeasurable sense of gratitude.

Guenter Schmidt, M.D.

Contributors

Barbara Beuscher-Willems, M.D.
Director
Klinikum Heilbronn GmbH
Department of Internal Medicine
Bethesda Hospital
Freudenberg, Germany

M.W. Max Brandt, M.D.
Director
St. Marienhospital
Department of Gastroenterology
Wesel, Germany

Christian Goerg, M.D.
Professor
Center for Internal Medicine
Department of Hematology/Oncology
University Hospital
Marburg, Germany

Lucas Greiner, M.D.
Professor and Director
Medical Clinic 2
Municipal Hospitals
Wuppertal, Germany

Christian Jakobeit, M.D.
Associate Professor and Director
Johanniter Hospital
Internal Medicine
Radevormwald, Germany

Johannes Mueller, M.D.
Klinikum Barmen
Medical Clinic A
Wuppertal, Germany

Dieter Nuernberg, M.D.
Associate Professor and Director
Ruppiner Kliniken GmbH
Medical Clinic B
Neuruppin, Germany

Contents

1 Vessels 1

Aorta, Vena Cava, and Peripheral Vessels 3
G. Schmidt

- **Aorta, Arteries 5**
  - Anomalies and Variant Positions 5
  - Dilatation 7
  - Stenosis 11
  - Wall Thickening 16
  - Intraluminal Mass 20
  - Perivascular Mass 22

- **Vena Cava, Veins 25**
  - Anomalies 25
  - Dilatation 26
  - Intraluminal Mass 28
  - Compression, Infiltration 31

Portal Vein and Its Tributaries 33
C. Goerg

- **Enlarged Lumen Diameter 35**
  - Portal Hypertension 35

- **Intraluminal Mass 43**
  - Thrombosis 43
  - Tumor 48

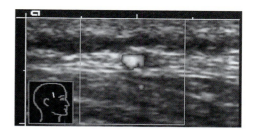

2 Liver 49
M. Brandt

- **Diffuse Changes in the Hepatic Parenchyma 61**
  - Enlarged Liver 62
  - Small Liver 67
  - Homogeneous Hypoechoic Texture 68
  - Homogeneous Hyperechoic Texture 70
  - Regionally Inhomogeneous Texture 71
  - Diffuse Inhomogeneous Texture 72

- **Localized Changes in Hepatic Parenchyma 74**
  - Anechoic Masses 76
  - Hypoechoic Masses 81
  - Isoechoic Masses 87
  - Hyperechoic Masses 89
  - Echodense Masses 94
  - Irregular Masses 97

- **Differential Diagnosis of Focal Lesions 98**
  - Diagnostic Methods 98
  - Suspected Diagnosis 99

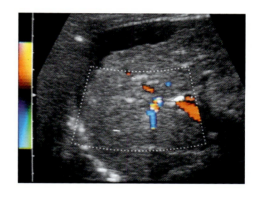

3 Biliary Tree and Gallbladder 101

Biliary Tree 103
L. Greiner and J. Mueller

- **Thickening of the Bile Duct Wall 105**
  - Localized and Diffuse 105

- **Bile Duct Rarefaction 106**
  - Localized and Diffuse 106

- **Bile Duct Dilatation and Intraductal Pressure 107**
  - Intrahepatic 108
  - Hilar and Prepancreatic 109
  - Intrapancreatic 111
  - Papillary 112

- **Abnormal Intraluminal Bile Duct Findings 112**
  - Foreign Body 112

- **Differential Diagnosis of Sonographic Cholestasis 114**
  - The Seven Most Important Questions 114

Gallbladder 119
C. Jakobeit

- **Changes in Size 122**
  - Large Gallbladder (> 10 cm) 122
  - Small/Missing Gallbladder 123

- **Wall Changes 125**
  - General Hypoechogenicity 125
  - General Hyperechogenicity 127
  - Focal Hypoechogenicity/Hyperechogenicity 128
  - General Tumor 129
  - Focal Tumor 131

- **Intraluminal Changes 134**
  - Hyperechoic 134
  - Hypoechoic 134

- **Nonvisualized Gallbladder 137**
L. Greiner and J. Müller
  - Missing Gallbladder 137
  - Obscured Gallbladder 137

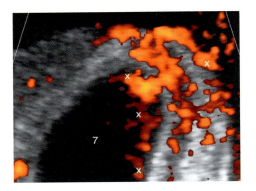

4 Pancreas 141
G. Schmidt

- **Diffuse Pancreatic Change 144**
  - Large Pancreas 144
  - Small Pancreas 145
  - Hypoechoic Texture 147
  - Hyperechoic Texture 148

- **Focal Changes 152**
  - Anechoic Lesion 152
  - Hypoechoic Lesion 154
  - Isoechoic Lesion 158
  - Hyperechoic Lesion 160
  - Irregular Lesion 163

- **Dilatation of the Pancreatic Duct 164**
  - Marginal/Mild Dilatation 166
  - Marked Dilatation 167

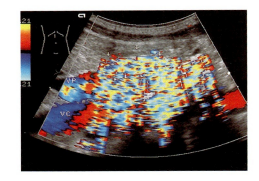

5 Spleen 171
C. Goerg

- **Nonfocal Changes of the Spleen 176**
  - Diffuse Parenchymal Changes 176
  - Large Spleen 177
  - Small Spleen 180

- **Focal Changes 182**
  - Anechoic Mass 182
  - Hypoechoic Mass 184
  - Hyperechoic Mass 193
  - Splenic Calcification 195

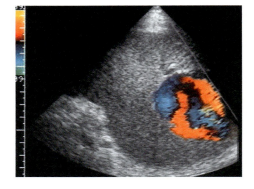

6 Lymph Nodes 197
C. Goerg

- **Peripheral Lymph Nodes 207**
  - Head/Neck 207
  - Extremities (Axilla, Groin) 210

- **Abdominal Lymph Nodes 212**
  - Hepatic Portal 212
  - Splenic Hilum 215

- Mesentery (Celiac, Upper and Lower Mesenteric Station) 216
- Retroperitoneum (Para-aortic, Paracaval, Aortointercaval, and Iliac Station) 219

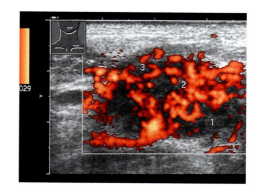

7 Gastrointestinal Tract 223
M. Brandt

- **Stomach 229**
  - Focal Wall Changes 229
  - Extended Wall Changes 232
  - Dilated Lumen 233
  - Narrowed Lumen 234

- **Small/Large Intestine 235**
  - Focal Wall Changes 236
  - Extended Wall Changes 241
  - Dilated Lumen 245
  - Narrowed Lumen 247

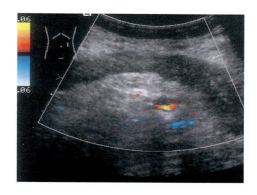

8 Peritoneal Cavity 249
D. Nuernberg

- **Diffuse Changes 254**
  - Anechoic Structure 256
  - Hypoechoic Structure 258
  - Hyperechoic Structure 261

- **Localized Changes 262**
  - Anechoic Structure 263
  - Hypoechoic Structure 264
  - Hyperechoic Structure 265

- **Wall Structures 266**
  - Smooth Margin 266
  - Irregular Margin 267

- **Differentiating Intra- and Extraluminal GI Tract Fluid 269**
  - Intragastric Processes 269
  - Intraintestinal Processes 270

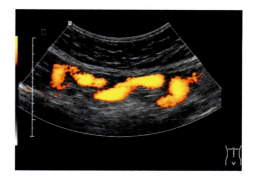

9 Kidneys 273
G. Schmidt

- **Anomalies, Malformations 276**
  - Aplasia, Hypoplasia 276
  - Cystic Malformation 277
  - Anomalies of Number, Position, or Rotation 278
  - Fusion Anomaly 280
  - Collecting System Anomaly 281
  - Vascular Anomaly 281

- **Diffuse Changes 282**
  - Large Kidneys 282
  - Small Kidneys 287

  - Hypoechoic Structure 289
  - Hyperechoic Structure 290
  - Irregular Structure 295

- **Circumscribed Changes 296**
  - Anechoic Structure 296
  - Hypoechoic or Isoechoic Structure 301
  - Complex Structure 307
  - Hyperechoic Structure 309
  - Echogenic Structure 311

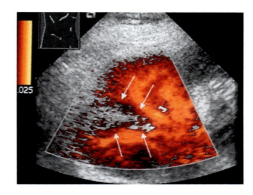

10 Adrenal Glands 315
D. Nuernberg

- **Enlargement** 318
  - Anechoic Structure 318
  - Hypoechoic Structure 320
  - Complex Echo Structure 324
  - Hyperechoic Structure 325

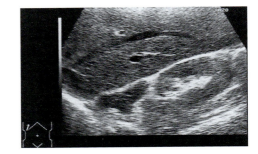

11 Urinary Tract 329
G. Schmidt

- **Malformations** 333
  - Duplication Anomalies 333
  - Dilatations and Stenoses 334

- **Dilated Renal Pelvis and Ureter** 336
  - Anechoic 336
  - Hypoechoic 342

- **Renal Pelvic Mass, Ureteral Mass** 344
  - Hypoechoic 344
  - Hyperechoic 345

- **Changes in Bladder Size or Shape** 348
  - Large Bladder 348
  - Small Bladder 349
  - Altered Bladder Shape 351

- **Intracavitary Mass** 352
  - Hypoechoic 352
  - Hyperechoic 355
  - Echogenic 358

- **Wall Changes** 359
  - Diffuse Wall Thickening 359
  - Circumscribed Wall Thickening 360
  - Concavities and Convexities 362

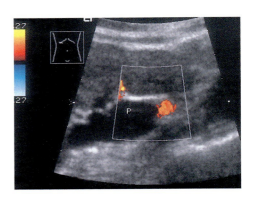

12 Prostate, Seminal Vesicles, Testis, Epididymis 365
G. Schmidt

The Prostate 367

- **Enlarged Prostate** 368
  - Regular 368
  - Irregular 370

- **Small Prostate** 371
  - Regular 371
  - Echogenic 372

- **Circumscribed Lesion** 372
  - Anechoic 372
  - Hypoechoic 373
  - Echogenic 375

Seminal Vesicles 376

- **Diffuse Change** 376
  - Hypoechoic 376

- **Circumscribed Change** 377
  - Anechoic 377
  - Echogenic 378
  - Irregular 378

- **Testis, Epididymis** 379
  - Anatomy and Topography 379

Testis, Epididymis 379

- **Diffuse Change** 380
  - Enlargement 380
  - Decreased Size 381

- **Circumscribed Lesion** 381
  - Anechoic or Hypoechoic 381
  - Irregular 383

- **Epididymal Lesion** 383
  - Anechoic 383
  - Hypoechoic 384

- **Intrascrotal Mass** 385
  - Anechoic or Hypoechoic 385
  - Echogenic 386

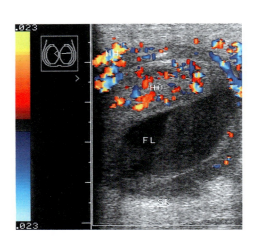

13 Female Genital Tract 387
B. Beuscher-Willems

- **Vagina** 390
  - Masses 390
  - Abnormalities of Size or Shape 391

- **Uterus** 392
  - Abnormalities of Size or Shape 393
  - Myometrial Changes 394
  - Intracavitary Changes 396
  - Endometrial Changes 398

- **Fallopian Tubes** 402
  - Hypoechoic Mass 402

- **Ovaries** 403
  - Anechoic Cystic Mass 404
  - Solid Echogenic or Nonhomogeneous Mass 407

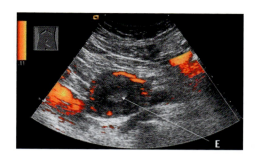

14 Thyroid Gland 415
G. Schmidt

- **Diffuse Changes** 419
  - Enlarged Thyroid Gland 419
  - Small Thyroid Gland 423
  - Hypoechoic Structure 427
  - Hyperechoic Structure 429

- **Circumscribed Changes** 429
  - Anechoic 429
  - Hypoechoic 431
  - Isoechoic 438
  - Hyperechoic 439
  - Irregular 441

- **Differential Diagnosis of Hyperthyroidism** 443
  - Types of Autonomy 443

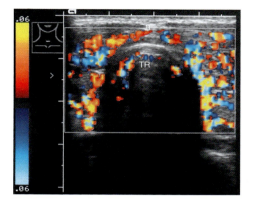

15 Pleura and Chest Wall 447
C. Goerg

- **Chest Wall** 451
  - Masses 451

- **Parietal Pleura** 456
  - Nodular Masses 456
  - Diffuse Pleural Thickening 459

- **Pleural Effusion** 462
  - Anechoic Effusion 463
  - Echogenic Effusion 464
  - Complex Effusion 466

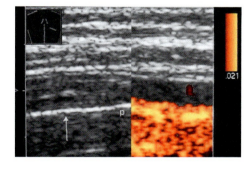

16 Lung 469
C. Goerg

- **Masses** 471
  - Anechoic Masses 472
  - Hypoechoic Masses 474
  - Complex Masses 483

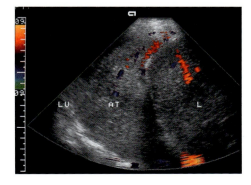

Index 489

1 Vessels

Aorta, Vena Cava, and Peripheral Vessels 1

▼ Aorta, Arteries — 5

▼ Anomalies and Variant Positions — 5
- Situs Inversus
- Aplasia, Hypoplasia, and Duplication of the Aorta
- Coarctation of the Aorta
- Oblique/Transverse Course of the Aorta
- Kinking of the Aorta
- Variant and Duplicated Arteries

▼ Dilatation — 7
- Aortic Ectasia
- True Aneurysms
- Dissecting Aneurysms
- False Aneurysms

▼ Stenosis — 11
- Aortic Stenosis
- Arterial Stenosis
- Aortic/Arterial Embolism
- Arteriosclerotic Aortic/Arterial Occlusion
- Anastomotic/Bypass Stenosis
- Tumor Stenosis/Infiltration

▼ Wall Thickening — 16
- Early Arteriosclerotic Lesions
- Advanced Arteriosclerotic Lesions
- Complex Arteriosclerotic Lesions
- Protruding Arteriosclerotic Lesions
- White Thrombus
- Arteritis
- Mönckeberg Arteriosclerosis
- Synthetic Grafts

▼ Intraluminal Mass — 20
- Aortic/Arterial Embolism
- Protruding Arteriosclerotic Plaques
- White Thrombi
- Endovascular Stent
- Intimal Dissection

▼ Perivascular Mass — 22
- Pseudoaneurysm
- Arteriovenous Fistula/Arteriovenous Malformation
- Suture-line Aneurysm
- Suture-line Breakdown, Graft Infection
- Hematoma, Abscess
- Lymphomas, Metastases
- Retroperitoneal Fibrosis
- Horseshoe Kidney
- Intestinal Loop

▼ Vena Cava, Veins — 25

▼ Anomalies — 25
- Anomalies/Duplication of the Inferior Vena Cava
- Anomalies of the Iliac Veins
- Duplication of Renal and Peripheral Veins

▼ Dilatation — 26
- Inferior Vena Cava Engorgement
- Prestenotic and Poststenotic Dilatation
- Thrombosis
- Venectasia
- Venous Insufficiency

▼ Vena Cava, Veins (Continue)

▼ Intraluminal Mass 28
- ▶ Venous Thrombosis
- ▶ Phleboliths, Calcification
- ▶ Venous Valves

▼ Compression, Infiltration 31
- ▶ Enlarged Caudate Lobe
- ▶ Budd–Chiari Syndrome
- ▶ Lymph Nodes, Cysts
- ▶ Other Masses
- ▶ Malignant Tumor
- ▶ Anatomy

Portal Vein and Its Tributaries 33

▼ Enlarged Lumen Diameter 35

▼ Portal Hypertension 35
- ▶ Prehepatic Block
- ▶ Intrahepatic Block
- ▶ Posthepatic Block

▼ Intraluminal Mass 43

▼ Thrombosis 43
- ▶ Portal Vein Thrombosis
- ▶ Splenic Vein Thrombosis
- ▶ Thrombosis of the Superior Mesenteric Vein

▼ Tumor 48
- ▶ Tumor Infiltration

1 Vessels

Aorta, Vena Cava, and Peripheral Vessels

G. Schmidt

Aorta: Anatomy and Topography

Microanatomy
- Intima (endothelial cells), media (smooth-muscle cells, elastic fibers), adventitia (fibrocellular connective tissue, vascular nerves)
- Intima-media thickness usually 0.4–0.7 mm

Retroperitoneal Branches of the Abdominal Aorta (incomplete)
- Lumbar arteries
- Left and right common iliac arteries

Splanchnic Branches of the Abdominal Aorta
- Superior suprarenal arteries
- Celiac axis
- Left gastric artery
- Splenic artery
- Common hepatic artery → gastroduodenal artery, right gastric artery, hepatic artery proper
- Middle suprarenal arteries
- Superior mesenteric artery
- Ovarian/testicular arteries
- Inferior mesenteric artery

Course of the Aorta
- Left of midline and approximately 5 mm anterior to the spine
- It enters the abdomen through the aortic hiatus at the level of the lower border of the 12th thoracic vertebra and runs for about 14 cm to the level of the fourth lumbar vertebra where it bifurcates into the common iliac arteries → in turn these bifurcate into the internal and external iliac arteries

Diameter of the Aortic Lumen
- Normal diameter of the aortic lumen immediately below the diaphragm is 25 mm, gradually tapering down to 20 mm at the infrarenal location

Microanatomy. The intima, the innermost layer of the aorta, comprises the luminal endothelium and a matrix of fibrils and fibers, while the media as the thickest layer is organized as concentric lamellae of elastin and collagen meshworks with embedded smooth-muscle cells. In the more peripheral arteries the media is characterized by a particular abundance of smooth-muscle cells. The adventitia of the aorta is composed of fibrocellular connective tissue and contains a network of vasa vasorum and vascular nerves. The arterial wall, and thus the aortic wall as well, is a key element in the context of atherosclerosis and its clinical manifestation of arteriosclerosis since the latter results in intimal and medial thickening that can be measured by ultrasonography (intima-media thickness). These pathological changes are due to lipid accumulation, proliferation of smooth-muscle cells, and fibroblastic connective tissue.

Ultrasonography depicts the arterial and aortic wall as a triple-layered structure with a hypoechoic layer sandwiched between two hyperechoic strata. The degree of atherosclerosis correlates quite well with the intima-media thickness, which can be measured using high-resolution scanners with high-frequency probes (7.5–10 Mhz). The changes in wall thickness are a function of both age and atherosclerosis; for example, the normal wall of the carotid artery is 0.4–0.7 mm thick (**Figs. 1.1** and **1.2**). The sonographic measurements match the thickness determined histologically.

Retroperitoneal branches of the abdominal aorta. The abdominal aorta gives off paired retroperitoneal as well as (mostly intraperitoneal) splanchnic branches. The retroperitoneal branches comprise the lumbar arteries, which are of no significance in ultrasonography, and the common iliac arteries, which are essential guideline structures and important in ultrasound pathology (**Fig. 1.3**).

Splanchnic branches of the abdominal aorta. With the advent of color-flow Doppler scans, imaging of the splanchnic branches of the aorta

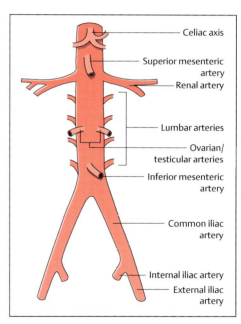

▲ **Fig. 1.3** The abdominal aorta with its branches.

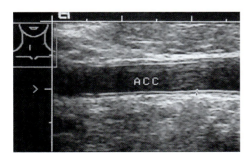

▲ **Fig. 1.1** Intima-media thickness of the right common carotid artery (ACC): regular arterial wall with triple layering as a result of reflection from the interfaces between intima, media, and adventitia. In this case the intima-media thickness is measured as 0.5 mm (cf. the calipers).

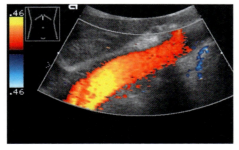

▲ **Fig. 1.2** Abdominal aorta—course and measurement of the wall thickness.
a The upper section of the abdominal aorta runs posterior to the liver. In the color-flow Doppler, laminar flow toward the probe is coded red.

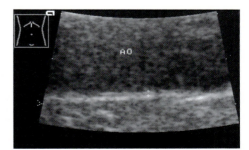

▲ ***b*** Same 73-year-old female patient: the thickness of the aortic wall with an intima-media thickness of 1 mm (calipers) is normal for this age. AO = aorta.

has played an increasingly important clinical role in organ studies and the detection of disease. Acute chronic intestinal ischemia is easily diagnosed using color-flow Doppler (**Fig. 1.29, p. 15**). All splanchnic branches (**Fig. 1.3**) are quite accessible to ultrasonography.

Course of the abdominal aorta. The abdominal aorta courses over a distance of about 14 cm from the aortic hiatus of the diaphragm at the level of the lower border of the 12th vertebra to the level of the fourth lumbar vertebra where it bifurcates into the common iliac arteries. In its beginning it passes anterior to the esophagus, which turns left toward the esophageal hiatus and is easily distinguishable by its target sign dorsal to the aorta. It then runs as a smooth straight band not more than 5 mm anterior to the spine, hugging its curvature; thus it follows the lumbar lordosis in an increasingly anterior direction.

Diameter of the aortic lumen. The maximum diameter of the upper intra-abdominal aortic lumen is 25 mm, tapering down to 20 mm at the infrarenal region; any larger diameter signifies ectasia (< 30 mm) or an aneurysm (> 30 mm) (**Figs. 1.14–1.16, ▣ 1.1 and ▣ 1.2**).

Inferior Vena Cava: Anatomy and Topography

Retroperitoneal and Splanchnic Branches
(except for: splenic vein, superior and inferior mesenteric vein, left and right gastric vein = tributaries to the portal vein)
▶ Left and right common iliac vein
▶ Lumbar veins
▶ Left and right renal vein
▶ Right ovarian/testicular veins (the corresponding left veins drain into the left renal vein)
▶ Hepatic veins

Course of the Inferior Vena Cava
▶ Right of the midline, anterior to the spine, and paralleling the aorta

Lumen Diameter of the Inferior Vena Cava
▶ Physiologic caliber changes
▶ Lumen fluctuates with respiration
▶ A diameter in excess of 20 mm is pathological: more precisely, it is pathological if the inferior vena cava shows a loss of kinetics—i.e., no change in caliber with respiration or on compression

Microanatomy. The venous wall is quite thin consisting of smooth-muscle cells and fibrocellular collagen bundles.

The low intrinsic pressure and the thin wall combine to make the inferior vena cava susceptible to caliber changes and extrinsic compression. Therefore, adjacent pathological processes may result in compression, impression, and displacement (**see Figs. 1.76, 1.78–1.80**).

Retroperitoneal and splanchnic branches. While all retroperitoneal branches mirror the arterial tree in that they are tributaries to the vena cava, only some of the splanchnic veins (renal, suprarenal, ovarian/testicular, and hepatic veins) drain into the inferior vena cava (**Fig. 1.4**) and the others into the portal vein (splenic, mesenteric, gastric, and pancreatic veins).

Course of the vena cava. The right and left common iliac veins join at the level of the fifth lumbar vertebra and thus give rise to the inferior vena cava. It courses right of the aorta and anterior to the spine hugging the lumbar lordosis. It passes along the posterior surface of the liver dorsal to the caudate lobe, receives the vein of the caudate lobe and at the 'bare area' the three hepatic veins as well. It then enters the thoracic cavity through the central tendon of the diaphragm, immediately terminating in the right atrium (**Fig. 1.5**).

Lumen diameter of the inferior vena cava. Since the inferior vena cava demonstrates physiological as well as respiration-induced caliber changes it does not exhibit a constant and precise lumen diameter. Nevertheless, a subphrenic diameter of more than 20 mm may be regarded as abnormal when associated with a lack of respiration induced changes in the lumen diameter and no compressibility.

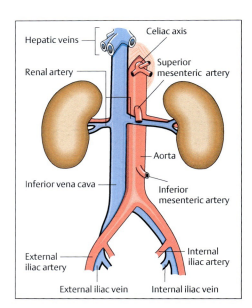

▲ **Fig. 1.4** Inferior vena cava and its branches.

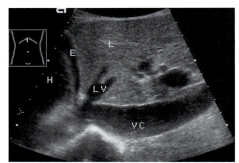

▲ **Fig. 1.5** Inferior vena cava and its branches.
a Upper section of the subphrenic inferior vena cava (VC): it courses posterior to the liver bordering the caudate lobe, just before it is joined by the hepatic veins (LV). H = right atrium; E = small pleural effusion; L = liver.

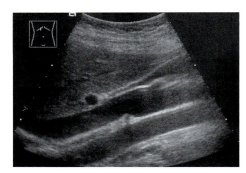

▲ **b** Longitudinal plane through the inferior vena cava with probe angled from right to left: In this image the vena cava is uppermost, being crossed posteriorly by the right renal vein. Since the aorta runs to the left of the vena cava in this image, it appears at the bottom (this atypical plane provides the best view of any lymphomas between aorta and vena cava). The cross-section of the portal vein with an oblique view through the gallbladder is anterior to the vena cava.

Aorta, Arteries

Anomalies and Variant Positions

- ▼ Aorta, Arteries
  - ▶ Anomalies and Variant Positions
  - ▶ Dilatation
  - ▶ Stenosis
  - ▶ Wall Thickening
  - ▶ Intraluminal Mass
  - ▶ Perivascular Mass
- ▶ Vena Cava, Veins

▶ Situs inversus
▶ Aplasia, Hypoplasia and Duplication of the Aorta
▶ Coarctation of the Aorta
▶ Oblique/Transverse Course of the Aorta
▶ Kinking of the Aorta
▶ Variant and Duplicated Arteries

▶ Situs Inversus

Anomalies of the aorta are quite rare; a situs inversus is the most likely reason for surprise but in most cases it is already known to the patient (**Fig. 1.6**).

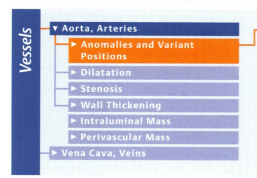

◀ *Fig. 1.6* Situs inversus viscerum: the aorta is on the right and the vena cava (not depicted) on the left; in most cases the diagnosis is clear-cut if both subcostal views demonstrate malrotation of the liver, i.e., it is located on the left.

▶ Aplasia, Hypoplasia, and Duplication of the Aorta

Aplasia, hypoplasia, and duplication of the aorta are extremely rare and in most cases they will have been diagnosed during the perinatal period. Usually an aplastic aorta results in a fatal defect and only two cases of aortic duplication have been described in the literature. Artifacts feigning duplication may arise in the transverse epigastric plane from the prismlike effects of the fatty tissue between the rectus abdominis muscles, which result in refraction artifacts[4a]. There is also the possibility of a misdiagnosis due to physical ultrasound if echo reverberation produces an image of multiple aortas. The preferred location of this mirroring is found at especially hard interfaces, e.g., plaque incrustation of the aortic wall; here,

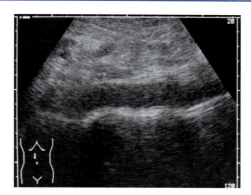

a kind of ping-pong effect at the echointensive reflectors increases the transit time, which in turn generates multiple images of the aorta (**Fig. 1.7**)

◀ *Fig. 1.7* Mirror imaging of the aorta (artifact) due to the parallel thin echogenic lines. AO = aorta.

▶ Coarctation of the Aorta

Congenital circumscribed circular narrowing of the aorta is known as aortic coarctation. It is found at several segments of the aorta: for the abdomen these are segments IV (from the subphrenium to below the renal arteries) and V (all the way to the aortic bifurcation). Sonographically these stenoses are best studied by color-flow Doppler imaging and analysis of the flow parameters (see below).

▶ Oblique/Transverse Course of the Aorta

In case of severe scoliosis or kyphosis of the spine, the aorta will follow this course; the usual longitudinal plane may result in a double lumen, while the transverse view would depict the aorta as a short bandlike structure (**Fig. 1.8**).

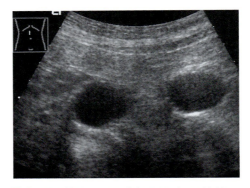
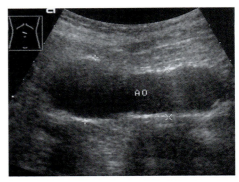

▲ **Fig. 1.8** Oblique course of the aorta due to kinking. **a** Longitudinal subxiphoid plane: because of its oblique course the aorta is visualized twice.

▲ **b** Oblique subxiphoid plane: the aorta (AO) has been insonated in an almost exact longitudinal direction. Calipers: aortic ectasia bordering on an aneurysm.

▶ Kinking of the Aorta

Hypertension and arteriosclerosis can lead not only to an ectatic but also tortuous aorta. Since the spine does not yield, the aorta becomes displaced in a lateral and/or anterior direction and escapes detection by the standard view in the paramedian plane. If the vessel does not follow a normal straight course, the probe should be angled and shifted laterally in order to demonstrate any kinking (**Fig. 1.9**).

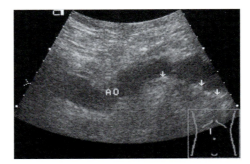

◀ **Fig. 1.9** Kinking of the aorta (AO) induced by hypertension and arteriosclerosis (arrows: arteriosclerotic lesions).

▶ Variant and Duplicated Arteries

The intraperitoneal and retroperitoneal vessels exhibit numerous variations in their branches and may course atypically or even become duplicated. Variants of clinical significance are found at the celiac axis and the renal arteries, as demonstrated by the following examples:
- ▶ Variants of the celiac axis (**Figs. 1.10 and 1.11**)
- ▶ Duplicated renal arteries (**Fig. 1.12**)
- ▶ Renal artery coursing anterior to the vena cava (**Fig. 1.13**).

Figure 1.10 is a schematic summary of the most important variants of the celiac axis (based on Netter). The most common variant anatomy is found in only 25% of cases: here, the left gastric, common hepatic, and splenic arteries arise from a common trunk, the so-called "Tripus Halleri." Quite often the left gastric artery branches off first, followed by the other two arteries.

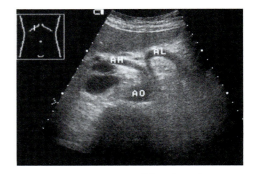

▲ **Fig. 1.11** Variant anatomy of the celiac axis. AO = aorta; AL = splenic artery; AH = hepatic artery. **a** Separate origins of the hepatic and splenic arteries from the aorta.

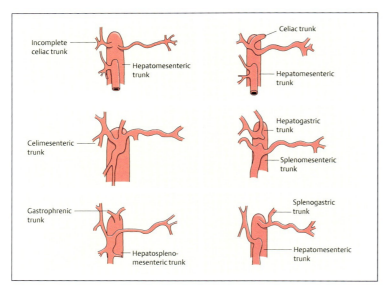

▲ **Fig. 1.10** Variant anatomy of the celiac axis (based on Netterq 9).

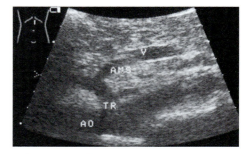

▲ **b** Atypical origin of the superior mesenteric artery (AMS) from the celiac trunk (TR): celiomesenteric trunk. V = superior mesenteric vein.

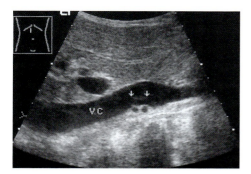 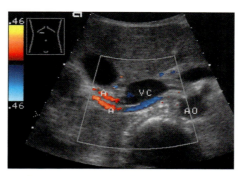 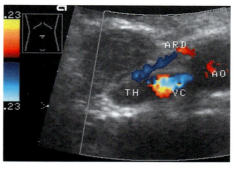

▲ **Fig. 1.12** Duplication of the renal artery.
a Longitudinal view: cross-section of two distinct arteries (arrows) posterior to the vena cava (VC).

▲ **b** Transverse view of the right upper quadrant, color-flow Doppler study. Both renal arteries (A) are depicted; if stenosis of the renal artery is suspected, possible duplication should be ruled out. AO = aorta.

▲ **Fig. 1.13** Irregular course of the right renal artery (ARD) anterior to the vena cava (VC). secondary finding: partial thrombosis (TH) of the vena cava. AO = aorta.

Dilatation

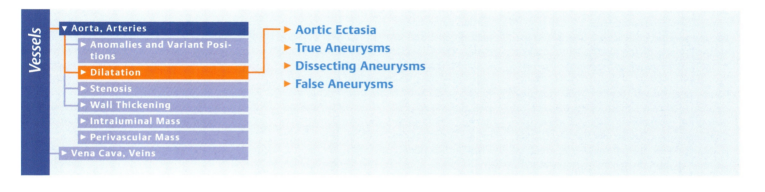

▶ Aortic Ectasia

A condition where the lumen diameter of the aorta expands to 25–30 mm is defined as ectasia. The primary trigger factors for this degeneration are hypertension and arteriosclerosis. In most cases an ectatic aorta also displays a tortuous course (**Fig. 1.14**).

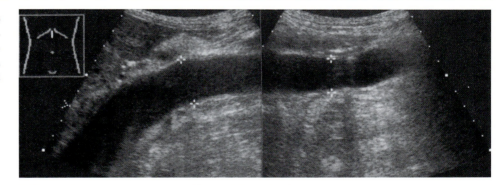

▲ **Fig. 1.14** Ectatic aorta with severe insufficiency of the aortic valve: tortuous ectatic aorta.

▶ True Aneurysms

An aneurysm is a localized dilatation of the arterial wall. Aneurysms may be classified as follows:
▶ Etiology
 – Congenital
 – Atherosclerotic
 – Dissecting
 – Inflammatory
 – Traumatic aneurysms
▶ Morphology
 – Fusiform
 – Pouch-shaped
 – Tortuous
 – Cylindrical
 – Saccular
 – Navicular aneurysms
▶ Pathogenesis
 – True
 – False (pseudo-)
 – Dissecting aneurysms

Aortic aneurysms. A practical working definition of abdominal aortic aneurysms is a transverse lumen diameter of at least 30 mm. Localized atheromatous lesions in the wall facilitate the dilatation of the vessel and impair its contractility, resulting in a weakened aortic wall with aneurysm formation. Small aneurysms do not usually have any thrombotic deposits. Larger aortic aneurysms are characterized by dilatation, arteriosclerosis, and white thrombi, each of these being identifiable by ultrasound. If all three signs can be demonstrated sonographically, the diagnosis of an aneurysm is confirmed.

Increased size. Aneurysms tend to expand in size over time. The larger the lumen becomes the less pressure the wall will tolerate before rupturing. According to Laplace's law the tension in the wall is directly proportional to the radius; thus, small aneurysms with a diameter

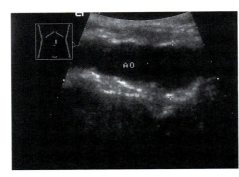
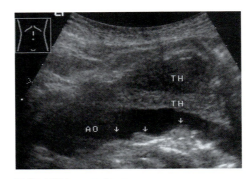
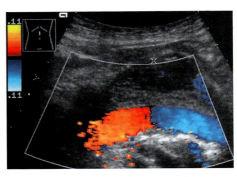

▲ **Fig. 1.15** Borderline aortic aneurysm: localized expansion of the ectatic aorta (AO) to 29.5 mm just cephalad of the bifurcation.

▲ **Fig. 1.16** Large aortic aneurysm.
a B-mode image: all criteria of a true aneurysm are fulfilled: widening of the vessel, sclerosis of the aorta (arrows), white thrombi (TH). AO = aorta.

▲ *b* Color-flow Doppler: the remaining perfused lumen is defined by the color-coded signal; the color change (from red through black to blue) signifies the change in the flow direction—the flow toward the probe is red, and away from the probe it is blue.

Formal and Causative Aneurysm Formation

In **true aneurysms** there is a localized dilatation of the entire wall, the most frequent cause being arteriosclerosis. Congenital aneurysms arise from defects in or fibromuscular dysplasia of the media. Most mycotic aneurysms are sequelae of systemic mycosis.

False aneurysms result from vascular trauma (nowadays most often because of diagnostic procedures, such as catheterization) leading to perivascular hematoma that is walled off by the surrounding tissue and quite often ends up becoming thrombosed.

Dissecting aneurysms occur spontaneously in middle-aged and older adults, with hypertension being one of the most common factors. Congenital (Marfan syndrome, idiopathic cystic necrosis of the media) and acquired (syphilis) etiology plays a minor role. The trigger event is a tear in the intima (entry point) with blood now forcing itself into the media. This results in a "pseudolumen" which rejoins the true lumen at a more caudad location through another tear in the intima (reentry point).

of less than 5 cm are not very likely to rupture while in aneurysms with a diameter of more than 7 cm the probability of rupture within one year approaches 50%. The aneurysm expansion rate can be monitored sonographically: aneurysms of more than 5 cm in diameter exhibit a mean annual increase in diameter of 0.6 cm, while for smaller aneurysms the corresponding value drops to 0.2 cm. Patients with diagnosed aneurysms should undergo follow-up scans every three to six months (**Figs. 1.15 and 1.16, 1.2a and b**).

1.1 The Shape of Aortic Aneurysms

▶ **Tortuous, berry-shaped, fusiform aneurysm**

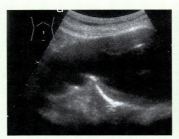
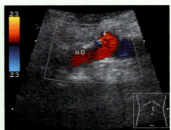
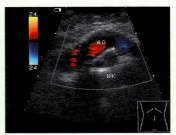

a Tortuous aortic aneurysm. These forms are difficult to define with ultrasound because the loops usually run sideways (see **1.2c**).

b Pouch-shaped aneurysm. Characteristic small asymmetric anterior bulge (arrow). AO = aorta.

c Fusiform aneurysm (AN): steadily increasing dilation of the aortic wall with subsequent reduction to the original diameter (here at the bifurcation into the iliac artery (AIS). AO = aorta; VC = vena cava.

▶ **Cylindrical, saccular, boat-shaped aneurysm**

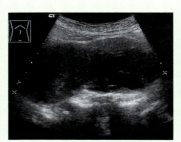
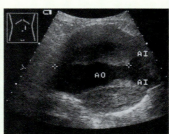
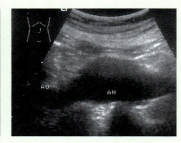

d Large cylinder-shaped aortic aneurysm extending over 13.2 cm, i.e., including the renal arteries (distance from aortic bifurcation is more than 9.5 cm!).

e Saccular aneurysm: remaining lumen (AO) in the center surrounded by a concentric thrombosis; the aneurysm ends where the aorta bifurcates into the iliac artery (AI). Characteristics: diameter 10 cm and more, balloonlike shape.

f Boat-shaped aneurysm (AN; cursors). The aneurysm projects anteriorly on one side.

1.2 Diagnosis in Aortic Aneurysm

▶ Aneurysm extent, aneurysm complications

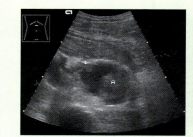

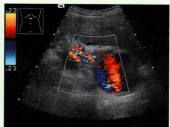

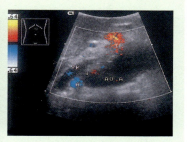

a and b Aortic aneurysm with open rupture, transverse subxiphoid scans.
a B-mode image: suprarenal aortic aneurysm (A) with partial thrombosis and anechoic band (arrow) extending to a subhepatic fluid pool.

b Color-flow Doppler image: rupture leaking blood; the turbulence produces this "confetti-like" phenomenon.

c Tortuous aortic aneurysm (AO A). Origin of the renal artery (A, arrow) and celiac trunk (TR, cut by the scan) from the aneurysm. VR = renal vein.

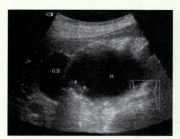

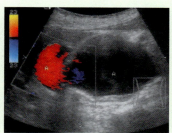

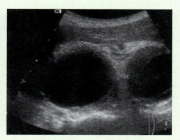

d Aneurysmosis of the aorta (A): the complete vessel has been turned into a succession of aneurysms. Right paramedian transverse subxiphoid view: crescent-shaped mass in the porta hepatis, initially misdiagnosed as gallbladder (GB).

e Color-flow Doppler: the anechoic masses in **d** are part of the aortic aneurysmosis (A); without the color-flow Doppler the anechoic crescent would be misdiagnosed as gallbladder.

f Longitudinal subxiphoid view in the median plane: adjacent saccular aneurysms.

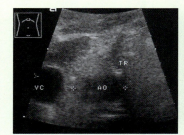

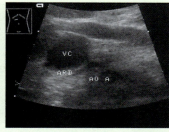

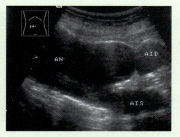

g and h Aneurysm extent:
g Origin of the celiac trunk (TR) from the aneurysm (AO).

h Origin of the right renal artery (ARD) from the aortic aneurysm (AOA). VC = vena cava.

i Aortic aneurysm (AN), junction with the aneurysmal right and left iliac arteries (AID, AIS). Longitudinal scan plane from right to left (to the origin of the inferior mesenteric artery, see **Fig. 7.45**, p. 243).

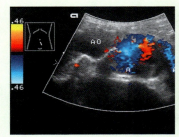

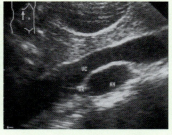

j In the color-flow Doppler there is turbulent blood flow with color changes. AO = aorta.

k Right subxiphoid view in the longitudinal plane: the vena cava (VC) is insonated through the oblique section of the aneurysm (AN). AR = renal artery.

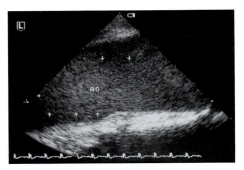

▲ **Fig. 1.17** Thoracic aortic aneurysm (AO), TEE: expansion of the aorta to 40 mm, floating thrombus within the lumen (red thrombus made up of fibrin and red blood cells; arrows). Massive thickening and sclerosis of the wall.

Aneurysm morphology. Ultrasound imaging depicts the different shapes possible in abdominal aortic aneurysms. Most often the fusiform, pouch-shaped, and tortuous aneurysms—and some of the saccular ones as well—are true aneurysms. Other saccular aneurysms and the unilateral navicular type may be classified as dissecting aneurysms. Cylindrical aneurysms start and end rather abruptly and therefore appear cylinder-shaped.

The various shapes of abdominal aortic aneurysms are illustrated in ▣ 1.1.

Diagnosis in abdominal aortic aneurysms. Aortic aneurysms command special interest because of their high propensity to rupture. In ultrasound studies the rupture appears as an echoic para-aortic band ("stable" rupture), and is confirmed for certain when the leak with its blood jet ("open" rupture) can be demonstrated (▣ **1.2a and b**). In most cases this life-threatening emergency, with its vital indication for emergency repair, does not leave much time for any detailed study.

Other essential parameters to note during ultrasound imaging of abdominal aortic aneurysms are location, length, and the possible involvement of the renal and iliac arteries (▣ **1.2c–h**).

Nonaortic aneurysms. Aneurysms are not limited to the aorta but may be found in other intra- and retroperitoneal or peripheral (subclavian artery) vessels as well. However, isolated iliac artery aneurysms without an associated abdominal aortic aneurysm are rare (▣ **1.2i–k**).

The images in ▣ **1.2** are a diagnostic summary of aortic and nonaortic aneurysms.

Thoracic aortic aneurysm. Most often a true aneurysm of the thoracic aorta is diagnosed first on plain chest films and then confirmed by TEE (transesophageal echocardiography) or CT (computed tomography) (**Fig. 1.17**).

▶ Dissecting Aneurysms

In ultrasonography, dissecting aneurysms are characterized by an echogenic intima floating in synchronous motion with the pulse, or this echogenic intima may be thickened and rigid because of atherosclerosis. The vessel itself may be dilated and display all other signs of an aneurysm; however, quite often the artery appears otherwise normal, and the diagnosis is confirmed only by demonstrating the sheared-off intima within the lumen generating the color-flow Doppler image of two distinct lumina.

In more than 90% of patients, dissection with its massive, sharp chest pain will commence as thoracic aneurysm and propagate to the abdominal aorta (Stanford classification type B: begins at the ascending aorta or the aortic arch with possible extension to the abdominal aorta). Thoracic aneurysms immediately distal to the aortic valve (Stanford classification type A: involving only the aortic arch and ascending aorta) are diagnosed sonographically by echocardiography or TEE (**Figs. 1.18 and 1.19**).

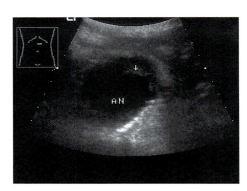

▲ **Fig. 1.18** Dissecting abdominal aortic aneurysm (AN), upper abdominal longitudinal scan (**a**) and transverse scan (**b**): intraluminal intimal flap (arrows).

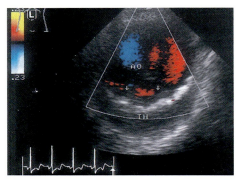

▲ **Fig. 1.19** Dissecting aortic aneurysm, Stanford type A. TEE demonstrates the intraluminal hyperechoic intima (arrows) and the thrombosed, nonperfused lumen of the dissected area. (Patient declined surgery, died suddenly 2 weeks later.) AO = aorta.

▶ False Aneurysms

Aorta. Compared with the false aneurysms (pseudoaneurysms) most common today, i.e., after puncture of the femoral artery, traumatic aneurysms of the aorta are quite rare. Sometimes false aortic aneurysms are seen as a result of suture-line leakage but these anastomotic pseudoaneurysms of the aorta are also rather infrequent. In ultrasound studies they appear as an anechoic periaortic mass, usually situated at the anastomosis and coursing with the aorta.

Femoral artery. Catheterization of the femoral artery is complicated by a fairly significant rate of pseudoaneurysm formation. The diagnosis is confirmed by color-flow Doppler, which shows blood spurting into the cavity of the aneurysm. This differentiates the diagnosis from other perivascular masses (see below). Quite often the leak is pinpointed precisely by the blood jet and may then be treated by compression of this area with the probe, resulting in thrombosis of the leak and thus closure (**Fig. 1.20**).

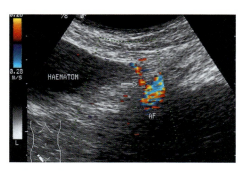

▲ **Fig. 1.20** False or pseudoaneurysm after catheterization of the femoral artery (AF): systolic jet (arrow) with leakage of blood and hematoma formation.

Stenosis

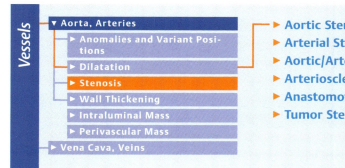

- Aortic Stenosis
- Arterial Stenosis
- Aortic/Arterial Embolism
- Arteriosclerotic Aortic/Arterial Occlusion
- Anastomotic/Bypass Stenosis
- Tumor Stenosis/Infiltration

▶ Aortic Stenosis

Stenosis of the aorta may be depicted directly in B-mode imaging, or it can be demonstrated by color-flow Doppler and spectral analysis of the blood flow. Apart from the congenital narrowing due to coarctation of the aorta (see above), most often these are multiple or extensive atherosclerotic stenoses. A peak systolic velocity of more than 200 cm/s in the Doppler spectral analysis is indicative of hemodynamically significant arterial stenosis[8].

Arteriosclerotic stenotic lesions also exhibit complex protuberances that produce luminal stenosis of varying significance. Generalized sclerosis of the aorta will lead to severe narrowing of the aortic lumen (**Figs. 1.21 and 1.22**).

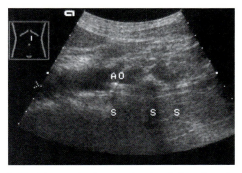

▲ **Fig. 1.21** Arteriosclerotic sclerosis of the aorta: severe narrowing of the distal aortic lumen (AO) due to complex calcified plaques with posterior shadowing (S).

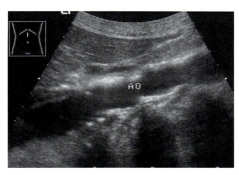

▲ **Fig. 1.22** Disseminated arteriosclerotic sclerosis of the aorta.
a Multiple stenoses of the aorta (AO) due to complex calcified plaques with posterior shadowing (S).

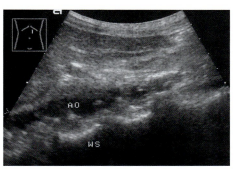

▲ ***b*** Paramedian view from the left with slightly angled probe, illustrating the plaques and thrombi protruding severely into the lumen.

▶ Arterial Stenosis

Splanchnic arteries. Although stenosis of the intraperitoneal and peripheral arteries is a quite common finding, the narrowing of the lumen tends to be of no hemodynamic significance. Usually even severe splanchnic artery stenosis does not result in clinical symptoms because these vessels are heavily interlinked via various branches (e.g., the arc of Riolan):

- Left gastric artery (celiac axis) → right gastric artery (common hepatic artery)
- Superior pancreaticoduodenal artery (celiac axis) → inferior pancreaticoduodenal artery (superior mesenteric artery)
- Middle colic artery (superior mesenteric artery) → left colic artery (inferior mesenteric artery)

Hemodynamically significant stenosis is confirmed by the increased systolic velocity in color-flow Doppler spectral analysis. In the branches of the celiac axis the regular systolic velocity is 138 ± 99 cm/s[6]. A peak systolic velocity of more than 220 cm/s in the celiac axis or superior mesenteric artery is indicative of arterial stenosis. In B-mode imaging these stenoses are seen as arteriosclerotic plaques with narrowing of the lumen. However, even if there is no inflow stenosis, this does not rule out intestinal ischemia since duplex scanning may easily miss the more peripheral stenosis or embolism. In this case the clinical symptoms and angiography settle the diagnosis (◨ **1.3a–g**).

Median arcuate ligament syndrome. Among the functional obstructions, the median arcuate ligament syndrome is a special case. The median arcuate ligament is a ligamentous arch across the surface of the aorta, interconnecting the crura of the diaphragm. Particularly in young women, postprandial epigastric pain mimicking ulcer may be due to compression of the celiac axis by the median arcuate ligament. Ultrasound confirms this diagnosis by color-flow Doppler with the non-respiration-dependent change in velocity: during expiration there is a clear-cut increase in velocity above 180 cm/s because of the stenosis, while during inspiration the velocity will drop. If the stenosis is fixated, the velocity increases during inspiration as well as expiration. Dissection of the ligament should eliminate the complaints (and the ultrasound pathology).

Renal artery stenosis. Arteriosclerosis is the underlying cause in most cases of renal artery stenosis, which is frequently found at the origin of the renal artery. Fibromuscular stenosis of the middle and peripheral segments of the renal artery is far less common.

The sonographic criteria of proximal renal artery stenosis are:

- Demonstration of a localized thickening of the wall, and in the B-mode image narrowing of the lumen (quite often not identifiable)
- Turbulence before and after the stenosis with color changes ("confetti phenomenon")

1.3 Splanchnic Artery Stenosis

▶ **Celiac trunk stenosis**

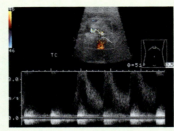 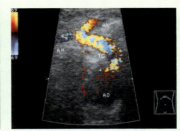 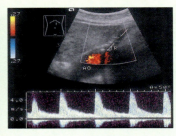

a and *b* **Stenosis of the celiac axis.**
a Penetration ~70 mm, color-flow Doppler velocity 46 cm/s. Despite baseline shift, the maximum velocity cannot be measured completely (> 300 cm/s).

b Magnified detailed view of *a*. Significant color changes indicating high speed turbulence induced by the stenosis (arrow). AH = common hepatic artery; AL = splenic artery; TC = celiac trunk; AO = aorta.

c High-grade stenosis of the celiac trunk, showing no detectable flow even at a low PRF. Doppler spectrum shows marked flow acceleration to (a velocity of) 400 cm/s. AO = aorta; TR = celiac trunk.

▶ **Mesenteric artery stenosis** (stenosis of the inferior mesenteric artery, see Fig. 7.45c).

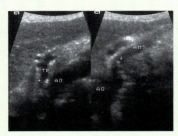 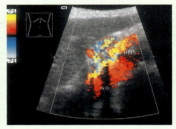 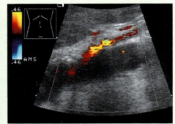

d B-mode image of vascular calcifications in the celiac trunk and superior mesenteric artery. AO = aorta; TR = celiac trunk; AMS = superior mesenteric artery.

e Color duplex: turbulent zones in both arteries, indicating significant stenosis. AO = aorta; TR = celiac trunk; AMS = superior mesenteric artery.

f Stenosis of the mesenteric artery. Color-flow Doppler: color change signifying stenosis induced turbulence.

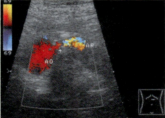

g Origins of the renal arteries (arrows, B-mode image); Penetration ~80 mm, color-flow Doppler velocity 69 cm/s. Severe stenosis (arrow) at the aortic origin (AO) of the renal artery (AR); the color changes signify increased velocity with turbulence.

▶ **Renal arteries**

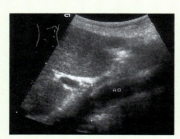 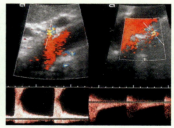

h and *i* **Stenotic renal artery.**

i Color duplex with spectral analysis: color reversals in the renal arteries plus flow acceleration to (a velocity of) 200 cm/s, indicating significant stenosis.

Table 1.1 Severity of stenosis—verified by B-mode imaging, spectral analysis, and color-flow Doppler scanning (modified after references 8, 11)

Severity of local stenosis	No stenosis (< 40%)	Slight (40–60%)	Moderate (60–70%)	Severe (about 80%)	Subtotal (> 90%)
B-mode image: quality of detection	+++	+++	++	+	+
B-mode image: findings	Slight plaque formation	Slight plaque formation	Moderate narrowing of the lumen	Severe narrowing of the lumen	Almost complete obstruction of the lumen
Spectral analysis	Unremarkable	Widening of the spectrum	Widening of the spectrum, larger fraction of lower frequencies	Inverse frequencies within the widened spectrum	Inverse frequencies within the reduced spectrum
Peak systolic velocity	< 120 cm/s	> 120 cm/s	> 120 cm/s	> 240 cm/s	Variable
Color-flow Doppler	No or just localized turbulence	Extended segmental systolic increase in velocity	Circumscribed segmental systolic increase in velocity	Tightly circumscribed segmental increase in velocity of high severity, with some backflow components	

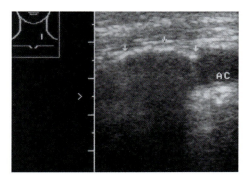

▲ Fig. 1.23a Conspicuous echogenic plaques in the internal carotid artery.

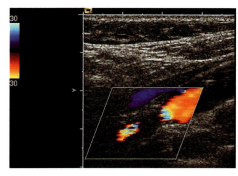

▲ b Turbulent zones and acoustic shadowing in the stenosis.

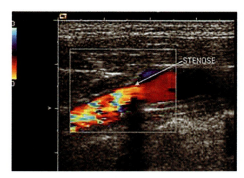

▲ c Vascular narrowing by hard plaque, with zones of turbulent flow.

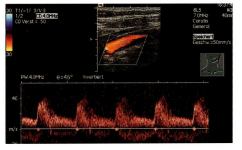

▲ Fig. 1.24a Decreased flow velocity proximal to the stenosis, with unchanged frequency spectrum.

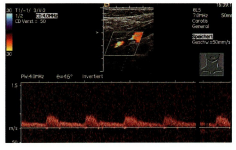

▲ b Doppler spectrum sampled just in front of the stenosis: marked decrease in flow velocity.

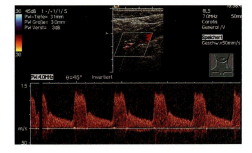

▲ c Doppler spectrum sampled in the stenosis: V_{max} is increased to 140 cm/s, indicating 50% stenosis.

- Increased velocity of more than 180 cm/s; increase in the end-diastolic velocity above 50 cm/s
- Poststenotic drop in the velocity
- Decrease in the resistance ratio below 0.5 when comparing both sides (poststenotic or at the intrarenal arteries)[1]

▣ 1.3 shows typical examples of splanchnic and renal artery stenosis.

Carotid artery. Ultrasonography of the carotid arteries and possibly the aortic arch may be of vital importance in internal medicine and neurology. B-mode imaging will demonstrate any stenosis and thrombosed plaques, while the severity is ascertained by duplex scanning. According to Widder, Neuerburg-Heusler, and Hennerici[8, 11], stenosis of the common, external, and internal carotids may be classified according to five possible degrees of severity (**Table 1.1, Figs. 1.23 and 1.24**).

Peripheral arteries. In the peripheral arteries the hemodynamic effects of a stenosis depend on its severity. B-mode imaging and color-flow Doppler scanning will directly demonstrate the stenosis of a peripheral artery. A peripheral artery in the extremities will be deemed to exhibit clinically significant stenosis (>50%, also known as *critical stenosis*), if the following criteria are present:
- Localized thickening of the vessel wall
- Reduction in the lumen diameter by more than 50%
- More than 2-fold increase in the peak systolic velocity

Certain locations of the iliac-femoral axis are predisposed to obstruction; these are: the bifurcation of the common femoral artery into the superficial and deep femoral arteries;

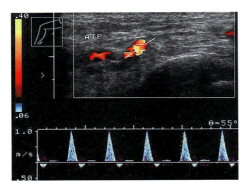
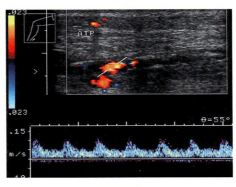
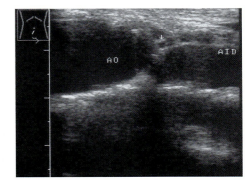

▲ **Fig. 1.25** Color-flow duplex scan with spectral analysis and measurement of the pulsatility index. ATP = posterior tibial artery.
a In a solely neuropathic foot (plantar ulcer): normal arterial spectral profile, pulsatility index 7.67.

▲ **b** For a neuroischemic foot (deep plantar ulcer Wagner grade II): marked decrease in the peak systolic velocity (10 cm/s), high diastolic plateau, pulsatility index 0.87; critical ischemia of the lower extremity.

▲ **Fig. 1.27** Stenosis (AID) of the right iliac artery. AO = aorta.
a B-mode image: severe narrowing of the origin (arrow) of the iliac artery.

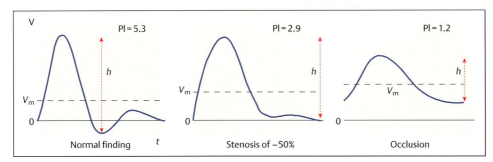

▲ **Fig. 1.26** Pulsatility index and velocity as a function of the severity of the obstruction in normal and pathological extremity flow pulses. The pulsatility index is computed by dividing the difference between peak and minimum flow velocity (h) by the mean flow velocity (V_m) (see reference 8).

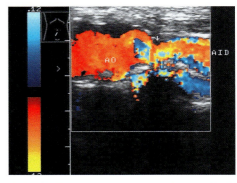

▲ **b** Color-flow Doppler scan: stenosis (arrow), the color changes signifying turbulent flow.

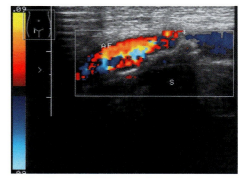

▲ **Fig. 1.28** Stenosis (arrow) of the femoral artery [AF], color-flow Doppler scan: prestenotic color changes denoting turbulence. The stenosis is due to a massive calcified plaque (note the shadowing, S) encroaching on the lumen.

Hunter's canal, where the tendon of the adductor magnus muscle crosses the superficial femoral artery; and the trifurcation of the popliteal artery. Even during routine ultrasound studies, it is usually possible to deliberately look for obstruction in the peripheral arteries of the limbs; clinical symptoms and the result of duplex scanning will be sufficient to indicate any need for angiography.

New modalities in ultrasonography with panoramic imaging of the vessel (e.g., SieScape) facilitate the search for stenosis in long peripheral arteries. One definite indication for detailed vascular work-up is the syndrome of the neuroischemic diabetic foot with its accompanying sclerosis of the media, where the pedal pulses are not palpable, even in the absence of any clinically significant obstruction, and the parameters generated by Doppler ultrasound are meaningless. Here, a subtle search for obstruction may be called for to differentiate and assess the status of the ischemic leg in the presence of any concomitant neuropathy. In our studies the diabetic foot, solely due to neuropathy and lacking any vascular obstruction, will yield a pulsatility index (PI) > 4, while in the neuroischemic foot PI lies between 4 and 1.2; in critical ischemia of the lower extremity the PI drops below 1.2 (**Fig. 1.25**)[2a].

Determination of the peak and minimum flow velocities as well as the pulsatility index of Gosling and King in the poststenotic segment of the artery is easier to perform. This will resemble the curves illustrated in **Fig. 1.26** (after Gosling as quoted in 8). **Figs. 1.27** and **1.28** are images of iliac and femoral artery stenoses, respectively.

▶ Aortic/Arterial Embolism

Acute aortic embolism (the same as in acute thrombosis of the aorta, aortic bifucation syndrome) is a rare event; however, acute embolism of the peripheral arteries is still common despite its incidence having decreased dramatically after the introduction of anticoagulant therapy for atrial fibrillation (see **Fig. 1.44**; the incidence of embolism at the various sites of the arterial tree is given in the schematic **Fig. 1.45**)[7].

▶ Arteriosclerotic Aortic/Arterial Occlusion

In ultrasound imaging, arteriosclerotic occlusion of the aorta and the other arteries is demonstrated by a complete loss of continuity in the lumen and no flow in color-flow Doppler scanning. Adjacent collateral vessels become visible. Spectral analysis identifies decreased systolic and diastolic flow velocity proximal to the occlusion, with no flow (or collaterals) or decreased systolic velocity combined with a high end-diastolic flow velocity distal to the obstruction (**Figs. 1.29 and 1.30**).

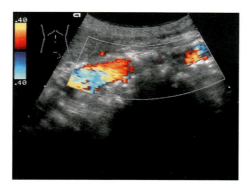

▲ **Fig. 1.29** Aortic occlusion.
a The interrupted color flow is caused by the shadowing due to wall calcification.

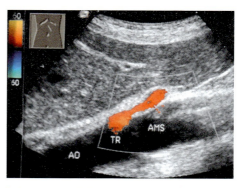

▲ **b** Occlusion of the superior mesenteric artery: no arterial flow. AO = aorta; TR = celiac trunk.

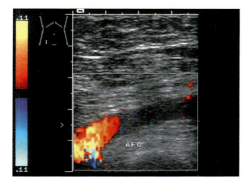

▲ **c** Acute thrombotic occlusion of the common femoral artery (AFC)

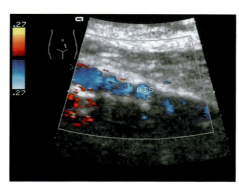

▲ **d and e** Chronic limb ischemia:
d High grade stenosis of the left iliac artery (AIS)

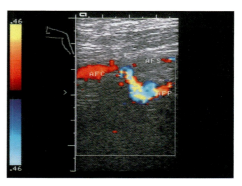

▲ **e** Following complete occlusion of the superficial femoral artery (AFS). Stenosis of the profound femoral artery (AFP)

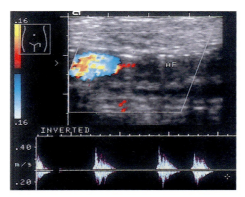

▲ **Fig. 1.30** Chronic long segment occlusion of the femoral artery (AF).
a Slowed preocclusive flow, absence of color flow distally, slight increase of echogenicity.

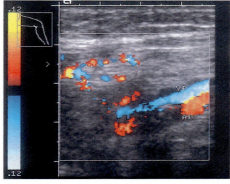

▲ **b** Collaterals refill the popliteal artery (AP). VP = popliteal vein.

▶ Anastomotic/Bypass Stenosis

Stenosis within a bypass, at its proximal segment, or at the anastomosis is easily identified sonographically by localized thickening of the wall with encroachment of the lumen, while color-flow Doppler scanning will demonstrate increased peak systolic velocity (**Fig. 1.31**).

▲ **Fig. 1.31** Stent insertion for carotid artery stenosis.
a Stent is clearly visible as a fragmentary echogenic band.

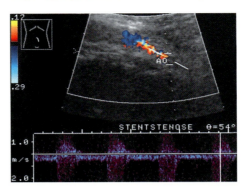

▲ **b** Carotid stent. Segments are devoid of color flow due to acoustic shadowing.

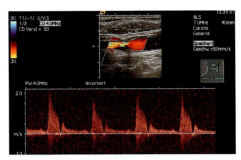

▲ **c** Carotid stent for external carotid artery stenosis. V_{max} indicates 70% stenosis.

▶ Tumor Stenosis/Infiltration

Malignant lymphomas tend to compress adjacent vessels (**Fig. 1.32**), while in carcinomas infiltration of the vessel wall is more common.

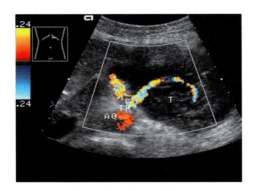

▲ **Fig. 1.32** Malignant lymphoma of the pancreas.
a Splenic artery coursing through the tumor (T), note the distinct compression of the vessel.

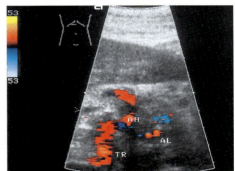

▲ **b** Invasion of the celiac trunk and its branches (common hepatic artery, hepatic artery and splenic artery [AL]) by inoperable pancreatic carcinoma: periarterial hypoechoic masses. AH = hepatic artery; TR = celiac trunk.

Wall Thickening

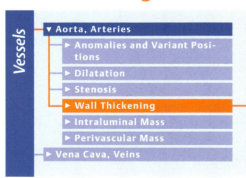

Vessels
- ▼ Aorta, Arteries
  - ▶ Anomalies and Variant Positions
  - ▶ Dilatation
  - ▶ Stenosis
  - ▶ **Wall Thickening**
  - ▶ Intraluminal Mass
  - ▶ Perivascular Mass
- ▶ Vena Cava, Veins

- ▶ Early Arteriosclerotic Lesions
- ▶ Advanced Arteriosclerotic Lesions
- ▶ Complex Arteriosclerotic Lesions
- ▶ Protruding Arteriosclerotic Lesions
- ▶ White Thrombus
- ▶ Arteritis
- ▶ Mönckeberg's Arteriosclerosis
- ▶ Synthetic Grafts

Most often thickening of the aortic and arterial walls is the result of arteriosclerosis, which in turn is rooted in atheromatosis and atherosclerosis. The WHO has defined atherosclerosis as follows:

WHO Definition of Atherosclerosis

"Atherosclerosis implies a fluid combination of intima changes in the arteries—as compared with the arterioles—comprising a focal accumulation of lipids, complex carbohydrates, blood and its components, fibrous tissue, and calcium deposits, accompanied by changes in the media."

► Early Arteriosclerotic Lesions

The early stages of arteriosclerotic lesions are characterized by lipid and cholesterol deposits (lipid plaques and "atheromas" or atherosclerotic plaques, respectively). Subsequently, these plaques may rupture (atherosclerotic ulcers) and become the focus for white thrombi (atherothrombosis).

The different phases and stages of arteriosclerosis result in a variety of sonographic structures in and at the wall of the vessels; however, this always will imply a thickening of the wall. The earliest morphological sign in ultrasonography of these alterations taking place within the intima and media is a widening of the intima-media complex (**Fig. 1.33**)[5].

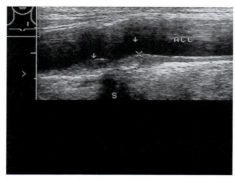

▲ **Fig. 1.33a** Soft plaques: small, soft, nonshadowing plaque (arrow) in the common carotid artery. Broadening of the intima-media complex, consistent with early atherosclerosis.

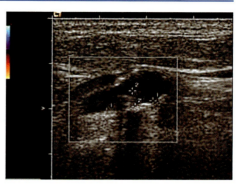

▲ **b** Hard plaques: calcified plaque in the carotid bulb. Complex atherosclerotic lesion with secondary calcification.

► Advanced Arteriosclerotic Lesions

The sonographic sign of advanced arteriosclerotic lesions is a thickened arterial wall. It may appear as a hypoechoic or—as in most cases—a hyperechoic structure. If there is no shadowing, this increased echogenicity could be explained by cholesterol deposits. On the other hand, in complex lesions there will be fibrosis leading to echogenic caps covering the plaques (**Fig. 1.34**).

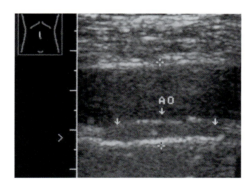

◄ **Fig. 1.34** Advanced arteriosclerotic lesion: localized thickening of the wall seen as a hypoechoic band covered by an echogenic (fibrous) cap (arrows). AO = aorta.

► Complex Arteriosclerotic Lesions

Secondary calcification, fibrosis, and plaque rupture (arteriosclerotic ulcer) with superimposed white thrombi lead up to a complex lesion.

The ultrasound image shows irregular wall thickening of a complex structure and protruding hypoechoic areas, or in the case of secondary calcification a severely hyperechoic area. Consecutive shadowing may block the lumen. Complex lesions protrude into the lumen to varying degrees and result in narrowing of the lumen (**Fig. 1.35–1.38**). Because of the tur-

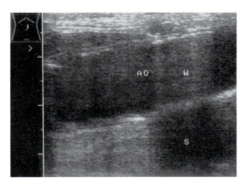

◄ **Fig. 1.36** Early stage of a complex arteriosclerotic lesion: nascent calcification at the anterior aortic wall, mirrored echo (W, resonance artifact). Compared to the remainder of the aorta (AO) this segment appears to generate an echo.

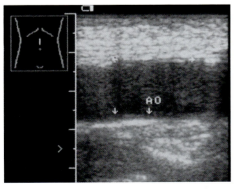

▲ **Fig. 1.35a** Complex arteriosclerotic lesion of the aorta; atheromatosis: echogenic thickening of the wall (arrows) without shadowing. AO = aorta.

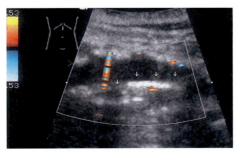

▲ **b** Advanced, complicated ("complex") atherosclerotic lesion: pronounced wall thickening (posterior) with a hypoechoic band of atheromatosis, bordered on the luminal side by hyperechoic plaque. "Stable plaque" with smooth margins. Note the twinkling artifact on the wall.

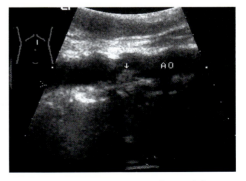

▲ **Fig. 1.37** Complex arteriosclerotic lesion of the aorta (AO): calcification of the aortic wall; shadowing. Protuberating soft plaque (arrow).

bulence, color-flow Doppler scanning produces numerous color changes from red to blue ("confetti phenomenon") (**Fig. 1.39, Fig. 1.24, and 1.2b**).

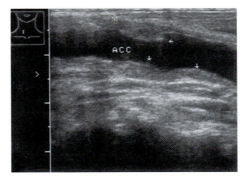

▲ **Fig. 1.38** Complex arteriosclerotic lesion of the common carotid artery (ACC): extensive white thrombi (arrows) feigning thickening of the wall but still resulting in significant narrowing of the lumen.

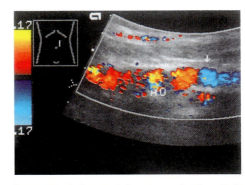

▲ **Fig. 1.39** Thickening of the aortic wall with multiple consecutive stenoses and turbulence-induced color changes. Arrow: color change at the origin of the iliac artery.

▶ Protruding Arteriosclerotic Lesions

Once the lesions become superimposed by white thrombi, the wall will bulge into the lumen, and these thrombi appear as hypoechoic intraluminal mass of sometimes irregular structure (**Fig. 1.40**).

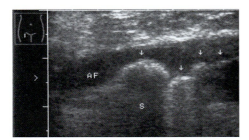

▲ **Fig. 1.40** Protuberant plaque with risk of embolization.
a Hyperechoic, well-circumscribed plaque (arrows), probably at low risk for embolization. (Femoral artery, AF). S = shadowing.

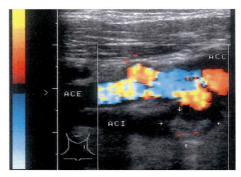

▲ *b* Hyperechoic plaque with a regular surface (arrows; internal carotid artery, ACI); mild to moderate embolization risk. ACE = external carotid artery.

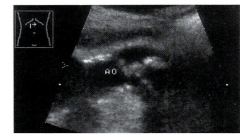

▲ *c* Complex structure with an irregular surface in the distal aorta (AO), presumably at greater risk for embolization.

▶ White Thrombus

Intraluminal white thrombi are most common in aneurysms. They do not represent a true thickening of the wall but nevertheless are a sequela of the underlying arteriosclerosis (**Fig. 1.16, Fig. 1.46**).

▶ Arteritis

There are clinical and histological differences between the various types of arteritis. **Figure 1.41** illustrates the sonographic characteristics of one such type. There are characteristic signs of temporal arteritis that can be visualized by color Duplex ultrasonography; the most specific sign is a dark halo on the artery wall, other signs are stenosis or occlusions of temporal-artery segments.

Classification and Histopathology of Arteritis [10]

- **Panarteritis nodosa.** Complex, aggressive autoimmune inflammation, particularly of the medium-sized arteries: intimal lesion with fibroid necrosis, superimposed thrombosis, granulation with localized nodular pouching; affects all layers of the wall, in particular the adventitia ("periarteritis").
- **Giant cell arteritis.** Giant-cell containing, aggressive autoimmune inflammation of the arteries, affecting primarily the temporal artery, with fragmentation of the tunica elastica and covered by lymphocytes, histiocytes, and giant cells; this results in "wormlike" thickening of the vessel and later in superimposed clot formation.
- **Mesoaortitis syphilitica.** Chronic bacterial (*Treponema pallidum*) inflammation of the aortic wall with granulomas, ulcerous destruction of the media, and aortic aneurysm formation; late sequelae are fibrosis and scarring.

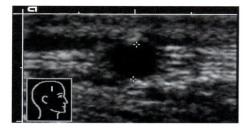 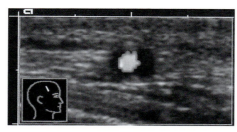 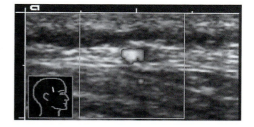

▲ **Fig. 1.41a, b and c** Temporal arteritis.
Hypoechoic wall thickening, regressed in response to treatment (**b, c**).

▶ Mönckeberg's Arteriosclerosis

This appears as a distinctive late effect of diabetes in large, medium-sized as well as small arteries, especially at the iliofemoral axis but also at the upper extremities (pseudohypertension). Mönckeberg's arteriosclerosis is a horseshoe-shaped calcification of the tunica elastica in the media and may be demonstrated as such on radiographic films and in ultrasonography. Because of the loss of elasticity in the arterial wall, the pedal pulses are no longer palpable and Doppler-controlled blood pressure measurements will yield extremely high values above 260 mmHg (this will also be true in case of upper limb involvement).

Ultrasound images will show beaded, hyperechoic thickening of the wall with incomplete shadowing. In color-flow Doppler scanning, it becomes evident that Mönckeberg's arteriosclerosis does not result in stenosis of the vessel (**Fig. 1.42**).

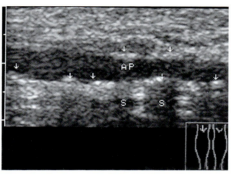

▲ **Fig. 1.42** Mönckeberg's arteriosclerosis. Clinical symptoms: diabetic neuropathic plantar ulcer, palpable pedal pulses, Doppler blood pressure above 300 mmHg. AP = popliteal artery.
a B-mode image: diffuse spots of calcification in the popliteal artery wall (arrows), sometimes with shadowing (S).

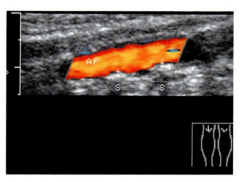

▲ **b** Color-flow Doppler scan: no significant stenosis. Strong reflections off the wall may account for segmental blanking of the color signals.

▶ Synthetic Grafts

Stents and synthetic grafts also exhibit the characteristics of wall thickening. However, their walls have such a unique corrugated echogenic appearance in ultrasound that they are easily identifiable (**Figs. 1.43, 1.31, and 1.50**).

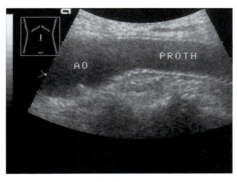

▲ **Fig. 1.43** Dacron graft (Prothesis).
a Synthetic aortoiliac bypass: echogenic, thickened corrugated wall of the graft. AO = aorta.

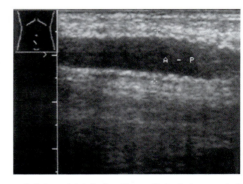

▲ **b** Enlarged detail of an iliac graft: typical corrugated appearance of the graft wall (in color-flow Doppler scanning and spectral analysis a peak systolic velocity above 300 cm/s implies a highly significant stenosis of the graft). A – P = artery graft.

Intraluminal Mass

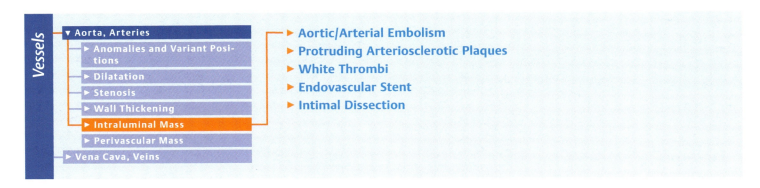

▶ Aortic/Arterial Embolism

Complete embolic obstruction of the aorta or of a major artery is always a serious, sometimes life-threatening, event. Duplex scanning is a rapid and precise imaging modality in the diagnosis of vascular occlusion (see below).

In B-mode imaging, the actual embolus is hard to see as an intraluminal mass since it lacks any impedance and thus is difficult to define within the low-level structures of the artery (in contrast to venous thrombosis) (**Fig. 1.44**). Knowing the clinical symptoms, it may be presumed as hypoechoic mass; this suspicion is confirmed by angiography and color-flow duplex scanning, where the decrease, and even cessation, in flow velocity becomes evident. **Figure 1.45**[7] shows the incidence of embolic events at the various locations of the arterial tree.

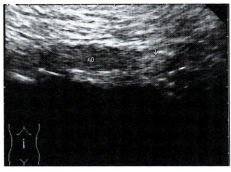

▲ **Fig. 1.44** Aortic saddle embolus (AO): weakly echogenic mass (arrow) cephalad of the aortic bifurcation. Clinical findings: mitral valve defect, acute pulmonary edema, pain in the lower extremities. Emergency operation without preoperative angiography.

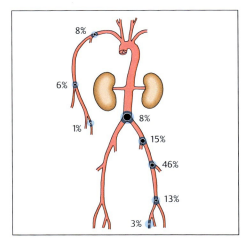

▲ **Fig. 1.45** Incidence of arterial embolism.

▶ Protruding Arteriosclerotic Plaques

Protruding arteriosclerotic plaques represent circumscribed thickening of the arterial wall (see above) but appear as an intraluminal mass. If a white thrombus becomes superimposed on a ruptured arteriosclerotic plaque, its sonographic appearance is that of a homogeneous, hypoechoic intraluminal mass. Such plaque–thrombus complexes increase the risk of arterial occlusion (myocardial infarction), rupture, and microembolism. They also make the vessels prone to sclerosis and calcification, in which case ultrasonography will demonstrate them as a heterogeneous irregular structure (**Figs. 1.46, 1.47 and Fig. 1.40**).

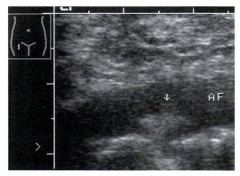

▲ **Fig. 1.46** Complex protruding lesion of the femoral artery (AF).
a B-mode image: echogenic white thrombus (arrow).

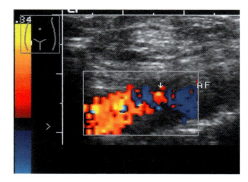

▲ **b** Color-flow duplex scan: there are blank areas within the flow; the "confetti phenomenon" indicates significant stenosis. Clinical diagnosis was a neuroischemic diabetic foot syndrome (in these lesions platelet inhibition is mandatory).

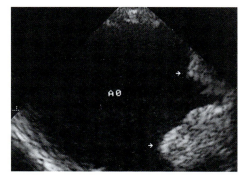

▲ **Fig. 1.47** Atheromatous plaques (arrows) protruding into the lumen, echogenic arteriosclerotic wall thickening of the descending aorta (AO); TEE search for source of embolism.

▶ White Thrombi

A white or pale thrombus arises from a lesion of the endothelium, leading to turbulence and decreased flow velocity. These clots spread in layers of "white" thrombi (platelets) and "red" thrombi (fibrin and red blood cells), and are found in atherosclerotic lesions and aneurysms.

In ultrasound they appear as layered hypoechoic bands. Sometimes they become reperfused again or they wall off anechoic spaces without flow in the interior or at the margin (serosanguineous fluid) (**Figs. 1.48 and 1.49**).

▲ **Fig. 1.48** White thrombus (TH) within a saccular aortic aneurysm: at first glance, the shape of the aorta (AO) seems to be regular while the vessels appears to be surrounded by a tumor; however, these are white thrombi within the aneurysmatic lumen.

▲ **Fig. 1.49** White thrombi within a saccular aortic aneurysm, staggered transverse views.
a Marginal layered thrombus (TH) and swirled thrombus (arrow) with the crescent-shaped anechoic remaining lumen; both clots are covered by an echogenic dissecting membrane (in aortic dissection this would be the intima).

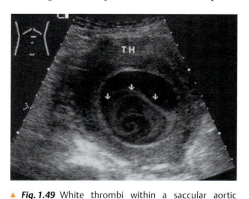

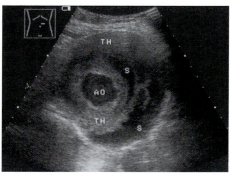

▲ *b* More caudad there is a regular, circular, central lumen of the aorta (AO). It is surrounded by alternating layers of white thrombi (TH) and serosanguineous fluid (S).

▶ Endovascular Stent

Depending on the situation involved, vascular grafts for aortic/arterial repair require open surgery or endovascular stenting. In the latter case, ultrasonography delineates these stents as echogenic reflecting bands (**Figs. 1.50, 1.43, and 1.31**).

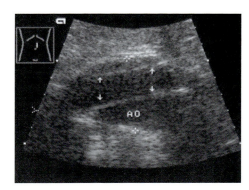

◀ **Fig. 1.50** Endovascular aortic stent; delicate echogenic wall of the intraluminal graft within an aortic aneurysm (transverse diameter 41 mm, calipers). AO = aorta.

▶ Intimal Dissection

Intimal dissection in the aorta or in aneurysms demonstrates a sonographic image similar to an endovascular stent; however, most often the patient's history is known, which then facilitates the differential diagnosis. Furthermore, the intima tends to be thicker and presents as a solitary echogenic intraluminal band. The origin of the dissection can be identified in only a few cases (**Fig. 1.51**).

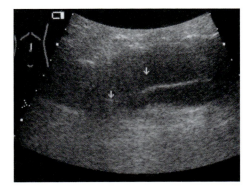

◀ **Fig. 1.51** Intraluminal structure almost identical to **Fig. 1.50**; dissection of the intima: in this case the origin of the dissection (arrows) is clearly visible.

Perivascular Mass

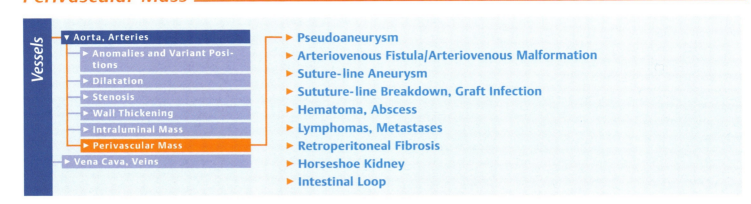

Perivascular masses may originate from the vessel itself (pseudoaneurysm, suture-line breakdown, graft infection) or arise completely independently of it. Ultrasound plays a vital role in the differential diagnosis of these diseases. The diagnosis cannot be confirmed in all cases; quite often the clinical picture will yield important clues, and sometimes additional imaging modalities are required or other diagnostic measures such as ultrasound-guided needle aspiration for cytology and histology.

▶ Pseudoaneurysm

A pseudoaneurysm (or false aneurysm) is a perivascular mass representing the extravasation of blood after iatrogenic or traumatic injury to the artery. This leads to a perivascular hematoma with either remaining blood flow or complete thrombosis. Ultrasonography will demonstrate a hypoechoic mass. In color-flow Doppler scanning the fistula with the perfused aneurysm and the degree of thrombosis can seen directly. After deliberate compression of the fistula with the ultrasound probe for about 20 minutes the canal of the fistula and the aneurysm should become thrombosed, thus making open surgery a thing of the past. This does not apply to arteriovenous fistulas (**Fig. 1.52**).

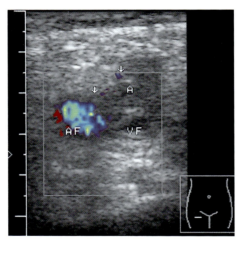

◀ *Fig. 1.52* Almost completely thrombosed pseudoaneurysm (A) of the femoral artery (AF) after catheterization. Red arterial Doppler signal. VF = thrombosed femoral vein.

▶ Arteriovenous Fistula/Arteriovenous Malformation

As is true for pseudoaneurysms, the most common cause of arteriovenous fistulas is iatrogenic (e.g., catheterization) while shrapnel injuries have become quite rare. The sonographic diagnosis is derived from the B-mode image and the arterial signal detected in the vein during duplex scanning (**Fig. 1.53**).

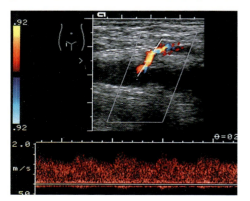 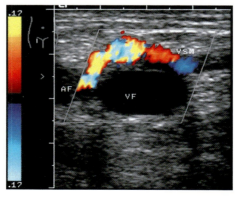 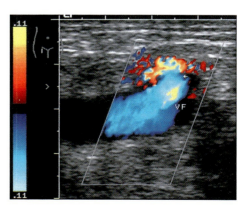

▲ *Fig. 1.53a,b and c* Arteriovenous fistula (F) between the femoral artery (AF) and the greater saphenous vein after catheterization *a* color flow doppler spectrum sampled in the fistula with a arterial signal *b,c* Fistula to the greater saphenous vein (VSM/arrow). VF = femoral vein.

An arteriovenous malformation is a congenital vascular anomaly in which an artery and vein are interconnected by undifferentiated vessels without a capillary network. The tangled vessels can be demonstrated by color duplex and spectral analysis only if a high shunt volume is present (**Fig. 1.54**).

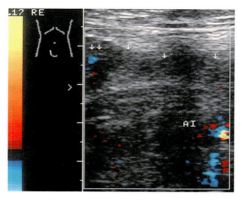
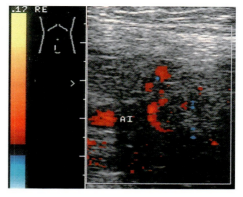

▲ *Fig. 1.54b* Arteriovenous malformation: **a** hypoechoic mass (arrows) anterior to and besides the iliac vessels (AI = iliac artery).

▲ **b** undifferentiated vessels with low flow in the color duplex scan.

▶ Suture-line Aneurysm

In a few cases bypass grafting may be complicated by the formation of a true or false aneurysm, the sonographic finding being the same as for the "normal" arterial system. The diagnosis is confirmed by color-flow duplex scanning.

▶ Suture-line Breakdown, Graft Infection

In most cases postoperative complications after bypass grafting manifest themselves immediately. A delayed onset combined with general symptoms, such as swelling, fever, or sepsis, may be difficult to diagnose.

The typical sonographic appearance of suture-line breakdown or graft infection is a hypoechoic perigraft mass; a local, walled-off mass tends to be a hematoma, while the band-like mass is more characteristic of purulent graft infection (**Figs. 1.55a and b**).

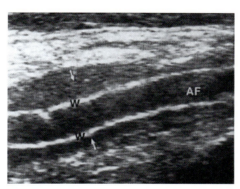
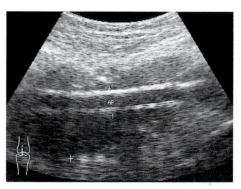

▲ *Fig. 1.55a* Leaking femoral graft and infected hematoma. The fluid surrounding the infected graft (arrows) permits excellent insonation of the graft wall (W). Longitudinal section. AF = left femoral artery.

▲ **b** Infected popliteal graft (arrows; AP) with extensive suppuration (calipers). Clinical signs were fever of unknown origin and possible thrombosis of the popliteal vein.

▶ Hematoma, Abscess

There is no clear-cut sonographic distinction between hematoma and abscess presenting as perivascular (aortic) mass, and the sonographer has to rely on the patient's history and the clinical signs. If the ultrasound findings are ambivalent, sonographically guided fine-needle aspiration may settle the diagnostic issue, possibly followed by therapeutic evacuation of the hematoma or abscess (**Fig. 1.56**).

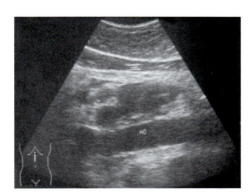

◀ *Fig. 1.56* Postoperative abscess anterior to the aorta after perforated appendicitis. (Clinical picture and possible echogenic gas bubbles, barely seen here, may point the way). AO = aorta.

▶ Lymphomas, Metastases

Malignant lymphoma may appear as hypoechoic para-aortic mass in 50% of cases. Malignant metastases usually are found along the lymphatics draining the tumor and thus may help pinpoint the primary. Whereas metastases are round, lymphomas tend to present a "sandwich" structure (**Fig. 1.57**).

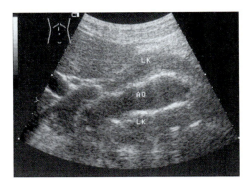

◀ **Fig. 1.57** A band of periaortic lymphomas (LK): "sandwich-like" appearance, highly malignant non-Hodgkin lymphoma. The sonographic finding could be confused with a partially thrombosed aortic aneurysm. AO = aorta.

▶ Retroperitoneal Fibrosis

In rare cases a hyperechoic periaortic and pericaval "encasing" mass may be due to retroperitoneal fibrosis, a disease associated with other manifestations (**Fig. 1.58**, also see Chapter 11 "Urinary Tract" **Fig. 11.28, p. 340**).

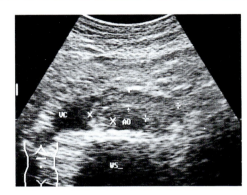

◀ **Fig. 1.58** Retroperitoneal fibrosis: hypoechoic masses (calipers) encasing the aorta (AO). WS = spine; VC = compressed vena cava.

▶ Horseshoe Kidney

A hypoechoic round or oval-shaped (in the transverse diameter) mass anterior to the aorta will confirm the diagnosis of a horseshoe kidney, if the study is continued into the flanks and a connection with the kidney becomes evident (**Fig. 1.59**).

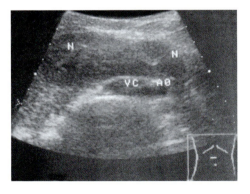

◀ **Fig. 1.59** Hypoechoic mass resembling lymph nodes anterior to the large abdominal vessels: horseshoe kidney (N). AO = aorta; VC = vena cava.

▶ Intestinal Loop

Differential diagnosis of a para-aortic mass has to include the possibility of a hypoechoic intestinal loop distended by fluid. If the mass is observed over a period of time and shows signs of peristalsis, this will settle any doubts (**Fig. 1.60**).

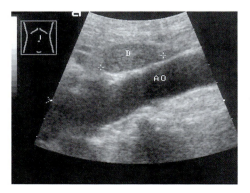

◀ **Fig. 1.60** Periaortic "mass": fluid filled intestinal loop, differentiation from a true intra-abdominal mass is possible only by its motion. AO = aorta; D = small bowel.

Vena Cava, Veins

Anomalies

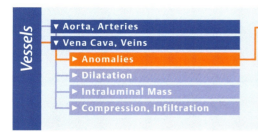

▶ Anomalies/Duplication of the Inferior Vena Cava

Anomalies. Anomalies of the vena cava are infrequent and most are incidental findings during ultrasonography, in which case they present problems regarding the differential diagnosis. Precise knowledge of the anatomy is invaluable in these instances. Agenesis is extremely rare and is usually associated with other clinically significant cardiovascular malformations during the prenatal and postnatal period. The situs inversus viscerum is discussed in the section on anomalies of the aorta.

Duplication. Quite often duplication of the vena cava is overlooked because it does not result in any symptoms—except for thrombosis.

According to Chuang (cited in 9), duplication of the inferior vena cava has an incidence of 0.05–3%, i.e., it is not especially rare. As part of complex embryonic disorders, such duplication develops from the embryonic post-, sub- and supracardinal veins, which comprise a primarily bilateral, symmetric, abdominal venous system fusing to the secondary dextroverted asymmetric system of the inferior vena cava. The classification is based on the three possible segments involved, and for the postrenal segment is subdivided into the four types A to BC. ▣ **1.4** shows examples of vena cava duplication.

> **Congenital Anomalies of the Inferior Vena Cava**
>
> ▶ **I Postrenal segment**
> Type A: persistent right postcardinal vein ("retro- or periaortic ureter")
> Type B: persistent right supracardinal vein ("normal inferior vena cava")
> Type C: persistent left supracardinal vein ("left inferior vena cava")
> Type BC: persistent left and right supracardinal veins ("duplicated inferior vena cava")
>
> ▶ **II Renal segment**
> Persistent ring of renal veins ("periaortic ureter")
>
> ▶ **III Prerenal or hepatic segment**
> Missing hepatic segment ("azygos or hemiazygos vein continuation")

▣ 1.4 Duplicated Inferior Vena Cava

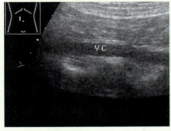 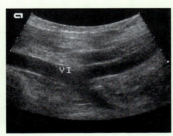 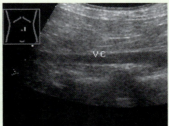

a Longitudinal right paramedian view of the abdomen: right iliac vein (VI) and inferior vena cava (VC).

b Longitudinal left paramedian view of the abdomen: left iliac vein (VI) and inferior vena cava (VC); partial view of the iliac artery (AI).

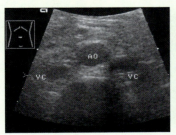 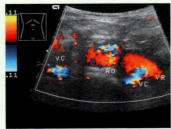 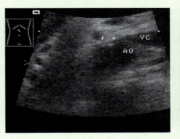 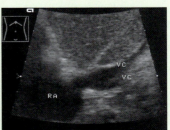

c Transverse view at the umbilicus, B-mode image and color-flow Doppler scan: there are two inferior venae cava (VC) with respective color signals. The left renal vein (VR) joins the left inferior vena cava and does not cross the aorta anteriorly in order to join the right vena cava as would be the case in normal anatomy. AO = aorta.

d Oblique subxiphoidal median view and longitudinal paramedian epigastric view: the left inferior vena cava (VC) crosses the aorta (AO) anteriorly and runs obliquely in a cephalad direction joining the right vena cava (VC) (other courses are possible) before entering the right atrium (RA).

▶ Anomalies of the Iliac Veins

Anomalies of the iliac veins are also known and may become a problem in surgery or thrombosis. In most cases it is an abnormal junction of the left iliac vein with the right common iliac vein or a true duplication.

▶ Duplication of Renal and Peripheral Veins

A retroaortic left renal vein, or duplicated renal veins, may become significant if there is thrombosis or the suspicion of tumor infiltration (**Fig. 1.61**). Duplication of the popliteal vein is a frequent variant of normal anatomy, while duplicated femoral veins are rare. Most of these cases are incidental findings in the work-up of deep venous thrombosis (see below).

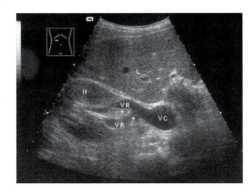

◀ **Fig. 1.61** Renal vein with partial duplication (VR), merging just before the junction with the inferior vena cava (VC). Arrows: partial view of the renal artery. L = liver; N = kidney.

Dilatation

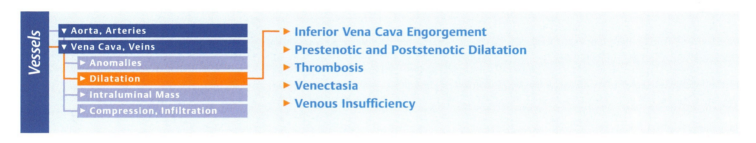

▶ Inferior Vena Cava Engorgement

The most common cause of an engorged inferior vena cava is cardiac congestion, which in turn may be due to right ventricular failure, pulmonary embolism, pericardial fibrosis (armored heart), or mitral valve disorders.

In ultrasonography, cardiac congestion is seen as engorgement of the right atrium and ventricle, inferior vena cava (beyond 20 mm), and hepatic veins (beyond 10 mm). The lack of physiological and respiration-induced variation in the caliber of the inferior vena cava and its incompressibility are vital diagnostic criteria and simply mirror the congestion of the vein. Engorgement of the inferior vena cava also implies enlarged venous tributaries (**Fig. 1.62**).

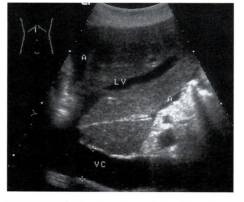

▲ **Fig. 1.62** Inferior vena cava and hepatic vein engorgement.
a Marked expansion of the vena cava to 27 mm (cursors), congested hepatic vein (LV), ascites (A).

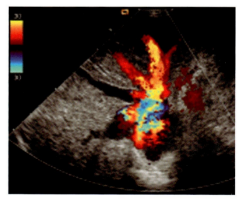

▲ *b* Subcostal section, color flow duplex scan: The red doppler signal of the liver veins marks the systolic reverse flow.

▶ Prestenotic and Poststenotic Dilatation

Stenosis of the inferior vena cava will result in prestenotic and poststenotic enlargement of the vein, this sometimes being the only sign of any obstruction (**Figs. 1.63 and 1.64**).

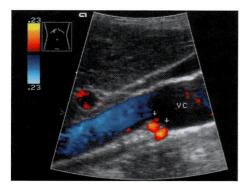

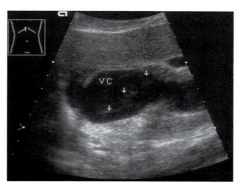

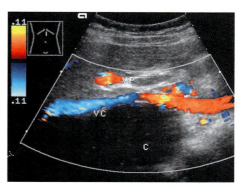

▲ **Fig. 1.63** Prestenotic enlargement of the inferior vena cava due to two renal arteries (arrows) crossing posteriorly. Color-flow Doppler scanning with fixed Doppler velocity of 23 cm/s. Because of decreased flow velocity there is no color signal in the vena cava segment (VC) proximal to the stenosis.

▲ **Fig. 1.64** Poststenotic enlargement of the inferior vena cava.
a Decreased flow velocity with turbulence ("RBC noise", arrows).

▲ **b** Slight prestenotic and poststenotic dilatation; color-flow Doppler scan: a 4-liter (!) liver cyst with hematoma, extending behind the vena cava (VC) with long-stretched indentation of the posterior wall of the vein. VP = portal vein. C = cyst.

▶ Thrombosis

Lesions in the vessel wall, venostasis, and hypercoagulability (Virchow's triad) will trigger venous thrombosis. The latter two also are causative factors in paraneoplastic thrombosis, which should always be included in the differential diagnosis.

In ultrasound imaging, the essential characteristics of venous thrombosis are a vein enlarged to more than 1.5 times the diameter of the respective artery[3] and the lack of compressibility (**Fig. 1.65; see Figs. 1.13, p. 7**) (also see "Intraluminal Mass," p. 28 ff.).

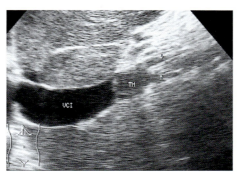

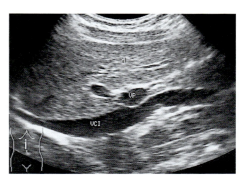

▲ **Fig. 1.65** Vena cava thrombosis (TH) in a patient with protein S and C deficiency, vena cava filter (arrows).
a Thrombotic (TH) and poststenotic enlargement of the vena cava (VCI).

▲ **b** After thrombolysis: complete recanalization, regular caliber of the vein. VP = portal vein; H = liver.

▶ Venectasia

Segmental dilatation of a vein may be physiological in nature or due to impaired outflow or anatomy: for example, a large vena cava lumen in adolescents, distended jugular veins, or physiological engorgement of the left renal vein when crossing the aorta. Venous aneurysms, e.g., in the popliteal vein, presenting with painful swelling may easily be differentiated from Baker's cyst, since in the latter case there will be no color signal in color-flow Doppler scanning (**Figs. 1.66 and 1.67**).

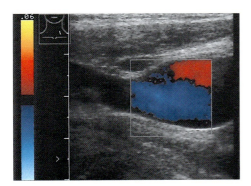

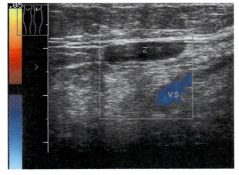

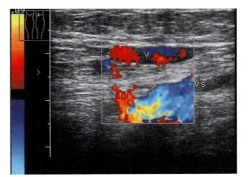

▲ **Fig. 1.66** Ectatic internal jugular vein: marked enlargement, slow turbulent flow demonstrated by the blue-red color signal; very low flow velocity (fixed low pulse repetition frequency, PRF, with corresponding maximum velocity of 6 cm/s).

▲ **Fig. 1.67** Presumed Baker's cyst. VS = lesser saphenous vein.
a Presumed cyst (Z) in the popliteal fossa.

▲ **b** After extrinsic compression of the lower leg, color-flow Doppler evaluation detects venectasia (V) with proven incompetence of the saphenopopliteal junction.

▶ Venous Insufficiency

Refluxing blood in a vein will lead to segmental dilatation, which in turn results in venous incompetence. Predisposed locations are:
- Saphenofemoral junction ("insufficient saphenous junction")
- Saphenopopliteal junction ("insufficient parva junction")
- Proximal femoral and popliteal vein
- Lower leg (varicosities, incompetent perforators)

The diagnosis is to be confirmed by color-flow Doppler scanning, and the severity can easily be graded according to the Hach classification[4] (**Figs. 1.68 and 1.69**).

Hach Classification of Greater Saphenous Insufficiency

- **Stage I**: Insufficient saphenous junction
- **Stage II**: Insufficient saphenous junction plus reflux to the distal thigh
- **Stage III**: Insufficient saphenous junction plus reflux to the proximal lower leg
- **Stage IV**: Insufficient saphenous junction plus reflux to the ankle

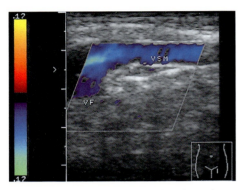
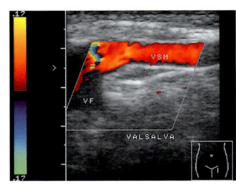
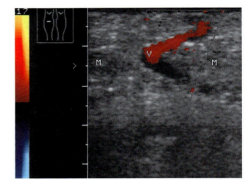

▲ **Fig. 1.68** Incompetence of the saphenofemoral junction.
a Junction of the enlarged greater saphenous vein (VSM) and the femoral vein (VF).

▲ *b* Valsalva maneuver: color change from blue to red, confirming venous reflux.

▲ **Fig. 1.69** Incompetent Cockett's perforators: venous runoff from the posterior tibial veins through the gastrocnemius muscle (M) to the superficial venous system.

Intraluminal Mass

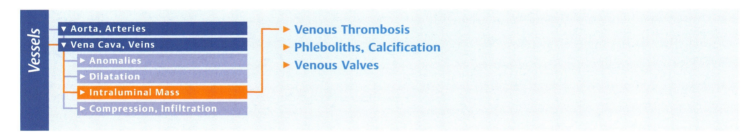

▶ Venous Thrombosis

The value of diagnostic ultrasound. Today, ultrasonography is the modality of choise thrombosis in case of suspected, and together with phlebography it has become the gold standard in the diagnosis of venous thrombosis. Color-flow Doppler scanning demonstrating little or no flow has expanded its diagnostic capabilities. Sonographic work-up for suspected venous thrombosis of easily accessible regions may be performed without difficulty and takes but a few minutes. It is more difficult to perform on the iliac veins, the lower leg, the periuterine venous plexus, or the ovarian vein, where it has a higher error rate. Phlebography only becomes necessary, if in case of strong clinical suspicion, the diagnostic findings are negative or ambivalent or if the conditions for the study are especially poor. Reliable sonographic diagnosis of venous thrombosis is even possible in the lower leg, although here usually only the posterior tibial veins can be imaged.

Venous filling. There may be problems if the deep veins are not filled enough, particularly in hypovolemia, in which case it may be helpful to evaluate the patient standing and with compression of the lower leg. On the other hand, marked venous engorgement will complicate the evaluation since the deep veins will come under pressure and this may mimic incompressibility.

Criteria of thrombosis. The surest sign of thrombosis is venous incompressibility. It is not possible to differentiate between old and fresh thrombi. Free-floating thrombus tail surrounded by blood flow, identification of the thrombus head, and discrete compressibility of the thrombus point to a soft thrombus. A normal venous lumen is seen only in old thrombosis. Extrinsic compression of the vein with the probe could shear off the thrombus in rare cases but would not result in any clinically evident embolism.

Ultrasonography of a thrombus surrounded by blood demonstrates an anechoic marginal lumen between thrombus and venous wall, the flow being confirmed by color-flow Doppler scan. Color-flow duplex evaluation is of vital importance for this type of thrombosis as well as for difficult sonographic conditions. Even if the vein is hardly visible in B-mode imaging, thrombosis can be definitively ruled out by color-flow duplex scanning. Compression ultrasonography is best suited for evaluating the treatment, making phlebographic controls unnecessary. There is no formal distinction between platelet- and tumor-induced thrombosis.

1.5 Sonographic Criteria for Assessing Venous Thrombosis

▶ Incompressibility (most important sign)

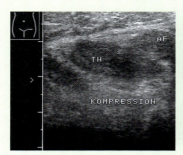
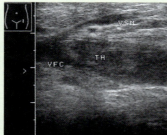
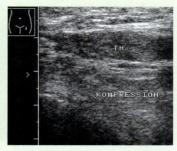

a–c Deep venous thrombosis (TH) of the thigh.
a Cross-section: this view permits better detection of the vein, which cannot be compressed because of the thrombosis.

b Longitudinal view: presentation of the patent proximal segment of the common femoral vein (VFC) as well as the thrombus (TH). The greater saphenous vein (VSM) is slender with no suspicion of thrombosis.

c Compression: under extrinsic compression there is complete collapse of the proximal femoral and the greater saphenous veins, while the thrombosed section is incompressible.

▶ Vascular enlargement (1.5 times the arterial diameter)

▶ Intraluminal echogenic structures

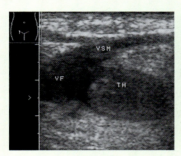
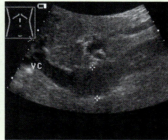
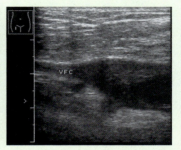

d Fresh venous thrombosis (TH), such as is imaged here, will always enlarge the diameter of the vessel. The lumen of the vein will remain normal only in cases of old thrombosis. VF = femoral vein; VSM = greater saphenous vein.

e Thrombosis of the vena cava (VC): localized engorgement of the vena cava (calipers). The thrombus itself hardly has any structural elements and therefore cannot be seen directly.

f Thrombosis of the common femoral vein (VFC): markedly dilated segment of the vein at the partial thrombosis (echogenic structures).

▶ No Doppler signals and flow or flow defects in color-flow Doppler scanning

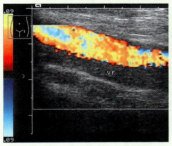
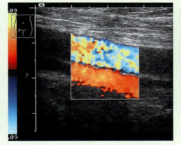
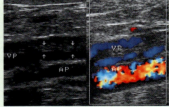

g and h Old thrombosis of the femoral vein (VF) in color-flow Doppler scanning.
g Since the vein is not dilated, there is no initial suspicion of thrombosis; no flow in color-flow duplex scanning.

h For comparison, the right femoral vein, which is not thrombosed.

i Partial thrombosis of the popliteal vein (VP). B-mode image: central thrombosis (arrows) of the vein. In color-flow Doppler imaging there is marginal flow. AP = popliteal artery.

1.5 gives examples of the sonographic criteria of thrombosis after Habscheid[3] (also see **Figs. 1.13 and 1.65**).

Crural thrombosis. Venous thrombosis in the calf is more difficult to image because the deep posterior tibial veins are hard to insonate, especially in hypovolemia and dialysis. In this case the lack of demonstrable veins almost *rules out* venous thrombosis since the latter would have resulted in easily viewed engorged veins (**Fig. 1.70**).

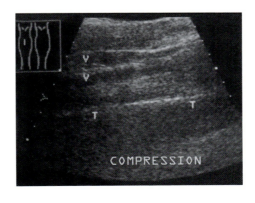

◀ **Fig. 1.70** Deep venous thrombosis of the calf affecting the posterior tibial group of veins (V, arrows). F = fibula; T = tibia.
a Longitudinal view of the calf.

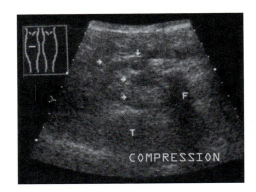
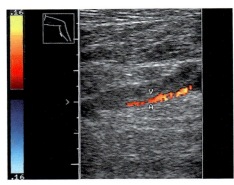

◄◄ **Fig. 1.70**
b Transverse view of the calf: incompressible veins (arrows).

◄ **c** Deep venous thrombosis of the calf, color-flow Doppler scan: enlargement of the vein (V) compared with the artery (A). Incompressibility.

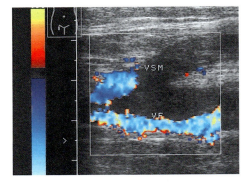
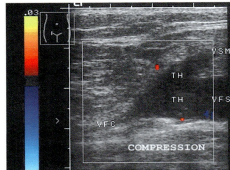

◄◄ **Fig. 1.71** Deep thrombosis of the superficial femoral and greater saphenous veins.
a No flow in the greater saphenous vein (VSM), with some flow in the superficial femoral vein (VF).

◄ **b** Compression: the remaining perfusion is blocked, while the thrombus (TH) is incompressible.

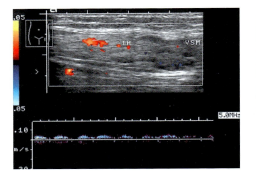
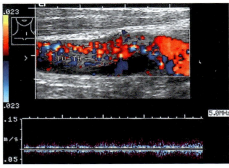

◄◄ **Fig. 1.72** Superficial venous thrombosis (TH).
a Thrombosis of the greater saphenous vein (VSM). Distended lumen, echogenic structures, low-level perfusion, spectral analysis.

◄ **b** Intensive spotty vascularization within a thrombus in the jugular vein: tumorous thrombus originating from thyroid metastasis of renal carcinoma.

Superficial venous thrombosis. Just as for the deep veins, superficial venous thrombosis fulfills the same typical sonographic criteria. In thrombosis of the greater and lesser saphenous vein, always insonate the saphenofemoral and saphenopopliteal junctions, respectively, to check the passage into the deep vein (**Figs. 1.71 and 1.72**).

▶ Phleboliths, Calcification

Phleboliths (also known as "vein stones") are calcified thrombi and appear as hyperechogenic masses, sometimes associated with shadowing. They may occur in focal fashion or as extended horseshoe-shaped calcifications, resulting in a bandlike structure within the vein with strong reflections (**Figs. 1.73 and 1.74**).

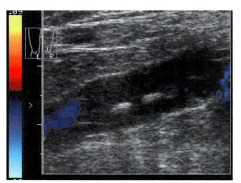

▲ **Fig. 1.73** Phleboliths with incomplete shadowing in a superficial vein of the calf, old thrombosis, flow defect in color-flow Doppler scanning.

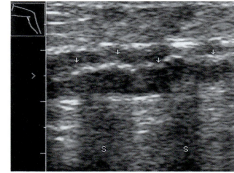

▲ **Fig. 1.74** Old calcified band-shaped thrombosis of the lesser saphenous vein, shadowing (S).

▶ Venous Valves

Venous valves are pocket-shaped intimal folds with check valve characteristics, permitting blood flow only toward the heart. Under excellent sonographic conditions they may be imaged as echogenic V-shaped intraluminal structures opening toward the heart (**Fig. 1.75**).

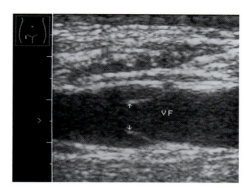

◀ **Fig. 1.75** Venous valves (arrows) within the femoral vein (VF).

Compression, Infiltration

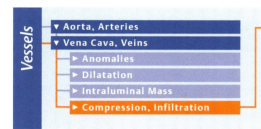

- ▶ Enlarged Caudate Lobe
- ▶ Budd–Chiari Syndrome
- ▶ Lymph Nodes, Cysts
- ▶ Other Masses
- ▶ Malignant Tumor

▶ Enlarged Caudate Lobe

The inferior vena cava arcs widely posterior to the caudate lobe. Because of this close anatomical relationship, it is more (tumorous infiltration) or less (long arced impression in case of cirrhotic enlargement of the caudate lobe) involved in any adjacent changes (**Fig. 1.76**).

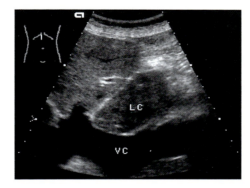

◀ **Fig. 1.76** Cirrhotic enlargement of the caudate lobe (LC): impressed and displaced Vena cava (VC).

▶ Budd–Chiari Syndrome

The most severe, and without treatment lethal, effect on the inferior vena cava is Budd–Chiari syndrome with thrombosis of all hepatic veins (young women on oral contraceptives) or tumorous occlusion (older patients with infiltration of the inferior vena cava at the junction of the hepatic veins). Ultrasonography, in particular color-flow duplex scanning with spectral analysis, is the imaging modality of choice in the diagnosis of a thrombotic or tumorous occlusion of the hepatic veins. It may also aid in the rapid diagnosis of the cause of lower venous congestion (as well as upper, e.g., with local metastasis of lung cancer) (**Fig. 1.77**).

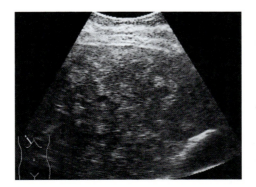
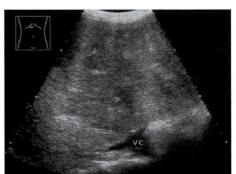

▲ **Fig. 1.77** Acute and chronic Budd–Chiari syndrome. *a* Acute Budd-Chiary-Syndrome: Occlusion of all three hepatic veins (infiltration of the vena cava by metastatic lymph nodes). Speckled liver structure, no visible veins. Clinical diagnosis was ovarian cancer; there was massive pain and the patient died after a few days.

▲ *b* Chronic Budd-Chiary-Syndrome: Diffuse metastatic infiltration with occlusion of the liver veins. VC = Vena cava.

▶ Lymph Nodes, Cysts

Compression of the vena cava and peripheral veins by lymph nodes and cysts is quite common. Because of their thin walls and low blood pressure, veins will yield to the pressure of an extrinsic mass and become indented according to its shape. The type of mass may be diagnosed on the basis of the patient's history and clinical symptoms, and occasionally by ultrasound-guided fine-needle aspiration biopsy.

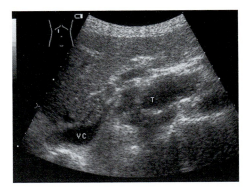

◀ **Fig. 1.78** Compression and displacement of the inferior vena cava (VC) by lymph nodes: relapse of a gastric MALT lymphoma post surgery. T = tumor.

▶ Other Masses

Retroperitoneal fibrosis is another, but rather uncommon, cause of impression of the vena cava. Aortic aneurysm or enlargement of the pancreatic head may also displace or severely compress the vena cava (**Figs. 1.79 and 1.80**).

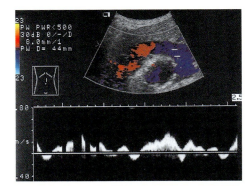

▲ **Fig. 1.79** Severe curved displacement of the vena cava by an aortic aneurysm: spectral analysis depicts the normal venous Doppler spectrum with cardiac modulation.

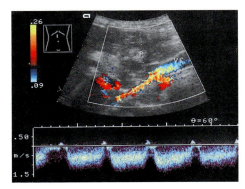

▲ **Fig. 1.80** Compression of the vena cava by the enlarged pancreatic head in an acute attack of chronic pancreatitis. The vena cava (VC) is markedly narrowed. Abnormal spectral waveform shows stenotic flow acceleration and a pulsatile flow pattern. P = pancreas.

▶ Malignant Tumor

Malignant tumors tend to infiltrate, whereas metastases compress. In both cases the end result may be occlusion of the vena cava with its prognostically poor sequelae (**Figs. 1.81, 1.82, and 1.97**).

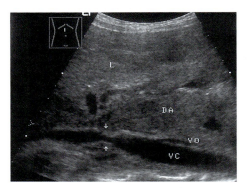

▲ **Fig. 1.81** Severe infiltration of the vena cava (arrows) by the caudate lobe metastasis of breast cancer. DA = small bowel; VO = ovarian vein; VC = vena cava; L = liver.

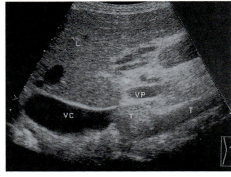

▲ **Fig. 1.82** Renal cell carcinoma. Upper abdominal longitudinal scan of tumor (T) infiltrating the vena cava (VC). L = liver; VP = portal vein.

References

1. Bönhof JA, Meairs SP, Wetzler H. Duplex- und Farbdoppler-sonographische Kriterien von Nierenarterienstenosen. Ultraschall Klin Prax 1990;5:187.s
2. Fellmeth BD, Roberts AC, Bookstein JJ et al. Postangiographic femoral artery injuries. Nonsurgical repair with US-guided compression. Radiology 1991;178:671.
3. Habscheid W, Landwehr P. Diagnostik der akuten tiefen Beinvenenthrombose mit der Kompressionssonographie. Ultraschall in Med 1990;11:268–73.
4. Hach W, Girth E, Lechner W. Einteilung der Stammvarikose der V. saphena magna in 4 Stadien. Phlebol Proktol 1977;6:116–23.
4a. Heyne, JP. Die doppelte Aorta-Rarität oder Artefakt im Ultraschall. Ultraschall in Med 2000; 21:145–148
5. Ludwig M, Kraft K, Rücker W, Hüther AM. Die Diagnose sehr früher arteriosklerotischer Gefäßwandveränderungen mit Hilfe der Duplexsonographie. Klin Wochenschr 1989;67:442–6.
6. Mallek R, Mostbeck G, Walter R, Tscholakow D. Duplexsonographie der Visceralarterien: Angiographische Korrelation. Ultraschall Klin Prax 1990;5:186.
7. Mörl H, Menges HW. Gefäßkrankheiten in der Praxis. 7th ed. Stuttgart: Thieme 2000.
8. Neuburg-Heusler D, Hennerici M. Gefäßdiagnostik mit Ultraschall. 2nd ed. Stuttgart: Thieme 1995.
9. Rettenmaier G, Seitz K. Sonographische Differentialdiagnostik. Stuttgart: Thieme 2000.
10. Riede UN. Taschenatlas der allgemeinen Pathologie. Stuttgart: Thieme 1998.
11. Widder B, von Reutern GM, Neuburg-Heusler D. Morphologische und dopplersonographische Kriterien zur Bestimmung von Stenosierungsgraden an der A. carotis interna. Ultraschall 1986;7.

Portal Vein and Its Tributaries

C. Goerg

The portal venous system comprises four regions: intrahepatic branches of the portal vein; portal vein at the porta hepatis; splenic vein; and splanchnic veins. Blood from the splanchnic region (including the spleen) normally flows in hepatopetal fashion.

Anatomy

Size
- Portal vein at the hilum: 1.0–1.5 cm
- Splenic vein at the hilum: 0.5–1.0 cm

Flow
- Mean flow velocity of the portal vein: 15–20 cm/s

Size and shape. The diameter of the portal vein displays a somewhat wider range between individuals (**see Fig. 1.93**). In fasting patients, a diameter of up to 15 mm is considered normal. Usually, the portal vein has an oval shape in the transverse plane. The mean portal flow velocity has been reported as 15–20 cm/s, with a wide range of values here as well.

Under normal conditions the diameter of the splenic vein at the hilum should be less than 7 mm (**1.6p and q**). The mesenteric vein is compressible and exhibits respiratory caliber variations of more than 15%.

Topography

The right gastric vein joins the trunk of the portal vein at the hepatic portal (**1.6a and b**). Within the liver the portal trunk divides like a "staghorn" into the left and right portal branches (**1.6c–f**). The main right portal branch gives off the anterior branch, which supplies segments V and VIII, while its posterior branch supplies segments VI and VII (**1.6g and h**). The left portal branch divides into the so-called horizontal and umbilical parts, supplying segments I, II, III, and IV (**1.6i–l**). The splenic vein is regarded as lead structure for the pancreas and can be followed into the splenic hilum. The superior mesenteric vein parallels the superior mesenteric artery and can be demonstrated, together with its branches, in the inferior parts of the mesentery (**1.6m–s, Fig. 1.83**). Anomalies of the intrahepatic branches of the portal vein are rare.

Position
- Splenic vein posterior to the pancreas
- Mesenteric vein parallel to the superior mesenteric artery
- Portal vein posterior to the bile duct and hepatic artery
- Intrahepatic bifurcation of the portal vein into left and right branch

Lead structure
- Posterior to the pancreatic head

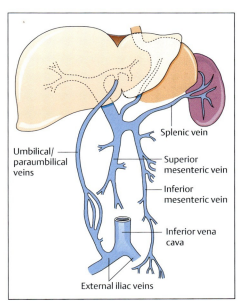

▲ **Fig. 1.83** Portocaval collaterals accessible to ultrasound in portal hypertension.

1.6 Topographic Anatomy of the Portal Vein and Its Tributaries

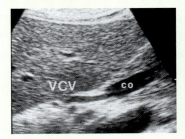 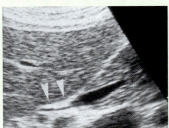 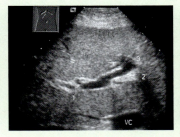 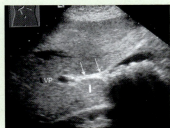

a and b Junction of the right gastric vein (VCV) with the confluence of the superior mesenteric and splenic veins (co); respiratory variation in the lumen diameter.
a Inspiration.

b Expiration (arrows).

c Subcostal view of the liver with left and right branches of the portal vein. VC = vena cava; 1, 2, 3 = segments I–III.

d Septum stretching between the right branch of the portal vein and the gallbladder. VP = portal vein.

1.6 Topographic Anatomy of the Portal Vein and Its Tributaries

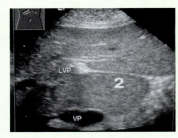
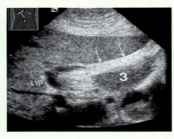
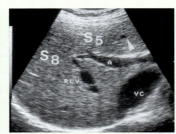
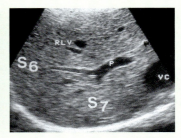

e The venous ligament runs from the left branch of the portal vein (2) to the posteroinferior aspect of the liver. LVP = left portal vein; VP = portal vein.

f The ligamentum teres stretches between the left branch of the portal vein (3) and the umbilicus. LVP = left portal vein.

g Right anterior branch of the portal vein (A) with branches supplying the anterior segments V (S5) (inferior) and VIII (S8) (superior). RLV = right hepatic vein.

h Posterior branch of the main right portal vein trunk (P) supplying the posterior segments VI (S6) (inferior) and VII (S7) (superior) of the right hepatic lobe. RLV = right hepatic vein; VC = vena cava.

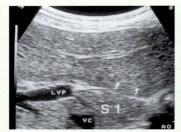
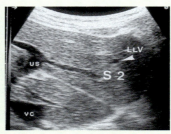
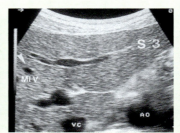
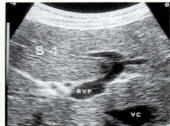

i–l The left branch of the portal vein (LVP) supplies segments I–IV (S1–S3) (VC = vena cava).
i Segment I.

j Segment II. US = umbilical segment, LLV = left hepatic vein.

k Segment III.

l Segment IV. RVP = right branch of portal vein).

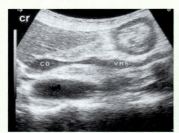
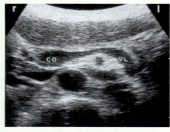
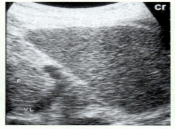
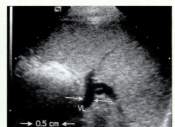

m Longitudinal subxiphoid view with superior mesenteric vein (VMS). CO = venous confluence.

n Transverse epigastric view with splenic vein (VL). CO = venous confluence

o Left intercostal plane with hilar view of the splenic vein (VL). P = pancreatic tail.

p Splenic vein (VL) with normal lumen diameter.

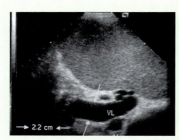
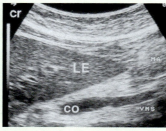

q Enlarged splenic vein (VL) in portal hypertension.

r and s Respiratory variation in the lumen diameter of the superior mesenteric vein (VMS). LE = liver. CO = venous confluence; MA = stomach.

Enlarged Lumen Diameter

Precise diagnosis of any enlargement of the portal vein diameter is one of the strong points of ultrasonography.

Portal Hypertension

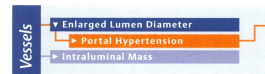

Portal hypertension is defined as a pressure of more than 10 mmHg in the portal vein. The pressure depends on the resistance of the run-off bed within the liver, the blood volume in the splanchnic vessels, and the pressure in the inferior vena cava. The etiology of its various types and causes is classified according to the location of the flow impediment. Accordingly, portal hypertension may be subdivided into prehepatic, intrahepatic, and posthepatic types, with the intrahepatic type being subdivided into postsinusoidal, sinusoidal, and presinusoidal forms (**Table 1.2**).

The pathophysiology of portal hypertension is characterized by a drop in flow velocity, enlarged vein diameter, sclerosis, opening up of collaterals, and flow reversal in the portal vein or its tributaries. The collaterals are differentiated by the direction of their drainage, i.e., they are subdivided into cephalad and caudad draining shunts (**Table 1.3**).

Sonographic studies in portal hypertension will yield presumed and rather firm findings. Images similar to ◨ 1.7 should raise the suspicion of portal hypertension:
▶ Enlarged vena cava and hepatic veins (◨ **1.7a and b**)
▶ Demonstration of ascites (◨ **1.7c and d**)
▶ Demonstration of liver cirrhosis (◨ **1.7a–d**)
▶ Thickening of the gallbladder wall (◨ **1.7e**)
▶ No respiratory variation in the diameter of the portal vessels (◨ **1.7f**)
▶ Thickening of the gastric/intestinal wall (◨ **1.7g–i**)
▶ Splenomegaly, splenic fibrosis (◨ **1.7j and k**)
▶ Enlarged lumen of the hepatic artery (◨ **1.7l**)

Table 1.2 Possible causes of portal hypertension

Posthepatic
 – Right-sided heart failure
 – Constrictive pericarditis
 – Tricuspid regurgitation
 – Membranous obstruction of hepatic segments of the vena cava

Intrahepatic
▶ Postsinusoidal
 – Liver cirrhosis
 – Budd–Chiari syndrome, venous occlusion
▶ Sinusoidal
 – Chronic hepatitis
 – Fatty liver
 – Liver cirrhosis
▶ Presinusoidal
 – Idiopathic portal hypertension
 – Hepatic fibrosis
 – Myeloproliferative disorders
 – Granulomatosis
 – Primary biliary cirrhosis
 – Severe splenomegaly without hepatic disease

Prehepatic
 – Portal vein thrombosis
 – Cavernous transformation of the portal vein
 – Segmental thrombosis of the splenic vein
 – Arterioportal fistula

Table 1.3 Formation of possible collaterals in portal hypertension (after reference 4)

Cephalad draining collaterals
▶ Right gastric vein
▶ Short gastric veins
▶ Periumbilical veins
▶ Portogastric collaterals
▶ Portorenal collaterals
▶ Hepatic, phrenic, and splenic capsule veins

Caudad draining veins
▶ Paraumbilical veins
▶ Gastrosplenic shunts
▶ Splenorenal shunts
▶ Splenolumbar shunts
▶ Hemorrhoidal plexus via the mesenteric veins

With the advent of color-flow Doppler imaging, the following are considered rather firm signs of portal hypertension:
▶ Flow reversal in the portal vein or some of its tributaries (**Fig. 1.84**)
▶ Oscillating flow in the portal vein or some of its tributaries (**Figs. 1.85–1.88**)
▶ No flow
▶ Demonstration of portosystemic collaterals

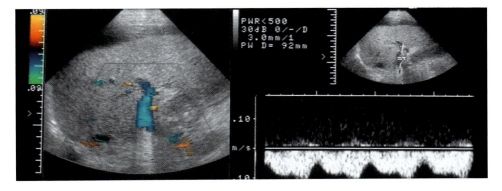

◀ **Fig. 1.84** Continuous flow reversal in the portal vein (hepatofugal flow) in a patient with liver cirrhosis.

1.7 Portal Hypertension: Suspect Findings

▶ Hepatic cirrhosis

▶ Contour signs

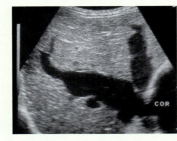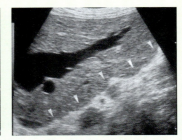

a and *b* Cardiac cirrhosis in tricuspid insufficiency. Massively dilated hepatic veins, the posteroinferior aspect of the liver has a corrugated appearance (arrows). COR = heart.

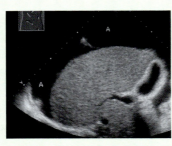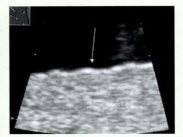

c and *d* Completely cirrhotic liver with ascites (A) and corrugated appearance (arrow) in a chronic alcoholic.

▶ Ascites, Thickening of the gallbladder, vascular change

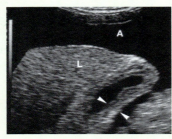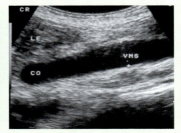

e Cirrhosis of the liver (L) with ascites (A) and thickened wall of the gallbladder (arrows).

f Markedly enlarged lumen of the mesenteric vein (VMS) and its confluence, with the splenic vein in portal hypertension without respiratory variation. LE = liver; CO = venous confluence.

▶ Thickening of the stomach, and bowel walls

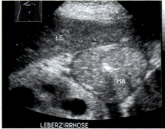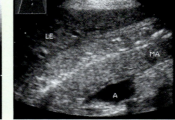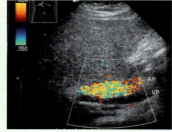

g and *h* Congested stomach with marked thickening of the gastric wall in cirrhosis of the liver and portal hypertension (A = ascites, MA = gastric wall; LE = liver).

i Pronounced intestinal wall in portal hypertension.

▶ Structural, vascular change, splenomegaly

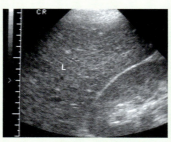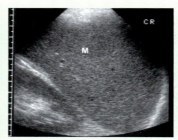

j Completely cirrhotic liver (L) with markedly coarse hepatic parenchyma.

k Portal hypertension with pronounced splenomegaly (M).

l Posthepatic cirrhosis of the liver with decreased portal blood flow and increased flow in the hepatic artery (AH). VP = portal vein.

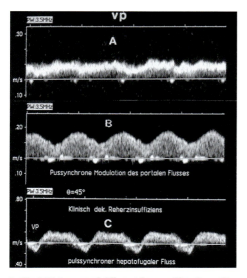
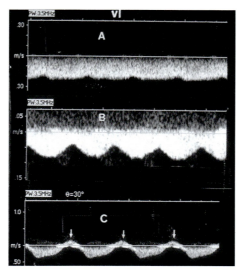
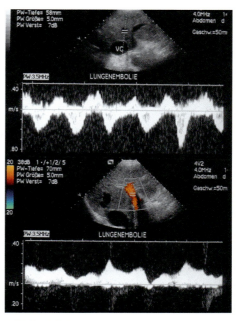

▲ *Fig. 1.85* Images of different flow profiles: **A**, continuous hepatopetal flow; **B**, pulsatile hepatopetal flow; **C**, pulsatile flow with brief pulse-synchronous flow reversal (arrows)
a In the portal vein.

▲ ***b*** In the splenic vein.

▲ *Fig. 1.87* Patient with clinically evident symptomatic pulmonary embolism.
a Flow profile of the hepatic veins with severe pulse-synchronous reflux.
b Flow profile in the portal vein with predominantly hepatopetal flow but also brief hepatofugal flow.

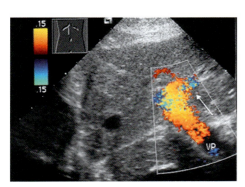
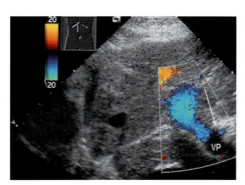
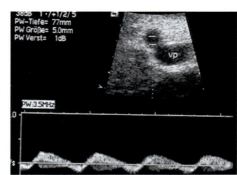

▲ *Fig. 1.86* Pulsatile portal flow with brief pulse-synchronous flow reversal in a patient with cardiac cirrhosis. VP = portal vein.

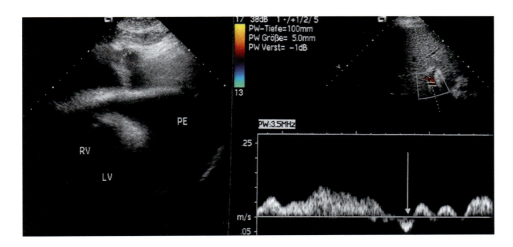

◀ *Fig. 1.88* Pericardial effusion.
a Patient with marked pericardial effusion (PE). RV = right ventricular; LV = left ventricular.
b The flow profile in the portal vein demonstrates a brief reflux episode (arrow).

▶ Prehepatic Block

In less than 20% of patients portal hypertension will be due to a prehepatic block. Important causes of prehepatic block are total or partial thrombosis of the portal, splenic, and mesenteric veins (**Fig. 1.89**). Extrinsic portal vein compression (**Fig. 1.90**), agenesis, or hypoplastic malformation also may result in portal hypertension (**Figs. 1.91 and 1.92**).

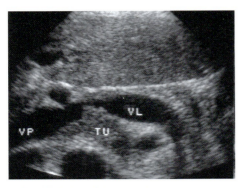
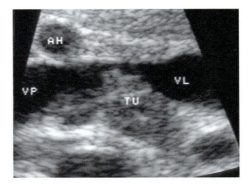
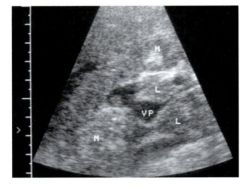

▲ **Fig. 1.89** Patient with pancreatic cancer.
a, b Tumor (TU) infiltrating the splenic vein (VL). VP = portal vein; AH = hepatic artery.

▲ **c** Color-flow Doppler scanning demonstrates turbulence, signifying a stenosis.

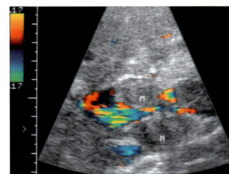
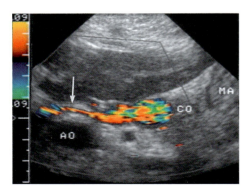

◀◀ **Fig. 1.90** Hepatic hilar lymph nodes in a patient with stomach cancer.
a Portal vein (VP) compression. M = spleen; L = liver.

◀ **b** Color-flow Doppler scanning demonstrates turbulence, signifying a stenosis.

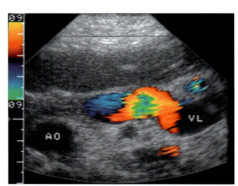
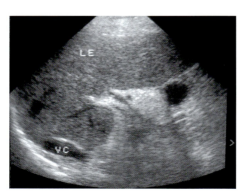

◀ **Fig. 1.91** Portal vein hypoplasia of unknown etiology, with severe compression of the vessel, prestenotic dilatation, and turbulence phenomena in color-flow Doppler scanning.

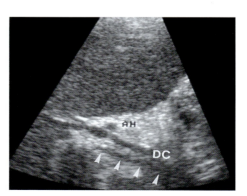

◀ **Fig. 1.92** Aplastic portal vein with collateralization, possibly due to old thrombotic and now fibrotic occlusion of the vein, in a 25-year-old woman. AH = hepatic artery; DC = D. hepatocholedochus; LE = liver; VC = vena cava.

▶ Intrahepatic Block

With ~80% of cases, intrahepatic block is by far the most common cause of portal hypertension. The most important factors are hepatic disorders, in particular cirrhosis of the liver.

Cirrhotic vascular changes. The sonographic criteria for transformation of the hepatic parenchyma should be noted since the cirrhotic vascular changes will point the way toward the diagnosis of portal hypertension:
- ▶ Enlarged diameter of the portal vein in the hepatic portal (**Fig. 1.93a**)
- ▶ Sudden diameter changes in the branches of the portal vein (**Fig. 1.93b**)
- ▶ Pronounced periportal encasement (**Fig. 1.94**)
- ▶ Rarified peripheral vascular tree in the liver

Collaterals. Demonstration of any collaterals is of particular interest, the following collateral systems being of primary importance:
- ▶ Enlarged right gastric vein with flow reversal (◨ **1.8a and b**)
- ▶ Demonstration of esophageal varices (◨ **1.8c and d**)
- ▶ Recanalization of the umbilical veins (inner and outer Medusa's head) (◨ **1.8e–i**)
- ▶ Demonstration of varicosities in the splenic hilum (short gastric veins) (◨ **1.8j–n**),
- ▶ Demonstration of splenorenal shunting (◨ **1.8o–q**)

Shunts. In rare cases, intrahepatic portocaval or intrasplenic cephalad draining varicosities may be demonstrated (◨ **1.8r and s**).

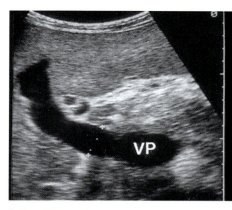
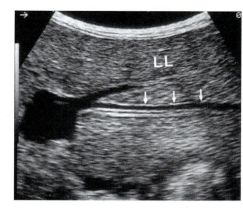

▲ **Fig. 1.93** Portal hypertension.
a Enlarged portal vein (VP).

▲ *b* Sudden caliber change in the portal branches of the left hepatic lobe (LL).

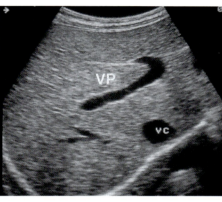
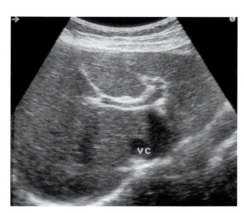

▲ **Fig. 1.94** Pronounced periportal echogenicity. VC = vena cava.
a Normal branching of the portal vein (VP).

▲ *b* Pronounced echogenic boundary of the portal vein (although this finding is also seen as a normal variant).

◨ 1.8 Collaterals in Intrahepatic Block

▶ **Coronary vein of stomach**

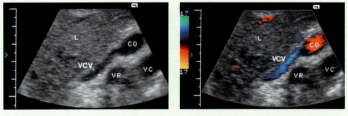

a Enlarged right gastric vein with normal flow into the portal vein. CO = confluence of superior mesenteric and splenic vein, VR = renal vein, VC = vena cava, L = liver.

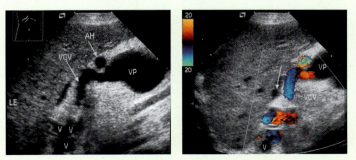

b Flow reversal in the right gastric vein (VCV) in portal hypertension. V = paraesophageal varices; AH = hepatic artery; VP = portal vein; LE = liver.

1.8 Collaterals in Intrahepatic Block

▶ **Paraesophageal varices**

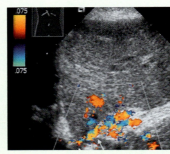
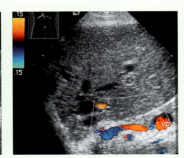

c Marked paraesophageal varices (arrow).

d The paraesophageal varices are supplied by the right gastric vein.

▶ **Recanalized umbilical vein**

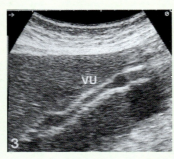
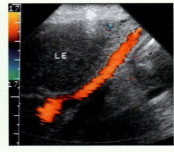
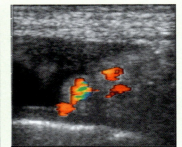

e Distinct recanalization of the umbilical vein (VU).

f and g **Recanalization of the umbilical vein in color-flow duplex scanning.**
f Longitudinal view. A = ascites.

g Transverse view.

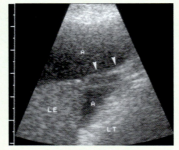

h Atypical course of a recanalized umbilical vein (arrows) (A = ascites, LE = liver, LT = ligamentum teres).

▶ **Tangled vessels, color-Doppler**

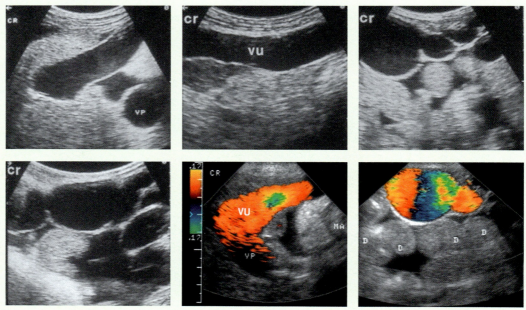

i Massively dilated umbilical vein. The other images (cephalocaudal view) demonstrate the varicosities of an inner Medusa's head. They could be mistaken for localized intra-abdominal fluid (caution: aspiration!). The last two images are color-flow duplex scans of the varicosities. VP = portal vein; VU = umbilical vein; MA = stomach; A = ascites; D = short bowel.

1.8 Collaterals in Intrahepatic Block

▶ Splenic hilum

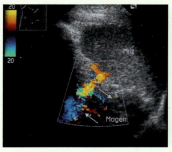 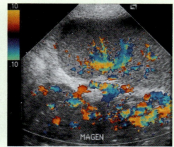

j Short gastric vessels (arrows) originating from the hilar vessels of the spleen (Milz) and draining into the stomach (Magen).

k Numerous collateral veins running from the splenic hilum to the gastric wall (Magen) in cirrhosis of the liver.

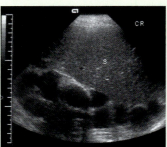 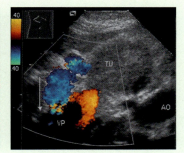

l Massive splenic varices in portal hypertension. S = spleen.

m Pancreatic cancer: Occluded splenic vein. TU = tumor; VP = portal vein; AO = aorta.

▶ Stomach wall, paragastric

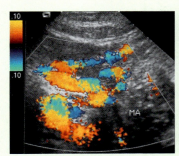 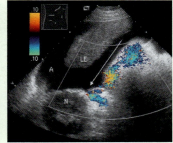

n Pancreatic cancer: Marked paragastric varices. MA = stomach.

o Retroperitoneal collaterals coursing toward the kidney (N) in liver cirrhosis and portal hypertension. A = ascites; LE = liver.

▶ Splenorenal

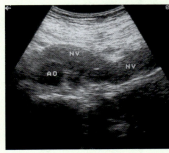 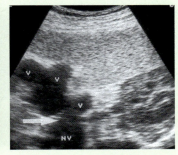

p and q Splenorenal shunt.
p Suspiciously dilated renal vein (NV). AO = aorta.

q Hilar splenic varices (V) draining into the renal vein (NV), resulting in a splenorenal shunt.

1.8 Collaterals in Intrahepatic Block

▶ **Intrasplenic**

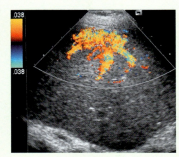

r Intrasplenic varicosity draining toward the surface of the spleen in myeloproliferative disorder and portal hypertension.

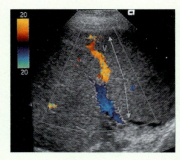 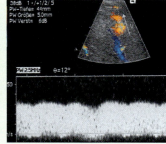 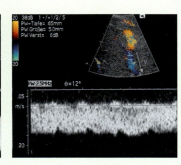

s Intrasplenic venous "watershed". The hilar splenic veins exhibit normal drainage into the hilum, whereas the cortical splenic veins drain toward the surface of the spleen (flow reversal).

▶ **Posthepatic Block**

Posthepatic block is quite rare and occurs in around 1% of all patients with portal hypertension. Budd–Chiari syndrome is really a thrombosis with occlusion of the major hepatic veins. The most important etiological factors are systemic hematological disease, disorders in hemostasis, and hepatic metastasis. In venous occlusive disease the major hepatic veins are patent while the small veins at the microscopic level are thrombosed. The primary etiological factor is graft rejection after allogeneic bone marrow transplant. Chronic constrictive pericarditis (armored heart) is a rare cause of posthepatic block, and another rare causative entity is primary tumor of the vena cava (**Figs. 1.95–1.97**).

Patients with posthepatic block usually exhibit thickening of the gallbladder wall, and sometimes it is possible to demonstrate intrahepatic venovenous collaterals or transdiaphragmatic veins draining in a cephalad direction. Flow reversal in the portal vein may also be seen[3]. Quite often in patients with cardiac decompensation, the portal vein will exhibit reduced blood flow with a pulsatile profile, which in some cases turns into full-fledged pulse-synchronous flow reversal.

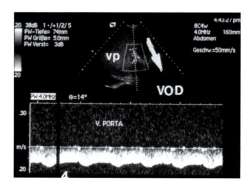 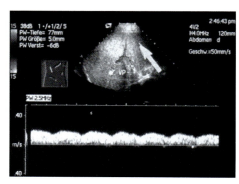

◀◀ *Fig. 1.95* A 23-year-old patient with ALL (acute lymphocytic leukemia) after allogeneic bone marrow transplantation.
  a Clinical diagnosis of hepatic veno-occlusive disease (VOD) with flow reversal in the portal vein (VP).

◀ *b* Posttherapy demonstration of normal direction of flow in the portal vein.

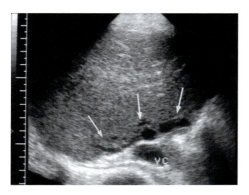 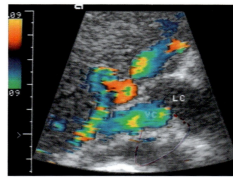

▸ **Fig. 1.96** A 24-year-old man with multiple drug dependence: old hepatic veno-occlusive disease (Budd–Chiari syndrome) with esophageal varices. Normal hepatic veins cannot be demonstrated; singular varicosities around the junction of the hepatic veins. VC = vena cava; LC = caudate lobe.

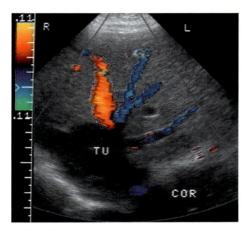 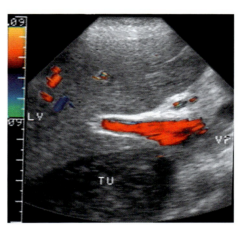 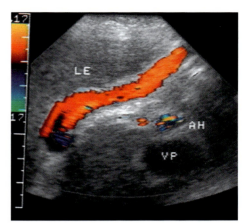

▲ **Fig. 1.97** Patient presenting with primary leiomyoma of the vena cava.
a Intracaval tumor mass (TU); flow reversal in the right hepatic vein. COR = heart.

▲ ***b*** Demonstration of the tumor and portal vein (VP) with normal direction of flow.

▲ ***c*** Marked recanalization of the umbilical vein in posthepatic block. LE = liver; AH = hepatic artery.

Intraluminal Mass

Thrombosis

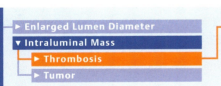

▸ Portal Vein Thrombosis

The etiology of portal vein thrombosis is rather varied (**Table 1.4**). Cirrhosis of the liver is by far the most common cause, although in fresh thrombosis hepatocellular carcinoma must be ruled out[3]. Portal vein thrombosis may be subdivided into partial intrahepatic thrombosis, complete or partial thrombosis of the portal trunk, and additional thrombosis of the tributaries (splenic and mesenteric veins).

Other less frequent collaterals may be seen alongside these cavernous transformations:
▸ Atypical paraportal collaterals (**Fig. 1.98**)
▸ Varices around the peribiliary vascular plexus (**Fig. 1.99**)

In addition, there may be hepatofugal collaterals via the right gastric vein or collaterals draining in a caudad direction[1].

Table 1.4 Etiology of portal vein thrombosis (after reference 1)

- ▸ Idiopathic
- ▸ Cirrhosis of the liver
- ▸ Malignancies
- ▸ Diseases of the pancreas
- ▸ Parainfectious
- ▸ Posttraumatic
- ▸ Collagen disorders
- ▸ Thrombophilia
- ▸ Myeloproliferative disorders

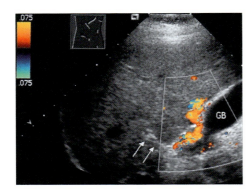 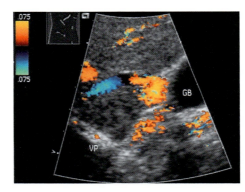

◄ **Fig. 1.98** A 3-year-old thrombosis of the portal vein with paraportal "recanalization" (collaterals). The portal blood drains toward the gallbladder (GB) and from there into the liver. VP = portal vein.

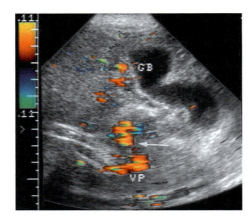 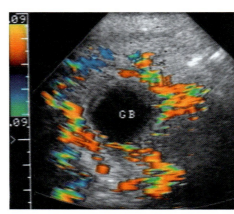

◄◄ **Fig. 1.99a** Patient with Klatskin tumor, stent palliation, and occlusion of the portal vein (VP).

◄ **b** Originating from the portal vein there are marked cephalad collaterals around the peribiliary venous plexus. GB = gallbladder.

1.9 Typical findings in portal vein thrombosis

▶ **Intrahepatic and extrahepatic**

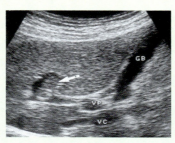 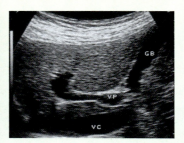

a and b A 71-year-old patient with cancer of the colon. GB = gallbladder; VC = vena cava; VP = portal vein.
a Incidental finding of partial thrombosis of the intrahepatic portal vein.

b Spontaneous lysis after two months.

▶ **Cavernous transformation of portal vein**

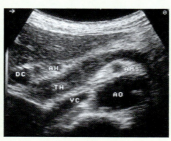 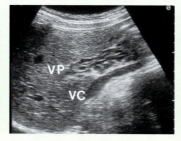 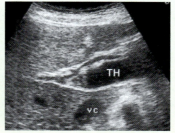

c Echogenic image of the portal vein in thrombosis. DC = D. hepatocholedochus; AH = hepatic artery; TH = thrombus; VC = vena cava; AO = aorta.

d A 24-year-old female with esophageal varices secondary to portal vein thrombosis. Varicosities along the portal vein as a result of cavernous transformation of the portal vein. VC = vena cava; VP = portal vein.

e–h Sonographic course of a fresh portal vein thrombosis (TH). VC = vena cava.
e Hypoechoic image of the thrombotic material.

1.9 Typical findings in portal vein thrombosis

▶ Cavernous transformation of portal vein

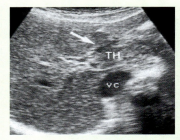

f Increasingly echogenic transformation of the thrombosis.

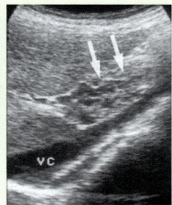

g Beginning recanalization after four months.

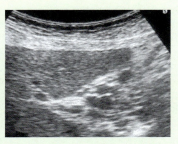

h Marked varicosities around the hepatic portal four years later.

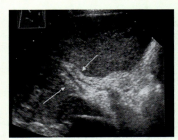
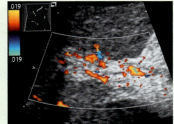

i Portal vein thrombosis, six years old. Fibrotic occlusion of the portal vein, no significant recanalization demonstrable.

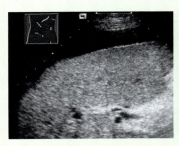
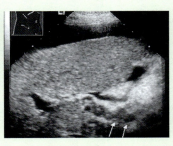
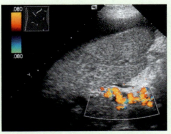

j–l Thrombosis of the portal vein with cavernous recanalization.
j Old portal vein thrombosis.

k Cavernous recanalization cephalad of the portal vein.

l Color-flow duplex scan of the cavernous recanalization.

▶ Splenic hilum collaterals

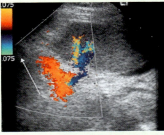

m Collateralization at the splenic portal.

▶ Splenic Vein Thrombosis

Complete or partial thrombosis of the splenic vein is a common complication of acute pancreatitis and cancer of the pancreas. It may also originate from portal vein thrombosis and grow by apposition.

The ultrasound image depicts a hypoechoic vascular lumen without any flow on color-flow Doppler scanning. Partial thrombosis of the splenic vein is sometimes observed. One of the sequelae of this vascular obstruction is "segmental" portal hypertension. Collateralization primarily opens the peripancreatic and perigastric veins draining cephalad via esophageal varices as well veins running in a caudad direction (omental veins draining into the mesenteric veins) (**Figs. 1.100–1.102**).

A finding of hepatosplenomegaly is not mandatory, and neither is the build-up of ascites. Over time, the splenic vein may become recanalized or undergo cavernous transformation, although quite often the collaterals will persist. In thrombosis of the splenic vein, one rare complication is splenic infarction or even rupture.

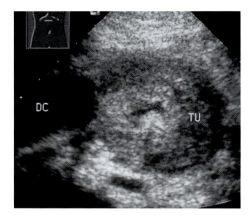
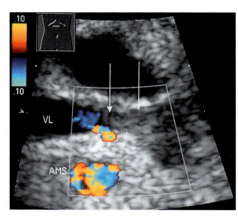

◂◂ **Fig. 1.100** Splenic vein thrombosis.
  a Cancer (TU) of the pancreatic head. DC = D. hepatocholedochus.
◂ **b** Demonstration of echogenic material in the splenic vein (VL). AMS = superior mesenteric vein.

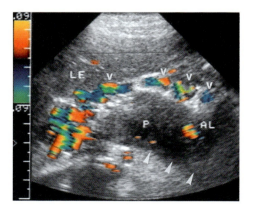
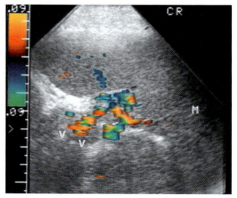

◂◂ **Fig. 1.101** Acute pancreatitis.
  a The splenic vein cannot be depicted. Marked varices anterior to the pancreas.
◂ **b** Demonstration of varicosities (V). M = spleen; LE = liver; P = pancreas; AL = splenic artery.

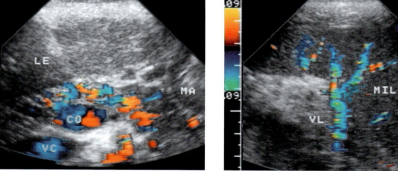

◂◂ **Fig. 1.102** Thrombosis of the splenic vein after mesenteric irradiation of a malignant lymphoma. LE = liver; MA = stomach; CO = venous confluence; VC = vena cava; VL = splenic vein; Milz = spleen.
  a The splenic vein cannot be imaged and there is marked peripancreatic collateralization.
◂ **b** Regular appearance of the splenic vein at the splenic portal.

▶ Thrombosis of the Superior Mesenteric Vein

Truly isolated thrombosis of the superior mesenteric vein does not result in portal hypertension. However, it may be associated with splenic and/or portal vein thrombosis. The etiology is primarily inflammatory, in particular acute pancreatitis (**Fig. 1.103**). During the acute phase, the clinical symptoms with severe abdominal pain are impressive (**Fig. 1.104**). On ultrasound the mesenteric vessels appear dilated and lined with echogenic structures. Color-flow Doppler scanning will not elicit any flow signals. Partial thrombosis is possible.

In rare cases there may be segmental infarction of the intestines. Usually this disorder does not require surgery, and quite often there will spontaneous recanalization.

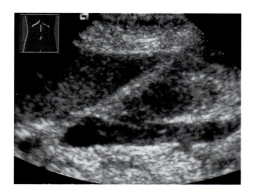
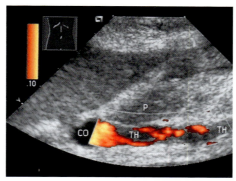

Fig. 1.103 Patient with acute pancreatitis.
a The tip of the thrombus within the superior mesenteric vein extends into the confluence of the mesenteric and splenic veins. Color-flow duplex scanning demonstrates echogenic thrombotic material.

b Color-flow duplex scanning depicts partial recanalization. P = tail of pancreas; CO = venous confluence; TH = thrombosis.

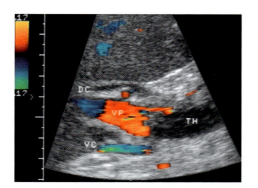
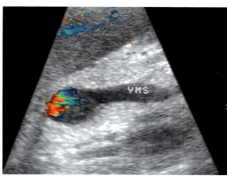
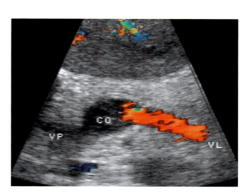

Fig. 1.104 A 50-year-old patient with acute abdomen.
a–c Color-flow duplex scanning demonstrates complete thrombosis of the superior mesenteric vein (VMS). DC = Common bile duct; TH = thrombosis; VP = portal vein; VC = vena cava; CO = venous confluence; VL = splenic vein.

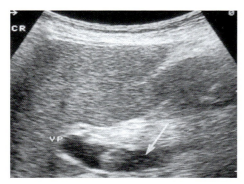
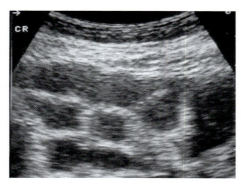
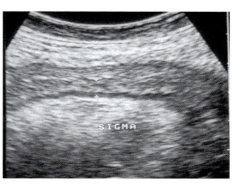

d–f B-mode imaging also depicts the thrombosis. Massive dilatation of the small intestine. There is thickening of the colonic wall at the level of the sigmoid and a lack of peristalsis (nonsurgical treatment proved to be successful).

Tumor

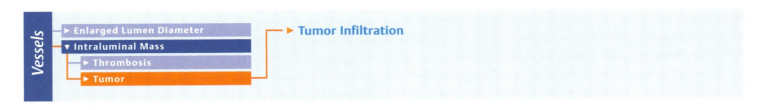

▶ Tumor Infiltration

Tumor infiltration into the portovenous system is not infrequent, and in primary hepatic malignancies it is observed quite often at the porta hepatis. Ultrasonography can differentiate between tumor infiltration and thrombosis of the portal vein, but may be difficult to perform for some segments. If color-flow Doppler imaging demonstrates tumor vessels within the "thrombotic material," this will confirm the diagnosis of tumorous thrombosis (**Fig. 1.105**).

At the confluence and along the splenic vein, tumor infiltration may be one complication of pancreatic cancer, with extensive infiltration of the tumor into the vessel usually being a sign of inoperability. Under good conditions in such cases, ultrasonography may be able to demonstrate direct infiltration of the portal vessels by continuity[3].

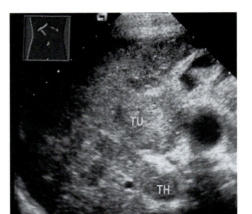
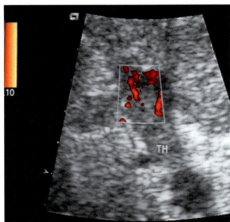

◀◀ **Fig. 1.105** Patient with hepatocellular carcinoma (TU). TH = thrombosis.
  a Demonstration of the tumor and the echogenic portal vein immediately adjacent to it.

◀ **b** Color-flow duplex scanning confirmed the diagnosis of portal vein thrombosis. The discrete flow signals within the thrombotic material raise the suspicion of a tumorous thrombus.

References
1. Furuse J, Matsutani S, Voskikawa M. Diagnosis of portal vein tumor thrombus by Pulsed Doppler Ultrasonography. JCU 1992;20:439–46.
2. Gaitini BD, Thaler I, Kaftori JK. Duplex sonography in the diagnosis of portal vein thrombosis. Fortschr Röntgenstr 1990;153(6):645–9.
2a. Janssen A. Pulsatility index is better than ankle-brachial Doppler index for non-invasive detection of critical limb ischaemia in diabetes. Vasa 2005;4 (accepted for publication).
3. Ochs A. Sonographie der Leber. Freiburg: Falk Foundation Freiburg 2000;1–115.
4. Seitz K, Wermke W, Haas K. Sonographie bei portaler Hypertension und TIPPS. Freiburg: Falk Foundation 1997;3–64.
5. Schmidt, WA, Kraft HE, Vorpahl K et al. Color Duplex Ultrasonography in the Diagnosis of Temporal Arteritis. NEJM 1997;337:1336–1342.

2 Liver

Liver 51

▼ Diffuse Changes in the Hepatic Parenchyma — 61

▼ Enlarged Liver — 62
- Congested Liver
- Fatty Liver
- Fatty Liver Hepatitis
- Fatty Cirrhosis
- Diffuse Infiltration

▼ Small Liver — 67
- Atrophy
- Cirrhosis
- Resection

▼ Homogeneous Hypoechoic Texture — 68
- Acute Liver Congestion
- Amyloidosis
- Acute Hepatitis

▼ Homogeneous Hyperechoic Texture — 70
- Fatty Liver
- Hemochromatosis
- Fibrosis

▼ Regionally Inhomogeneous Texture — 71
- Focal Fatty Infiltration
- Necrosis
- Portal Venous Gas Embolism

▼ Diffuse Inhomogeneous Texture — 72
- Chronic Hepatitis
- Cirrhosis
- Diffuse Tumor Growth

▼ Localized Changes in Hepatic Parenchyma — 74

▼ Anechoic Masses — 76
- Cysts
- Polycystic Liver Disease
- Hemorrhage/Hematoma
- Bilioma
- Abscess
- Hydatid Cysts
- Osler Disease/Hepatic Peliosis
- Lipoma
- Lymphoma
- Metastases
- Vessels/Bile Ducts

▼ Hypoechoic Masses — 81
- Metastasis
- Lymphoma
- Abscess
- Hematoma
- Complicated Cyst
- Adenoma
- Focal Nodular Hyperplasia (FNH)
- Hepatocellular Carcinoma (HCC)
- Lipoma
- Atypical Hemangioma
- Focal Fatty Change
- Bile Ducts/Vessels

Localized Changes in Hepatic Parenchyma (Continue)

Isoechoic Masses — 87
- Focal Nodular Hyperplasia (FNH)
- Adenoma
- Hepatocellular Carcinoma (HCC)
- Metastasis
- Atypical Hemangioma
- Hematoma
- "Hepatized" Gallbladder
- Bile Ducts/Vessels

Hyperechoic Masses — 89
- Hemangioma
- Bile Duct Hamartomas
- Porphyria
- Regenerative Nodules
- Hepatocellular Carcinoma (HCC)
- Focal Nodular Hyperplasia (FNH)
- Metastasis
- Abscess
- Necrosis
- Diaphragmatic Slips
- Ligamentum teres Hepatis
- Focal Fatty Change
- Bile Ducts/Vessels

Echogenic Masses — 94
- "Comet-Tails"
- Calcification
- Calculus
- Foreign Body
- Air

Irregular Masses — 97
- Hepatocellular Carcinoma (HCC)
- Thorotrastosis
- Diffuse Metastasis
- Alveolar Hydatid Disease

Differential Diagnosis of Focal Lesions — 98

Diagnostic Methods — 98

Suspected Diagnosis — 99

2 Liver

M. Brandt

The liver is the largest gland as well as the largest single organ in the human body, weighing 1500–1800 g (accounting for about 2.3–3% of body weight). Blood, primarily from the splanchnic region, flows through the liver, where numerous substances are recovered and metabolized. Apart from breaking down and synthesizing substances, the liver is a key element in storage pathways (glycogen, fat). It either releases these metabolites directly into the bloodstream or excretes them via the bile (1500 ml/day). In addition, the liver is characterized by its organ-specific macrophages (Kupffer cells), which are an integral part of the human macrophage system (reticuloendothelial system, RES). In summary, this organ plays a vital role not only in metabolic detoxification but also in the synthesis de novo and storage of proteins, sugar molecules, and fat as well as in the secretion of digestive juices.

In order to realize these varied functions, the anatomy of the liver is based on the so-called hepatic lobules with their functional unit, the hepatic acinus according to Rappaport (**Fig. 2.1**). Splanchnic blood flowing through a branch of the portal vein passes three successive metabolic zones where the substances transported by the blood are metabolized. All products synthesized by the liver are passed into the bloodstream through the central vein or excreted via a countercurrent mechanism into the bile ducts that parallel the terminal portal branches (**Fig. 2.2**).

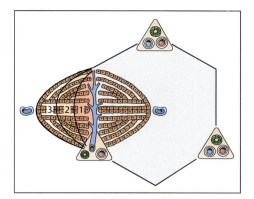

▲ **Fig. 2.1** Hepatic lobule and acinus according to Kiernan and Rappaport. The gray hepatic lobule of Kiernan is characterized by its central vein and the peripheral portal areas; the colored hepatic acinus of Rappaport has a terminal branch of the portal vein in its center while the central veins (of the hepatic lobule) are on its periphery, and in between there are three distinct metabolic zones: zone 1 rich and zone 3 poor in nutrients.

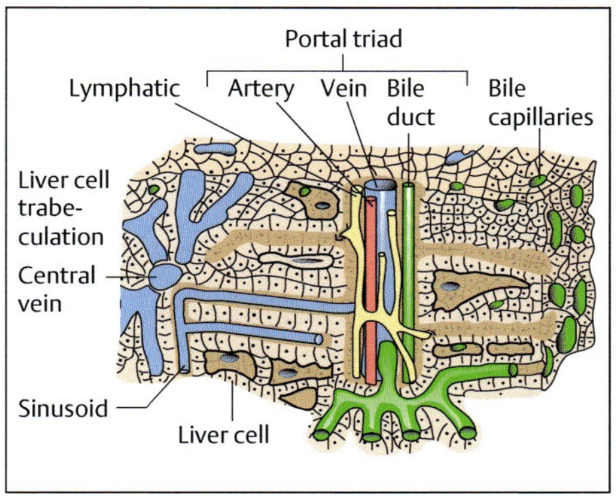

▲ **Fig. 2.2** Schematic diagram of a hepatic sinusoid together with a portal triad. In the sinusoids, blood from the terminal branch of the portal vein (joined in the portal triad by the artery and the bile duct) flows through the three successive metabolic zones into the central vein. Excretion into the bile ducts paralleling the branches of the portal vein is by countercurrent principle.

Topography

The liver is located in the right hypochondrium, protected by the ribs (**Fig. 2.3**). Its general shape is that of a pyramid, with the base pointing to the right side of the body. The average transverse diameter is 25–30 cm, the cephalocaudal length is 12–20 cm, and the normal anteroposterior diameter is 6–10 cm. The superior aspect borders the diaphragm (facies diaphragmatica hepatis) and is composed of a fixed and a mobile part; parts of the anterior aspect are in contact with the abdominal wall. The inferior surface of the liver points in a posterocaudal direction; on the left and in the middle the inferior aspect is in contact with the gastric wall, while on the lateral right side it borders the hepatic flexure of the colon. The gallbladder is attached to the inferior surface of the liver in the midclavicular line. The right dorsal aspect of the liver is anterior to the upper pole of the right kidney. The hepatic portal is situated in the middle of the inferior surface, anterior to the caudate lobe (see below) and the dorsal vena cava (**Fig. 2.4**); the porta hepatis comprises the portal vein, hepatic artery, bile duct, lymphatics, and nerves.

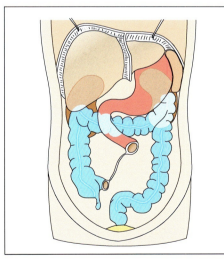

▲ **Fig. 2.3** Topography. Location of the liver in the right hypochondrium, protected by the lower right ribs; note the relationship with the diaphragm, right kidney, major retroperitoneal vessels, colon, and stomach.

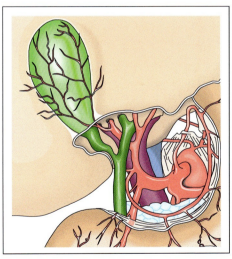

▲ **Fig. 2.4** Schematic anatomy of the hepatic portal. Aorta and vena cava are posterior; the portal vein is on the right coursing obliquely and anteriorly to the vena cava. The portal vein is posterior to the hepatic artery and medial to the extrahepatic bile duct.

Table 2.1 Hepatic segments

Segment	Location	Topography, boundary	Name	Tributary
I	Left medial, posterior, anterior to vena cava	Anterior to vena cava, posterior to seg. IVa	Caudate lobe	Left portal vein branch PVS I
II	Left lateral, superior, subcardial	Superior to seg. I, medial to seg. IVa, forms superior left medial margin	Superior part is anatomical left lobe	Left portal vein branch PVS II
III	Left lateral, inferior	Inferior to seg. II, medial to seg. IVb, forms inferior left medial margin	Inferior part is anatomical left lobe	Left portal vein branch III
IV	Left medial, anterior	Right lateral to lig. teres and lateral to seg. II/III, medial to seg. V	Quadrate lobe	Left portal vein branch IV
V	Right medial, inferior	Medial to seg. VI/VII, superior to gallbladder	Forms gallbladder fossa	Right portal vein branch PVS V
VI	Right lateral, inferior	Inferior to seg. VII, lateral to seg. V, forms right lateral margin		Right portal vein branch PVS VI
VII	Right lateral, superior, subphrenic	Superior to seg. VI, lateral to seg. VIII, subphrenic, forms right lateral superior margin		Right portal vein branch PVS VII
VIII	Right medial superior, subphrenic	Superior to seg. V, medial to seg. VII, subphrenic		Right portal vein branch PVS VIII

Anatomy

From a macroscopic anatomical point of view, the liver is subdivided into a larger right lobe (representing the base of the pyramid) and a smaller left hepatic lobe (the apex of the pyramid), with the falciform ligament (containing the ligamentum teres) dividing the two lobes (**Fig. 2.5**). In terms of its microanatomy, the liver is composed of eight functionally separate segments that follow the vascular tree (**Fig. 2.6; Table 2.1**). If circumscribed masses or pathological findings can be correlated to a specific segment, this is extremely helpful in preoperative and intraoperative diagnosis as well as for possible resectability or any planned interventional angiographic procedures. However, since the numerous anatomical variants are not particularly infrequent, segmental correlation is not always certain and thus may be of only limited value in some cases.

Couinaud's Segmental Anatomy of the Liver

The microanatomy of the liver is composed of eight functionally different segments; when viewed from the front/below they are counted clockwise: the left hepatic lobe comprises segments I–IV and the right lobe segments V–VIII. Compared to the anatomical division of the liver along the falciform ligament (including the ligamentum teres) into a smaller left lobe (only segments II and III) and a larger right lobe (segments V–VIII plus segments I and IVa/b), Couinaud's segmental anatomy follows the vascular tree (**Fig. 2.6**). Here the branches of the portal vein (accompanied by the branches of the hepatic artery and the bile ducts = portal triad) are the central structures of each segment, while the hepatic veins running between the segments drain the blood. There are three major hepatic veins—right (lateral right), middle, and left (medial)—all joining the vena cava posteriorly at the bare area of the superior aspect of the liver below the diaphragm. The middle hepatic vein divides the angiographic right hepatic lobe from the left lobe. The left hepatic vein drains between double segments II/III as well as IVa/IVb of the left lobe. The right hepatic vein drains between double segments VI/VII and V/VIII. Segment I is the caudate lobe and is part of the left hepatic lobe. Segment IV corresponds to the quadrate lobe, while segment V forms the base of the gallbladder fossa.

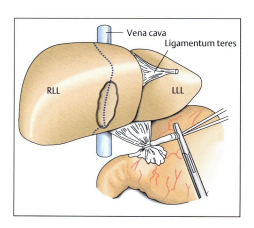

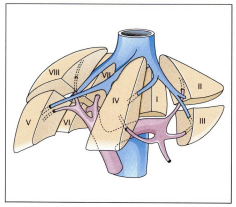

◂◂ *Fig. 2.5* Liver anatomy. Inferior view: the ligamentum teres (falciforme) separates the anatomical left hepatic lobe (LL) from the lateral anatomical right lobe, which is larger and is shown with the gallbladder fossa on its inferior aspect. The vena cava can be seen posteriorly. The dotted line marks the imaginary plane running through the gallbladder fossa and vena cava, which is considered the dividing line between the vascular tree of the left and right branches of the portal vein.

◂ *Fig. 2.6* Segmental hepatic anatomy according to Couinaud. Schematic diagram of the hepatic segments I (caudate lobe) to IV (quadrate lobe) of the left lobe as well as segments V–VIII of the right lobe; the gallbladder fossa is posteroinferior to segment V.

Sonographic Morphology

Extrinsic Criteria

Size—depends on the patient's build (Table 2.2)
- Pyknic: 80 mm
- Regular build: 120 mm
- Asthenic: 150 mm
- Caudate lobe: around 50 × 20 mm
- Left hepatic lobe < right lobe

Shape
- Left hepatic lobe (viewed anteriorly to the aorta): convex/concave
- Right hepatic lobe (viewed laterally right): biconvex

Surface
- Smooth

Contour
- Sharply angled configuration, 30° (asthenics)
- < 45° (pyknic)

Anomalies
- Situs inversus
- Accessory lobe

Normal Variants in Liver Anatomy

Normal variants may impact on position and shape of the liver and/or its microanatomy (hepatic segmental anatomy) and vascular supply.
One normal variant of position would be situs inversus.
Accessory hepatic lobes (the so-called Riedel's lobe) (**Figs. 2.7 and 2.8**) are most often found around segment VI, less often around segments IV or V, appear as large fingerlike projections, and are normal variants in segmentation and shape. They differ from malignant masses in their regular parenchymal architecture with its smooth surface and a normal vascular supply, i.e., a central branch of the portal vein paralleled by a branch of the hepatic artery, a bile duct, and a single accessory central vein which drains the blood separately from the portal branch.
The most common normal variants in the vascular supply are found in the hepatic artery (right hepatic artery originating from the superior mesenteric artery) and the hepatic veins (additional hepatic veins or accessory hepatic veins not terminating at the common venous junction but directly at the vena cava).

Table 2.2 Assessment of liver size (longitudinal view in right MCL)

Build of patient	Normal values
Asthenic (slim, long-limbed)	< 15 cm
Normal	< 12 cm
Pyknic (squat, short-limbed)	< 10 cm

Ultrasonography of the liver has to assess numerous criteria. Only by putting together these pieces of the puzzle will the sonographer come up with a well founded diagnosis. The following paragraphs will consider extrinsic, intrinsic, and dynamic criteria, including adjacent findings. Routine study of the sonographic characteristics of the liver is performed with the patient in the supine position (sometimes supplemented by the left lateral decubitus position or with the patient standing). The organ is imaged in the longitudinal and transverse planes and along the lower right costal margin of the ribs, as well as in planes parallel to the intercostal spaces, by sweeping the probe in fanlike fashion during inspiration, expiration, and breath-holding. The examination is completed by specific localized palpation with the probe, if needed.

Extrinsic criteria (■ 2.1; Table 2.3). The size of the liver, its superior and inferior aspect, its shape, its caudal edge, and any normal variants are assessed on the basis of the following extrinsic criteria.

The *size* of the liver is determined along the midclavicular line and is given in centimeters; to a large extent this parameter depends on the build of the patient (**Table 2.2**). In addition, the dimensions of the caudate lobe and the distribution of mass between left and right hepatic lobe have to be assessed.

Usually, the *surface* of the liver is smooth; during routine studies its appearance is better visualized at the inferior aspect of the liver since, owing to the physics of the ultrasound beam, the image is blurred at the near field. Another alternative is to switch to a higher-frequency probe.

The *shape* takes into account the distribution of mass between the right lobe and the left as well as the caudate lobe; in addition, the inferior aspect of the organ is assessed in longitudinal views, with the left lobe being imaged in the midline anterior to the aorta (the anterior aspect is convex and the posterior one concave), while the right hepatic lobe is scanned in the right axillary line (biconcave).

The inferior *contour* of the liver is examined, too; for the left lobe it is sharply angulated at 30–45°, while the lateral edge of the right hepatic lobe is blunt (60°).

Normal variants are uncommon and, apart from the variant position (situs inversus), the sonographer has to keep accessory lobes in mind (so-called Riedel's lobe) (**Figs. 2.7 and 2.8**).

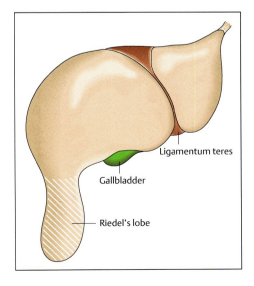

◄ **Fig. 2.7** Schematic anatomy of Riedel's lobe. Accessory hepatic lobes are normal variants and may appear at various locations of the liver. The most common form is the so-called Riedel's lobe, corresponding to a long projection of the right hepatic lobe around segment VI and possessing a regular architectural structure.

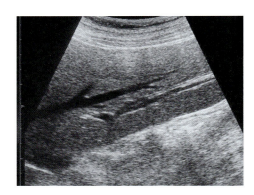
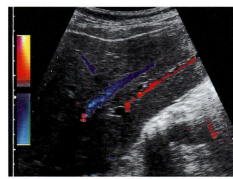

Fig. 2.8 Riedel's lobe.
a Lateral longitudinal view: image of Riedel's lobe with absolutely normal structural architecture of hepatic veins and portal areas, normal parenchyma.

b Color-flow duplex scan.

Table 2.3 **Extrinsic criteria**

Criterion	Normal	Pathological	Example
Size	▶ 12 cm in right MCL	▶ Bigger, smaller	▶ Fatty cirrhosis, atrophic cirrhosis
Shape	▶ Convex/concave	▶ Biconvex, rounded	▶ Fatty liver, infiltration
Surface	▶ Smooth	▶ Irregular, localized bulging, pitting	▶ Chronic hepatitis, focal mass, metastasis; status post hepatitis
Contour	▶ Angulated	▶ Blunt, rounded, beaklike	▶ Fatty liver, cirrhosis
Normal variants	—	—	▶ Riedel's lobe

Intrinsic Criteria

Parenchymal echotexture
▶ homogeneous, finely dispersed, medium-sized, moderately bright, individual echoes

Conduction
▶ Normal

Hepatic veins
▶ Draining between segments
▶ Common junction at the vena cava ("venous star")
▶ Running straight, sharply angulated branching
▶ No wall echoes
▶ Typical signal on duplex scanning

Portal vein branches
▶ Originating at the hepatoduodenal ligament (bifurcation of the portal vein) and coursing in the center of the segments
▶ Periportal encasement
▶ Sufficient duplex signal for analysis

Hepatic artery
▶ Paralleling the branches of the portal vein

Bile ducts
▶ Paralleling the branches of the portal vein

Lymphatics
▶ Paralleling the branches of the portal vein
▶ At this time without clinical significance
▶ Pathological lymphadenopathy at the hepatic portal

Intrinsic criteria (Table 2.4). The intrinsic criteria deal with the actual parenchymal echotexture of the liver, organ-induced attenuation of the ultrasound beam, and in particular the demonstration of and changes in the venous vessels and portal triads with portal vein, bile duct, branches of the hepatic artery, and the lymphatics.

The echotexture of the hepatic *parenchyma* (■ 2.2) comprises numerous individual echoes. Assessment of these individual echoes has to consider size (graininess), brightness, uniformity (homogeneity) as well as distribution and position (density). The parenchyma of a normal liver will present as finely dispersed, moderately bright, homogeneously and uniformly distributed individual echoes of moderate echogenicity. With normal presettings of the equipment, no relative amplification or attenuation will be seen: both criteria are highly dependent on the type of equipment used and the presets (time gain compensation, TGC).

The *hepatic veins* (■ 2.3 and ■ 2.4) converge on the so-called venous star (**Fig. 2.9**), which terminates at the vena cava; they drain the blood from the periphery of the liver, run in straight lines between the segments with sharply angled branching, are smoothly lined, and do not demonstrate any wall echoes. The blood flow within the hepatic veins may be assessed qualitatively and quantitatively by duplex and color-flow duplex scanning.

The *portal vein* (■ 2.5) enters the liver at the termination of the hepatoduodenal ligament, bifurcates at the hepatic portal (**Fig. 2.10**) into the left and right branch, and supplies the center of the individual hepatic segments via its respective segmental branches. The portal vein branches are characterized by echoes in the wall (periportal reinforcement), and the blood flow in the portal vein and its branches may be assessed and quantified by duplex and color-flow duplex scanning. The portal veins regularly are paralleled by branches of the *hepatic artery* and *bile ducts*; these three vessels form the so-called hepatic triads. Blood flow in the various segments of the hepatic artery may also be assessed and quantified by duplex and color-flow duplex scanning. The intrahepatic lymphatics are too small to be assessed with today's equipment, and all extrahepatic lymph nodes at the hepatic portal visualized by ultrasound are pathological.

Dynamic criteria (Table 2.5). The dynamic criteria take into account the respiratory motion of the liver, its consistency, and its (possible) tenderness on palpation.

Supplementary findings. Any pathological findings in other organs and structures of the abdomen also must be noted, for instance in the gallbladder (wall thickening, visible blood vessels within the wall), spleen (splenomegaly), pancreas (cysts, pancreatitis), and portal vessels (varicosities, collaterals), as well as any free intra-abdominal fluid (amount, type).

Table 2.6 is a summary of the criteria used in sonographic assessment of the liver.

2.1 Extrinsic Criteria

▶ **a–c** Surface, angle, and consistency.

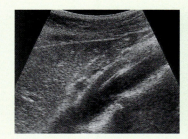
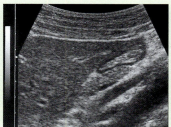
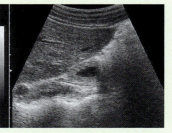

a In the median line the liver is convex/concave and sharply angled.

b Misinterpretations may be due to deformation of the surface with indentation of the anterior surface by the pressure of the probe pushing down on the abdominal wall.

c On the lateral aspect the liver is biconvex or convex/concave and obtusely angled.

▶ **d–l** Changes in the hepatic surface.

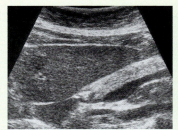
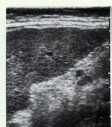
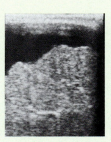

d Usually, the surface of the liver is smooth (most often best assessed at the inferior aspect).

e Inflammatory disorders will result in diffuse changes in the entire surface of the liver with an irregular wavy contour, here in chronic autoimmune hepatitis.

f Irregular nodular hepatic surface in cirrhosis; imaging is facilitated by the presence of ascites.

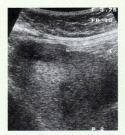
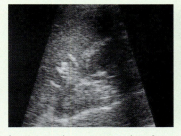
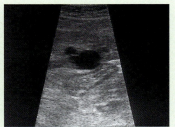

g Localized changes in the surface due to scarring after bypass surgery with subsegmentation in the left lobe.

h Traumatic lesions: scar at the inferior aspect of segment VI after blunt abdominal trauma with ruptured liver, which was sutured.

i Intrahepatic masses can bulge the surface of the liver and indent adjacent organs: here, a unilocular cyst at the inferior aspect of segment III indenting the gastric wall.

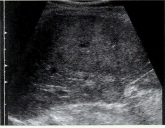
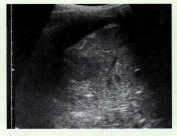
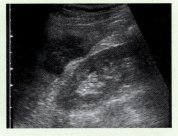

j Circumscribed changes in the surfaces due to a bulging colon cancer metastasis.

k Gastric cancer metastasis infiltrating and penetrating into the diaphragm with concomitant pleural effusion.

l Cancerous impression at the inferior aspect of segment VI of the right hepatic lobe with central pit and bulging wall.

2.2 Assessing the Hepatic Parenchyma

▶ **a–c** Compared with the kidney, the regular parenchyma of the liver is slightly more echogenic, finely grained, and homogeneous; in normal sonography there is no ultrasound attenuation; other organs used for comparison are the spleen, pancreas, and psoas muscle.

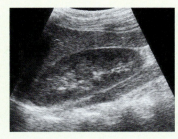

a Regular hepatic parenchyma.

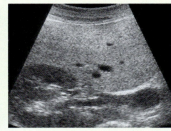

b Simple fatty degeneration, easily recognized by the increased echogenicity when compared with the (healthy!) kidney.

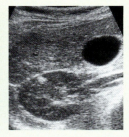

c Comparison of hepatic parenchyma with other structures: anechoic (cystic, transverse view of gallbladder) and hyperechoic mass (small angiolipoma in the cortical parenchyma of the kidney).

▶ **d–f** Parenchymal changes in fatty degradation. Characteristic increased echogenicity, and despite the excellent conduction of sound in fat, there is definite attenuation in the parenchyma because of the increased number of boundaries, diffraction, and dispersion of the sonic beam, and runtime artifacts.

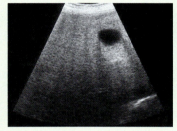

d Blurred contour and boundaries.

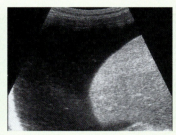

e The surface becomes rounded (fatty cirrhosis of the liver).

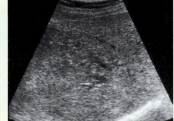

f Inhomogeneous parenchyma due to irregular fat deposits and inflammatory reaction (fatty liver hepatitis caused by diabetes, alcoholism, or nonalcoholic steatohepatitis).

▶ **g–i** Fatty degradation may lead to regional, segmental, or focal differences in the parenchymal changes. Preferred locations are the base of segment IV proximal to the hepatic bifurcation and the gallbladder fossa in segment V.

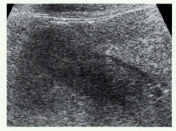

g As in this case, quite often focal differences in parenchymal changes are found around the veins and below the capsule as well as around the teres ligament.

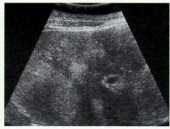

h Maplike circumscribed pseudotumorous parenchymal changes in fatty degradation.

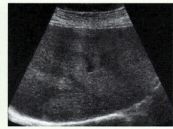

i Splotchy changes induced by fatty degradation of the parenchyma.

▶ **j–l** Inflammatory parenchymal changes and cirrhosis of the liver. Acute inflammation does not present with any changes; because of the transformation and the infiltration of the inflammatory cells, only chronic inflammation with its inhomogeneous and coarsened parenchymal structures will be visualized. However, this is a nonspecific sign.

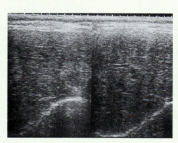

j Autoimmune hepatitis.

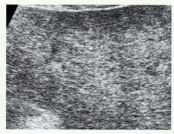

k Chronic toxic fatty liver hepatitis/cirrhosis.

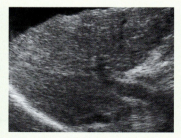

l Primary biliary cirrhosis.

2.2 Assessing the Hepatic Parenchyma

▶ **m–o** Noninflammatory diffuse parenchymal changes: diffuse coarse inhomogeneities of the hepatic parenchyma are also seen in numerous other diseases and can only be recognized when many other criteria are looked at as well.

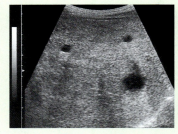
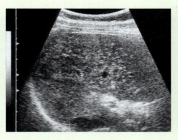
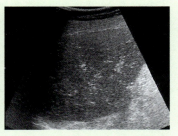

m Fibrosis of the liver with unilocular cysts in Caroli disease.

n Cholangiofibromatosis = von Meyenburg complexes.

o Portovenous gas embolism with small gas bubbles deposited in the periportal hepatic parenchyma.

Table 2.4 Intrinsic criteria

	Normal	Pathological	Example
Parenchyma	▶ Homogeneous, finely dispersed	▶ More echogenic ▶ Less echogenic ▶ Inhomogeneous	▶ Fatty liver ▶ Congestion ▶ Hepatitis, cirrhosis
Conduction	▶ Normal	▶ Attenuated ▶ Enhanced	▶ Fibrosis ▶ Edema
Hepatic veins	▶ Straight, sharply angulated branching ▶ Sharply delineated, no wall echoes ▶ Unobstructed lumen	▶ Rounded, obtusely angled branching ▶ Diffuse delineation ▶ Irregular contour ▶ Rarefied ▶ Occluded	▶ Fatty liver ▶ Fatty liver ▶ Chronic hepatitis ▶ Cirrhosis ▶ Veno-occlusive disease, Budd–Chiari syndrome
Portal veins	▶ Sharply delineated, wall echoes	▶ Scabby ▶ Sudden alteration in caliber	▶ Cirrhosis ▶ Cirrhosis + portal hypertension

Table 2.5 Dynamic criteria

Criterion	Normal	Pathological	Example
Respiratory motion	▶ 2–3 fingerbreadths or 4–6 cm (about 2 inches)	▶ Missing	▶ Abscess, adhesions
Consistency	▶ Soft	▶ Increased, hardened	▶ Infiltrative changes, cirrhosis
Tenderness	▶ None	▶ Tender on palpation	▶ Capsular tension

Table 2.6 Sonographic criteria for assessing the liver

Extrinsic criteria	Intrinsic criteria	Dynamic criteria	Supplementary criteria
Size Shape Surface Inferior margin Angle Normal variants	Parenchymal structure Conductivity of sound Hepatic veins Hepatic arteries Portal veins (bile ducts) (lymphatics)	Respiratory motion Consistency, malleability Tenderness	Changes in neighboring organs and vessels, free fluid

Venous Flow Pattern

There is a distinct difference between the flow patterns in the hepatic and the portal veins.

Hepatic veins. Here, blood flow is characterized by a physiological triple-peak/triphasic curve resembling the pulse curve in the jugular vein; it mirrors the pressure situation in the right heart.
- **Phase I**: first part of the blood flow is toward the heart; at the latter, it corresponds to the mechanical displacement of the valve plane (systolic phase)
- **Phase II**: second part of the blood flow is toward the heart; at the latter, it corresponds to the opening of the atrioventricular valve (diastolic phase)
- **Phase III**: regurgitation (back flow) is from the right atrium; it results from the contraction of the right atrium and the bulging of the tricuspid valve.

Measurements are taken at all three major hepatic veins. The flow pathology concerns the make-up of various phases (increased regurgitation in right ventricular failure, vena cava engorgement, tricuspid insufficiency) or the number of phases (biphasic pattern or monophasic pattern in cirrhosis of the liver). A ribbonlike flow profile, solely back flow, or no flow at all are found in Budd–Chiari syndrome or veno-occlusive disease (VOD).

Portal veins. These exhibit a ribbonlike flow profile with arterial modulation by the pulsations of adjacent arteries or propagated through the liver; there is
- Physiological hepatopetal flow (anterograde into the liver)
- Pathological hepatofugal flow (retrograde out of the liver)
- No flow or oscillating flow
and
- Thrombosis of the portal vein.

Measurements of the flow direction and the flow velocity are taken at the trunk of the portal vein as well as its left and right branches.

Dynamic Criteria

Respiratory motion
- During inspiration 2–3 fingerbreadths or 4–6 cm (~2 inches) caudad

Consistency
- Squeezable like a wet sponge
- Returns to its original shape once the pressure is released

Tenderness
- None

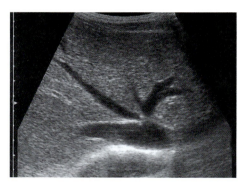

▲ **Fig. 2.9** View parallel to costal margin: regular hepatic parenchyma with the starlike junction of the hepatic veins.

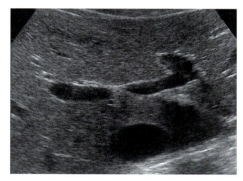

▲ **Fig. 2.10** Portal veins. View parallel to right costal margin: regular hepatic parenchyma with portal vein bifurcating into the left and right branches.

2.3 Hepatic Veins

- **Right, middle, and left hepatic veins, venous confluence**

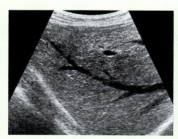 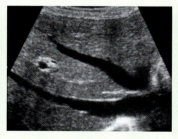 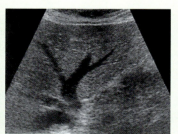

a Right hepatic vein. The major hepatic veins run in a straight or slightly curved line, and their margins are smooth without any wall echoes.

b Right and middle hepatic veins. Wall echoes are found at the portal vessels (transverse view) and wherever the sound waves strike the hepatic veins at right angle (large drop in impedance).

c Middle/left hepatic vein.

2.3 Hepatic Veins

▶ **Flow parameters**

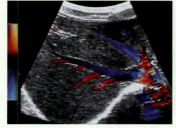
d Hepatofugal flow in the hepatic veins.

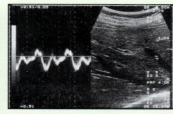
e Regular triphasic duplex signal of a normal middle hepatic vein.

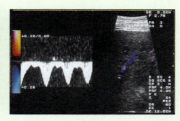
f Abnormal monophasic duplex signal of a hepatic vein in cirrhosis of the liver.

▶ **Bifurcation**

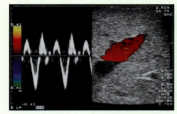
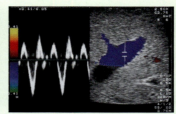
g and h Chronic liver congestion. Same duplex signal on the left, while the signal on the right varies with time.
g Hepatopetal flow reversal.

h Hepatofugal flow toward the heart.

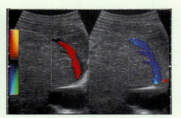
i Hepatofugal and hepatopetal flow at different times in the same hepatic vein.

▶ **Structural parameters**

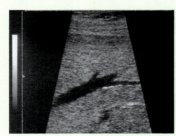
j Usually, the hepatic vein branches at sharp angles.

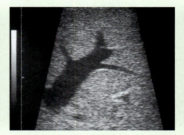
k Increased volume of the hepatic parenchyma (e.g. in fatty liver) results in obtuse angle branching (chronic liver congestion).

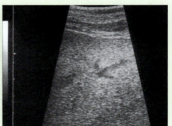
l In hepatosteatosis and inflammation, the contour of the veins becomes blurred and irregular.

2.4 Pathologic Liver Findings

▶ **Stasis**

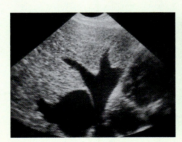
a–c Chronic liver congestion. Rigid engorged hepatic vein.

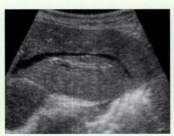
b In vena cava congestion, the hepatic vein becomes visible well into the (subcapsular) periphery of the liver.

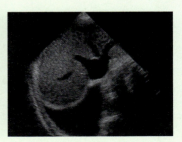
c Vena cava congestion with enlarged junction of the hepatic veins and right pleural effusion.

2.4 Pathologic Liver Findings

▶ Rarefaction

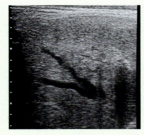 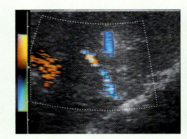 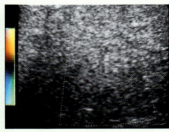

d Irregular contour of the hepatic vein with pitting and scarred indentations in inflammatory disease.

e Scarred irregular contour of the vascular wall with obstruction of the lumen resulting in local flow disturbances, visualized in color-flow duplex scanning as aliasing.

f–h Progress of the destructive inflammatory changes leading to the appearance of the so-called "rarefied hepatic vein": typical finding in cirrhosis.
f Rarefied hepatic vein, sonographic imaging not possible because of the parenchymal changes.

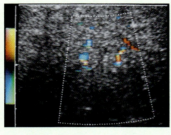 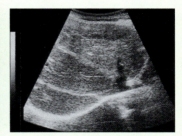

g Only color-flow duplex scanning of the same area delineates the hepatic vein by its disturbed flow.

h Differential diagnosis: hepatic vein with fibrous occlusion in veno-occlusive disease.

▶ Displacement and Infiltration

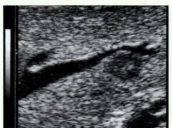

i and j Perivascular infiltration, impression, displacement, and vascular infiltration in malignancies.
i Breast cancer metastasis indenting the hepatic vein.

j Diffuse metastasis of gastric cancer infiltrating the wall of the hepatic vein

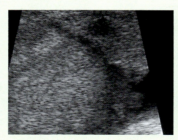 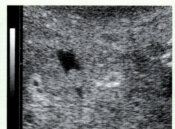 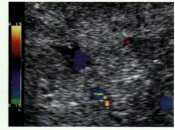

k–m Hepatocellular carcinoma (HCC) with typical infiltration of the hepatic vein.
k Lengthy wall infiltration of the hepatic vein and vena cava.

l Tumor thrombus of an HCC obstructing the lumen of the hepatic vein.

m Color-flow duplex scan: the tumor thrombosis does not occlude the lumen recognizable by the local flow acceleration with aliasing.

2.5 Portal veins

Bifurcation

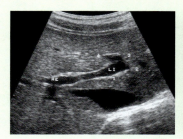
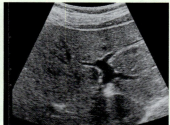
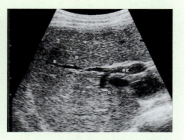

a–c Bifurcation of the portal vein.
a Left (LI) and right (RE) branch of the portal vein. Liver segments 1, 2, 3, 4.

b With the branches for segments I–IV of the left hepatic lobe.

c With the branches for segments V–VIII of the right hepatic lobe. RE = liver segments; 5, 6, 7, 8 = right.

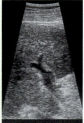
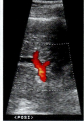

d Appearance of "amputated" lateral and terminal branches.

Flow parameters

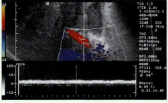
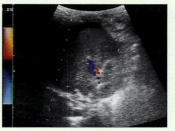

e–f Color-flow duplex scan of the portal vein in cirrhosis.
e Hepatopetal flow in atrophic cirrhosis of the liver.

f Hepatofugal flow; the arterial compensation is easily recognized. Cirrhosis of the liver in an infant before transplantation.

Diffuse Changes in the Hepatic Parenchyma

The settings of the equipment used will have a deep impact on the sonographer's ability to recognize and assess diffuse changes in the hepatic parenchyma. Apart from a careful analysis of the actual shape, texture, echogenicity, and distribution of the individual echoes representing the parenchyma, a successful overall assessment of the liver has to include as many additional criteria as possible (**Table 2.6**). Only by putting together the various criteria like pieces of a puzzle will a reliable assessment of this organ be achieved. One possibility, although to be used with caution, is a comparison of the hepatic parenchyma with that of other organs (kidney, spleen, pancreas, psoas muscle) (**2.2a**). This caveat has to do with the fact that apart from disease one has to take into account that aging will alter the characteristics of the different parenchymas differently (**Table 2.7**).

Thus, assessment of diffuse changes in the hepatic parenchyma is still influenced by any number of subjective aspects, and to a large extent depends on the sonographer's experience. Early results of studies using parametric ultrasound are encouraging and give rise to the hope that this might open up the possibility of objective findings and their assessment.

> ### Parametric Ultrasonography
>
> Parametric ultrasonography does not generate images but rather numbers. This is supposed to neutralize any subjective bias on the part of the sonographer as well as any possible objective bias due to the presettings and/or equipment used. Not only can tissues be detected and described objectively, but it is also possible to quantify and document the brightness and homogeneity. These digital signals are then processed and compared by various statistical computer programs, and the result opens up the possibility of noninvasive classification of diffuse tissue changes in ultrasonography, objective quality control in ultrasound equipment, and improved imaging.

Table 2.7 Comparison of hepatic parenchyma with other organs

Criterion	Liver	Spleen	Kidney	Pancreas	Psoas muscle
Single echo size	++	+	+++	+	++
Echogenicity	++	+++	+	+ – +++	+ – ++
Brightness	++	+	++	+	++
Distribution	Homogeneous	Homogeneous	Inhomogeneous	Homogeneous	Structured
Age-dependent changes	Slight	Yes	Slight	Distinct	Slight
Function-dependent changes	-	-	Yes	-	Distinct
Disease-dependent changes	++	+	++	+++	+

Enlarged Liver

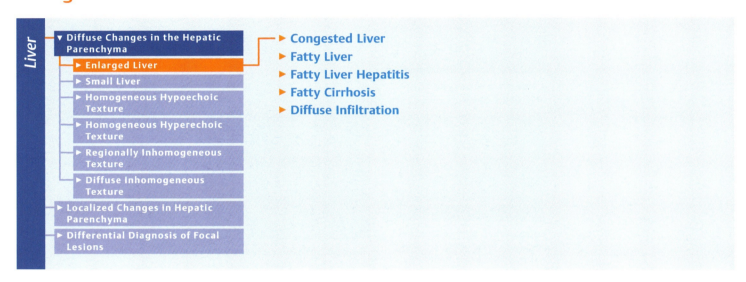

When the liver increases in volume, this does not necessarily become evident on a quantitative level because of the distinct interpersonal variability of this organ or because the change may be compensated by a change in shape. Sometimes the increase is noticed and documented only during follow-up studies. Enlargement of the liver is therefore an unrecognized finding that is often overlooked and becomes evident only in its more advanced stages.

Determining the Size of the Liver

Sonographic assessment of the size of the liver is fraught with problems.
Volumetric measurements yield a value of around 1/40 of the body weight (2.3–3%); for the adult male this would mean 1500–1800 ml and for the adult female 1200–1500 ml.
Organ measurements yield a width (right–left) of 25–30 cm, a length (cephalocaudad) of 12–20 cm, and a sagittal depth (anteroposterior) of 6–10 cm. Different shapes are encountered depending on the build: in asthenic persons the liver expands mostly in the longitudinal direction, while in pyknics the largest dimension is in the sagittal plane. Therefore, the build alone will account for different normal values of size.
In *ultrasonography* the size of the liver is determined in the right midclavicular line (MCL), a normal value being 12 cm (9 cm in pyknics, up to 15 cm in asthenics). Assessment of the superior diaphragmatic aspect is critical, since ultrasound may not be able to clearly delineate the boundary because of superposition of the phrenicocostal sinus, and percussion is rather imprecise. One option would be assessment of the inferior border at the costal margin; however, this value also varies widely depending on the build of the patient (normal: inferior edge at the costal margin), and cannot be relied on because of the respiratory motion of the liver or abnormal position of the diaphragm (emphysema, phrenic nerve palsy). Sagittal measurements also display a rather wide margin of error since there are no fixed markers to be used in reconstruction.
Determining the size of the caudate lobe, either in absolute terms or in relation to the right hepatic lobe, may aid in the presumed diagnosis of cirrhosis or Budd–Chiari syndrome.
When assessing the size of the liver, the intersegmental comparison and the relation between right and left hepatic lobe (normal: left < right) have to be considered as well. Should the left hepatic lobe slide in between the spleen and the diaphragm, displacing the spleen inferiorly, this would be the firm sign of an enlarged left hepatic lobe.

▶ Congested Liver

Acute congestion of the liver (Figs. 2.11 and 2.12). In cases of acute liver congestion the liver is usually characterized by a significant increase in size; this is due to congestion of the vena cava, normally caused by cardiac insufficiency, which leads to blood backing up into the liver, thus increasing its volume (edema) and providing the explanation for the decreased echogenicity as well as the improved ultrasound image of the organ. On the other hand, quite often this will lead to capsular tension and pain. The liver has a smooth surface; the inferior margin is obtusely angled or round. The organ is tightly elastic/firm and quite tender (on palpation); sometimes an expansive hepatic pulse may be palpated. The hypoechoic parenchyma has a "fluffy" appearance with improved conduction of the ultrasound beam. Characteristic sign are the distended hepatic veins, which can be visualized all the way into the periphery of the liver, and the engorged junction of the hepatic veins at the vena cava ("venous star"). Regular B-mode imaging already displays real-time turbulent flow in the hepatic veins, which presents rather impressively in duplex and color-flow duplex scanning with an increased percentage of flow reversal and the typical change in the pulsed Doppler curve (see "Venous Flow Pattern", p. 58).

The diagnosis of acute congestion of the liver, suspected on abdominal ultrasound, is firmed up by additional findings, such as ascites, pleural effusion, incompressible enlarged lumen of the vena cava, and congestion-induced sequelae in other organs (kidneys, spleen, stomach).

Chronic congestion of the liver (Figs. 2.13 and 2.14, ▣ 2.4a and b). Although chronic congestion of the liver also may present as substantial enlargement of the organ, it is primarily characterized by extended fibrotic changes; in other words, the increase in size may not be quite apparent or it might be pretended by a low position of the liver in the abdomen without any actual increase in size (e.g., in emphysema). These fibrotic changes ("cardiac cirrhosis") may result in the organ becoming smaller and would explain the distinct increase in consistency as well as the increasing echogenicity. The hepatic surface is smooth, possibly slightly

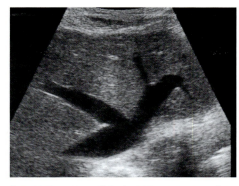

▲ **Fig. 2.11** Junction of the hepatic veins in acute hepatic congestion. Hypoechoic homogeneous parenchyma of the liver resulting from the edema: rigid engorged hepatic veins and vena cava signifying congestion of the vena cava; other criteria are: increased size and consistency, possibly tenderness on palpation.

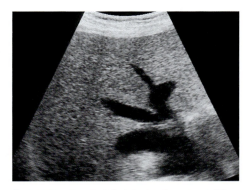

▲ **Fig. 2.12** Junction of the hepatic veins in acute failure of preexisting chronic hepatic congestion. Homogeneous parenchyma with an increased number of diffusely dispersed, finely grained echoes; rigid engorged hepatic veins and vena cava.

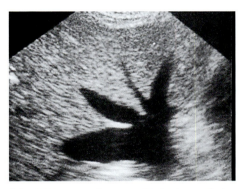

▲ **Fig. 2.13** Chronic congestion of the liver with distinctly engorged rigid junction of the hepatic veins, and a homogeneous hyperechoic parenchyma.

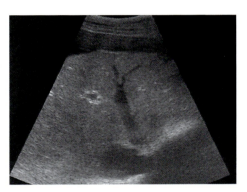

▲ **Fig. 2.14** Cardiac cirrhosis. Irregular surface and homogeneous parenchyma; the engorged hepatic vein is visible far into the periphery. Signs of ascites and right pleural effusion (not seen here).

irregular because of the ongoing fibrosis, the inferior margin is blunt or sharply angled. Sometimes an expansive hepatic pulse may be palpated. Capsular tension with concomitant pain would be unusual for chronic hepatic congestion, as it is more characteristic of acute decompensation of the underlying congestion of the vena cava. As is the case in acute hepatic congestion, too, the engorged hepatic veins can be visualized far into the periphery of the liver, and also the junction of the hepatic veins at the vena cava is enlarged.

Just as in acute congestion of the liver, duplex and color-flow duplex scanning demonstrates the impressive flow changes. The cardiac modulation may affect the duplex curve of the portal system. Sometimes there may be additional findings, such as ascites, pleural effusion, rigid enlarged lumen of the vena cava, and congestion induced changes in other organs (kidneys, spleen, stomach). **Table 2.8** is a summary of the criteria relevant in acute and chronic congestion of the liver.

Table 2.8 Sonographic diagnostic criteria used in acute/chronic congestion of the liver

Criterion	Acute hepatic congestion	Chronic hepatic congestion
Size	Enlarged	Normal or enlarged
Shape	Biconvex	Biconvex
Surface	Smooth	Smooth/irregular
Contour of margin	Blunt	Blunt
Parenchymal structure	Hypoechoic, homogeneous	Hyperechoic, homogeneous
Ultrasound conduction	Improved	Normal
Hepatic veins	Engorged, can be imaged far into the periphery	Engorged, can be imaged far into the periphery
Portal veins	(Marked)	(Marked)
Hepatic artery	No characteristic change	No characteristic change
Respiratory motion	Present or lessened	Present or lessened
Consistency	Tightly elastic	Firm
Tenderness	Marked	None
Other	Ascites/pleural effusion/pericardial effusion, rigid engorged vena cava	Ascites/pleural effusion/pericardial effusion, rigid engorged vena cava

▶ Fatty Liver (◧ 2.6)

Extrinsic and dynamic criteria. Fatty infiltration of the hepatic parenchyma is a frequent but nonspecific finding, increasing the volume of the liver and thus its size. Initially, this increase in total organ volume manifests itself by a change in the shape; the increased size of the liver as such becomes evident and can be quantified only in the more advanced stages. But even then the organ will still have a smooth surface and exhibit a normal soft consistency. The inferior margin of the liver becomes more and more blunt while the angle increases. The left hepatic lobe becomes biconvex and the inferior margin almost round (so-called rounding of the organ).

Intrinsic criteria. Since fatty infiltration of the cells goes hand in hand with an increased volume of the liver, the vessels are pushed apart, the hepatic veins take a somewhat curved course, and their branching no longer is sharply angled but obtuse. The regular well-defined contour of the hepatic veins becomes blurred: this artifact is due to the increased refraction and scattering of the ultrasound waves at the numerous boundaries of the individual fatty vesicles within the hepatocytes and can be demonstrated at all contours.

This increase in boundaries is also the reason for the typical increased echogenicity and degraded ultrasound conduction (i.e., attenuation) (**Fig. 2.15**). The degree of fatty infiltration, the type of fatty deposits in the hepatocytes (large vesicles = few additional boundaries; or small vesicles = numerous additional boundaries), the type of fat, and additional factors (severity of any concomitant inflammation, degree of fibrosis) will define any changes in the echotexture, in particular any changes in the number, size, and density of the echoes as well as in the degree of attenuation (**Fig. 2.16**). The homogeneous distribution of the echoes may vary between segments or regions but still remains one of the basic characteristics of fatty liver.

Causes. By itself, the sonographic finding of fatty liver cannot tell anything about the underlying cause. Nutrition may be assumed as probable cause if there are also fatty changes in other organs (abdominal wall, pancreas, body mass index BMI > 24), in which case the fatty changes in the liver could be regarded as "normal" findings. However, if a slim patient with a thin abdominal wall (BMI < 24) exhibits fatty liver whose consistency is significantly softer or harder than normal, this finding would have to be assessed as pathological and would mandate further work-up.

Fatty Change of the Liver

Definition. Fatty liver or steatosis hepatis is present if the moist mass of the liver contains > 10% fat, or if more than 50% of the hepatic cells display medium- or large-sized lipid vacuoles and there is a diffuse pattern of distribution.

Pathogenesis. The causes of underlying fatty change may be *exogenous*:
▶ Increased fat transport
▶ Increased carbohydrate intake
or *endogenous*:
▶ Increased peripheral mobilization of fat
▶ Inhibited intracellular utilization of fat in the hepatic cells
▶ Increased fat synthesis in the hepatic cells
▶ Decreased removal of fat.

Morphology. Morphology differentiates between small-, medium-, and large-sized lipid vacuoles with low (5% of the moist mass of the liver), moderate (6–8%), and marked (8–9%) involvement of the liver. The distribution pattern of the fatty change can be classified as peripheral, centroacinar, zonal, or diffuse.

Etiology. In terms of etiology, fatty liver is encountered as nonspecific reaction in numerous diseases and conditions; these include:
▶ Nutrition
▶ Metabolic disorders
▶ Alcohol
▶ Medication
▶ Chemical substances
▶ Phytotoxins and mycotoxins
▶ Infection
▶ Hypoxia
▶ Endocrine disorders
▶ Pregnancy

2.6 Fatty Liver, Fatty Liver Hepatitis and Focal Fatty Infiltration

▸ Increased structural density

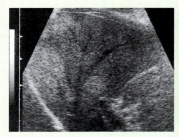 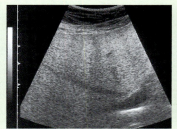 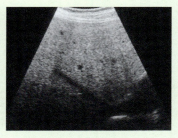

a–c Fatty liver.
a The displaced hepatic veins no longer course in a straight line but are slightly curved and are poorly delimited.

b Because of the increased refraction and scattering at the boundaries and the runtime artifacts, the contours as well as the boundaries are poorly delimited.

c Fatty liver/fatty liver hepatitis: increasing fatty infiltration will diminish the echodensity and increase the attenuation.

▸ Regional differences in fatty infiltration: focal

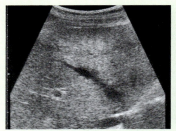 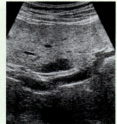 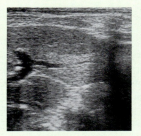

d The additional inflammatory changes in diabetic or toxic fatty liver or non-alcoholic steatohepatitis induce irregular margins of the hepatic veins; here, a case of diabetic fatty liver hepatitis with focal inhomogeneous fatty infiltration.

e–g Focal fatty infiltration (FFI).
e Focal non-steatosis in loco typico at the inferior aspect of segment IV in the left hepatic lobe anterior to the portal bifurcation.

f FFI of segment II in the left hepatic lobe; the parenchyma with its increased fatty infiltration appears hyperechoic.

▸ Regional differences in fatty infiltration: bizarre, maplike

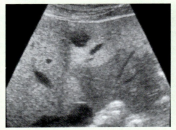 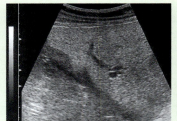 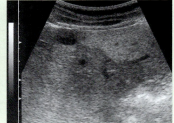

g–i FFI may parallel the vessels and display a map of bizarre irregular margins.

▸ **Fatty Liver Hepatitis (◨ 2.6)**

In fatty liver hepatitis (**Fig. 2.15–2.18**) (e.g., alcoholic hepatitis, nonalcoholic steatohepatitis, diabetic fatty liver), the fatty infiltration is accompanied by necrosis and inflammatory changes with fibrosis. Apart from the sonographic signs of fatty deposits discussed above, this results in increased consistency of the liver and a decreased plasticity. The surface still remains smooth.

The decisive aspect is the changes in the hepatic veins: contrary to their somewhat curved course in simple fatty liver, they now appear as an entire network but can only be imaged in a disjointed fashion, with some fragments visible while whole other segments are missing. Artifacts will blur the contours of the hepatic veins and ultrasonography will show irregular walls due to perivenous inflammation. Ultimately, increasing fibrosis and scarring will lead to fatty cirrhosis, the transition between these states being fairly fluid.

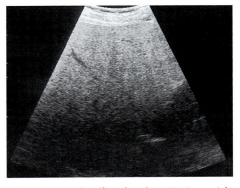

▲ **Fig. 2.15** Fatty liver/fatty liver hepatitis. Large right hepatic lobe with a diffuse increase in the delicate to moderate echotexture, which appears more densely packed, with slightly irregular graininess, and signals fatty infiltration; apart from the coarser graininess of the parenchyma, the inflammation is characterized by the irregular contour of the hepatic veins. There is marked attenuation of the ultrasound waves.

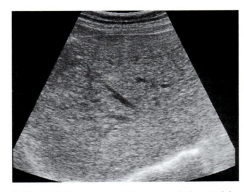

▲ **Fig. 2.16** Fatty liver hepatitis. Large right hepatic lobe with a diffuse increase in the delicate and particularly the moderate echotexture, which appears more densely packed and with irregular graininess; the hepatic veins exhibit a networklike and disjointed appearance, the fatty infiltration and inflammation blurring their contours.

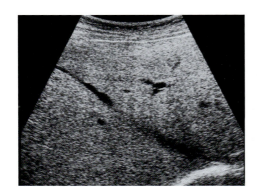
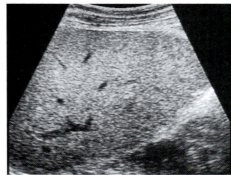

◄◄ **Fig. 2.17** Fatty liver hepatitis. Large right hepatic lobe with a diffuse increase in the moderate echotexture, which appears more densely packed and with irregular graininess; the hepatic veins exhibit markedly irregular contours, signifying perivascular inflammation; the fatty liver aspect is recognizable by the blurred contours and the echo density, the inflammatory reaction being the most important aspect (surface no longer totally smooth, increased consistency at one-finger palpation).

◄ **Fig. 2.18** Chronic toxic fatty liver hepatitis. Large right hepatic lobe with a marked diffuse increase in the moderate echotexture, which appears more densely packed and with irregular graininess. The hepatic veins present as a network and appear irregular; the surface shows fine irregularities as well, and there is a marked increase in volume and consistency.

▶ Fatty Cirrhosis

In fatty cirrhosis (**Fig. 2.19**) the liver has turned into a densely firm organ. In many cases there is a distinct shift in the mass relation of the lobes from right to left, with a more significant increase in the mass of the left lobe, and the right hepatic lobe even appearing smaller than normal. The caudate lobe may become quite prominent. The fine nodular surface in fatty cirrhosis can only be visualized by high-resolution probes; during routine studies the liver presents with a smooth surface. The individual echoes of the hepatic parenchyma are coarse, hyperechoic, and arranged as a homogeneous texture. One of the typical findings is the beginning rarefication of the hepatic veins; however, in contrast to posthepatitic cirrhosis, they still are easily recognized. The portovenous system is prominent and exhibits distinct so-called periportal reinforcement, a scabby knotted bifurcation of the portal vein, enlarged central aspect of the vascular tree, and distinct caliber changes at the more peripheral segments. Other criteria of cirrhosis may also be evident: e.g., ascites, splenomegaly, thickening of the gallbladder wall, and collaterals in portal hypertension.

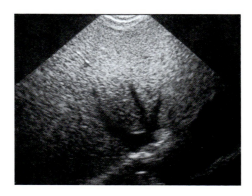

◄ **Fig. 2.19** Fatty cirrhosis. Liver with marked diffuse increase in moderately and coarsely textured echoes, which display irregular graininess and are more densely packed; the junction of the hepatic veins appears stunted, and the peripheral segments of the hepatic veins seem rarefied; obvious evidence of attenuation of the ultrasound beam.

▶ Diffuse Infiltration

Diffuse infiltration with an increased size of the liver may be the result of extracellular or intracellular substrate deposits.

Intracellular deposits. Apart from fatty infiltration as discussed above, these deposits are also encountered in other storage diseases such as hemochromatosis and the glycogen storage diseases. Just as in fatty liver, not only does the echogenicity of the parenchyma increase but so also does the consistency of the liver. The vascular architecture, particularly that of the hepatic veins, remains unchanged for a long time.

Extracellular infiltrations. These may be caused by fluid (edema) or cellular mechanisms (e.g., chronic lymphocytic leukemia) and lead to increased size and consistency of the organ, with a typical decrease in parenchymal echogenicity but improved conduction. In many cases the echoes display a homogeneous/diffuse distribution, though regional differences (perivenous) or segmental patterns are also quite common.

Small Liver

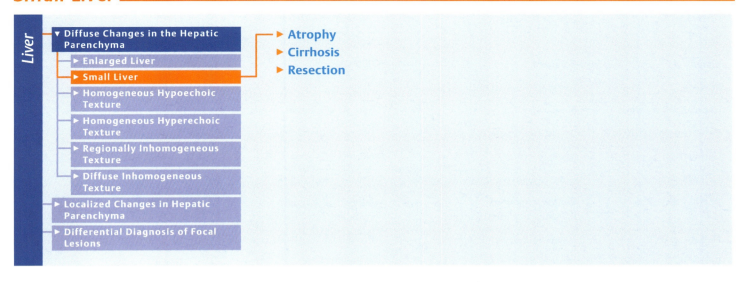

A small liver is a rather infrequent finding and becomes evident only if the decrease in size is substantial. Owing to the small probe contact area and the hidden position below the ribs, the conditions for ultrasound studies of the liver are less than ideal.

▶ Atrophy

Hepatic atrophy is a rather rare finding and may pertain to the entire organ or just individual segments. Its possible causes comprise vascular disorders or chronic inflammatory disease, the most common being chronic atrophic cirrhosis.

▶ Cirrhosis

Apart from the decrease in size, the cirrhotic liver is characterized by certain typical criteria (**Table 2.9**). Quite often there is a substantial amount of ascites, in which the small organ seems to float like a wooden block in water and thus can still be insonated well despite its lack of size (**Figs. 2.20 and 2.21**). Also, there are clear-cut signs of portal hypertension, with a drop in flow velocity within the portal vein, even all the way down to no flow and sometimes a hepatofugal flow.

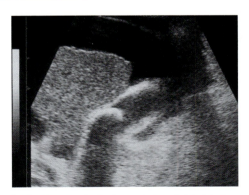

▲ **Fig. 2.20** Atrophic cirrhosis. Grainy, slightly inhomogeneous hepatic parenchyma, irregular surface, rarefied vasculature; the liver floats like a wooden block in the ascites. Ancillary finding: thickened gallbladder wall, gallstone evident within the lumen of the gallbladder.

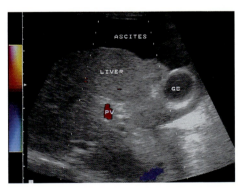

▲ **Fig. 2.21** Completely atrophic cirrhosis of the liver with irregular surface, rarefied intrahepatic vasculature, and marked ascites; demonstration of hepatopetal flow in the portal vein (PV) on color-flow duplex scanning. Ancillary finding: thickened gallbladder (GB) wall.

Table 2.9 **Diagnostic criteria in cirrhosis of the liver**

Criterion	Fatty cirrhosis	Posthepatitic cirrhosis	Cardiac cirrhosis
Size	+++	Normal–smaller	Normal
Shape	Rounded	Beaklike	—
Surface	Comparatively smooth	Irregular	Smooth
Contour of margin	Blunt/rounded	Sharply angulated	Sharply angulated/blunt
Parenchymal structure	Dense, homogeneous	Coarse, inhomogeneous	Coarse, inhomogeneous
Conduction	Attenuated	Normal	Increased
Hepatic veins	Narrow, blurred, beginning rarefaction	Marked rarefaction	Engorged
Portal veins	Center: engorged Periphery: caliber change	Center: engorged Periphery: caliber change	Engorged
Hepatic artery	No characteristic change	Prominent due to compensation	No characteristic change
Respiratory motion	Normal	Normal	Normal
Consistency	Firm	Hard	Hard
Tenderness	Possible	No	In acute decompensation

▶ Resection

Usually, the status post resection of any parts of the liver is hard to recognize just by looking at the size of the organ since the liver has an enormous capacity for regeneration, and any surgical reduction in volume will be compensated for by hypertrophy of the remaining tissue. A postresection liver is best assessed by the change in vascular architecture, but one has to remember that the numerous normal variants of the vascular system and the congenitally different sizes of the various liver segments (smaller left lobe) may make this an impossibility. Quite often, right hemihepatectomy will produce an anomalous position of the remaining liver with tilting, rotation, and twisting around the portal axis. Apart from the usual small contact area at the right thoracic wall, these factors will hamper orientation about the anatomy even further.

Homogeneous Hypoechoic Texture

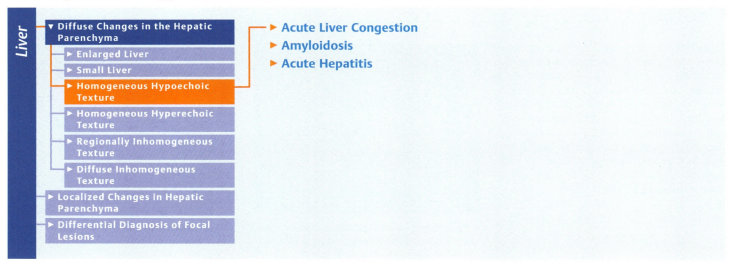

A hypoechoic homogenous echotexture within the liver is due to a decrease in the number of echoes per unit area because of fluid accumulation on the intracellular level (edema), or the extracellular/intracellular/sinusoidal level (hypervolemia, congestion), or both (right sided heart failure, renal failure, hemodialysis).

▶ Acute Liver Congestion

Congestion of the inferior vena cava will increase the volume load of the liver (edema) and explains the lessened echogenicity but heightened conduction of the organ; on the other hand, such typical criteria as the significant capsular tension with its concomitant pain and the tightly elastic/firm consistency of the liver on palpation with marked tenderness will be hard to miss. The hypoechoic coarse parenchyma may be quite discrete and become masked by previous chronic congestion of the liver aggravated by acute right ventricular failure; however, sonographic findings of improved ultrasound conduction of the organ, engorged hepatic veins easily followed far into the periphery, and a dilated junction of the hepatic veins remain the characteristic sonographic signs of an acutely congested liver (**Figs. 2.11 and 2.12**).

▶ Amyloidosis

Amyloidosis is characterized by a homogeneous increase in the size of the liver, with regular architecture and a homogeneous hypoechoic parenchyma of coarse consistency.

▶ Acute Hepatitis

Since acute hepatitis is accompanied by edema and the infiltration of inflammatory cells, one would expect a hypoechoic organ that is easy to insonate; unfortunately, a liver such as this is rarely encountered in acute viral hepatitis. Ultrasonography is therefore not the modality of choice in the work-up of acute hepatitis, especially since there are far more characteristic findings suggesting the diagnosis of acute viral hepatitis: even if shape, size, and echotexture of the liver appear absolutely normal, quite often an increasing resemblance of the parenchymal splenic and hepatic echotextures (possibly with homogeneous enlargement) becomes evident (**Figs. 2.22–2.24**). A thickened striated gallbladder wall of up to 20 mm (no tenderness!) and hypoechoic, pathologically enlarged hilar lymph nodes can also frequently be demonstrated (**Figs. 2.25 and 2.26**). Parenchymal hypoechogenicity in acute viral hepatitis is an incidental finding in fulminating necrosis of the liver; in this case, the organ is surprisingly small, displays a markedly soft consistency, and is characterized by a hypoechoic to splotchy/inhomogeneous parenchymal echotexture.

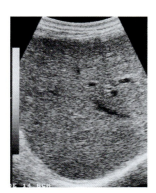

▲ *Fig. 2.22* Acute hepatitis in mononucleosis.

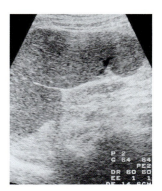

▲ *Fig. 2.23* The spleen of the same patient as in **Fig. 2.22**. Compare spleen/liver: in acute hepatitis the parenchymal texture of the liver and spleen may start resembling each other.

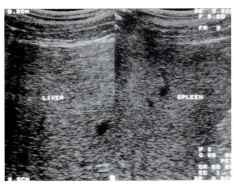

▲ *Fig. 2.24* Acute hepatitis. Compare spleen/liver: in this case of acute viral hepatitis the hepatic and splenic parenchyma begin to resemble each other. This is a case of acute hepatitis A.

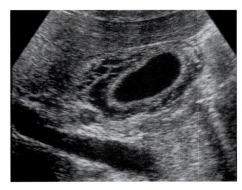

▲ *Fig. 2.25* Gallbladder in acute hepatitis. Marked thickening and striation of the wall > 20 mm without any tenderness in a case of acute hepatitis A; positive demonstration of hypoechoic enlarged lymph nodes in the duodenal ligament. The parenchyma itself and the ultrasound conductivity of the liver are normal (smooth surface, normal/soft consistency as seen by the impressions formed on palpation with the probe).

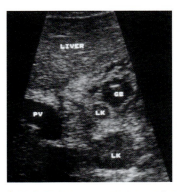

▲ *Fig. 2.26* Gallbladder (GB) in acute hepatitis A. Here, too, there is marked thickening and striation of the gallbladder wall > 20 mm. No tenderness; demonstration of hypoechoic enlarged lymph nodes (LK) in the hepatoduodenal ligament; normal parenchyma and ultrasound conductivity of the liver. PV = portal vein.

Homogeneous Hyperechoic Texture

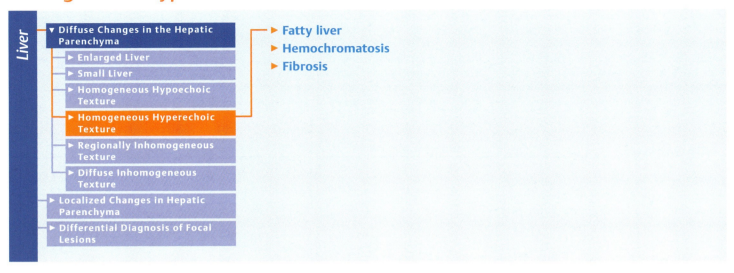

A hyperechoic homogeneous texture of the liver may be the result of an increased number of echoes/boundaries per unit area, which in turn may be traced back to intracellular or interstitial deposits of foreign substances (e.g., fat or iron, and fibrosis, respectively).

▶ Fatty Liver

In principle, fatty tissue lends itself quite well to insonation: it is characterized by a low density and impedance and conducts ultrasound better than water or hepatic parenchyma. It is the increase in the number of boundaries that is responsible for the typical hyperechogenicity and attenuation encountered in fatty liver. The severity of the steatosis, the type of fatty deposits within the hepatocytes (large vesicles = few additional boundaries; small vesicles = numerous additional boundaries), the type of fat, and other factors (severity of any concomitant inflammation or fibrosis) predetermine the change in the echotexture, i.e., the number, size, and density of the individual echoes and the degree of attenuation. But one aspect remains constant: even if the overall echotexture varies between segments or regions, within any such affected area the individual echoes still exhibit the homogeneous appearance (**2.6**).

▶ Hemochromatosis

Although iron deposits in the hepatocytes result in a homogeneous increase in the echogenicity as well as attenuation, this finding is nonspecific, making ultrasonography an unsuitable modality in the early diagnosis. Only inflammatory changes and cirrhotic transformation of the hepatic parenchyma will then characterize the disease (**Fig. 2.27**).

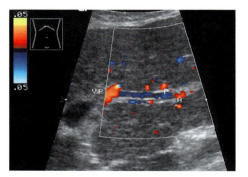

◀ *Fig. 2.27* Hemochromatosis with subsequent cirrhosis of the liver: coarse hyperechoic texture due to the fibrosis; prominent hepatic artery (A). P = pancreas; VP = portal vein.

▶ Fibrosis

Fibrosis of the liver may be a primary hepatic disorder, a sequela to a previously overcome bout of hepatitis, or a chronic vascular disease. Typical ultrasound findings are the homogeneous, if somewhat coarsely grained, echogenicity of the liver, demonstration of a slightly undulating surface, firm consistency, and quite often a still evident vascular and hepatic architecture (**Fig. 2.28**).

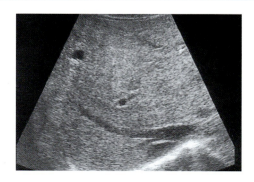

◀ *Fig. 2.28* Fibrosis; in this case, Caroli syndrome with slightly inhomogeneous, coarsely grained, hyperechoic hepatic parenchyma; demonstration of a small cyst, still present hepatic vein taking a mildly arced course.

Regionally Inhomogeneous Texture

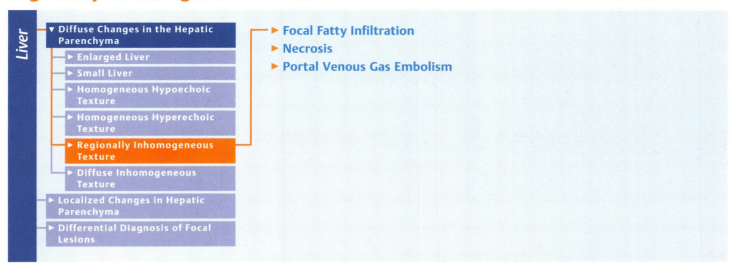

The sonographic texture of the hepatic parenchyma is determined by the size, density, brightness, and distribution/arrangement of the individual echoes. In other words, irregular ultrasound texture is the sequel to changes in one or more of these echo characteristics. These changes may pertain uniformly to the entire organ or just to a segment, region, or zone.

In parenchyma with limited segmental, regional or zonal irregularities (parenchyma with circumscribed "splotches") one has to differentiate between changes found in one or more segments (**Fig. 2.29**), or developing in typical perivascular fashion or along the portal structures (**2.2g and h**), and those whose distribution appears without any semblance of order. In the latter case, it becomes rather difficult to distinguish these changes from infiltrating metastatic changes (**Fig. 2.30**).

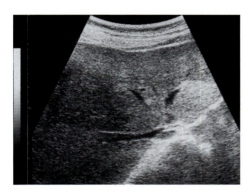

▲ **Fig. 2.29** Example of segmental inhomogeneity: varying degree of fatty infiltration limited to one segment (segment II).

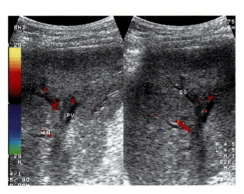

▲ **Fig. 2.30** Example of periportal inhomogeneity: periportal infiltration in metastatic pancreatic cancer. AH = hepatic artery; PV = portal vein; GG = bile duct.

▶ Focal Fatty Infiltration

Focal fatty infiltration of the liver (FFI) appears as a mass within the classic findings of fatty liver (**2.6, Figs. 2.29 and 2.31–2.33**) (see above). It is a rather common finding, characterized by the juxtaposition of two different areas of the parenchyma with echoes of the same size/brightness, which may be densely (hyperechoic) or more loosely (hypoechoic) packed but always displaying a homogeneous arrangement. There are a number of prime locations for focal fatty infiltration (posteriorly in segment IV, at the gallbladder fossa, around the veins, left > right). Quite often they exhibit a maplike delineation toward the neighboring parenchyma but still fit in harmoniously with the hepatic architecture, i.e., they do not deform any boundaries nor do they change the surface or alter the course of any vessels. Focal fatty infiltration seems to take place more frequently in certain situations, such as severe nutritional steatosis or after anesthesia. If ultrasonography is the only diagnostic modality used, it is sometimes impossible to differentiate between focal infiltration and diffuse metastasis, in which case abdominal CT or hepatobiliary scintiscanning would have to be employed.

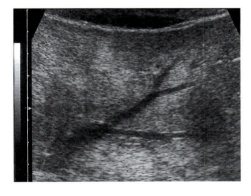

◀ **Fig. 2.31** Focal fatty infiltration. Inhomogeneous splotches of hyperechoic/hypoechoic parenchyma in the left hepatic lobe without involvement of the vessels.

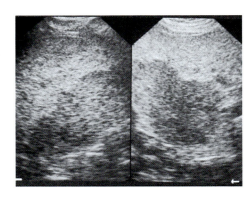
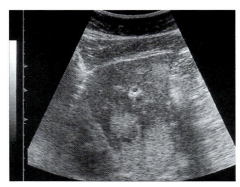

◀◀ *Fig. 2.32* Segmental fatty infiltration. Hypoechoic parenchyma with fatty infiltration of varying degree along segment II of the left hepatic lobe; tonguelike delineation of the fatty infiltration without any changes in the surface or the course of the vessels.

◀ *Fig. 2.33* Segmental fatty infiltration. Pseudotumorous pseudonodular hyperechoic areas respecting the boundaries and surfaces of vessels and segments.

▶ Necrosis

Segmental necrosis requires a break in the blood supply from the corresponding branch of the portal vein as well as from the hepatic artery. The early phase usually evades detection and is characterized by swelling and edema, with a hypoechoic somewhat broken-up parenchyma. Older necrosis presents as segmental coarse changes in the parenchymal texture, with an irregular arrangement of echoes of varying coarse graininess and brightness.

▶ Portal Venous Gas Embolism

Necrotizing intra-abdominal disease (e.g., acute mesenteric ischemia, pancreatitis), diseases with a breakdown in the barrier between the intestinal lumen and the portal venous system (e.g., penetrating GI ulcer, diverticulitis), and septic conditions with gas-producing pathogens from the portal run-in areas may sweep gas bubbl, es into the liver via the portal vein. In ultrasound, these bubbles appear as coarse turbulent echoes within the portal vein; in the hepatic parenchyma they are deposited first in the periportal regions and there present as coarse echoes (**Fig. 2.34**). Eventually, these coarse echoes will spread across the entire parenchyma, and within just a few hours portal venous gas embolism can develop into life-threatening acidosis (Kussmaul respiration) and fatal hepatic failure.

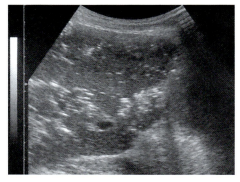

▲ *Fig. 2.34* Portal venous gas embolism. Initial periportal deposits of gas bubbles.

Diffuse Inhomogeneous Texture

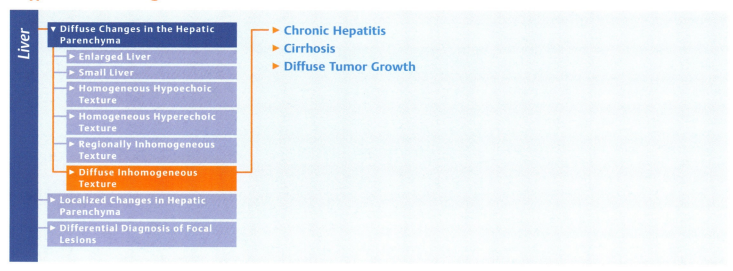

▶ Chronic Hepatitis

During the course of hepatitis there will be periportal and parenchymal inflammation, accompanied by edema and necrosis. As a result size, density, brightness, and distribution of the individual echoes within all of the hepatic parenchyma will exhibit coarse inhomogeneity of varying degree. The surface becomes increasingly irregular and displays fibrotic dimpling, which also will be found along the hepatic veins where it leads to irregular margins ("nibbling away"). Eventually the veins will become tortuous and increasingly rarefied in the periphery. The branches of the portal veins present with multiple periportal echoes, while the consistency of the liver becomes increasingly firm and in the end hard (**Figs. 2.35 and 2.36**). The extent of the sonographic changes depends not so much on the possible etiology of chronic hepatitis but rather on its duration and severity. Any pathological enlarged lymph nodes at the hepatic portal will correlate with the severity and activity of chronic hepatitis. There is a fluid transition between the sonographic findings of chronic hepatitis and cirrhosis of the liver.

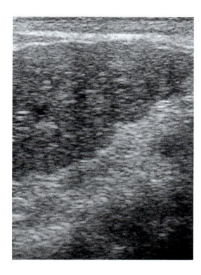

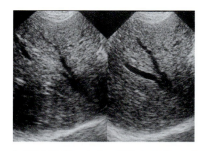

▲ *Fig. 2.36* Chronic hepatitis. Irregular surface, inhomogeneous parenchyma, irregular corkscrewlike hepatic vein with so-called "nibbling away." Other criteria: increased consistency.

◄ *Fig. 2.35* Chronic autoimmune hepatitis: Irregular surface, inhomogeneous and coarse parenchyma. Hepatic veins already rarefied. Other criteria: increased consistency, splenomegaly.

▶ Cirrhosis

In a liver with cirrhotic changes, the diffuse irregular parenchymal echotexture by itself is a rather poor criterion for the presence or absence of any cirrhosis. Irregular surface, typical changes in the shape, firm/hard consistency of the organ, rarefied hepatic veins, splenomegaly, and collateralization in portal hypertension are much more reliable indicators of any cirrhotic transformation (**Figs. 2.37–2.39, Fig. 2.20, ▣ 2.2l, ▣ 2.4f–h, and ▣ 2.7**). The types of parenchymal disturbance may differ: a relatively homogeneous hy-

▣ 2.7 Cirrhosis of the Liver

▶ Surface and Structure

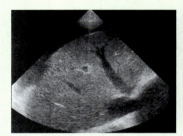

a Cardiac cirrhosis with engorged hepatic vein visible far into the periphery; homogeneous dense parenchyma with subtly irregular surface, ascites.

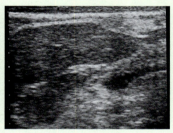

b In the longitudinal view at the midline, typical beak-like/dolphin-nosed appearance, large caudate lobe.

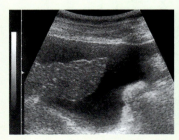

c Rigid inferior right lobe with coarsely irregular surface, ascites.

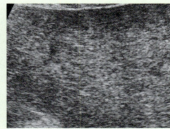

d Inhomogeneous coarse parenchyma, subtly irregular surface, the rarefied hepatic veins cannot be visualized.

▶ Extrahepatic findings: portal vein and gallbladder

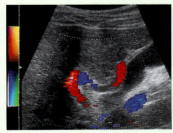

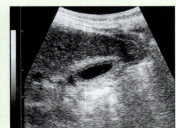

e and f Extrahepatic findings in cirrhosis.
e Occlusion of the intrahepatic segment of the portal vein, with collateral varicosity in the gallbladder fossa.

f Thickening of the gallbladder wall.

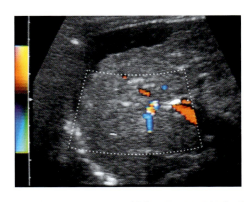

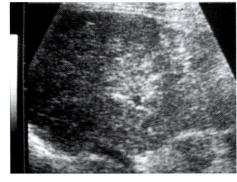

Fig. 2.37 Cirrhosis of the liver. Irregular surface, ascites, coarse inhomogeneous parenchyma, rarefied hepatic veins, irregular lumen, and in color flow scanning demonstration of localized increased flow velocity. Other criteria: increased consistency at one-finger palpation.

Fig. 2.38 Cirrhosis of the liver. Small organ with coarse inhomogeneous parenchyma, change in caliber of the portal vessels, and rarefied hepatic veins.

perechoic texture would be more typical of fatty cirrhosis, while a parenchymal change characterized by large nodules would most probably be due to chronic inflammatory disease. The vascular architecture could also provide clues about the possible etiology: rarefied vessels are typical of inflammation, while in toxic cirrhosis quite often the vessels still can be imaged, and in cardiac cirrhosis the hepatic veins will always be easy to visualize.

▶ Diffuse Tumor Growth

Diffuse infiltration of the liver by a tumor is an infrequent finding; in rare cases, it may simply lead to an increased size of the liver and to coarse hypoechoic parenchyma (e.g., in chronic lymphocytic leukemia), but more often it is seen as an irregular region within the liver (e. g., breast cancer) (**Figs. 2.39–2.41**). The decisive diagnostic aspect is the presence of criteria for malignancy (see below).

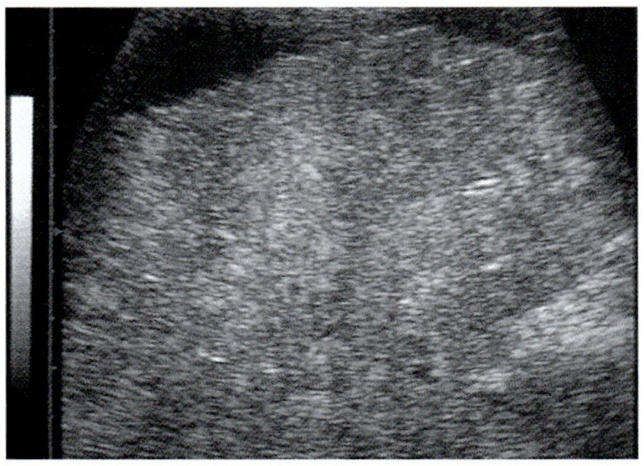

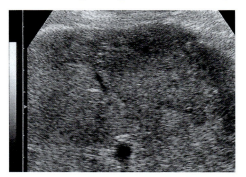

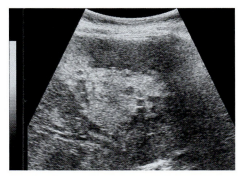

▲ **Fig. 2.39** Differential diagnosis of irregular parenchymal echotexture; in this case, hepatocellular carcinoma (HCC) in underlying cirrhosis.

▲ **Fig. 2.40** Differential diagnosis of irregular parenchymal texture; in this case, diffuse infiltration by a carcinoma of the gallbladder.

▲ **Fig. 2.41** Differential diagnosis of irregular parenchymal texture; in this case, diffuse breast cancer metastasis.

Localized Changes in Hepatic Parenchyma

The detection and identification of focal masses in the liver largely depends on their size, the difference in echogenicity and echotexture compared to the adjacent hepatic parenchyma, the location of the mass within the liver, and the diligence with which the sonographer studies the organ.

It is vital to cover all views possible (longitudinal, transverse, along the costal margin, intercostals, and those adapted to the particular findings) in order to image the liver completely. Despite all efforts, there remain some problem areas where focal masses might be missed owing to location, technical reasons, or the finding itself (**Table 2.10**).

Despite this caveat, ultrasonography is the prime diagnostic modality of choice when it comes to imaging focal masses in the liver, particularly when one takes into account its easy availability and only minor discomfort for the patient.

After the mass has been detected, its analysis, characterization, and assessment according to predefined criteria is of vital importance (**Fig. 2.42**).

Sonographic criteria. The following criteria are used.
▶ **Number**. The quantity is detailed as "solitary", a number (e.g., "4") or as "multiple". It is useful to specify the estimated volume of the mass as a percentage of the whole liver.

Table 2.10 Detection of intrahepatic masses–problems and possible solutions

Problem	Example	Solution
Location	▶ Anterior subphrenic ▶ At the ligamentum teres ▶ Posterior in the caudate lobe	▶ Examine in inspiration/expiration ▶ Use sector probe
Technical	▶ Mass outside the focal range ▶ Frequency dependent resolution of the probe ▶ Noise	▶ Alter the focal range ▶ Use high-frequency probes ▶ Tissue harmonic imaging
Finding	▶ Small mass ▶ Isoechoic mass	▶ Use high-frequency probe ▶ Contrast harmonic imaging

- **Location.** For solitary masses or a small number of masses, their location is specified. The distinction is made between central masses and those that have reached the surface of the liver. If at all possible, the segment involved is noted and whether or not the margins of the segment are clear; at minimum, it must be stated whether the mass is in the left or right lobe.
- **Distribution.** Masses may be disseminated or focal (periportal, perivenous, at the porta hepatis, subcapsular).
- **Size.** In solitary masses it is quite useful to specify the size, particularly in follow-up studies. The size is defined by two orthogonal diameters and given in centimeters or millimeters; it is better to measure a mass in all three planes (longitudinal, transverse, sagittal). To compare the findings for future reference, reproducible reference structures should be included in the image. Multiple masses are characterized by descriptive terms (e.g., small nodular, large nodular).
- **Shape.** A mass may be round, oval, bizarre, or maplike; only the shape of solitary masses should be described.
- **Margin.** This term specifies how the mass is delineated against the surrounding tissue; it may be sharp, smooth, and easily detectable, or blurred and irregular, or perhaps even undetectable.
- **Center/edge.** Masses may possess a capsule, a hypoechoic ring of parenchyma ("halo"), and peripheral vasculature. Others present with an anechoic, hypoechoic, or hyperechoic center signifying central necrosis, liquefaction, or hemorrhage.
- **Interrelationship with adjacent tissue.** The surface may be respected or it may undergo local bulging or protrusion, while other masses may produce localized indentation of their surface. Vessels may be indented, compressed, or locally displaced. Masses may grow infiltratively into vessels or infiltrate the adjacent tissue with podlike offshoots.
- **Changes in the surroundings.** It is not always possible to differentiate between marginal changes of a mass and reaction of the adjacent parenchyma. However, hypoechoic coarse parenchyma (usually caused by inflammation/edema) or hyperechogenicity are typical such changes.
- **Echogenicity.** Masses may be anechoic, hypoechoic, isoechoic, or hyperechoic compared to the surrounding parenchyma. It should be noted that this is no definite absolute measure and does not characterize the properties of the mass on a concrete level, but specifies them relative to the surrounding tissue without taking into account that the echogenicity of this parenchyma is by itself not a constant but may vary substantially depending on numerous factors (e.g., disease, nutrition, age).
- **Texture.** Assessment of the echotexture of a mass is based on its size, brightness, and echogenicity and the distribution/layout of the individual echoes within the mass.
- **Architecture.** The architecture of a mass takes into account structural changes caused by reaction at the margins, formation of a capsule, peduncle, etc.
- **Consistency.** Although often the consistency of a mass may not be amenable to direct examination, sometimes it can be assessed by one-finger palpation or by observing the resilience of the liver to vascular pulsation. The terms used are firm, tightly elastic, and soft/pliant.
- **Tenderness.** Rapid growth of a mass may be painful. The reason may be tension in the wall/capsule or pressure on adjacent tissue by cysts, bleeding, or abscess.
- **Vascularization.** Vascularization is assessed in the static state as well as dynamically after administration of a contrast agent. Apart from the quantitative aspect, the sonographer has to evaluate the blood flow qualitatively by looking at the flow direction, the type of vascularization (arterial, venous, shunting), and the timing of the circulation in the mass compared with the surrounding parenchyma. In the future, the interaction between contrast agent and tissue, and also between contrast agent and ultrasound beam (energy), will yield further criteria for assessing masses and parenchyma in the liver.
- **Extrahepatic factors.** Proper assessment of a mass has to include any changes in other organs (primary tumor? lymphadenopathy?) and clinical parameters (e.g., fever, night sweat).
- **Change in or activity of the mass.** In follow-up studies the sonographer can track any changes taking place spontaneously, under an antibiotic regimen, or with chemotherapy (**Figs. 2.43–2.45**).

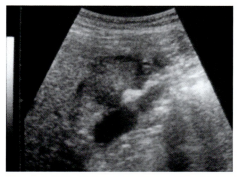

▲ **Fig. 2.42** Criterion: location of the mass/its relation to the surface; in this case a hypoechoic metastasis with central necrosis and breaking through the posterior surface of the right hepatic lobe at segment V (to the gallbladder fossa). Ancillary criterion: superficial lesion with the typical central depression.

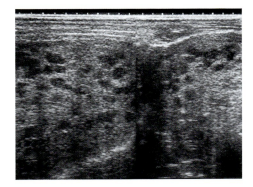

▲ **Fig. 2.43** Criterion: change/activity of a mass; in this case, a small cell lung cancer at the time of the original diagnosis—diffuse micronodular metastasis of the liver with demonstration of numerous hypoechoic, irregularly shaped masses.

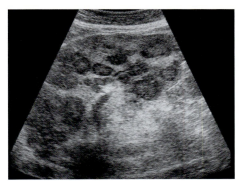

▲ **Fig. 2.44** Criterion: change/activity of a mass; in this case, the same small cell lung cancer after two cycles of chemotherapy with the ACO protocol; the metastases have grown in size and have a distinct halo (zone of active tumor growth) and echogenic material (necrosis) in the center. Note the increased echogenicity of the hepatic parenchyma resulting from the toxic steatosis induced by the chemotherapy.

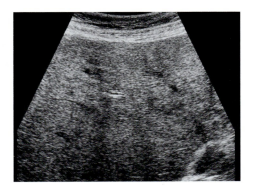

▲ **Fig. 2.45** Criterion: change/activity of a mass; in this case, the same small cell lung cancer after four cycles of chemotherapy with the ACO protocol; there is an inkling of diffuse infiltration although no definite focal metastatic transformation can be seen except in a few questionable places; complete remission clinically.

Anechoic Masses

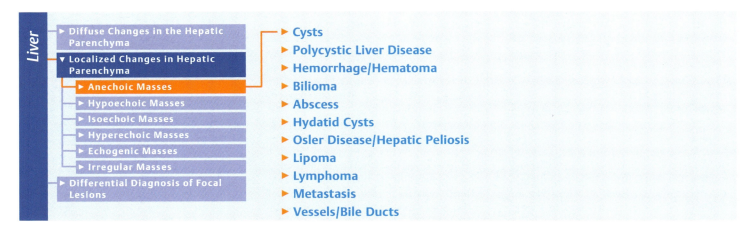

Anechoic masses in the liver are either pure fluid-filled cavities or masses with very few or weakly reflecting (hardly discernible) boundaries. The sonographer should always bear in mind the possibility of inadequate presettings of the equipment (insufficient gain)—one option would be comparison with the vascular lumen.

▶ Cysts

Intrahepatic cystic masses (**Figs. 2.46 and 2.47**, ▣ **2.8d**) may be unilocular or multiple, may vary in size (a few millimeters to > 10 cm), and may be found anywhere in the liver.

Unilocular cysts are round and smooth, and the lumen is absolutely without any echoes. Since the lumen of the cyst does not attenuate the ultrasound beam, unilocular cysts demonstrate posterior enhancement that is not always easy to detect in the near field, at large depths, and in very small masses. The walls of unilocular cysts do not exhibit any echotexture, and they may elevate a surface or protrude above it, but do not cross segmental boundaries. They are not vascularized and the adjacent parenchyma of the liver appears absolutely normal. In cases of multiple true cystic masses, the differential diagnosis of polycystic liver disease should not be overlooked.

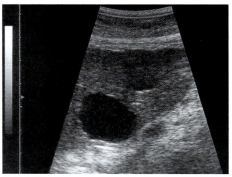

▲ **Fig. 2.46** Solitary cysts; here, there are two solitary cysts in the right hepatic lobe: one reaching the surface, anechoic, and with characteristic posterior enhancement; the other central within the parenchyma, significantly smaller, and hard to differentiate from the adjacent liver tissue, recognizable by its clearly delimited posterior wall.

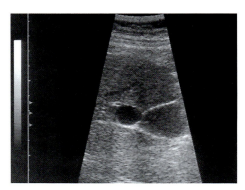

▲ **Fig. 2.47** Cysts and gallbladder. Compared with the gallbladder wall, the cystic masses in polycystic liver disease do not display any echotexture in the wall.

▶ Polycystic Liver Disease

This autosomal dominant disease may be limited just to the liver but can involve the kidneys and/or the pancreas as well. With age, the liver is permeated by an uncountable number of cystic masses in the liver (**Figs. 2.48–2.50**, ▣ **2.8e and g**). Initially, the cysts may be quite small but vary in size later. In the end, this leads to an enormous increase in the size of the organ (all the way into the small pelvis). The liver is firm, tightly elastic, and tender (capsular tension) and its surface is marred by a myriad protruding cysts. Regular segmental anatomy and the shape of the liver have disappeared altogether. The image is dominated by the cysts, and in the terminal stage of the disease hardly any parenchyma can be demonstrated. The gallbladder is differentiated (best after a meal) from the cysts by its triple-layered

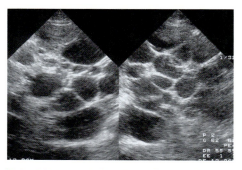

▲ **Fig. 2.48** Polycystic liver disease. The hepatic parenchyma is permeated by numerous cysts; typical "blooming" of the meager remaining parenchyma, caused by the diminished attenuation.

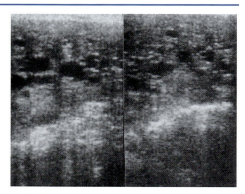

▲ **Fig. 2.49** Polycystic liver disease. The hepatic parenchyma is permeated by numerous very small cysts; these are recognizable not only by their better conduction but also by the marked boundaries of the cyst walls.

wall since, although the cysts are lined by a simple columnar epithelium, they do not exhibit any wall structures. Complications may arise from hemorrhage into or infection of the cysts; apart from the clinical sign of local tenderness it may alter/increase the echogenicity of the pathological cystic contents.

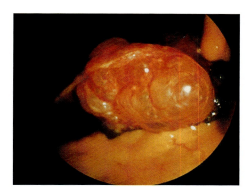

◄ *Fig. 2.50.* Polycystic liver disease. Finding during laparoscopy.

▶ Hemorrhage/Hematoma

Hemorrhage or localized hematoma (**Fig. 2.51, 2.8j–l**) may be due to local trauma, e.g., needle biopsy, stab wound, or rupture of healthy adjacent tissue, and is different from bleeding into an existing lesion (e.g., adenoma, metastasis, q.v.). Typically, a recent hematoma would be anechoic and exhibit a smooth boundary with the surrounding tissue; in cases of major parenchymal rupture, the shape could become irregular and even bizarre. Subcapsular hemorrhage may lift the capsule off the liver like a tent. The bleeding is characterized by a less than optimal posterior enhancement, and frequently the adjacent parenchyma displays a slight increase in echodensity due to compression artifacts. Older hemorrhages/hematomas lose their anechogenicity: the bleeding becomes organized, first with hypoechoic and later with hyperechoic intraluminal thrombi, which may appear in bizarre lumps and strands.

Hemorrhage/Hematoma

Hemorrhage. Bleeding in the liver may be due to inadvertent trauma, iatrogenic injury (needle biopsy, drainage), coagulation disorder, or it may complicate a preexisting mass (e.g., adenoma). The typical finding would be a hypoechoic to anechoic liquid mass; in rare cases (due to compression) it is homogeneously hyperechoic. The mass caused by a hemorrhage is sharply delimited and sometimes of irregular shape; the surrounding tissue is compressed (increased echogenicity), and quite often the patient is in pain (capsular tension).

Older hemorrhage. Apart from irregular liquid regions, these demonstrate inhomogeneous echogenic areas corresponding to clots, strands of fibrin, and different stages of organization in the hemorrhage. Subcapsular bleeding may come from ruptured parenchyma with irregular borders and end up as perforation and massive hemorrhage into the abdominal cavity (demonstration of free fluid in the abdominal cavity).

Capsule injuries. In ultrasonography, injuries solely to the capsule of the liver are detected as gaps in the hepatic contour; however, frequently this direct sign is impossible to demonstrate and the sonographer has to rely on the indirect sign of free fluid in the abdominal cavity increasing in volume during frequent follow-up scans.

▶ Bilioma

It is not possible to differentiate between acute bleeding and collections of bile that may also gather as a result of liver trauma and display the same sonographic characteristics (**Fig. 2.51, 2.8j**).

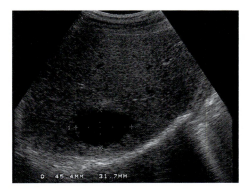

◄ *Fig. 2.51* Hemorrhage/hematoma/bilioma in the right hepatic lobe after unguided needle biopsy in chronic CMV hepatitis.

▶ Abscess

An abscess may present as anechoic mass with distinct posterior enhancement (**Fig. 2.52, 2.8g and i**).

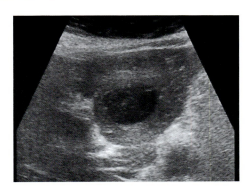

◄ *Fig. 2.52* Abscess. Not quite anechoic, slight posterior enhancement; the adjacent parenchyma appears coarse and hypoechoic.

2.8 Cysts

▶ Primary cysts/polycystic syndrome

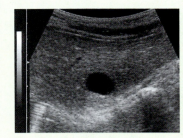

a Typical unilocular cyst with anechoic lumen, smooth margin without any structures: so-called posterior enhancement.

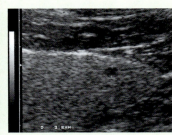

b Tiny unilocular cyst anteriorly in segment III of the left hepatic lobe; owing to its small size, definite assessment as cyst is not possible.

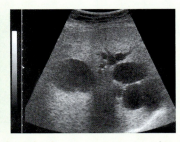

c Unilocular cysts may occur in multiples, or clusters, or are disseminated.

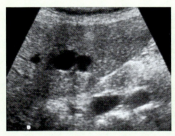

d Septated unilocular cyst in the left hepatic lobe.

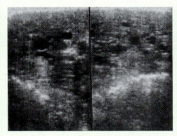

e and f Polycystic liver disease.
e Easy to diagnose owing to the number of cysts and the disturbed architecture of the organ.

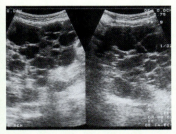

f Polycystic liver disease with medium-sized cysts.

▶ Secondary Cysts

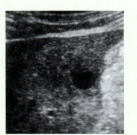

g–k Differential diagnosis of cystic mass.
g Small abscess in left hepatic lobe; hypoechoic reaction of the adjacent parenchyma.

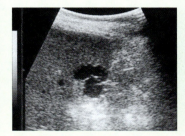

h Septated cyst, posterior cyst not quite anechoic—complication?

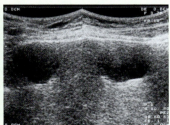

i Amebic liver abscess confirmed by fine-needle aspiration; note the unusual posterior enhancement.

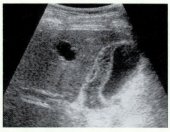

j Accumulation of fluid along the intrahepatic canal of the fresh knife wound (history): Hemorrhage? Bilioma? Involvement of the gallbladder wall.

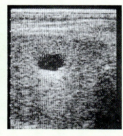

k Bleeding after unguided needle biopsy: hyperechogenicity of the adjacent parenchyma as a result of compression.

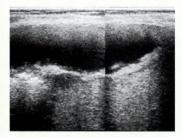

l Differential diagnosis of hypoechoic mass. Large subcapsular hematoma/hemorrhage in HELPP syndrome with the capsule "sort of torn off" the parenchyma.

2.8 Cysts

▶ Hydatid disease

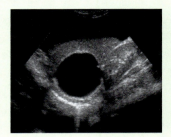 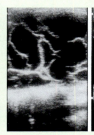 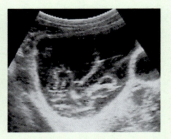

m–q **Hydatid cyst.**
m Cystic Echinococcosis Type I WHO

n Heavily encapsulated polycystic lesion with numerous septa and minor calcification, type IIB according to Koischwitz.

o Cystic Echinococcosis Type III WHO

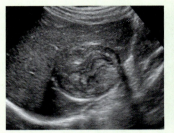 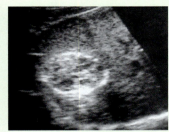

p Cystic Echinococcosis Type IV WHO

q Cystic Echinococcosis Type V WHO

▶ Osler disease; peliosis

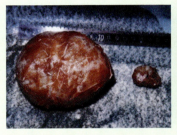 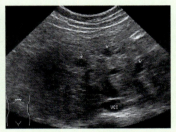

r Resection specimen of the two hydatid cysts.

s Peliosis hepatis. The features resemble a cystic liver (left), but the hepatic structure is irregular with patchy low echogenicity and multiple anechoic cystic masses up to 10 mm in size (arrows). Magnified view shows a relationship of the cysts to portal vessels. VCI = inferior vena cava.

▶ Hydatid Cysts

Hydatid cysts are parasitic cysts of *Echinococcus granulosus* and may be present in the liver as solitary or multiple cysts. Their typical appearance is that of cyst-within-cyst or as a conglomerate of cysts (**Fig. 2.53**, **2.8m–r**). The lumen of the hydatid cyst is anechoic, and a layered cyst wall, akin to a capsule, is a typical finding. Demonstration of marginal daughter cysts (cyst-within-cyst) and calcification in the wall is pathognomonic for hydatid disease. Because of the wall thickness, posterior enhancement is less marked or may even be absent, and calcifications result in posterior shadowing. The morphological classification of hydatid disease is summarized in **Table 2.11**.

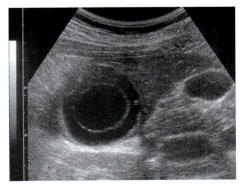 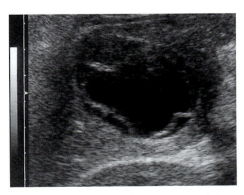

▲ **Fig. 2.53 a und b** Hydatid cyst.
a Typical cyst-within-cyst image in *Echinococcus granulosus* infection; located in segment VI of the right hepatic lobe; vital cyst, Koischwitz type IIA. Note the normal gallbladder.

▲ *b* Disintegrated cyst in *q* after two courses of albendazole.

Table 2.11 Morphological WHO classification of cystic echinococcosis (CE)[1,2]

Type	Characteristics
CE 1	unilocular anechoic
CE 2	multivesicular, multiseptated
CE 3	floating laminated membrane, daughter cysts, hyperechoic mass
CE 4	heterogeneous, degenerative content, hyper-/hypoechoic, or mixed structure
CE 5	arch-shaped image, cone-shaped shadow, calcified

Echinococcus Infection

This tapeworm infection may be due to *Echinococcus granulosus* resulting in cystic echinococcosis (Echinococcus Granulosus, parasitic in canines), also known as unilocular hydatid disease, or alveolar Echinoccocosis (*Echinococcus multilocularis*), (parasitic in foxes and small rodents) terminating in alveolar hydatid disease.

Ultrasonography of **cystic echinococcosis** demonstrates the characteristics of a complex cyst: thickened, sometimes layered cyst wall, akin to a capsule, with marginal daughter cysts (cyst-within-cyst) and calcification in the wall (pathognomonic). Because of the wall thickness, posterior enhancement is less pronounced or may even be absent, and in calcification there will be posterior shadowing. Old and no longer vital hydatid cysts may present with different degrees of lumen degradation, bizarre membrane formation, irregular hyperechoic compaction, and also central calcification, or they may exist just as calcified remnants.

In multilocular hydatid disease there is diffuse poorly delimited infiltration of the hepatic parenchyma with inhomogeneous coarse texture, whose more advanced stages involve the vessels and bile ducts, may demonstrate calcification, and can spread from the liver to destroy the diaphragm, lungs, hepatic portal, retroperitoneum, duodenum, and pancreas.

▶ Osler Disease/Hepatic Peliosis

Osler disease is also associated with the presence of arteriovenous malformations in the liver, which yield a corresponding Doppler signal. This finding is absent in peliosis, which is characterized by blood-filled lacunae separate from the portal circulation (**2.8**).

▶ Lipoma

Smooth margins and anechogenicity are not characteristic of lipomas, and posterior enhancement is not very marked. Most lipomas are found around the ligamentum teres.

▶ Lymphoma

Sometimes hepatic involvement in systemic lymphatic malignancy may result in anechoic masses in the liver. The intrahepatic masses accompanying lymphomas are frequently multiple, vary in size, and tend to be of irregular rather than round or oval shape (**Fig. 2.54**). One typical feature is the simultaneous presence of the various stages of lymphatic infiltration: apart from solitary anechoic masses (no or slight posterior enhancement), there are often irregular areas of varying size with hypoechoic infiltration of the parenchyma. In addition, extrahepatic criteria such as splenomegaly with infiltrative changes and lymphadenopathy may be seen.

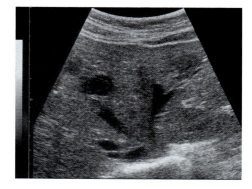

◀ *Fig. 2.54* Lymphoma of the liver. Non-Hodgkin lymphoma with multiple hypoechoic masses and one almost completely anechoic lesion.

Infiltrating Lymphoma

Involvement of the liver is seen in about 50% of lymphoma cases (Hodgkin disease and non-Hodgkin lymphoma). Particularly the more advanced stages will demonstrate hepatic involvement with circumscribed malignant lymphadenopathy. Diffuse, miliary, or periportal infiltration of the parenchyma is primarily found in early stages of the disease and usually escapes ultrasound detection. In diffuse nonspecific parenchymal changes, the presence of splenic pathology and lymphadenopathy may warrant the presumed diagnosis of diffuse infiltrative lymphoma of the liver. This suspicion must then be confirmed by needle biopsy.

▶ Metastases

Hypoechic/anechoic malignant lesions or deposits within the liver are highly suspicious for a tumor with a high degree of malignancy and a low degree of differentiation (see below) (**Fig. 2.55**). Diffuse metastasis of the small nodular type may present as numerous anechoic masses that differ from polycystic liver disease by their irregular shape and diffuse margin. There is no posterior enhancement.

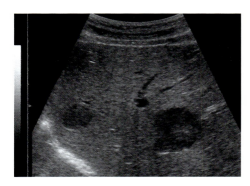

◀ **Fig. 2.55** In some cases the metastases of neuroendocrine tumors may present as almost anechoic lesions.

▶ Vessels/Bile Ducts

Any differential diagnosis of anechoic masses in the liver has to include the possibility of vessels or bile ducts being viewed in cross-section. In this case, the characteristic aspects are the tubular shape of the lesion when imaged in the second plane, and its course, which can be traced all the way back to the originating vessel/duct. In addition, vessels may be identified by duplex or color-flow duplex scanning. For reasons of clarity, these anechoic "masses" are listed here.

▶ **Bile ducts.** Bile ducts appearing as anechoic masses in the liver have to be pathologically enlarged/engorged (e.g., Caroli disease). These cases are characterized by their periportal location and identification of the so-called hepatic triad, i.e., delineation of a branch of each of the proper hepatic artery and the portal vein as well as the enlarged bile duct.

▶ **Portal vein branches.** Being part of the hepatic triad, the branches of the portal vein course through the periportal area as well. Venectasia, varicosities, and collaterals in case of portal hypertension will all be imaged as enlarged segments of the intrahepatic tree of the portal venous system.

▶ **Hepatic vein branches.** They are easily identified by their typical course terminating at their stellate junction with the vena cava. The sonographer should keep in mind the possible venectasia and anomalies of the Budd–Chiari syndrome.

▶ **Hepatic artery aneurysms, shunts, and vascular malformation.** These may be identified by color-flow duplex scanning.

Hypoechoic Masses

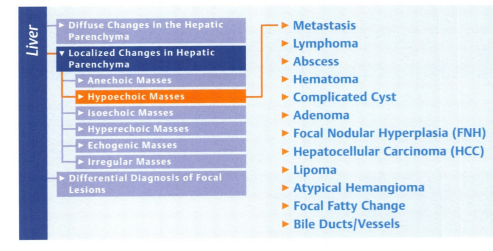

The typical lesions of liver pathology within the hepatic parenchyma are hypoechoic masses. However, the operator should always be aware of possible "technical glitches" (e.g., improper presettings with the gain too high), when noise will turn anechoic masses into echogenic lesions and thus result in misinterpretation.

▶ Metastasis

Numerous tumors will deposit hypoechoic metastatic masses in the liver (**Figs. 2.56–2.58**). These lesions may differ in size and distribution, but in most cases they are small and tend to have an irregular/diffuse margin. Although one cannot, in principle, deduce the type of tumor from the sonographic image alone, these hypoechoic metastatic deposits are quite frequent in undeveloped, undifferentiated, and actively growing malignancies. The finding of hypoechoic metastasis is rather common (but *not* pathognomonic) in breast cancer, in small cell lung cancer, and in endocrine tumors. Numerous tumors exhibit this hypoechogenicity when initially invading the liver with these small focal metastases. The growing size of the lesion will lead to complications of tumor growth, such as central necrosis, hematoma, etc., and eventually the original hypoechoic appearance will be found only along the active outer rim (so-called "halo sign"). Thus, in cases of rapid tumor growth quite often one will discover small hypoechoic masses next to large lesions with a halo.

Hepatic Metastases

Primary tumors. The incidence of hepatic metastasis of nonhepatic primaries is about 50 times higher than that of primary cancer of the liver; and in autopsies of patients who have succumbed to nonhepatic malignancies, these metastases are found in 36–40% of cases. The most common primaries are cancer of the lung, colon, stomach, breast, and pancreas as well as renal cell carcinoma, malignant melanoma, and neuroendocrine tumors of the gastrointestinal tract.

Metastatic spread. The tumors metastasize primarily via the venous system, most often taking the portal route with periportal deposits, and far less frequently via the arterial tree; spread via the lymphatics tends to be the exception. Decreased portal blood flow and the decrease in the number of lectin receptors, which are needed if the tumor cells are to bind to the hepatocytes, are common findings in chronic liver disease and have helped to explain, especially in cirrhosis of the liver, why metastases of nonhepatic primaries are a rather infrequent finding. Therefore, any mass detected in a cirrhotic liver has to raise a very high level of suspicion of hepatocellular carcinoma (HCC) or granulomatous regeneration.

Echogenicity. The echogenicity of hepatic metastases does not depend very much on the type of primary malignancy but rather on their activity and rate of growth: rapidly growing tumors and the metabolically active rims (halo) of metastases tend to present as hypoechoic images, while slowly growing tumors are inclined toward hyperechogenicity. While small hepatic lesions tend to be hypoechoic as well, their growth is accompanied by the sequelae of complications such as central necrosis, hematoma, liquefaction, calcification, etc.

Vascularization. In primary and secondary tumors of the liver, 90–95% of the blood supply arises from the hepatic artery. In color-flow Doppler scanning, metastases tend to be hypovascular (except for the neuroendocrine tumors), while contrast-enhanced imaging depicts a bizarre/chaotic irregular vascular bed. Although it is not possible yet to identify hepatic metastases on the basis of their vascular bed, this technique has improved the differentiation of benign lesions and malignant metastases of the liver. But contrast-enhanced imaging studies and special ultrasound techniques[4,5] have resulted in dramatically improved detection rates for solid focal liver lesions with an overall diagnostic accuracy from 49% to 88% and with a sensitivity for metastases from 60% to 88%.

Further diagnostic modalities. Suspicious lesions in the liver may be subjected to further diagnosis by specific indirect modalities such as CT, MRI, PET, scintigraphy, or angiography, while in the end metastases have to undergo aspiration cytology—but only if it results in clinical/therapeutic consequences.

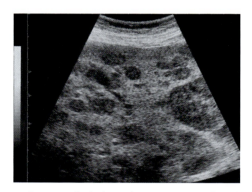

▲ *Fig. 2.56* Multiple hypoechoic metastases of small cell carcinoma of the lung.

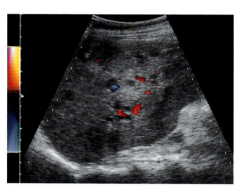

▲ *Fig. 2.57* Diffuse and fine nodular hypoechoic metastases of breast cancer in the liver.

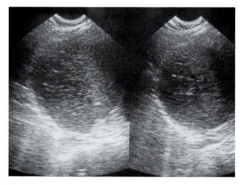

▲ *Fig. 2.58* Large solitary metastasis of squamous cell carcinoma of the esophagus.

▶ Lymphoma

Hepatic spread of a systemic lymphatic malignancy typically presents as hypoechoic lesions (**Fig. 2.59**). Quite often these are numerous, vary in size, and are neither spherical nor ovoid in shape but exhibit irregular margins. The difference in the degree of lymphatic infiltration is rather characteristic: apart from solitary, seemingly anechoic lesions (little or no posterior enhancement), there are often irregularly shaped areas, differing in size, of hypoechoic parenchymal infiltration. It is common in these cases to encounter extrahepatic involvement as well, such as splenomegaly with infiltrative changes and lymphadenopathy.

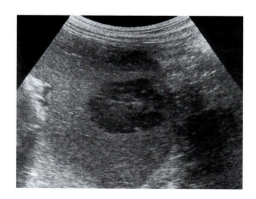

◀ *Fig. 2.59* Hypoechoic infiltration of a non-Hodgkin lymphoma.

▶ Abscess

Abscess-forming lesions (☐ **2.8g**) start as hypoechoic masses, usually with an ill-defined margin. They are located either within the parenchyma or in close proximity to bile ducts. The liver tissue surrounding an abscess is characterized by distinct hypervascularization. As the abscess increases in size this may produce a more hypoechoic, and even anechoic, liquid center, or there may be hyperechoic changes in the center because of necrosis and the formation of gas. Such an abscess will present with a wide, ill-defined hypoechoic halo.

> **Liver Abscess**
>
> **Location.** Usually, a liver abscess has a diffuse margin and is secondary to bacterial or parasitic infection, which may be unifocal or multifocal. If blood-borne, these abscesses may be found anywhere within the parenchyma; if arising from the biliary tree, they will form close to the bile ducts. If they are the sequelae of interventional procedures, they appear along the drainage or biopsy canal.
>
> **Appearance.** An acute inflammation may appear as hypoechoic edema surrounding the intraparenchymal abscess, accompanied by inflammatory hypervascularization, while the abscess itself will present as a completely avascular lesion. No matter what the clinical symptoms (fever, septicemia, disseminated intravascular coagulation [DIC], etc.), acute pyogenic abscesses under close follow-up demonstrate a change in shape and increase in size and possibly number, and exhibit definite coarse intrinsic echoes. Gas formation may herald complications.

▶ Hematoma

Hemorrhage/hematoma is usually characterized by anechogenicity, but as time goes by and the blood coagulates/becomes organized the image becomes less and less anechoic; quite often compression will produce a hyperechoic halo.

▶ Complicated Cyst

Cysts may be complicated by hemorrhage or infection, or they may be scanned in an oblique plane resulting in a hypoechoic rather than anechoic image; in these cases ultrasound morphology would suggest hemorrhage/hematoma or an abscess, and not a cyst (**Fig. 2.60**).

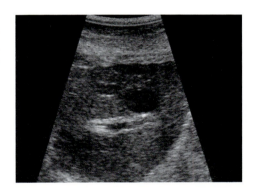

◂ **Fig. 2.60** Cyst. Obliquely imaged and complicated cysts may yield the image of a hypoechoic rather than an anechoic cyst.

▶ Adenoma

Adenomas of the liver are uncommon lesions and they usually exhibit the same texture as the regular parenchyma, but slightly less echogenicity (**Fig. 2.61**).

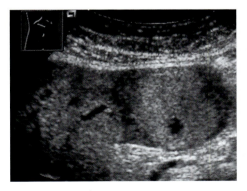

▴ **Fig. 2.61** Liver adenoma.
a Isoechoic tumor with focal anechoic necrosis/hemorrhage.

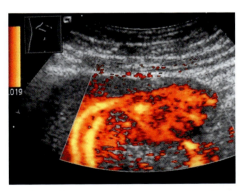

▴ *b* Power Doppler: distinctive vascularization with arterial supply. Histology: hepatocellular adenoma.

Liver Adenoma

Pathophysiology. Adenomas of the liver are uncommon tumors; since they may be hormone induced, young women are most at risk. In most instances the lesions will be solitary, with a diameter between 2 and 30 cm or more. Histologically, these are hepatocytes arranged in orderly fashion but lacking any sign of portal areas. The typical complications arising from these adenomas stem from the increased internal pressure, which eventually will lead to pain, central necrosis/hemorrhage (peliosis hepatis), and rupture. Apart from these common complications, there is firm evidence of the adenoma → malignancy sequence.

Ultrasound. Liver adenomas do not exhibit a specific sonographic appearance. Smaller lesions tend to have a somewhat hypoechoic texture, while larger tumors display a coarser echotexture, probably due to the degenerative changes in the tissue, and possibly a hypoechoic rim (target lesion). Complications (central liquefaction/calcification) may also be present. Color-flow Doppler imaging demonstrates the distinct venous vascularization at the margin.

▶ Focal Nodular Hyperplasia (FNH)

Focal nodular hyperplasia may exhibit all the characteristics of a hypoechoic mass, especially in a hyperechoic fatty liver. However, hypoechogenicity of the lesion is not the most important criterion but rather the textural characteristics of the parenchyma (inhomogeneous, coarse), the architecture of the mass (central stellate scar radiating fibrous septa, characteristic vascular tree), and the blood supply (hypervascularization) (◾ 2.9).

FNH Gross Anatomy and Microanatomy

Focal nodular hyperplasia is the second most common benign tumor of the liver, with a diameter mainly about 5 cm (1–15 cm). The lesion is characterized by a distinct vascular pedicle and hypervascularization. Histologically, it resembles liver parenchyma with circumscribed cirrhotic transformation. The architecture demonstrates the typical stellate scar tissue with a vessel at its center radiating arteries in the fibrous septa that course toward the periphery of the lesion, while being accompanied by lymphocytic infiltration and proliferating bile ducts. The hepatocytes between the fibrous septa form sinusoids with Kupffer cells and make up the bulk of the lesion. The mass is not encapsulated but is delineated by compressed hepatic parenchyma, where distinct hypervascularization may be found. Significant growth under estrogen replacement therapy has been reported in the literature; malignant transformation remains a controversial issue but this risk appears to be negligible.

Detection of FNH by the various imaging modalities rests on its structural characteristics (vascular pedicle, stellate scar tissue), its typical mulberry-like hypervascularization with a pedicle, central artery radiating centrifugal blood flow, as well as the cellular differentiation of the tumor with the presence of Kupffer cells and proliferating bile ducts.

▶ Hepatocellular Carcinoma (HCC)

One third of all hepatocellular carcinomas will exhibit hypoechogenicity. They have ill-defined margins and typically are found in a cirrhotic liver (**Fig. 2.62**, ◾ 2.10). On color-flow duplex imaging they demonstrate a distinctly hypervascularized blood supply of bizarre irregular outline.

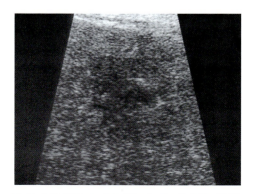

▲ **Fig. 2.62** HCC growing diffusely. The ill-defined infiltration raises the suspicion of HCC and would call for ultrasound-guided biopsy.

Hepatic Carcinomas

Cause. HCC is the most common hepatic malignancy. Although HCC may be found in healthy livers as well, the most prevalent risk for the development of HCC is cirrhosis of the liver due to chronic alcoholism, viral infection (hepatitis B and C), storage diseases such as hemochromatosis or α_1-antitrypsin deficiency, and exposure to aflatoxins.

Histology. The tumor may grow as solitary focal mass, but in 18–38% of cases it will appear as a multifocal malignancy. The grading includes highly differentiated (fibrolamellar), moderately differentiated, and anaplastic HCC. The differential diagnosis must include cholangiocellular carcinoma as well.

Sonographic image. The differences in the histological findings also help to explain the varied sonographic appearance, with hyperechoic, hypoechoic, and isoechoic (compared with the surrounding hepatic parenchyma) masses. In an otherwise healthy liver it is impossible to differentiate between solitary HCC and other tumors; however, one characteristic of HCC is its tendency to invade the vascular system, which may be demonstrated quite well by ultrasound imaging. The observation that malignant metastases are infrequent findings in a cirrhotic or diseased liver also serves to reaffirm the suspicion that any mass detected in a cirrhotic liver has to be regarded as HCC, unless proven otherwise. In color-flow Doppler scans, HCC quite often exhibits irregular hypervascularization.

2.9 Focal Nodular Hyperplasia (FNH)

▶ FNH is a benign hepatic lesion, its histology corresponding to circumscribed cirrhotic transformation: there is a central vessel where the radial strands of scar tissue terminate; at the rim, increased circular vascularization can be demonstrated.

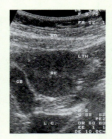

a FNH (RF) in segment IV of the left hepatic lobe. BD = abdominal wall; LTH = round ligament of liver; GB = gallbladder; L.C. = caudate lobe.

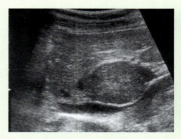

b Spokelike appearance of a hydatid cyst.

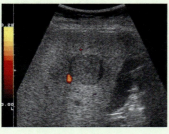

c Isoechoic mass in a fatty liver. Even color-flow Doppler imaging was unable to ascertain its character.

▶ B-mode: stellate scar

▶ Color duplex: peripheral vascularity, central vessel, spoked-wheel pattern

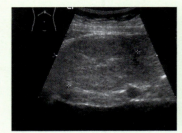

d Isoechoic mass in segment IV a (cursors; echogenic stellate scar, suggestive of FNH).

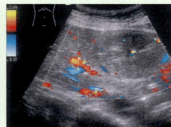

e The same mass as in *d*, demonstrating a central vessel and subtle peripheral vascularity.

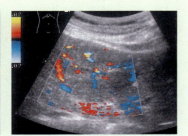

f Additional presence of a typical circular, spoked-wheel vascular pattern confirms FNH.

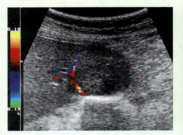

g Distinctive afferent vascular pedicle and circular vascularization at the rim.

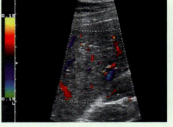

h Increased vascularization at the margin and barely visible vascular star radiating vessels; as a snapshot for documentation purposes it is possible proof, but during real-time imaging this type of vascularization is definite proof.

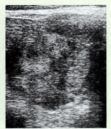

i With this B-mode image alone differential diagnosis is difficult. Spokelike metastasis of cancer of the colon.

▶ Differential diagnosis: metastasis, hydatid disease

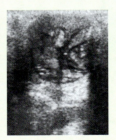

j Spokelike representation of a hydatid cyst.

▶ ## Lipoma

Lipomas are rare. They are encapsulated, smooth, almost anechoic masses with only faint posterior enhancement and are frequently found close to the ligamentum teres.

2.10 Hepatocellular Carcinoma (HCC)

▶ **a–c Hypoechoic HCC.** One-third of all HCC present as hypoechoic lesions, and they may infiltrate the parenchyma diffusely (quite often in previously existing cirrhosis) or appear as circumscribed masses.

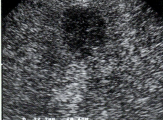 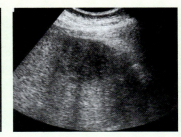 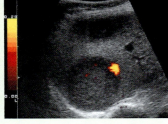

a Ill-defined infiltration.   *b* Ill-defined infiltration.   *c* Circumscribed mass.

▶ **d–f Isoechoic HCC.** About one-third of all HCC are isoechoic to the surrounding liver tissue and may only be detected by their complications or circumscribed irregularities in the texture

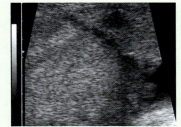 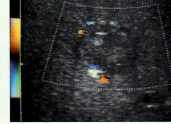

d Ill-defined invasion of a hepatic vein by HCC.   *e* Ill-defined invasion of a portal vein by HCC.   *f* Isoechoic HCC with halo sign and bizarre irregular hypervascularization.

▶ **g–i Hyperechoic HCC.** About one-third of all HCC are hyperechoic to the surrounding liver tissue and may easily be mistaken for hemangiomas, although HCC is characterized by a more pronounced attenuation of the signal.

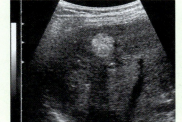 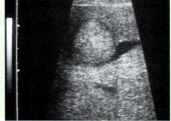 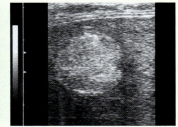

g Hyperechoic HCC.   *h* HCC invading a vessel.   *i* Hyperechoic HCC with signal attenuation.

▶ **Vascular complications in HCC**

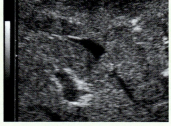 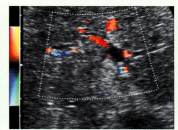 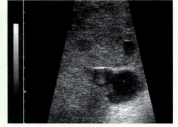

j HCC invading a hepatic vein.   *k* HCC invading a portal vein   *l* HCC invading a hepatic vein and the vena cava.

▶ ## *Atypical Hemangioma*

Approximately 5% of all hemangiomas do not exhibit the characteristic hyperechoic parenchyma but are less echogenic than the adjacent hepatic tissue (**Fig. 2.63**). This may be due to increased echogenicity of the parenchyma in the vicinity of the mass, e.g., as part of fatty changes; in rare cases, one is dealing with rather hypoechoic hemangiomas of slightly inhomogeneous texture and frequently ill-defined margins.

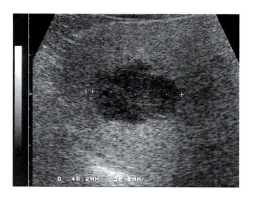

◀ **Fig. 2.63** Atypical hemangioma in the right hepatic lobe.

▶ Focal Fatty Change

If a hypoechoic lesion is due to focal fatty change, it will typically be found at certain locations: at the inferior aspect of segment IV, near the bifurcation of the portal vein; in the fossa of the gallbladder; and around the hepatic veins (**Figs. 2.64 and 2.65**). Characteristic features are the frequently maplike appearance of the mass, the fact that it respects segmental interfaces and surfaces, the lack of tissue reaction at the margin, and the undisturbed course of the blood vessels.

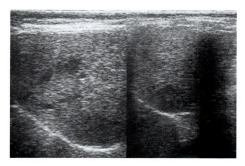

▲ *Fig. 2.64* Focal fatty change.

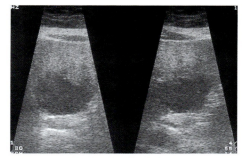

▲ *Fig. 2.65* Differential diagnosis in focal fatty change: metastasis, in this case cancer of the colon.

▶ Bile Ducts/Vessels

Bile ducts may be dilated and contain hypoechoic sediment or tumor tissue. The portal and hepatic veins may also be clogged by this hypoechoic thrombotic material (**Fig. 2.66**). Imaging in the orthogonal plane will confirm the lesion to be a pathological vessel.

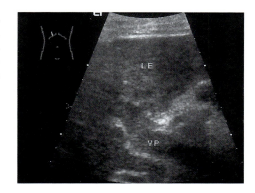

◄ *Fig. 2.66* Portal vein thrombosis in HCC. VP = portal vein; LE = liver.

Isoechoic Masses

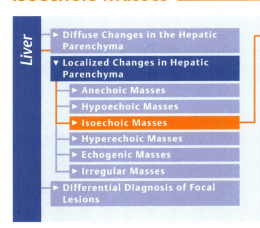

Detection of isoechoic masses in the liver is rather difficult and hinges on the slight differences in texture. The most important diagnostic signs are surface and contour changes at the segmental and vascular interfaces.

▶ Focal Nodular Hyperplasia (FNH)

In terms of histopathology, FNH is defined as circumscribed cirrhosis of the liver. Thus, there are FNH variants that hardly differ from the surrounding hepatic parenchyma and may only be detected because of the circumscribed inhomogeneity of their texture (▣ **2.9a**) and their vascular characteristics (if visible at all): in the latter cases, color-flow Doppler scanning will unmask these lesions.

▶ Adenoma

Sometimes it is almost impossible to distinguish between normal parenchyma and adenoma of the liver.

▶ Hepatocellular Carcinoma (HCC)

One-third of all HCC are isoechoic and may be difficult to detect, particularly when superimposed upon underlying cirrhotic liver disease; this corresponds to the diffuse infiltrative type of hepatocellular carcinoma. In these cases, extra care should be given to the typical changes induced by the tumor invading vessels. In isoechoic HCC, color-flow Doppler scanning will yield bizarre irregular hypervascularization (**Figs. 2.67, 2.62,** ▣ **2.10d–f and 2.10j–l**).

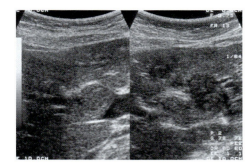

◀ **Fig. 2.67** HCC invading a portal vein in cirrhosis of the liver.

▶ Metastasis

Small hepatic metastases in particular may escape detection because of their possible Isoechogenicity. However, when scrutinized more closely their parenchymal texture is somewhat coarser and more echogenic. It is vital to check for any changes in contour at the surfaces and vascular interfaces. Isoechoic metastases are quite typical in diffuse metastasis of gastric and pancreatic cancer (**Fig. 2.68**), and after successful chemotherapy as remnants of previously confirmed metastases (**Fig. 2.45**).

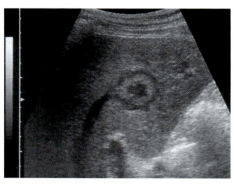 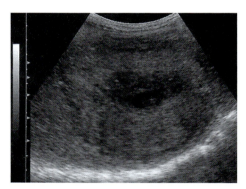

▲ **Fig. 2.68 a** Isoechoic metastasis of pancreatic cancer; the lesion is identified by its vascular invasion, halo sign, and the central necrosis.

▲ **b** Large isoechoic metastasis of cancer of the colon; note the central liquefaction and the delicate hypoechoic halo with its irregular margin.

▶ Atypical Hemangioma

Detection and differentiation of hemangiomas depends not only on the texture and echogenicity of the surrounding parenchyma but also on the direction and angle of insonation. This explains why hemangiomas can be detected quite easily at one time but may remain undetected during follow-up studies, and in the more echogenic fatty liver hemangiomas may be masked altogether (**Figs. 2.69 and 2.70**).

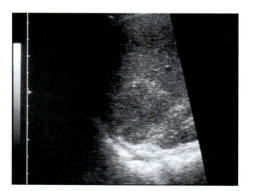 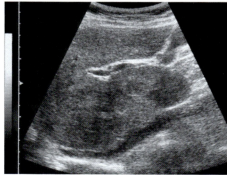

▲ **Fig. 2.69** Atypical hemangioma. Isoechoic mass in the right hepatic lobe, subphrenic segment, with marginal echo enhancement.

▲ **Fig. 2.70** Giant hemangiomas. They can be demonstrated in all of segments IV and I as isoechoic masses.

▶ Hematoma

Organized hemorrhage and hematoma may appear as isoechoic lesions.

▶ "Hepatized" Gallbladder

Viscous bile, rich in cholesterol, within the lumen of the gallbladder may mimic the texture of parenchymal tissue. The typical location and recognition of the gallbladder wall as a continuous margin will prevent the sonographer from misinterpreting this mass as an accessory lobe; this presumed hepatic parenchyma also lacks any kind of vascularization (**see Fig. 3.36 b, p. 122**).

▶ Bile Ducts/Vessels

Sediments within dilated bile ducts, thrombosis of branches or the trunk of the portal vein, as well as branches of the portal vein invaded by tumor may appear isoechoic to the surrounding parenchyma of the liver.

Hyperechoic Masses

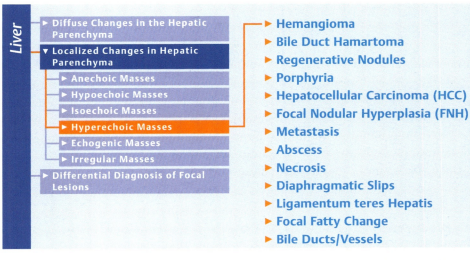

Hyperechoic liver masses are the typical target structures when diagnosing parenchymal liver pathology. Differential diagnosis is based on essential criteria such as echotexture, delineation, the always present through-transmission of a hyperechoic mass, the interaction of the lesion with vessels and the surface, and the reaction of the surrounding parenchyma.

▶ Hemangioma

The typical hemangioma is a hyperechoic mass with a diameter of 10–30 mm, a smooth clearly-defined margin, and good transmission; it appears as a solitary lesion or comes in multiples, and will always be found next to a vessel. Although the round margin may displace vessels, and give the surface a nodular appearance, hemangiomas respect adjacent structures. An afferent vessel can often be identified. Large hemangiomas display an increasingly inhomogeneous echotexture with a nodular hypoechoic center. Palpation with the bare fingertips and the effects of transmitted pulsation will evidence their soft nature. In CT imaging the slow blood flow in hemangioma results in the so-called filling-in phenomenon, and this helps to explain why most of these hypervascular tumors cannot be detected by color-flow Doppler imaging (2.11 and 2.12).

Liver Hemangioma

Pathology and histology. Hemangioma is the most frequently encountered benign liver tumor, occurring in 0.4–7.3% of autopsies. Most often they are solitary (90%), are between 1 and 3 cm in diameter, while 7% are classified as giant hemangioma (> 4–5 cm). They consist of interconnected cavernous vascular spaces, whose walls are lined with a fibrous matrix and delicate epithelium, the spaces being filled with blood and clots. Hemangiomas are soft, compressible tumors that may grow in size by enlargement of their spaces. Such enlargement has been reported for estrogen replacement therapy and pregnancy. Degenerative changes will result in fibrosis of the connective-tissue septa and calcification.

Ultrasound. The typical (95%) sonographic image of a hemangioma is a hyperechoic mass measuring 10–30 mm in diameter, with a smooth, clearly-defined margin and good through-transmission. The fact that the echogenicity may vary, depending on the plane of scanning, is another typical characteristic. Hemangiomas always arise in the vicinity of a vessel, which their bulge may displace. In many cases an afferent vessel can be demonstrated. In CT imaging the slow blood flow in the hemangioma results in the so-called filling-in phenomenon, and this helps to explain the paradox that usually color-flow Doppler scanning will not detect these hypervascular tumors. Contrast enhanced sonographic studies are required to demonstrate the filling-in effect and to better characterize the lesion by taking advantage of stimulated acoustic emission (SAE).

Atypical variants. Atypical hemangiomas (about 5%) exhibit an inhomogeneous echotexture in many cases, while others demonstrate hyperechoic textural changes and ultrasound signal attenuation due to increased fibrosis and calcification.

2.11 Hemangiomas

▶ Sharply circumscribed hyperechoic mass

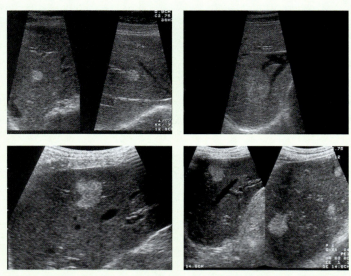

a–d Typical hemangiomas: hyperechoic, smooth contour and clearly-defined, good through transmission, frequently in contact with vessels.

▶ Color duplex findings

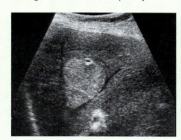 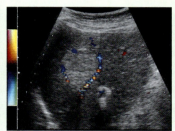 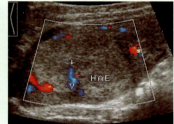

e–g Demonstration of the vascular pedicle; curved displacement but no further interference with the other vessels.

f Color-flow Doppler scanning cannot identify the blood-filled cisterns because the flow is too slow.

g Intratumoral vessel (V, arrow). HAE = hemangioma

▶ Atypical hemangiomas

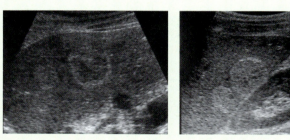

h and i The same hemangiomas displaying varying degrees of echogenicity depending on the time as well as plane of scanning.

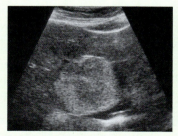 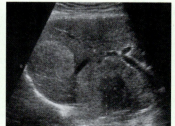 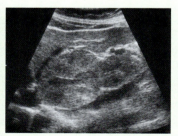

j–l Giant hemangiomas. Their characteristics resemble those of the smaller variant: hyperechoic, smooth contour and clearly-defined, good through transmission; the small hypoechoic centers and nodules within are quite typical. Frequently, these hemangiomas will break the surface of the liver, and their soft texture can be demonstrated on palpation or compression.

2.12 Atypical hemangiomas and differential diagnosis

▶ **Atypical hemangiomas**

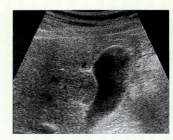 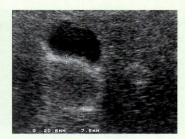

a* and *b Atypical isoechoic hemangioma in segment V of the right hepatic lobe in the gallbladder fossa. In ***b*** there is another small hemangioma.

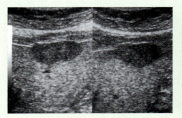 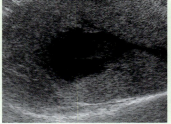 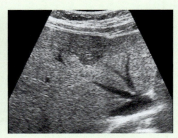

c–e Atypical hypoechoic hemangiomas. In ***c*** note the unusual buckling of the liver surface.

▶ **Differential diagnosis: angiosarcoma, cholangiofibroma, porphyria, gastrointestinal metastases**

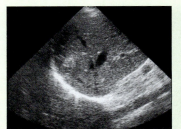 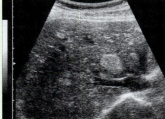 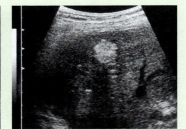

f–i Differential diagnosis of hemangiomas.
f Metastasis of myosarcoma.

g Hemangioma adjacent to multiple small cholangiofibromas.

h HCC; note the distinctive signal attenuation of the lesion.

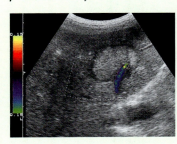

i Metastasis of esophageal cancer.

▶ Bile Duct Hamartomas

Bile duct hamartomas (so-called Meyenburg complexes) appear as very small hyperechoic nodules, diffusely and unevenly distributed in the parenchyma, usually <5 mm in diameter (**Fig. 2.71**). (The echogenic masses in porphyria are similar; see below.)

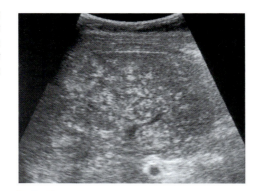

▲ *Fig. 2.71 a* Bile duct hamartomatosis.

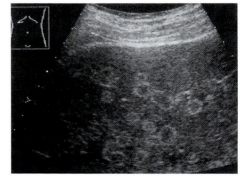

▲ *b* Differential diagnosis of hepatic hemangioma. Multiple round "masses" with hypoechoic centers, initially misinterpreted as multiple hemangiomas: chronic hepatic porphyria. Color duplex image shows vessels passing freely through the lesions (which resolved completely in six years!).

▶ Porphyria

In hepatic porphyria, hyperechoic lesions may be seen in an otherwise normal parenchyma. These pseudo tumors are characterized by the fact that they do not induce changes in the texture of the tissue or the course of vessels, contours, segmental interfaces, and surfaces (**Fig. 2.71b**).

▶ Regenerative Nodules

In cirrhotic or inflammatory parenchyma, there may be nodular zones that could be either slightly hyperechoic, isoechoic, or even hypoechoic to the surrounding tissue. They should be kept in mind as a rare, but significant, differential diagnosis when considering hyperechoic masses (**Fig. 2.72**).

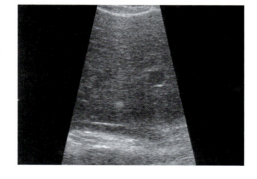

◀ *Fig. 2.72* Regenerative nodule.

▶ Hepatocellular Carcinoma (HCC)

Any hyperechoic mass in a cirrhotic liver must be suspected of HCC, since about 1/3 of all HCC will present as such a hyperechoic lesion (◨ **2.10g**). Frequently these lesions attenuate the through-transmission and exhibit posterior shadowing. Color-flow Doppler imaging shows these masses to have a significant hypervascularization. Contrast-enhanced imaging results in an improved detection of HCC from 52 to 67%.

▶ Focal Nodular Hyperplasia (FNH)

Although focal nodular hyperplasia may be more echogenic than the surrounding parenchyma, the most important criteria are structural changes, such as the spokelike architecture with its central vessel, and its vascularization (enhanced marginal vascularization, radial centrifugal flow, central vessel, vascular pedicle of the mass).

▶ Metastasis

Hyperechoic metastatic masses in the liver vary in size and may occur in any segment; they are characterized by the changes in texture and contour of the normal parenchyma. If the metastatic mass presents as a hyperechoic lesion, the tumor activity in the lesion may be regarded as low (**Fig. 2.73**); only a hypoechoic rim indicates the zone of active growth.

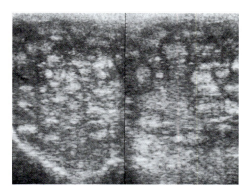

◀ **Fig. 2.73** Colon cancer metastases, note the "moth-eaten" appearance.

▶ Abscess

The hyperechoic image of an abscess is due to the textural transformation and organization. Usually, this type of abscess is found as a solitary mass and lacks the typical concomitant clinical symptoms (**Fig. 2.74**).

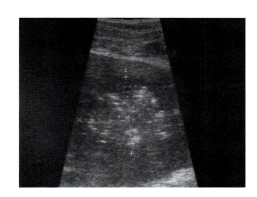

◀ **Fig. 2.74** Abscess.

▶ Necrosis

Tumor- or inflammation-induced necrosis may yield a coarsely inhomogeneous and hyperechoic mass. The increased echogenicity may also be due to local compression. Apart from this hyperechoic necrosis, additional complications can induce liquid areas that in turn may be due to sequestered bile, hemorrhage, or liquefaction of necrotic material.

▶ Diaphragmatic Slips

Diaphragmatic incisures at the dome of the liver may present as hyperechoic curved or triangular lesions. They will always demonstrate a connection with the diaphragm and may be more or less pronounced, depending on the respiratory motion.

▶ Ligamentum teres Hepatis

In cross-sectional views of the upper quadrants, usually the teres ligament will appear as a more or less hyperechoic lesion (**2.12h and i**). The decisive aspect for differentiating this spherical hyperechoic lesion from a true mass is scanning in the sagittal plane, and its characteristic location between segments II and III on the left and segment IV on the right.

Anatomy of the Ligamentum teres Hepatis

The ligamentum teres hepatis is a fibrous septum separating the double segments II/III medially on the left from the double segments IVa/IVb laterally on the right, thus splitting the liver into the anatomical left and right lobes. The obliterated umbilical vein ascends in this fibrous cord from the umbilicus to end in the left branch of the portal vein. In portal hypertension, varicose collaterals are opened up along the obliterated umbilical vein (which may become patent again), shunting blood from the portal venous system of the liver to the convoluted cutaneous varicosities around the umbilicus (caput medusae) (see also Cruveilhier–Baumgarten syndrome, **1.8i**).

▶ Focal Fatty Change

Increased fatty infiltration in individual segments or certain areas of the liver parenchyma may mimic an echogenic mass. The lack of texture-induced changes in the surface, the preservation of segmental interfaces, and course of vessels usually points the way toward diagnosing this parenchymatous lesion as focal fatty change.

▶ Bile Ducts/Vessels

Dilated bile ducts may be filled with sediment, sludge, or viscous bile (**Fig. 2.75**). Past thrombosis of the portal vein may appear as mass of moderate echogenicity.

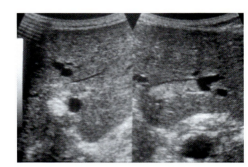

◀ **Fig. 2.75** Sediments in the bile duct.

Echodense Masses

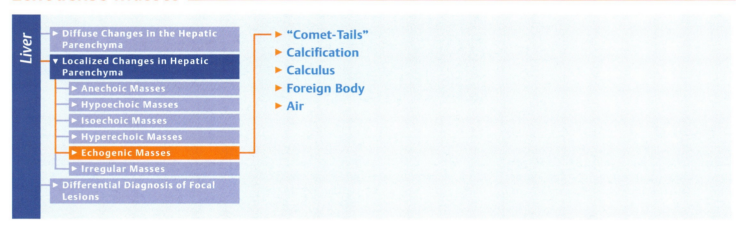

The echogenic appearance of a mass in the liver is due to changes that result in total reflection of the signal, complete absorption of the ultrasound energy, and in consequence posterior shadowing. Since in many cases the texture of the mass itself cannot be evaluated, any further differentiation has to rely on the type of shadowing encountered.

▶ "Comet-Tails"

Very small but powerful reflectors produce impressive comet-tail–like artifacts. The most frequent location of the reflectors is periportal, but they may also be found within the parenchyma. By themselves, the reflectors are hard to detect and differentiate, but their comet-tails, which sparkle in real-time studies, make them hard to miss (**Figs. 2.76 and 2.77**). These impressive comet-tail–like artifacts are the sequelae of changes induced by inflammation of the liver or bile ducts.

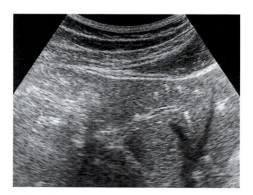

▲ **Fig. 2.76** So-called "comet-tails." Coarse reflectors within the hepatic parenchyma, characterized by their strong intrinsic echo and the posterior reverberation artifacts.

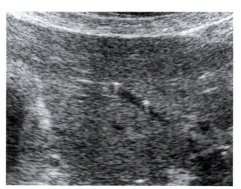

▲ **Fig. 2.77** "Comet-tails." Coarse perivenous reflectors; note the characteristic posterior reverberation artifacts.

▶ Calcification

Calcifications present as echogenic masses that, depending on their size, will always lead to posterior shadowing. They may be found in the parenchyma, around the portal veins, and even within hepatic masses. The calcifications in hydatid cysts, hepatocellular carcinoma, and metastases (**Figs. 2.78 and 2.79**) are such typical examples. Differential diagnosis of echodense periportal masses has to include the possibility of calculi in the intrahepatic bile ducts as well as phleboliths in branches of the portal vein.

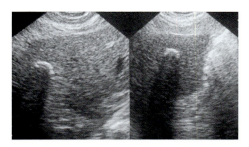

▲ **Fig. 2.78** Calcification in an old *Echinococcus* infection.

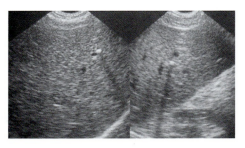

▲ **Fig. 2.79** Small periportal calcification.

▶ Calculus

Gallstones in the intrahepatic bile ducts are a characteristic finding in Caroli disease (**Fig. 2.80**). They may obstruct the duct completely and thus mimic an intrahepatic echodense mass. Frequently, these changes are limited to individual segments of the liver, in which case these echodense masses are grouped like beads on a string. To confirm the suspected diagnosis, the sonographer has to pin-point a fluid-filled/congested bile duct.

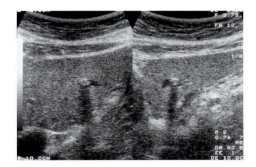

◀ **Fig. 2.80** Calculus within a bile duct.

▶ Foreign Body

Iatrogenic foreign bodies in the liver (drains, stents, clips) are detected as echodense hepatic masses of varying shape with relative ease because of their typical texture and the patient's history (**Figs. 2.81–2.83**). Metallic splinters and projectiles will also be imaged as echodense masses with posterior shadowing. Depending on the time since they penetrated the liver, they may be surrounded by hypoechoic liquid lesions (hemorrhage, biliary leak) or hyperechoic repair areas with organization/granulation and the formation of scar/fibrous tissue.

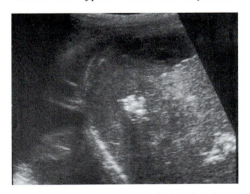

▲ **Fig. 2.81** Foreign body—here the basket of an abscess drain.

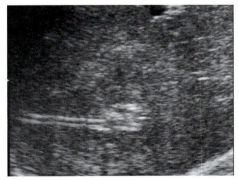

▲ **Fig. 2.82** Foreign body—here abscess drain with basket.

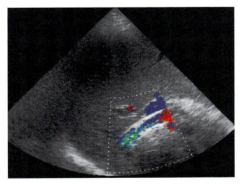

▲ **Fig. 2.83** Foreign body—transjugular intrahepatic portosystemic shunt (TIPS).

▶ Air

Gas will produce hyperechoic reflections, and sometimes even brilliant sparkles. There is an eminent difference between the sonographic appearance of small individual gas bubbles and large areas containing gas. The latter result in the characteristic total reflection and posterior shadowing with its ill-defined margin, while small individual gas bubbles will not generate posterior shadowing. The acoustic stimulation triggers natural oscillation, which in turn produces an ill-defined posterior tail, a hum, and may therefore be identified by real-time scanning. Gas pockets can be found in bile ducts and portal vein branches or they may be part of complications within a hepatic mass (tumor, metastasis, abscess) (◻ 2.13).

2.13 Intrahepatic Accumulation of Gas

▶ **Pneumobilia**

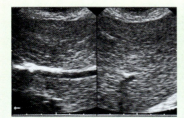

a Pneumobilia: periportal echoes.

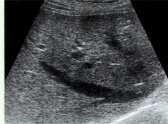

b Periportal echoes in discrete pneumobilia after Whipple procedure; no comet-tails.

▶ **Gas formation**

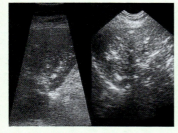

c Portovenous gas embolism. *Left:* Early stage with initial gas deposits in the parenchyma. *Right:* Late stage with advanced confluent accumulation of gas in the parenchyma.

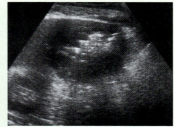

d Abscess with central necrosis and gas formation.

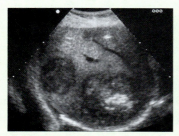

e Necrosis, after percutaneous ethanol injection, with gas formation in HCC.

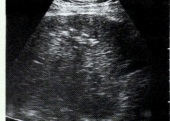

f Necrosis with gas formation in HCC, after transarterial chemoembolization.

Intrahepatic Accumulation of Gas

Any accumulation of gas detected in the liver has to be regarded as a serious complication unless it is due to iatrogenic intervention.

Mass. Gas accumulated in a mass points to an infection with gas-forming bacteria, usually Gram-negative pathogens; another alternative would be necrosis with or without complications.

Diffuse. Diffusely distributed gas in the hepatic parenchyma is found in portovenous gas embolism, initially as coarse periportal echoes (■ 2.13c). Real-time ultrasound scanning can demonstrate gas bubbles being swept into the liver via the portal vein. If the barrier between the intestinal lumen and the mesenteric vascular system is impaired due to necrotic inflammation or ulcers, or because of endoscopic/radiological procedures, the result may be this potentially life-threatening pathological finding.

Aerobilia. In the case of portovenous gas embolism, the detection of immobile sessile echoes in the hepatic parenchyma and the hepatopetal flow of gas bubbles within the portal vein rules out the differential diagnosis of pneumobilia (■ **2.13a and b**). In the latter case, the air in the bile ducts will shift, and when the patient is repositioned the gas will accumulate at the highest point; the acoustic energy may induce reverberation in the gas, making it "hum".

Irregular Masses

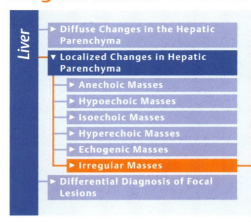

The texture of the hepatic parenchyma can be inferred from the size, density, brilliance, and distribution/pattern of the individual echoes. Textural irregularities result from changes in one or more of the characteristics of the individual echo. If hepatic lesions are distributed more or less evenly and affect the entire organ, they may be very hard to detect as circumscribed lesions or at all. The following entities are characterized by precisely such textural changes.

▶ Hepatocellular Carcinoma (HCC)

Diffuse HCC cannot be differentiated from the coarse echotexture of cirrhosis. Tell-tale signs of malignancy are typical complications of HCC, such as invasion of the vascular system, and the diffuse irregular hypervascularization that may be demonstrated on color-flow Doppler imaging (**Fig. 2.84** and ▣ **2.10f, k,** and **l**).

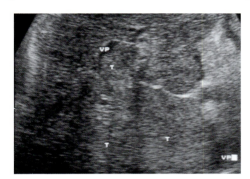

◀ **Fig. 2.84** HCC with diffuse invasion of the portal vein (VP). T = tumor.

▶ Thorotrastosis

This tumor is hardly ever seen now and is also characterized by diffuse changes of the entire hepatic parenchyma (**Fig. 2.85**).

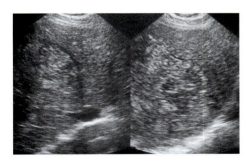

◀ **Fig. 2.85** Thorotrastosis.

▶ Diffuse Metastasis

Although diffuse metastasis of the liver may involve the entire organ, it may be impossible to delineate individual lesions as metastases with any certainty. Such changes are quite frequent in cancer of the breast, stomach, and pancreas (**Figs. 2.86** and **2.87**).

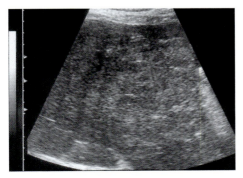

▲ **Fig. 2.86** Diffuse liver metastasis of pancreatic cancer.

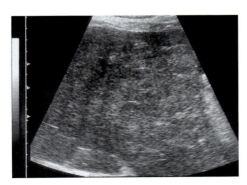

▲ **Fig. 2.87** Diffuse liver metastasis of carcinoid tumor.

▶ Alveolar Hydatid Disease

Infection with *Echinococcus multilocularis* yields images similar to invasive tumor growth and cannot be distinguished from a malignancy by sonography alone **(Table 2.12)**.

Table 2.12 Alveolar hydatid disease. Sonographic classification after Wechsler and Kern[3]

Stage	Characteristic
I	Circumscribed inhomogeneous changes in the liver; ill-defined margin; mostly hyperechoic with a hypoechoic rim; calcification; no invasion of the portal vein, bile ducts, and hepatic veins
II	Appearance of hypoechoic cystic areas with ill-defined margins; invasion of bile ducts, branches of the portal vein, and hepatic veins; increasing calcification
III	Marked infiltration of the liver with complications due to invasion of bile ducts and vessels; extensive calcification at the inhomogeneities; increasingly cystic hypoechoic areas
IV	Crossing the organ boundary of the liver and invasion of the porta hepatis, diaphragm, retroperitoneum, head of the pancreas, and the duodenum

Differential Diagnosis of Focal Lesions

Diagnostic Methods

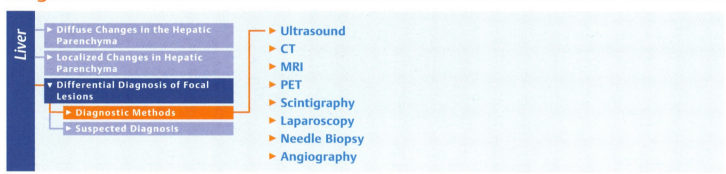

Apart from the patient's history, clinical findings, and laboratory parameters, the differential diagnosis of focal liver lesions can draw on other technical modalities that permit study of the mass either directly by cytology/histology and function testing, or indirectly by diagnostic imaging. The importance of each modality depends not only on the physical/technical limits but, owing to rapid technical advances, also on the model of the equipment used, the actual performance of the study, and the personal expertise of the clinician. It is essential to regard the different diagnostic modalities as being complementary rather than rivals, and to employ them as efficiently as possible to maximize the return for the patient. The importance of diagnostic ultrasound within this group of diagnostic modalities still has to be defined.

Undoubtedly, abdominal sonography is the imaging modality of choice in the detection and diagnosis of hepatic disorders. Not only is it the most widely available alternative of all the imaging modalities, but it can be performed at any time, with a high degree of sensitivity and specificity, it does not endanger the patient, and it can be repeated as often as needed. However, since not all lesions are amenable to sonographic diagnosis, it has to be supplemented by other specific diagnostic methods.

The actual application of each modality depends not only on the indication and issue at hand but to a large extent also on its availability, expenditure of diagnostic resources, and cost; its invasiveness and the stress/danger for the patient should also be considered. Therefore, the differential diagnostic aspects of the various modalities summarized below cannot hope to be exhaustive; they are listed only in terms of their importance as supplementary measures to diagnostic ultrasound.

Alternative Modalities in the Differential Diagnosis of Focal Liver Lesions

Ultrasonography. Routine abdominal sonography can be supplemented by special ultrasound techniques that can help in the further diagnosis of a mass; primarily, this would involve contrast-enhanced studies, qualitative and quantitative studies of the vascularization of the lesion, as well as the various possibilities of guided needle biopsy and intervention.

Computed tomography (CT). The primary drawback of abdominal CT scanning is the radiation exposure; furthermore, it only permits static cross-sectional images. Its advantages are in terms of documentation and the imaging of masses in locations that might be hard to study by ultrasound (subphrenic, in massive obesity, etc.). The limits of detection are about the same in both modalities (CT and US); the sensitivity of each method in detecting focal liver lesions is about 90%, which increases to about 95% if both modalities are combined.

Magnetic resonance imaging (MRI). The most rapid advances in the imaging of focal liver lesions have taken place in the field of MRI, which nowadays plays an important role in the detection and differential diagnosis of these lesions. Because of the significant cost and expenditure of resources and its lack of widespread availability, MRI is not regarded as a primary imaging modality but rather as an important adjunct in the specific differential diagnosis of lesions detected by routine sonography. Suspected hemangiomas lend themselves particularly well to confirmation by MRI.

Positron emission tomography. The importance of PET in the diagnostic armament is still the subject of clinical studies; at present, it cannot be regarded as a routine measure.

Scintigraphy. Because of the significant logistics and radiation exposure involved, scintigraphic studies are also regarded as second-line options. However, blood-pool scintigraphy is quite important when it comes to confirming focal lesions suspected of being hemangiomas. The same holds true for the diagnosis of FNH by hepatobiliary scintiscan (HIDA scan), which specifically detects the proliferating bile ducts of this disorder.

Laparoscopy. Laparoscopy is a minimally invasive procedure that permits assessment of the hepatic surface, precise guided biopsy of circumscribed lesions, and, with the option of an ultrasound scanner, a high-resolution study of the liver. It is used primarily for unknown diffuse disorders of the parenchyma, and in the preoperative work-up of malignant disease when the transabdominal ultrasound finding is negative.

Needle biopsy with cytology/histology/bacterial culture. Needle biopsy always is an invasive procedure and can only be justified if it might lead to changes in the treatment—in which case it becomes a necessity.

Angiography. Today, angiography does not play any primary role in the diagnostic work-up of the liver. It is of limited value in the preoperative assessment of hepatic lesions.

Suspected Diagnosis

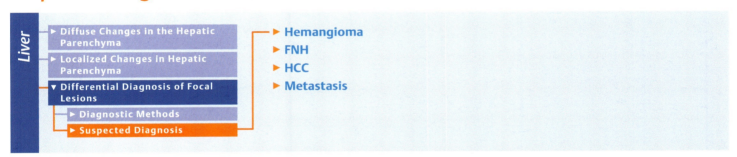

If the sonographic findings are tentative, the sonographer has the following options to confirm or rule out the suspected diagnosis. **Table 2.13** summarizes the significance of the various diagnostic modalities.

Hemangioma. If contrast enhancement is available, it can be used during the same study to demonstrate the so-called filling-in phenomenon by color-flow Doppler scanning, or the pooling of the contrast agent within the hemangioma by other imaging techniques (stimulated acoustic emission, SAE).

The pooling of tracer-marked red blood cells is also the basis for confirming a hemangioma by blood-pool scintiscanning. The confirmation of hemangiomas by CT also has its roots in the filling-in phenomenon. In MRI, hemangiomas are characterized by their typical behavior in T1- and T2-weighted sequences.

Since hemangiomas are prone to hemorrhaging, they should not be needle-biopsied. Unknown lesions breaking the surface of the liver should be needle-biopsied in such a fashion that the canal passes through a thick enough stretch of normal hepatic parenchyma. One characteristic of hemangiomas is a gush of blood on aspiration.

Focal nodular hyperplasia. The diagnosis of FNH is based on its architecture, with a thick vascular pedicle, central stellate scar and radiating fibrous septa, thick central blood vessel, and radial centrifugal blood flow as well as mulberry-like vascular tree. These characteristics are easily demonstrated by abdominal color-flow Doppler imaging (improved by contrast enhancement), angio CT, and special MRI studies.

FNH is confirmed by HIDA scanning since the tracer is secreted into the bile ducts, whose detectable presence is pathognomonic for this disease (compared to adenoma, HCC, and metastasis). However, this statement has to be viewed in the light of recent studies that have also demonstrated positive HIDA scans for some adenomas.

Needle biopsy requires a tissue cylinder of sufficient diameter; the procedure should allow for the hypervascular nature of this tumor (possible hemorrhage), which is characterized by its firm consistency.

Hepatocellular carcinoma. Any focal mass in a cirrhotic liver should be suspected of HCC and calls for further work-up and confirmation by ultrasound guided needle biopsy (only if it results in clinical consequences for the patient).

Noninvasive color-flow Doppler scanning may be able to demonstrate vascular invasion of the tumor or its bizarre irregular hypervascularization. HCC is delineated by its filling defect on gadolinium-enhanced MRI.

Metastasis. Numerous proven methods can detect hepatic metastases, including transabdominal ultrasound (particularly effective with contrast enhanced imaging) and the equally effective modalities of CT and MRI. Laparoscopy is the method of choice in the detection of small superficial metastases since it bests all other measures. At this time, typing a metastasis in terms of its primary can only be achieved by cytology/histology. However, confirmation by ultrasound-guided needle biopsy after color-flow Doppler study is called for only if it would result in clinical consequences. The canal of the biopsy should always run through a stretch of healthy parenchyma long enough to prevent hemorrhage. Lesions with a sonographic halo sign should be biopsied at the hypoechoic rim.

References

1. WHO Informal Working Group. International classification of ultrasound images in cystic echinococcosis for application in clinical and field epidemiological settings. Acta Tropica 2003;85:253–261.
2. WHO Informal Working Group on Echinococcus (WHO-IWGE). WHO/CDS/CSR/APH 2001.
3. Kern P, Wechsler, Lauchart W, Kunz R. Klinik und Therapie der alveolären Echinokokkose. Deutsches Ärzteblatt 91:2494–2501, 1994.
4. Albrecht T, Blomley MJ, Bam PN, et al. Improved detection of hepatic metastasis with pulse inversion US during the liver-specific phase of SHU 508 A: multi-center study. Radiology 2003;227:361–370.
5. Quaia. E, F. Calliada, M. Bertolotto, S. Rossi, L. Garioni, L. Rosa, R. Pozzi-Mucelli Characterisation of Focal Liver Lesions with Contrast – Spezific US Modes and a Sulfur Hexalfluoride-filled Microbubble Contrast Agent: Diagnostic Performance and Confidence. Radiology 2004;232:420–430.
6. Becker D, Günter E, Hahn EG, Heyder N. Imaging tumor vascularisation of hepatocellular carcinoma with ultrasound angiography. Ultraschall Med 1995;16:109–112.

Table 2.13 The importance of additional diagnostic modalities

Suspected sonographic diagnosis	Additional diagnostic modality	Importance
Hemangioma	Contrast enhanced color-flow Doppler imaging	++
	MRI	+++
	Blood-pool scintigraphy	++
	Angio-CT	+
	!Caution: needle biopsy!	
FNH	Contrast enhanced color-flow Doppler imaging	++
	Hepatobiliary BIDA-imaging	+++
	CT	+
	MRI	++
	Needle biopsy	+
HCC	Contrast enhanced color-flow Doppler imaging	++
	MRI	++
	Needle biopsy	+++
Metastasis	Contrast enhanced sonography with contrast harmonic imaging (CHI)	++
	Needle biopsy	+++

3 Biliary Tree and Gallbladder

Biliary Tree 51

Thickening of the Bile Duct Wall — 105
Localized and Diffuse — 105
- Benign Thickening of the Bile Duct Wall
- Malignant Thickening of the Bile Duct Wall

Bile Duct Rarefaction — 106
Localized and Diffuse — 106
- PSC and Cirrhosis of the Liver

Bile Duct Dilatation and Intraductal Pressure — 107
Intrahepatic — 108
- Intrahepatic Gallstones
- Hepatocellular Carcinoma (HCC)/Cholangiocellular Carcinoma (CCC)

Hilar and Prepancreatic — 109
- Benign Causes of Obstruction
- Malignant Tumors

Intrapancreatic — 111
- Benign Intrapancreatic Stenosis
- Cancer of the Pancreatic Head

Papillary — 112
- Benign Periampullary Obstruction
- Cancer

Abnormal Intraluminal Bile Duct Findings — 112
Foreign Body — 112
- Pneumobilia/Stent
- Uncommon Causes

Differential Diagnosis of Sonographic Cholestasis — 114
The Seven Most Important Questions — 114
- Anatomy
- Topography

Gallbladder 67

Changes in Size — 122
Large Gallbladder (> 10 cm) — 122
- Asymptomatic (Functional)
- Asymptomatic (Pathological)
- Symptomatic (Pathological)

Small/Missing Gallbladder — 123
- Asymptomatic (Functional)
- Asymptomatic (Pathological)
- Symptomatic (Pathological)

Wall Changes — 125
General Hypoechogenicity — 125
- Acute Cholecystitis
- Special Cases
- Wall Thickening in Hepatic/Pancreatic Disorders and Trauma

General Hyperechogenicity — 127
- Chronic Cholecystitis
- Porcelain Gallbladder

Focal Hypoechogenicity/Hyperechogenicity — 128
- Focal Inflammation
- Gallbladder Varicosity

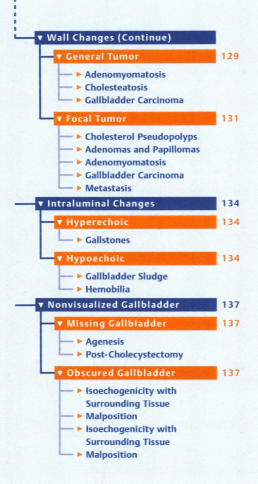

3 Biliary Tree and Gallbladder

Biliary Tree

L. Greiner and J. Mueller

The intrahepatic and extrahepatic bile ducts are delicate tubular structures without the stratified appearance so typical of smooth-muscle walls—the epithelium of the bile ducts lies directly adjacent to the outermost connective-tissue layer. Any rise in pressure within the ducts results in immediate dilatation of those parts of the ducts (and possibly also of the gallbladder and/or cystic duct) upstream of the obstruction. This facet of dilatation may be detected quite easily by ultrasound and is the most important aspect in the differential diagnosis of (obstructive) cholestasis (with or without jaundice). The changes in wall thickness, intraluminal matter, and adjacent structures form the basis for the sonographic assessment of the level and cause (benign or malignant) of biliary obstruction.

Anatomy

When viewed in the direction of bile flow, the anatomy of the biliary tree may be subdivided into an intrahepatic as well as an extrahepatic compartment, the gallbladder appearing to be "just" a dilated dead-end. The extrahepatic course of the bile ducts can be broken down further in to the hilar, prepancreatic, and intrapancreatic segments (ultrasound cannot differentiate between a (rare) true intrapancreatic course and the duct running in a "groove"). Only in rare instances does another anatomical landmark become visible by sonography—the union of the cystic duct with the common hepatic duct. In ultrasound nomenclature this then becomes DHC or "ductus hepatocholedochus," i.e., the common hepatic and hepatocystic ducts (CBD, "common bile duct").

Diameter. Differential diagnosis in the ultrasound of the biliary tree relies much more on the shape of the ducts than their "actual" or "identifiable" diameter, since the precise measurement of biological structures is characterized by numerous variables: the definition of the distances to be measured—which diameter at which organ/tubule border and at which position—is arbitrary and therefore not precise. In addition, this issue becomes even more complex when taking into account the typical changes seen in the extrahepatic biliary tree, where the diameter of the ducts increases with advancing age. Localized increases in the prepancreatic duct diameter without a concomitant rise in the intraductal pressure ("cholangiectasia") do not depend on age and are a frequent finding **(see Fig. 3.3)**. Careful studies have not been able to confirm the prevailing concept that the diameter of the common duct increases after cholecystectomy (taking into account age adjusted cholangiectasia).

There are no systematic ultrasound studies correlating bile duct diameter and patient position, and neither have there been any studies on the (possible) changes in bile duct diameter after meals or pressure relief, e.g., by endoscopic intervention.

Thus, any statement of "standard values" for the diameter of the intrahepatic and extrahepatic bile ducts carries quite a large degree of uncertainty.

Shape. Under normal pressure conditions (< 20 cmH$_2$O), the intrahepatic and extrahepatic biliary tree is slender, particularly so upstream of where the hepatic artery crosses the common duct. The hepatic duct confluence is very difficult to visualize on ultrasound (▪ **3.1d**). Even minor increases in intraductal pressure will change the morphology of the confluence **(Fig. 3.1b)**, i.e., it appears to become visualized more easily rather than there being any actual changes in the measurements themselves, and the differentiation between the intrahepatic and extrahepatic segments of the biliary system improves almost excessively **(Fig. 3.1c)**. Those segments close to the hepatic duct confluence and the latter itself can be differentiated immediately and the intrahepatic bile ducts become dilated, resulting in the well known "double-barrel shotgun sign" **(Figs. 3.1b and 3.2)**.

Diameter (Figs. 3.1 and 3.2)
▶ Barely visible interlobar branches
  – Right/left hepatic duct: 1–2 mm
  – Hilar common hepatic duct: 1–2 mm/ detection limit
  – Prepancreatic CBD: 3–7(9) mm

Shape
▶ Slender interlobar segment/close to the hepatic duct confluence
  – Hepatic duct confluence not or barely visualized
  – Slender hilar segment
  – Slender/slightly ectatic prepancreatic segment
  – Intrapancreatic segment not or barely visualized

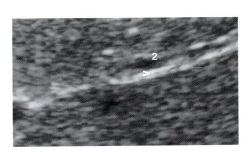

▲ **Fig. 3.1** Diameter of the intrahepatic biliary tree.
a Slender intrahepatic bile duct (>) (segment II), accompanying branch of the portal vein (2).

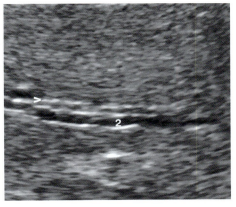

▲ **b** Slightly dilated intrahepatic bile duct (>) (segment III), accompanying branch of the portal vein (2).

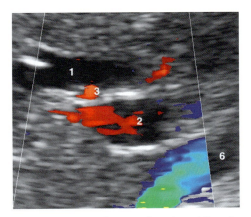

▲ **c** Hepatic duct confluence with moderate biliary obstruction. Hepatic duct confluence (1) and portal vein (2), branch of the hepatic artery (3), inferior vena cava (6).

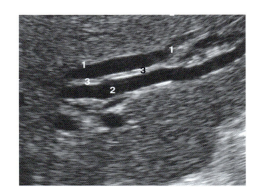
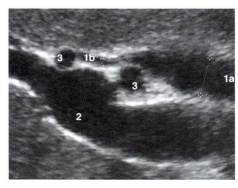

◄◄ **Fig. 3.2** Dilated intrahepatic bile duct (1), accompanying branch of the portal vein (2), and hepatic artery (3) (segment III).

◄ **Fig. 3.3** Prepancreatic cholangiectasis with ampullary CBD (1a) and slender segment near the hepatic duct confluence (1b); early branching of the hepatic artery as a regular variant (3); portal vein (2).

Topography and Ultrasound Morphology

Both other vessels of the hepatic triad, the trunks and branches of the portal vein and the hepatic artery, can be considered mandatory and highly reliable sonographic landmarks accompanying the intrahepatic and extrahepatic biliary tree.

Intrahepatic biliary tree. Ultrasound visualization of the intrahepatic biliary tree (**Figs. 3.1 and 3.2**) is facilitated by the fact that the regular vascular branching of the hepatic triad ("vascular architecture") at all levels results in multiple, ever-smaller branches coursing parallel to the surface of the probe, which makes for optimum detection. The best resolution of details, almost resembling that of a magnifying glass, is seen in the portal vein branches (up to the intralobular level), followed by the small branches of the bile ducts. Normally, only the large intrahepatic branches of the hepatic artery can be seen (with color-flow Doppler scanning even more peripheral branches may be visualized).

Extrahepatic biliary tree (■ **3.1**). The hilar/prepancreatic course of the extrahepatic biliary tree is also well defined in terms of ultrasound anatomy by the vascular triads originating here. The portal vein always runs posterior to the more slender common duct (■ **3.1 a–f**). The relationship of the portal vein with the hepatic

Topography
► Hepatic triads:
Branches of the bile ducts, hepatic artery, and portal vein running in parallel
► Intrahepatic:
Interlobular sheaths of connective tissue
► Extrahepatic:
Between segments I (caudate lobe) and IVb then posterior to the duodenum and head of the pancreas/intrapancreatic caudad to the gastroduodenal artery

Sonographic landmarks
► Intrahepatic:
Typical topography of the branching structures accompanying the portal vein (segments II + III !)
► Extrahepatic:
Portal vein to the posterior
Hepatic artery from the left running between portal vein and common duct, denting the latter

artery and its variant extrahepatic hilar branches is somewhat more complex (**Fig. 3.4c, d**). The hepatic artery always enters the hepatic portal from the left (■ **3.1 f**) and therefore initially lies to the left of the common duct; it (or its main right branch) then crosses behind the common duct (■ **3.1c**). Thus, it courses anterior to the portal vein and posterior to the common duct (■ **3.1a–c, Fig. 3.1c**), and in scans of the hepatic portal (■ **3.1f**) it appears as a round tubular cross-section. Infrequently—only in about 5%—this cross-section of the hepatic artery may progress into its intrahepatic course anterior to the common duct (**Fig. 3.4a, b**). Owing to the pressure of the adjacent pancreatic parenchyma, the intrapancreatic segment of the CBD is almost impossible to visualize; it is best seen in sections orthogonal to its anatomical course (■ **3.1f**).

Clinical Notes

The structures of the hepatic portal are best imaged with the patient in left lateral decubitus position and inhaling deeply: this moves the liver caudad and to the left, thereby providing an excellent "sono-optical" window.

Previous operations in the upper abdomen often lead to significant scarring with a subsequent left shift of the intestinal organs (including the common duct) since the adhesions tend to shrink.

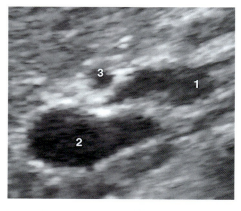
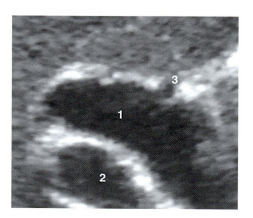
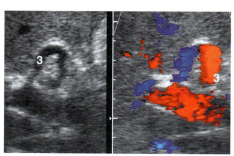

▲ **Fig. 3.4** Hepatic artery. **a and b** Variants in the position of the hepatic artery (3); here, it is anterior to the dilated common duct (1); portal vein (2).

▲ **c and d** Kinking of the hepatic artery (3).

3.1 Anatomy of the Extrahepatic Biliary Tree

▶ Common duct (1), portal vein (2), hepatic artery (3), pancreas (4), liver (5), inferior vena cava (6), left and right hepatic ducts (7), splenic vein (8), right renal artery (9), abdominal aorta (10), crura of diaphragm (11), superior mesenteric artery (12), left renal vein (13), posterior wall of the gastric antrum (14), anterior wall of the gastric antrum (15).

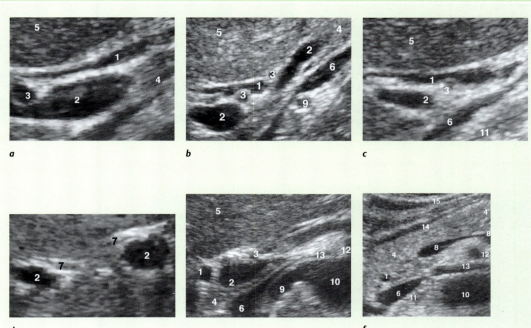

Thickening of the Bile Duct Wall

Localized and Diffuse

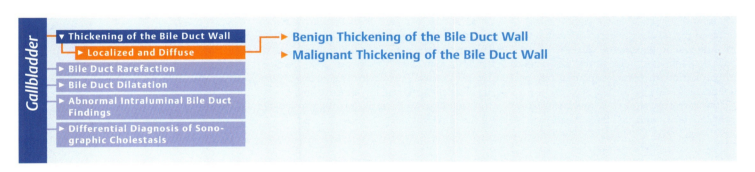

▶ Benign Thickening of the Bile Duct Wall

Transcutaneous ultrasonography can assess localized benign thickening of the bile duct wall in two disorders of the biliary system: intrahepatic and extrahepatic presentation of primary sclerosing cholangitis (PSC) (**Fig. 3.5**), and the solely extrahepatic manifestation of (severe) suppurative cholangitis (**Fig. 3.6**). Except for a few cases, in both instances the sonographic morphology cannot be considered as primary proof but rather "suggests" the suspected diagnosis, with a greater or lesser degree of probability, which then will have to be confirmed by other means (clinical findings, blood chemistry, and endoscopic retrograde cholangiography).

The prolonged course of chronic inflammatory bowel disease (Crohn disease, ulcerative colitis) is often accompanied by the sonographic telltale signs of PSC, from segmental diffuse bile duct wall thickening all the way to complete obstruction of the lumen, alternating with dilated/ectatic bile duct segments; ducts may also appear simply to break off, and intraductal sludge is a frequent finding. It is not possible to rule out early cholangiocellular carcinoma (CCC), and even fine-needle aspiration cytology has its problems. PSC-like changes have been described for HIV infections with manifest AIDS symptoms.

Acute suppurative cholangitis may result in thickening of the common duct wall, which can be demonstrated for the extrahepatic segment. This thickening of the wall becomes particularly evident if endoscopic intervention (endoscopic papillotomy = EPT) has provided pressure relief by removing or bypassing the biliary obstruction (**Figs. 3.22 and 3.27**): the dilated bile duct walls, originally thinned out by their distension, collapse and their inflamed and swollen true structure becomes exceptionally well visualized (**Figs. 3.6 and 3.28**).

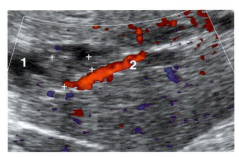
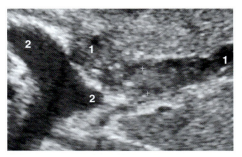
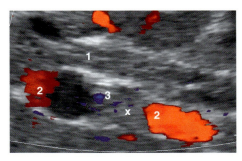

▲ **Fig. 3.5** Primary sclerosing cholangitis.
a Dilatation and wall thickening (calipers) of the intrahepatic bile duct (1) in segment III. Accompanying branch of the portal vein (2).

▲ **b** Dilatation and wall thickening (calipers) of the intrahepatic bile duct (1) in segment II/III.

▲ **c** Wall thickening ("sclerosis") of the common duct (1); hepatic artery (3) crossing in between.

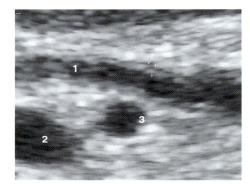

◄ **Fig. 3.6** Suppurative cholangitis, subsiding after endoscopic papillotomy and extraction of calculi, with thickened wall (calipers) of the common duct (1); portal vein (2); hepatic artery (3) crossing in between.

▶ Malignant Thickening of the Bile Duct Wall

Malignant bile duct wall thickening may be localized as in CCC or infiltrating as in HCC (hepatocellular carcinoma), and in both cases ultrasound detects these changes solely in terms of the resulting biliary obstruction with its subsequent prestenotic dilatation of the duct. Consequently, these entities are discussed in the section on pressure-induced bile duct dilatation.

One rare special case is mucinous biliary papillomatosis with its fluent transition to well-differentiated cholangiocarcinoma (**Fig. 3.7**). The ultrasound findings show a nonexpansile solid mass originating in but well defined and demarcated from the surrounding bile duct wall, which it dilates to sometimes bizarre shapes; complete biliary obstruction tends to occur late in the disease. It has a rather indolent course (over many years), and treatment is characterized by effective long-term interventional endoscopy (stenting, removal of the tumor masses).

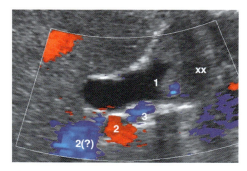

▲ **Fig. 3.7** Obstruction of the common duct (1) in intraductal spread of cholangiocarcinoma (xx); portal vein (2); hepatic artery (3).

Bile Duct Rarefaction

Localized and Diffuse

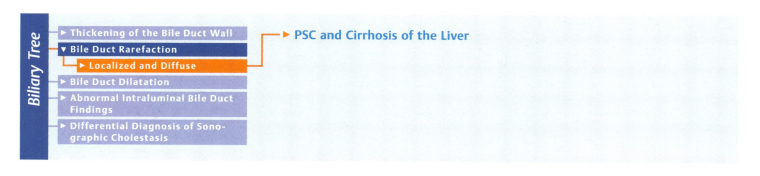

PSC and Cirrhosis of the Liver

Visualization of a rarefied biliary tree, be it localized or diffuse, by ultrasound plays a role of its own only in pediatrics (except for the segmental bile duct rarefaction sometimes seen in PSC). However, in the diagnostic work-up of the cirrhotic liver the indirect criterion of an "abnormal vascular architecture" (◨ 3.3f) also ties in with the rarefied intrahepatic bile ducts. By analogy, this concept applies to all types of cirrhosis as the common end point of severe chronic hepatobiliary disorders, and thus also to cirrhosis in PSC and in primary biliary cirrhosis (PBC), for example.

Bile Duct Dilatation and Intraductal Pressure

No intraductal pressure increase. Dilatation of the bile ducts without concomitant rise in intraductal pressure can be classified into two entities: for the intrahepatic bile ducts this would correspond to Caroli disease (**Fig. 3.8**), and for the extrahepatic biliary tree the underlying disorder would be congenital cystic malformation of the common duct. It is not true that cholecystectomy always results in a dilated common duct.

With acute pressure increase. Any acute rise in intraductal pressure within the biliary tree, which has to drain about 700 ml of bile per day, will lead to immediate dilatation of the bile ducts (**Figs. 3.1 b and 3.9**): the intrahepatic and extrahepatic bile ducts are tubes of connective tissue lined with epithelium but lacking any muscle fibers in the wall, and therefore they cannot resist the pressure increase (this observation becomes obvious during any retrograde injection of contrast media into bile ducts with an initially regular diameter). In acute biliary obstruction, the sonographic finding of bile duct dilatation is the first reproducible indication of this rise in pressure, since in intermittent obstruction the biochemical markers (gamma-glutamyltransferase [α-GT], alanine transaminase [ALT], aspartate transaminase [AST]) will not change or will rise to abnormal values only hours later (6–24 hours). One rather subtle but convincing sonographic sign of the increased pressure in postcholecystectomy patients is the visualization of the cystic duct remnant (**Fig. 3.9**).

The more pronounced the acute rise in pressure (for instance, in status post cholecystectomy there is no possibility of pressure compensation by the gallbladder), the more pronounced the changes become in the intrahepatic biliary tree (**Fig. 3.1 b**)—dilatation ("double barrel shotgun sign") that can be demonstrated quite well at the sonographically easily accessible segments II and III, since there the hepatic triads branch in a plane paralleling the probe; (**Fig. 3.2**). However, this is true only if the tissue surrounding the bile ducts is elastic enough to allow this dilatation; in bile ducts passing through cirrhotic parenchyma, even high intraductal pressure may not result in dilatation.

With chronic pressure increase. Chronic pressure-induced dilatation of the bile ducts (**Figs. 3.2, 3.7, 3.10–3.13**) is characterized by maximal dilatation of the ducts involved; descriptive terms (the image of the "exfoliated oak tree") for the intrahepatic bile duct dilatation convey the situation quite accurately (as long as they trigger the corresponding associations in the mind of the sonographer).

Long-term biliary obstruction with borderline nonicteric compensation is typical of localized intrahepatic obstruction (**Fig. 3.12**), for instance in CCC (particularly in unilateral Klatskin tumors). If the biliary obstruction is incomplete and takes place over a long period, just 20–25% of parenchyma with regular drainage will still be adequate to avoid any manifest jaundice. Biliary obstruction arising at the lower levels and being compensated over a long period is a common finding in well-differentiated periampullary carcinoma (in which case the pancreatic duct will be dilated as well—twin-duct stenosis; **Fig. 3.13**) and the somewhat rare truly benign stenosis of the papilla of Vater.

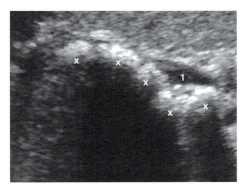

▲ **Fig. 3.8** Dilated intrahepatic bile duct (1) with multiple calculi (xx); Caroli disease.

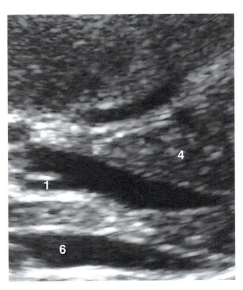

▲ **Fig. 3.9** Dilated cystic duct (1) in pancreatitis of the pancreatic head (4); inferior vena cava (6); portal vein (2).

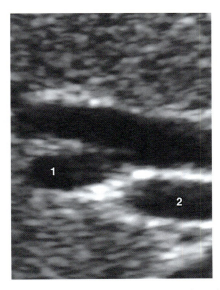

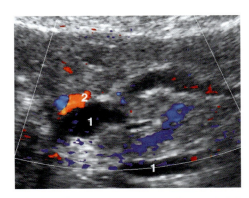

▲ **Fig. 3.10** Extensive dilatation of the intrahepatic bile duct (1) with accompanying portal vein (2).

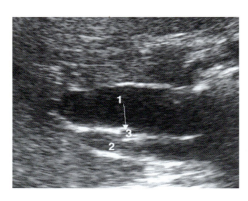
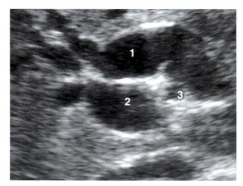

◂◂ **Fig. 3.11** Dilated common duct.
a Extensive dilatation of the common duct (1); portal vein (2); hepatic artery (3).

◂ **b** Kinking of the common duct (1) in long-term pressure increase within the biliary tree; portal vein (2); hepatic artery (3).

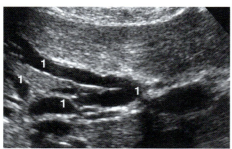
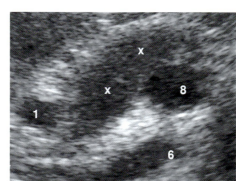

◂◂ **Fig. 3.12** Extensive dilatation of the intrahepatic branches (1) of just the right hepatic lobe in Klatskin tumor.

◂ **Fig. 3.13** Twin-duct stenosis in periampullary carcinoma: dilated intrapancreatic CBD (1) and maximum dilatation of the pancreatic duct (xx); inferior vena cava (6); splenic vein (8).

Intrahepatic

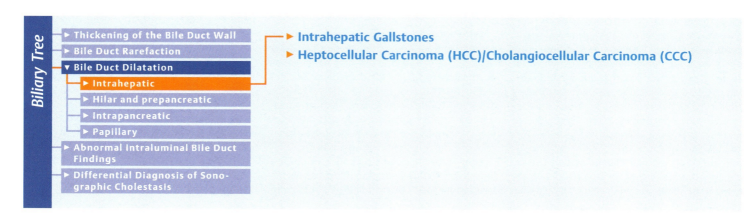

▶ Intrahepatic Gallstones

In most cases benign obstruction of the intrahepatic bile ducts is caused by intrahepatic biliary calculi (cholangiolithiasis and hepatolithiasis) (**Fig. 3.14**).

Focal liver lesions usually do not affect the intrahepatic bile ducts, or at most they displace them without any significant biliodynamic consequences. This is also true for (very) large benign and malignant focal lesions (e.g., voluminous hemangiomas, cysts, or metastases of colorectal cancer).

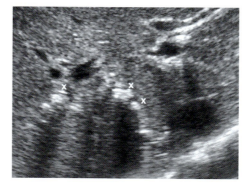

◂ **Fig. 3.14** Multiple intrahepatic biliary calculi (hepatoliths) (xx).

▶ Hepatocellular Carcinoma (HCC)/Cholangiocellular Carcinoma (CCC)

Even aggressive metastatic spread within the liver usually respects the structures of the biliary tree. HCC may be the one exception, since it is known to invade not only the blood vessels but the bile ducts as well; tumor thrombi in the venous (**Fig. 3.15**) and biliary vessels (**see Figs. 3.19–3.21**) are pathognomonic for HCC. As a possible cause of pressure-induced malignant dilatation of intrahepatic bile ducts, its incidence is well above that of the (quite rare) true CCC (**Fig. 3.16**); however, in undifferentiated tumors even pathological histomorphology and/or cytomorphology will sometimes be unable to diagnose precisely whether one is dealing with HCC or CCC.

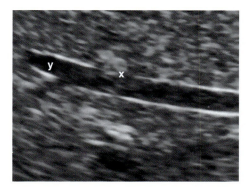

▲ **Fig. 3.15** Small hepatocellular carcinoma (x) invading a hepatic vein (y).

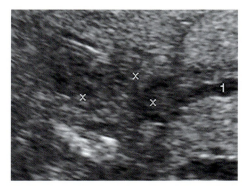

▲ **Fig. 3.16** Cholangiocellular carcinoma (x) with localized intrahepatic biliary obstruction(1) (segment II).

Hilar and Prepancreatic

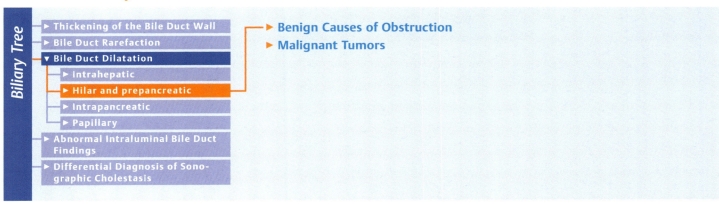

▶ Benign Causes of Obstruction

Gallstones. The primary cause of benign bilio-dynamic obstructions in the hepatic portal and the prepancreatic CBD are biliary calculi (☐ **3.2**), which may differ significantly in terms of shape, size, and number. Gallstones at the hepatic duct confluence and in the CBD will be easier to detect by ultrasound the bigger they are and the more they are encased by fluid. In addition, "young" calculi made up of pure cholesterol (☐ **3.2c**) display a higher impedance than old pigmented gallstones of low reflectivity (☐ **3.2d**). Direct detection of intrahepatic and common duct biliary calculi may also depend on the quality of the ultrasound platform employed and, primarily, on the diligence and experience of the sonographer. Sonographic visualization of small and minute gallstones ("microlithiasis") (☐ **3.2h**) is particularly challenging, since their passage through the papilla of Vater appears to be the underlying cause in most cases of so-called idiopathic pancreatitis. When considered in the context of a typical history and clinical findings, ultrasound can detect the presence of such microliths only indirectly by demonstration of the dilated bile ducts. Even in endoscopic retrograde cholangiopancreatography [ERCP] studies there is sometimes lingering doubt about the possible presence of microliths, which may be screened out by the contrast agent. In these cases it pays to insonate the gallbladder immediately after endoscopic retrograde cholangiographic [ERC] cystography: these minute calculi may now be seen in the boundary layer between the (heavier) contrast agent and the (lighter) bile, although they may have escaped detection in previous studies despite patient positioning (☐ **3.2h**). When dealing with small CBD calculi, posterior shadowing may facilitate detection much better than actually looking for the biliary calculus itself (☐ **3.2b and e**).

Intraductal gallstones without any clinical or biochemical findings are quite rare and should always be treated by interventional endoscopy (while silent calculi in the gallbladder may be left alone).

A special case of calculus-induced inflammatory bile duct obstruction is Mirizzi syndrome (which can be difficult to visualize on ultrasound) (**Fig. 3.17**).

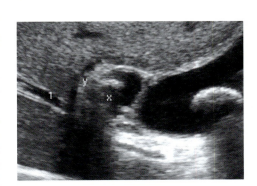

▲ **Fig. 3.17** Mirizzi syndrome with cholecystolithiasis in typical infundibular position (x), with hydrops and inflamed thickened wall (y) and biliary outlet obstruction (1).

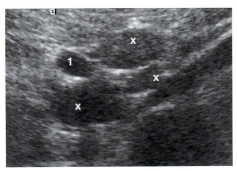

▲ **Fig. 3.18** Hodgkin lymphoma (x) with dilatation of the CBD (1).

▣ 3.2 Choledocholithiasis

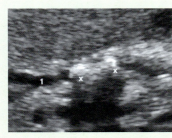 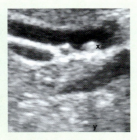 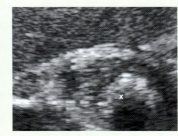 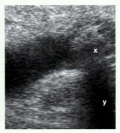

a Two calculi (xx) in the dilated CBD (1).

b Small calculus (x) in the CBD with faint but definite posterior shadowing (y).

c Hyperechoic (cholesterol?) CBD stone (x) with surface defects after extracorporeal shock-wave lithotripsy (ESWL).

d Hypoechoic (pigmented?) CBD stone (x and arrows) with posterior shadowing (y).

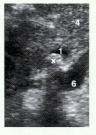 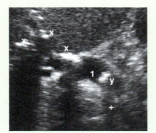 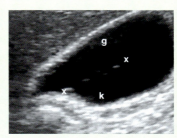

e Preampullary hyperechoic (cholesterol?) CBD stones (x); CBD (1); inferior vena cava (6); pancreatic head (4).

f Floating intraductal gas bubbles = pneumobilia (x) and CBD calculi (y) with posterior shadowing (+); dilated CBD (1).

g After ERC and with the patient supine: floating microliths (xx) marking the boundary layer between the lighter bile (g) and the more viscous contrast agent (k).

Hemobilia. In most cases hemobilia is iatrogenic; because of the highly thrombolytic activity of bile, biliary obstruction is the exception rather than the norm.

Cicatricial stenosis. Only rarely is stenosis of the hilar biliary tree and common duct due to scarring the sole cause of the obstruction—most often they will be compensated for a considerable time, and additional factors, such as (micro-)lithiasis, are required for fully blown cholestasis to develop.

Because of their propensity for scar contraction, bilioenteric anastomoses may, however, decompensate without any additional lithic obstruction. The short length of these strictures does not make them amenable to direct sonographic visualization.

Vascular causes. Intramural venous malformations have been described as a vascular cause underlying common duct obstruction.

Lymph node enlargement. Differential diagnosis should always include mechanical cholestasis by lymph node enlargement, no matter what the etiology.

▶ Malignant Tumors

Once again, when viewed in the direction of bile flow, malignant obstruction at the level of the hilar hepatic confluence or the prepancreatic common duct is due to CCC of the Klatskin type, and in the case of CBD involvement it is the invasive carcinoma of the gallbladder or HCC infiltrating the biliary tree (**Figs. 3.19–3.21**). Most of these masses are isoechoic with the adjacent hepatic parenchyma and their only evidence is obstruction of the biliary vessels resulting in bile duct dilatation.

Cholangiocellular carcinoma of the Klatskin type, obstructing just one of the two hepatic ducts, is characterized by the difference in echogenicity of the two hepatic lobes, which is due to the different amounts of fluid in the parenchyma.

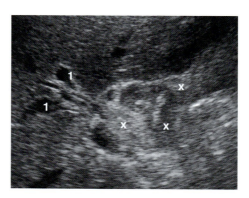 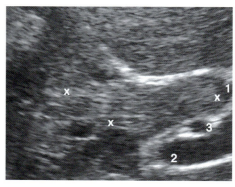

▲ **Fig. 3.19** Cholangiocellular carcinoma (x) with enlarged lymph node (y) and tumor projecting into the CBD (1).

▲ **Fig. 3.20** Carcinoma of the gallbladder (x) invading the hepatic portal, dilatation of the intrahepatic bile ducts (1).

▲ **Fig. 3.21** Hepatocellular carcinoma (x) with peg-shaped invasion of the CBD (1); portal vein (2), hepatic artery (3).

Classification of Klatskin Tumors

Klatskin tumors[24] is a collective term for bile-duct adenocarcinomas located at the bifurcation of the hepatic duct. They were subdivided into three types by Bismuth and Corlett in 1975.[3a] *Type I* tumors involve the common hepatic duct, with no involvement of the right and left secondary ducts. *Type II* tumors involve the hepatic duct bifurcation, without involving the secondary intrahepatic ducts. *Type III* tumors involve the hepatic duct bifurcation, infiltrate the common hepatic duct, and also involve one or both hepatic ducts toward the liver or second-order bile ducts. The different types are easily identified by ultrasound.

Intrapancreatic

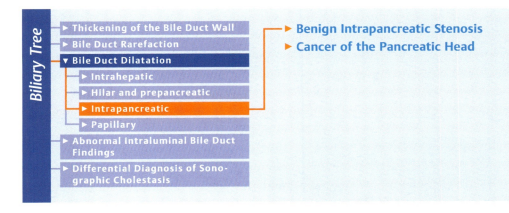

▶ Benign Intrapancreatic Stenosis

One of the most common causes of benign intrapancreatic stenosis, apart from the acute passage of gallstones, is marked chronic pancreatitis: in the presence of the typical sonographic signs (**Figs. 3.22 and 3.23**) and the pointed cone shaped obstructed CBD (compared with the more plump cut-off appearance in malignancies) (**Fig. 3.24**), this preliminary diagnosis is well founded. Biliary obstruction may also be caused by pseudocysts and acute (segmental cephalic) pancreatitis. Other rare causes described in the literature are benign pancreatic masses along the line of focal mesenchymal lesions.

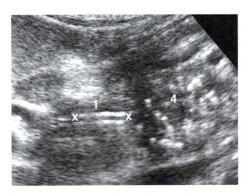

▲ **Fig. 3.22** Hepaticoduodenal stent (x) draining the CBD (1); reduced pancreatic parenchyma with multiple small hyperechoic lesions (probably corresponding to calcium deposits).

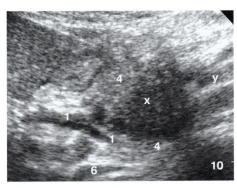

▲ **Fig. 3.23** Chronic pancreatitis (4), with pseudocyst (x) obstructing the CBD (1); dilated pancreatic duct (y); inferior vena cava (6); abdominal aorta (10).

▶ Cancer of the Pancreatic Head

Most cases of malignant intrapancreatic obstruction (**Fig. 3.24**) are due to ductal carcinoma of the pancreatic head. But at times (undifferentiated carcinoma), even histology may not be able to differentiate between ductal pancreatic carcinoma and CCC of the intrapancreatic CBD. Pancreatic metastases are rare by themselves and will hardly result in obstruction of the biliary passage.

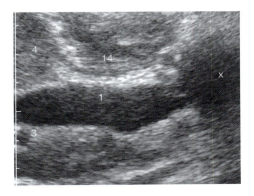

◀ **Fig. 3.24** Cancer of the pancreatic head (x), obstructing the CBD (1); hepatic artery (3); liver (4); posterior wall of the gastric antrum (14).

Papillary

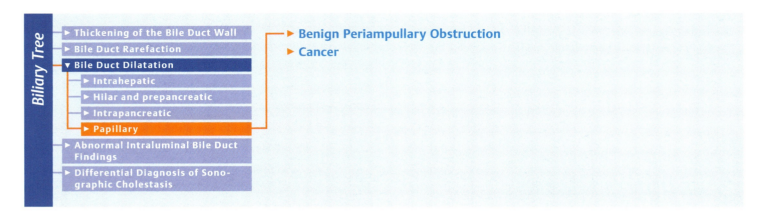

▶ Benign Periampullary Obstruction

The periampullary duodenal diverticulum is very hard to visualize on ultrasound, and its role as a benign obstruction of the biliary tree remains unclear. True sclerosis of the papilla of Vater is also quite rare. Sonography can hardly ever demonstrate calculi impacted in the papilla of Vater. Other benign obstructions at the level of the papilla, such as cysts of the duodenal wall and intramural duodenal heterotopic pancreatic remnants, also escape sonographic detection.

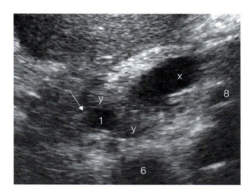

◀ **Fig. 3.25** Periampullary cancer (y) obstructing the CBD (1) and pancreatic duct (x); inferior vena cava (6), splenic vein (8).

▶ Cancer

In characteristic sonomorphology, periampullary and true papillary carcinomas result not only in biliary but also pancreatic obstruction, with the "double duct dilatation" of both duct systems (**Figs. 3.13 and 3.25**). In cases of painless jaundice, this sonographic picture raises the hope of possible curative surgery.

Abnormal Intraluminal Bile Duct Findings

Foreign Body

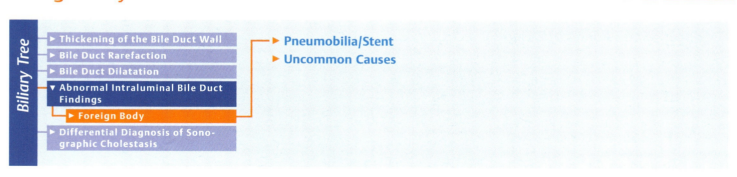

▶ Pneumobilia/Stent

Intraductal gas or pneumobilia (**Fig. 3.26**) after endoscopic papillotomy (or hepatoenteric anastomosis) is a clear sign of unobstructed bile flow; here, too, sonography and endoscopy of the abdomen are complementary rather than competing modalities. The same holds true when checking the function and position of biliary stents (**Fig. 3.27**). Compared with computerized tomography, sonographic real-time scanning can differentiate, without problems, between pneumobilia and the pulsatile snow-shower–like inflow of portal gas bubbles (**Fig. 3.26**).

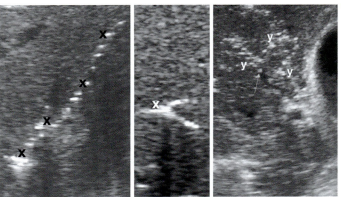

◀ *Fig. 3.26* Pneumobilia (x) of the intrahepatic bile ducts, on the left in "string of beads" configuration and in the middle image filling a small duct completely. On the right: small and minute pulsatile inflow of brightly echogenic gas bubbles in the portal vein (y)

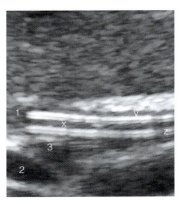

▲ *Fig. 3.27* Hepatoduodenal stents (x).
a Satisfactory drainage. Anterior (y) and posterior walls (z) of the stent; portal vein (2). 1 = common duct; 3 = bile duct.

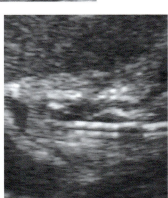

▲ **b** Dysfunctional stent with dilated CBD and sludge.

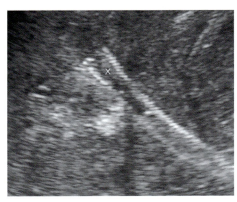

▲ **c** Lumen (x) of a self-expanding hepatoduodenal stent with satisfactory drainage.

▶ Uncommon Causes

Numerous other intraluminal foreign bodies of the bile duct have been described, mostly in the literature on endoscopy; the common characteristic of these uncommon findings is their unfailing *lack* of detection by ultrasound. They are listed here simply to round out this discussion of differential diagnosis:
- Metal fragments after gunshot injuries
- Clips after surgery (**Fig. 3.28a**)
- Sutures and parts of T-tube drains
- Food particles (after choledochoduodenostomy)
- Parasites (*Echinococcus, Ascaris, Opisthorchis sinensis*, and others) (**Fig. 3.28b–d**).

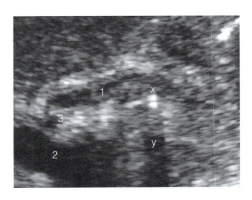

◀ *Fig. 3.28 a* Clip (x), with posterior shadowing (y), close to the CBD after laparoscopic cholecystectomy; portal vein (2); hepatic artery (3); CBD (1) with residual inflammation of the wall (after endoscopic papillotomy).

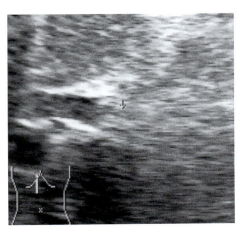

▲ **b** Ascariasis: oval-shaped hyperechoic voids, slightly distended duct (arrow) (clinical diagnosis: acute necrotizing pancreatitis).

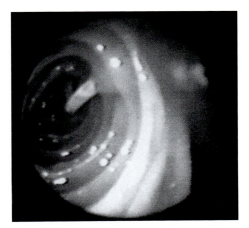

▲ **c** ERC photograph: ascaris, emerging from the papilla of Vater.

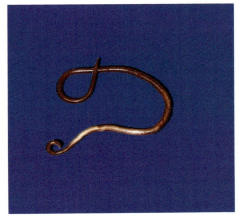

▲ **d** "Recovered" ascaris.

Differential Diagnosis of Sonographic Cholestasis

In today's age of imaging modalities, the term cholestasis—meaning "stoppage of the bile flow"—is equated with mechanical obstruction of the bile flow. Thus, the differentiation of this term with respect to parenchymal cholestasis (3.3) in acute hepatitis (3.3a), hepatic congestion (3.3b), veno-occlusive disease (3.3c), cholangitis with abscess formation (3.3d), diffuse metastasis (3.3e), or in cirrhosis has become an issue of minor importance. This is understandable because the extent and duration of the ductal distension, and the type and anatomical location of the obstruction with its possible impact on bile flow dynamics, can be visualized so easily by means of ultrasonography.

As in all other fluid-filled tubular systems, any pressure increase in the bile-filled vessels will increase their diameter, pressure in the adjacent tissue permitting, and thus result in distension. Therefore, the leading differential diagnostic sign in the sonographic morphology of cholestasis is distension of the intrahepatic and/or extrahepatic bile ducts, with or without clinical symptoms and rarely without concomitant rise in the blood level of bilirubin and/or the other enzymes characteristic of cholestasis.

The Seven Most Important Questions

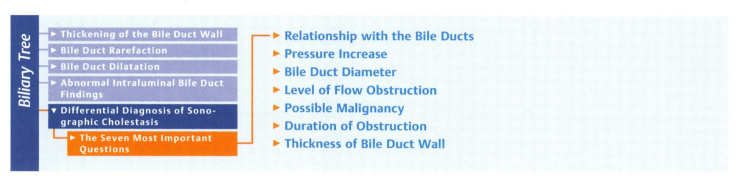

1. Are the vascular structures in question truly part of the biliary tree?

The first step in the differential diagnosis of vascular distension within the liver parenchyma or at the hepatic portal is to ascertain whether the vessels are truly part of the biliary tree. Intrahepatic arteries or the arteries and veins of the porta hepatis are typical examples of such misdiagnosed structures (3.3f, i, j). Even without the capabilities of color-coded Doppler scanning of the flow, precise knowledge of the anatomy with its numerous variants is essential for this first step in the differential diagnosis.

2. Are there signs of a (segmental or general) pressure increase in the biliary tree?

The second aspect to be addressed when considering dilatation of the biliary tree is to resolve the issue of a pressure-independent increase in the diameter ("ectasia") (3.4d)

Practical Considerations

The differential diagnosis of "sonographic cholestasis"—more precisely, the question of obstructive nonparenchymatous cholestasis—is the prime example of a medical problem where ultrasonography (the Italians prefer the much more descriptive and pertinent term of echoscopy) and endoscopy are the perfect diagnostic as well as interventional/therapeutic partners, preferably performed by one and the same physician. Other diagnostic modalities such as CT or MRI would usually not be needed at all.

or true dilatation by increased tubular pressure—be it within individual segments ("levels") (3.4h–j, k, q) or the entire biliary tree (3.4k–p, r–u). Congenital malformations such as choledodochal cysts or Caroli disease and the age-dependent increase in the ductal diameter, particularly that of the prepancreatic CBD, are not pressure-dependent (3.4d). The prevailing concept that the diameter of the common duct increases after cholecystectomy does not hold true.

3. What is the diameter of the bile ducts—subjectively and measured?

The third question deals with the determination of the bile duct diameter. These millimeter values measured at ill-defined locations are diagnostically inferior to the morphological appearance of the biliary tree, since the latter allows much better conclusions to be drawn regarding the actual cause of the increased pressure within the bile ducts (3.4d–g). Vessels distended owing to increased pressure are more or less dilated along their entire prestenotic course; it should be noted that in case of extrahepatic obstruction the hepatic duct confluence is easily differentiated from its surroundings. Only ectatic segments of the bile tree (preferably in the prepancreatic region of the CBD) with slender segments upstream (3.4d) do not exhibit any intraductal pressure increase, i.e., no cholestasis.

It stands to reason that in cases of intraductal pressure increases the possibility of ductal dilatation depends on the pressure of the surrounding tissue: for instance, if the intrapancreatic course of the CBD becomes visible this is (almost) proof of a significant pressure increase in the prepapillary segment which must more than negate the compression exerted by the head of the pancreas. Cirrhosis of the liver will not result in dilatation of the intrahepatic biliary tree even if the pressure increases significantly.

4. At what level of the biliary tree is the obstruction located?

5. Is the obstruction malignant or benign?

The fourth question concerning the "level" and the fifth question dealing with the nature (malignant or benign) of the biliary obstruction are discussed in detail elsewhere in this chapter in the section on "Bile Duct Dilatation and Intraductal Pressure."

6. How long has the biliary tree been obstructed/dilated (acute—hours/days, or chronic—weeks/months)?

The sixth issue focuses on the duration of the cholestasis and has to be resolved in the context of the patient's history and laboratory work-up. Lacking any muscle layers, the walls of the bile ducts are quite thin, and therefore any pressure increase will result in immediate expansion of their diameter. In acute obstruction from calculi, e.g., impacted in the papilla of Vater, bile duct dilatation is the first detectable symptom (3.4g) and can be demonstrated several hours before any rise in the cholestatic enzymes.

Compensated chronic (weeks or months) obstruction in the intrahepatic or extrahepatic segments of the biliary tree (3.4g, i, q–u) can lead to bizarre bile duct dilatation (3.4o) and tortuosity.

7. Is there localized or diffuse thickening of the bile duct walls?

The seventh aspect to be considered in the differential diagnosis of cholestasis concerns the thickness of the bile duct walls. If the obstructed bile flow is accompanied by cholangitis, quite often thickening and layering can be demonstrated in the bile duct walls, in particular after successful relief by interventional endoscopy. Irregular wall thickening, with juxtaposed segmental narrowing and dilatation of the bile ducts, is characteristic of primary sclerosing cholangitis (PSC) (**Fig. 3.5**).

3.3 Parenchymatous Cholestasis

▶ Viral hepatitis, congested liver, portal vein thrombosis

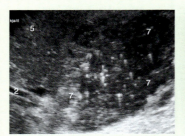
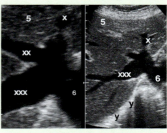

a Gallbladder, with a lot of sludge but little fluid and ill-defined wall (7), in acute hepatitis A. 2 = branch of the portal vein; 5 = liver.

b Congested liver (5). *Left:* with dilated inferior vena cava (6), and congested middle (xx) and right (xxx) hepatic vein. *Right:* same constellation, plus gas filled parts of the lung (y).

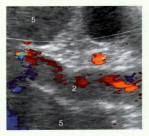
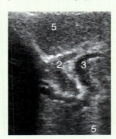

c Left: thrombosis of the portal vein (2); hepatic artery (3). *Right:* thrombosis of the intrahepatic portal veins (2) with concomitant dilatation of the intrahepatic bile ducts (3).

▶ Abscess, metastases

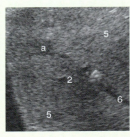
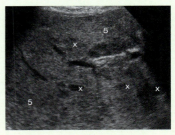

d Cholangitis with intrahepatic (5) abscess (a). 2 = branch of the portal vein; 6 = hepatic vein.

e Diffuse liver (5) metastases (x).

▶ Cirrhosis

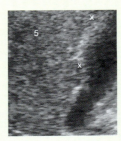
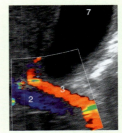

f Left: macronodular (x) cirrhosis of the liver (5). *Right:* rather pronounced hepatic artery (3) in known cirrhosis. 2 = portal vein.

3.3 Parenchymatous Cholestasis

▶ Cirrhosis

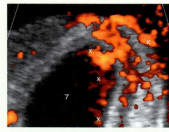 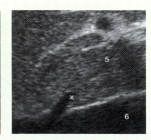

g Portal hypertension with convoluted varicosities (x) in the wall and lumen of the gallbladder (7).

h Segment I vein (x) of the caudate lobe (5). 6 = inferior vena cava.

▶ DD fluid-filled structures

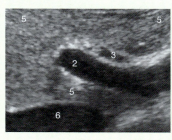 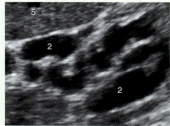 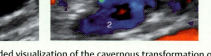

i Portal vein (2); variant course of the hepatic artery (3). 6 = inferior vena cava.

j B-mode image and color-coded visualization of the cavernous transformation of the portal vein (2).

3.4 The Diagnosis of "Sonographic Cholestasis"

▶ Bile duct dilatation: shape, location, degree, origin

Pancreas (4), liver (5), inferior vena cava (6), gallbladder (7)

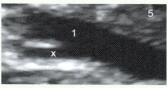 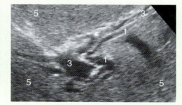 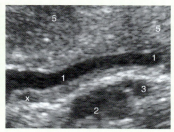

a Dilated CBD (1) with distended cystic duct (x).

b Characteristic "double-barrel shotgun" sign with intrahepatic branches of the bile ducts (1) and portal veins (3).

c Dilated prepancreatic CBD (1) with small (inflammatory?) lymph node (x). 2 = portal vein; 3 = hepatic artery.

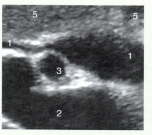 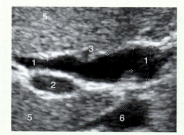 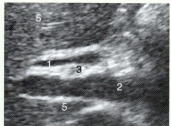

d Cholangiectasia with slender CBD (1) upstream and prepancreatic distension. 2 = portal vein; 3 = hepatic artery.

e Subjective morphological dilatation of the CBD (1) with various possible errors in measurement. 2 = portal vein; 3 = hepatic artery (variant position).

f Acutely congested CBD (1) (erroneously normal diameter on measurement). 2 = portal vein; 3 = hepatic artery.

3.4 The Diagnosis of "Sonographic Cholestasis"

▶ **Bile duct dilatation: shape, location, degree, origin**

Pancreas (4), liver (5), inferior vena cava (6), gallbladder (7)

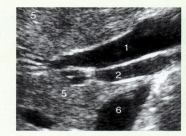

g Significantly (chronic) dilated intrahepatic and extrahepatic biliary tree (1). 2 = portal vein.

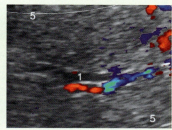

h Dilated intrahepatic bile duct (1).

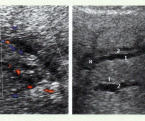

i Dilated intrahepatic bile ducts (1). *Left:* in CCC (confirmed by needle aspiration biopsy). *Right:* adjacent branches of the portal vein (2) in CCC (x).

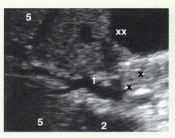

j Dilated intrahepatic and extrahepatic biliary tree (1) in stenosis (x) due to tumor (CCC?). 2 = portal vein; xx = liver cysts.

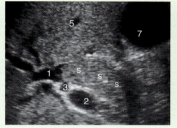

k Dilated intrahepatic and extrahepatic bile ducts (1) due to sludge (s) after extracorporeal shock-wave lithotripsy of a CBD gallstone. 2 = portal vein; 3 = hepatic artery.

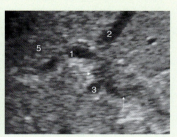

l Obstruction of the main right (1) and left (2) bile ducts (→) due to tumor, probably CCC. 3 = hepatic artery.

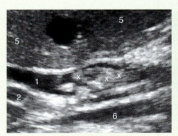

m Dilated CBD (1) due to fragmentation (x) of an intraductal calculus by extracorporeal shock wave lithotripsy. 2 = portal vein.

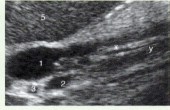

n Dilated CBD (1) due to nonfunctional stent; "anterior" (x) and "posterior" (y) wall of the stent. 2 = portal vein; 3 = hepatic artery.

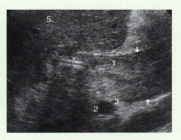

o Well-differentiated cholangiocarcinoma (initially biliary papillomatosis) with pronounced dilatation of the CBD (→ ←). 2 = portal vein; 3 = hepatic artery; x = biliary stent.

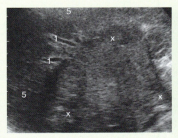

p Dilatation of the intrahepatic biliary ducts (1) in a large CCC (x).

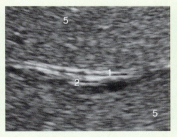

q Moderate "double-barrel shotgun sign" with dilatation of the intrahepatic bile ducts (1). 2 = branches of the portal vein.

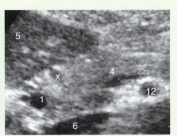

r Dilated intrahepatic CBD (1). 12 = superior mesenteric artery; x = gastroduodenal artery.

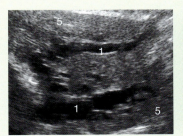

s Significant (chronic) dilatation of the intrahepatic bile ducts (1).

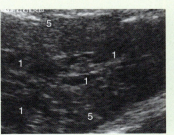

t Maximum dilatation of the intrahepatic biliary tree (1) with almost lacunar transformation.

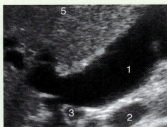

u Maximum (long-term chronic) dilatation of the CBD (1). 2 = portal vein; 3 = hepatic artery.

References

1. Akhan O, Demirkazik FB, Ozmen MN, Ariyurek M. Choledochal cyst: Ultrasonographic findings and correlation with other imaging modalities. Abdom Imaging 1994;19:243–7.
2. Baltazar U, Dunn J, Gonzalez-Dias S, Browder W. Agenesis of the gallbladder. South Med J 2000;93(9):914–5.
3. Bismuth H, Majno PE. Hepatobiliary surgery. J Hepatol 2000;32(1):208–24.
3a. Bismuth H, Nakache R, Diamont T. Management Strategies in Resection for hilar Cholangiocarcinoma. Ann Surg 1992;215:31–38.
4. Börsch G, Wedmann B, Brand J, Zumtobel V. The significance of preoperative and postoperative sonography for biliary tract surgery. Dtsch Med Wochenschr 1985;110(36):1359–64.
5. Braun U, Pospischil A, Pusterla N, Winder C. Ultrasonographic findings in cows with cholestasis. Vet Rec 1995;137(21):537–43.
6. Campbell WL, Ferris JV, Holbert BL, Thaete FL, Baron RL. Biliary tract carcinoma complicating primary sclerosing cholangitis: evaluation with CT, cholangiography, US and MR imaging. Radiology 1998;207(1):41–50.
7. Carlo I, Sauvanet A, Belghiti J. Intrahepatic lithiasis: a Western experience. Surg Today 2000;30(4):319–22.
8. Contractor QQ, Boujemla M, Contractor TQ, el-Essawy OM. Abnormal common bile duct sonography. The best predictor for choledocholithiasis before laparoscopic cholecystectomy. J Clin Gastroenterol 1997;25(2):429–32.
9. Gebel M, Wagner S, Meier P, Bleck J, Manns M. IDUS-Differentialdiagnose von Gallenwegsstenosen. Ultraschall in Med 1995;16:49.
10. Greiner L, Schulz HJ. Sonographie und Endoskopie bei Cholostase. Endoskopie heute 1999;12:24–8.
11. Greiner L, Münks C, Heil W, Jakobeit C. Gallbladder stone fragments in feces after biliary extracorporeal shock-wave lithotripsy. Gastroenterology 1990;98(6):1620–4.
12. Greiner L. Die Weite des D. hepatocholedochus bei Zustand nach Cholezystektomie: Ultraschalldiagnostik 84. Stuttgart: Thieme 1985; p. 448.
13. Greiner L. Sonographische Kontrollen nach endoskopischen Papillotomien sowie internen und externen Gallenwegsdrainagen. In: Riemann JF, Demling L (eds.). Endotherapie der Gallenwegserkrankungen. Stuttgart: Thieme 1985; p. 146–50.
14. Greiner L, Pilger HJ. Sonographische Kontrolle nach EPT, PTD und endoskopisch implantierten Gallenwegsprothesen. Leber Magen Darm 1983;13:113–6.
15. Greiner L, Prohm P. Differentiating sonographic diagnosis of cholelithiasis. An operation controlled study. Med Welt 1983;34(27):769–72.
16. Hou MF, Ker CG, Sheen PC, Chen ER. The ultrasound survey of gallstone diseases of patients infected with Clonorchis sinensis in southern Taiwan. J Trop Med Hyg 1989;92(2):108–11.
17. Iida F, Kajikawa S, Horigome N. Evaluation of imaging examination for hepatic invasion of carcinoma of the gallbladder and postoperative patient outcome. J Am Coll Surg 1995;180(1):72–6.
18. Ikematsu Y, Eto T, Tomioka T, Matsumoto T, Tsunoda T, Kanematsu T. Biliary diverticulum with pancreaticobiliary maljunction. Hepatogastroenterology 1994;41(1):70–2.
19. Jakobeit C, Greiner L. Ultrasonography and biliary extracorporeal shock-wave lithotripsy. J Clin Ultrasound 1993;21(4):251–64.
20. Jakobeit C, Rebensburg S, Greiner L. Sonographische Gallensteinmorphologie. Z Gastroenterol 1992;30:594–7.
21. Jansen S, Jorgensen J, Caplehorn J, Hunt D. Preoperative ultrasound to predict conversion in laparoscopic cholecystectomy. Surg Laparasc Endosc 1997;45(3):307–9.
22. Johanns W, Greiner L. Stellenwert der Farbdopplersonographie beim Budd-Chiari-Syndrom. Ultraschall 1995;16(1):43.
23. Khan AN, Wilson I, Sherlock DJ, De Krester D, Chisholm RA. Sonographic features of mucinous biliary papillomatosis: a case report and review of imaging findings. J Clin Ultrasound 1998;26(3):151–4.
24. Klatskin, G. Adenocarcinoma of the hepatic duct at its bifurcation within the porta hepatis: An unusual tumor with distinctive clinical and patholocial features. Am J Med 1965;38:241–56.
25. Kuo CM, Kuo CH, Changchien CS. Sequential sonographic changes of the gallbladder in hemobilia: case report patient with intrahepatic duct stones. Changgeng; Yi; Xue; Za; Zhi 1999;22(3):541–5.
26. Laing FC, Frates MC, Feldstein VA, Goldstein RB, Mondro S. Hemobilia: sonographic appearances in the gallbladder and biliary tree with emphasis on intracholecystic blood. J Ultrasound Med 1997;16(8):537–43.
27. Leopold GR. Ultrasonography of jaundice. Radiol Clin North Am 1979;17(1):127–36.
28. Miller WJ, Sechtin AG, Cambell WL, Pieters PC. Imaging findings in Caroli's disease. Am J Roentgenol 1995;165:333–7.
29. Naganuma S, Ishida H, Konno K et al. Sonographic findings of anomalous position of the gallbladder. Abdom Imaging 1998;23(1):67–72.
30. Pezzilli R, Billi P, Barakat B, Dimperio N, Miglio F. Ultrasonographic evaluation of the common bile duct in biliary acute pancreatitis patients: comparison with endoscopic retrograde cholangiopancreaticography. J Ultrasound Med 1999;18(6):391–4.
31. Rettenmeier G, Seitz KH. Ultrasonic diagnosis in jaundice. Dtsch Med Wochenschr 1977;102(43):1559–60.
32. Sharma MP, Ahuja V. Aetiological spectrum of obstructive jaundice and diagnostic ability of ultrasonography: a clinican's perspective. Trop gastroenterol 1999;20(4):167–9.
33. Wagner S, Maschek H, Meier PN, Nashan B, Manns MP. IDUS improves ERC in the diagnosis of bile duct stenosis. Dtsch Med Wochenschr 1998;123:291–5.
34. Wetter LA, Ring EJ, Pellegrini CA, Way LW. Differential diagnosis of sclerosing cholangiocarcinomas of the common hepatic duct (Klatskin tumors). Am J Surg 1991;161(1):57–63.
35. Whitaker AJ. Agenesis of the gallbladder: case report and review of the literature. J S C Med Assoc 1981;77(10):503–4.
36. Willi UV, Reddish JM, Teele RL. Cystic fibrosis: its characteristic appearance on abdominal sonography. Am J Roentgenol 1980;134(5):1005–10.

Gallbladder

Ch. Jakobeit

Anatomy

Size
- Length 10 cm and diameter 4 cm max., when fasting

Shape
- Quite variable (depends on the constitution of the patient; also numerous variants)
- Fasting: ovoid, pear-shaped
- Visualization of fundus, body, and neck

Wall thickness
- Fasting 2–4 mm
- Postprandial 4–8 mm
- Single-layered wall when fasting, triple-layered postprandially

The gallbladder is assessed according to criteria of location, size, shape, echogenicity, and intraluminal material.

Size. Since the size of the gallbladder depends on its filling volume and on stimulation by the possible presence of food, it should be measured in the fasting state. The most reliable measurement of the length is obtained in the longitudinal view at the edge of the liver (in inspiration), while the subcostal oblique view (also in inspiration) yields the best measurement for the diameter. In healthy adults, the normal size of the gallbladder is up to 10 cm in length and up to 4 cm in diameter. A postprandial study yields excellent results for gallbladder function: after stimulation the volume may be calculated as an ellipsoid of rotation: 0.5 × (length × width × height). The data for the volume measurements should be obtained 20, 40, and 60 minutes after stimulation by oral intake (**Fig. 3.29**).

Shape. The shape of the gallbladder depends on the filling volume and thus varies widely. Shape and contour of the gallbladder are closely tied to the constitution of the patient and the state of filling of the adjacent organs (e.g., the intestines). With the patient fasting, the gallbladder is most often visualized as an ovoid or pear-shaped organ. Ultrasound can delineate reasonably well the anatomical divisions into fundus, body, and infundibulum. The wall of the gallbladder can easily be demonstrated as a single-layered lamina with an approximate thickness of 2–4 mm (**Fig. 3.30**). Since the gallbladder does not possess any true histological tunica submucosa and tunica muscularis, the wall in the fasting gallbladder will appear as a single layer. Postprandial contraction alters the appearance of the gallbladder wall into triple-layering (hyperechoic inner, hypoechoic center, and hyperechoic outer layer), and the wall thickness may be up to 4–8 mm (**Fig. 3.31**).

Variant shapes (3.5). The shape of the gallbladder is intimately tied to its degree of filling. The most important criterion denoting a healthy gallbladder is a wall smoothly and clearly demarcated from the hepatic fossa as well as the lumen. In many instances, precise measurements of the wall can only be taken on the hepatic side. Changes in shape and contour may be focal (more frequent) or diffuse. Position-induced foldover (**3.5a**) will recede when being checked with the patient in a different position or while standing and can therefore be separated from true septation (**3.5b–e**). Most true septa are found in the neck and fundus, and the caplike septation in the latter is called "Phrygian cap" (**3.5f**).

This region may be difficult to assess because of the proximity of the intestines. A subtle ultrasound study employing views of different orientation (during inspiration and after patient repositioning) is vital if any calculi hidden here are to be demonstrated. Tortuous or corkscrew-like gallbladders are known congenital variants. Multiple septa of the gallbladder are infrequent findings, and so are diverticula and doubling (**3.5g–i**).

Cystic duct. Demonstration of the cystic duct is easiest during deep inspiration (supine or left lateral decubitus). With subtle shifts of the probe, the cystic duct is visualized beginning from the infundibulum of the gallbladder. The distal segment of the cystic duct, most often joining the hepatic duct at the posterior aspect, is best demonstrated (by compression technique) with the patient supine in the plane through the hepatic portal, where it is anterior to the portal vein. The cuspidal junctional folds primarily found at the infundibulum are without pathology and are known as the spiral valve of Heister (**Fig. 3.32**).

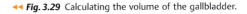

◂◂ **Fig. 3.29** Calculating the volume of the gallbladder.

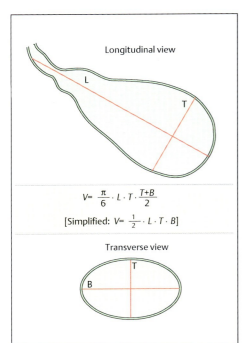

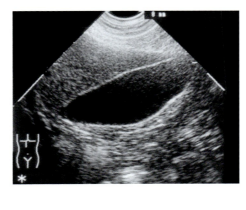

◂ **Fig. 3.30** Longitudinal section through a typical gallbladder in the fasting state. The wall is well demarcated from the liver as a 2 mm single-layered lamina.

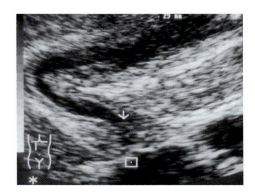
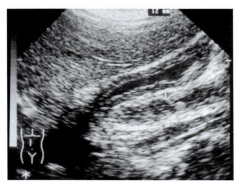

◄◄ **Fig. 3.31** Contracted gallbladder.
a Characteristic postprandial visualization.

◄ **b** Checking the gallbladder function (after oral intake). Very well contracted, triple-layered postprandial wall, clearly demarcated from the liver and the lumen.

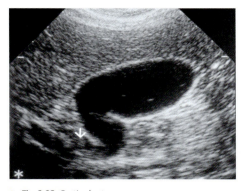
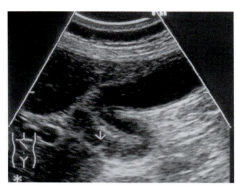
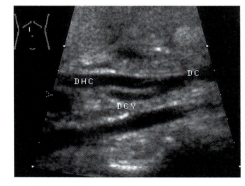

▲ **Fig. 3.32** Cystic duct.
a Spiral valve of Heister at the junctional segment of the cystic duct origin.

▲ **b** Optimized visualization of the cystic duct with the spiral valve of Heister.

▲ **c** Junction of the cystic duct at the posterior aspect of the common hepatic duct. DHC = common hepatic duct; DC = distal bile duct; DCY = cystic duct.

Topography

When looking for the gallbladder, useful landmarks are the hepatic portal and the edge of the right hepatic lobe (paramedian view) (**Figs. 3.33 and 3.34**). During deep inspiration the gallbladder may easily be demonstrated anterior to the vena cava (the probe being tilted somewhat to the median plane). In the subcostal oblique view the landmark structure to be used is the interlobar fissure, which can be visualized in almost all patients, and the gallbladder will be found by aligning the probe with the fissure and then tilting it caudad. The gallbladder will be located inferior or lateral to the fissure (between liver segments IV and V).

Landmark structures
► In the paramedian view: hepatic portal and the edge of the right hepatic lobe
► In the subcostal oblique view: interlobar fissure

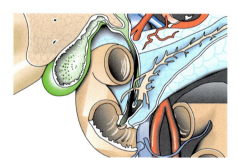
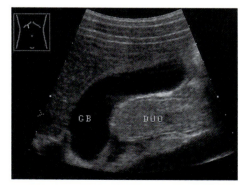
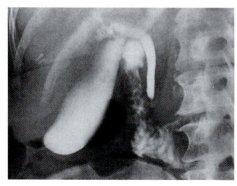

▲ **Fig. 3.33** Schematic illustration of the relationship between the gallbladder and its adjacent organs.

▲ **Fig. 3.34** Relationship of the gallbladder (GB) to the duodenum.
a The posterior wall of the body of the gallbladder is indented by the distended atonic duodenal bulb (DUO).

▲ **b** ERCP image of the bile duct, gallbladder, and duodenum. The longitudinal axis of the gallbladder is directed inferiorly and slightly to the right.

3.5 Variant Shapes of the Gallbladder

▶ Septations, kinking

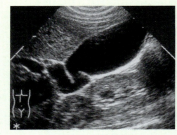 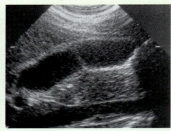

a Foldover (pseudo-septation): in supine position a seeming septation in the body is seen as a normal body demonstration in a left lateral decubitus position.

b and c True septation: even after repositioning into left lateral decubitus, the septum in the neck of the gallbladder persists.

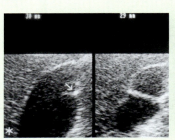 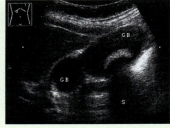 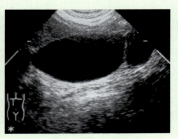

d Furrow: when supine (right), a seeming septum in the body, which recedes almost completely in left lateral decubitus position (left); now, only a slight furrow (arrow) with pseudoseptum remains.

e Septation of the gallbladder. Longitudinal scan through the upper abdomen shows an echogenic ridge (arrow) dividing the gallbladder (GB) into two incomplete compartments. Septation makes the gallbladder prone to lithiasis, as in this case. D = duodenum.

f Phrygian cap.

▶ Torsion, malformation, doubling

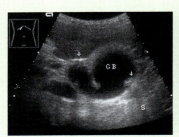 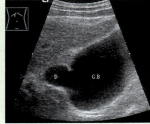

g Torsion and lateral displacement of the gallbladder (GB); stones (arrows). S = acoustic shadow (harmonic imaging).

h Diverticula (D). GB = gallbladder.

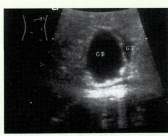 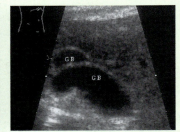

i Duplicated gallbladder (GB). Longitudinal scan: longitudinal septation.

Transverse scan: gallbladder (GB) is completely divided in two. The small second gallbladder has a separate duct (arrows, left).

Changes in Size

Large Gallbladder (> 10 cm)

Biliary Tree
- ▼ Changes in Size
  - ▶ Large Gallbladder
    - ▶ Asymptomatic (Functional)
    - ▶ Asymptomatic (Pathological)
    - ▶ Symptomatic (Pathological)
  - ▶ Small/Missing Gallbladder
- ▶ Wall Changes
- ▶ Intraluminal Changes
- ▶ Nonvisualized Gallbladder

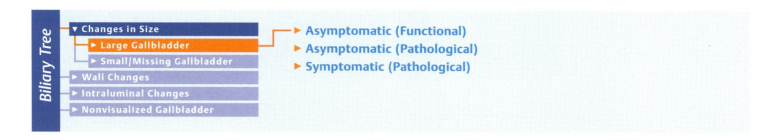

▶ Asymptomatic (Functional)

A large flaccid gallbladder with normal wall (and a large volume of fluid) may be demonstrated as a variant in the asthenic patient or as an atonic sequel of long-term total parenteral nutrition **(Fig. 3.35)**. Long periods of fasting may also result in a large, functionally flaccid gallbladder, not infrequently with intraluminal sludge (viscous bile or microliths) **(Fig. 3.36a)**. Passing, and in case of permanent dysfunction of the gallbladder even persistent, sludge formation may be demonstrated in patients with atonic/hypotonic gallbladder function after abdominal surgery as well as in abdominal disorders accompanied by various organ dysfunctions (e.g., GI tract infection, hepatitis, pancreatitis, peritonitis, ileus). Metabolic disorders with abdominal manifestation (for instance, diabetes mellitus, polyneuropathy) may also effect large atonic gallbladders with or without sludge **(Fig. 3.36b)**. In contrast to inflammatory gallbladder disease, here the gallbladder does not exhibit any tenderness on palpation (negative ultrasonic Murphy's sign), and on ultrasound the wall appears normal. Another important criterion for differentiation from cholecystitis is the lack of tense gallbladder distension (hydrops).

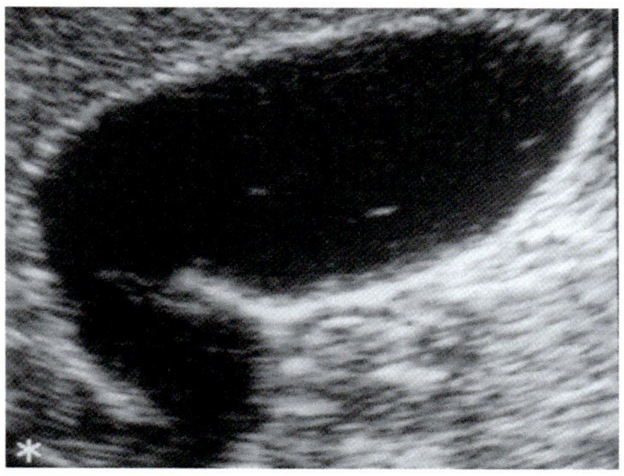

▲ ***Fig. 3.35*** Large flaccid gallbladder (congenital variant). Characteristic: normal wall and texture, anechoic intraluminal material.

▲ ***Fig. 3.36*** Flaccid gallbladder.
a After parenteral nutrition: normal wall, possibly intraluminal sludge.

▲ ***b*** Flaccid gallbladder in diabetes mellitus with concurrent polyneuropathy. Afunctional gallbladder filled with sludge ("hepatized gallbladder").

▶ Asymptomatic (Pathological)

The large still-functional gallbladder has to be differentiated from the large pathological specimen. Gallbladder size alone is insufficient to differentiate between dysfunction and pathological outflow obstruction. One such classic criterion in this differential diagnosis is the tense distension of the gallbladder, or hydrops. The nature of the outflow obstruction (obstruction of the cystic duct due to, e.g., calculus or tumor of the cystic duct, CBD, or pancreas) with enlarged palpable hydropic gallbladder (Courvoisier's sign) can be differentiated by subtle ultrasound study (**Figs. 3.37 and 3.38**). For optimum visualization of the cystic duct the patient should be supine, while the proximal CBD is best demonstrated in the left lateral decubitus position.

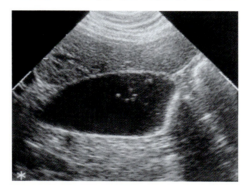

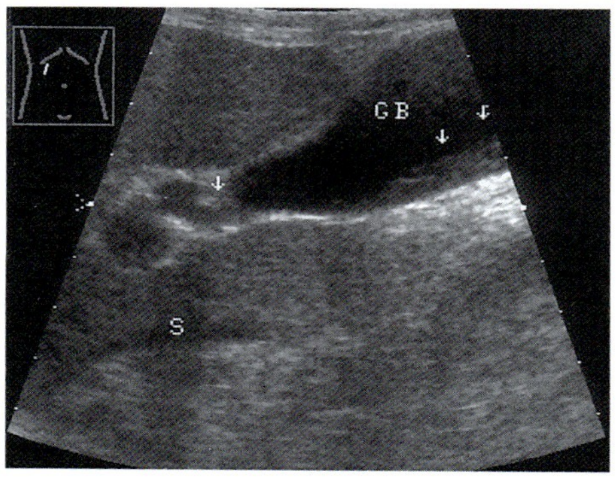

▲ ***Fig. 3.37*** Hydropic gallbladder (GB) (with dependent sedimentation; S hepatic artery) in cystic duct obstruction. Gallbladder wall normal.

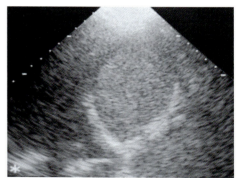

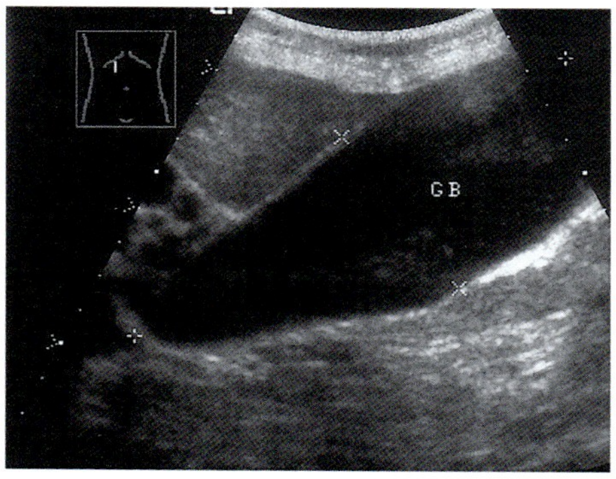

▲ ***Fig. 3.38*** Gallbladder hydrops associated with a tumor of the pancreatic head/common bile duct. The Courvoisier's sign is typical: palpable, tense, nontender gallbladder.

▶ Symptomatic (Pathological)

Symptomatic hydrops of the gallbladder is one of the main criteria in cystic duct obstruction due to gallstones and is characterized by a tensely distended gallbladder tender on palpation. In the early phase of acute calculous cystic duct obstruction, the concurrent cholecystitis may not be manifest (**Fig. 3.39**). However, the classic case does exhibit the combination of cholecystolithiasis and cholecystitis (**Fig. 3.40**). The sonographic Murphy's sign (gallbladder tender on palpation under ultrasonic guidance during inspiration) is quite characteristic. After oral intake the gallbladder does not contract.

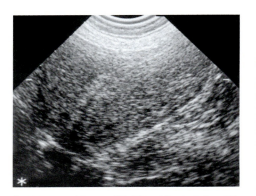

▲ **Fig. 3.39** Hydropic gallbladder without cholecystitis in calculous obstruction of the cystic duct/CBD.
a Major criterion of floating gallstone with intermittent impaction, no wall thickening.

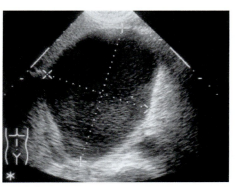

▲ **b** Calculus obstructing the cystic duct not visible; normal gallbladder wall, gallbladder tensely distended, round, tender on palpation, partially filled with sludge.

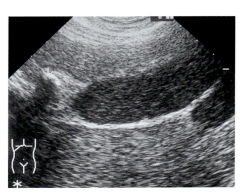

▲ **Fig. 3.40** Hydropic gallbladder with cholecystitis in cholecystolithiasis/cholangiolithiasis. Typical sonographic Murphy's sign: distended gallbladder tender on ultrasound guided palpation.

Small/Missing Gallbladder

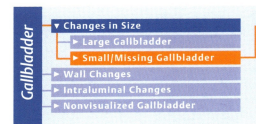

▶ Asymptomatic (Functional)

Agenesis of the gallbladder is an extremely rare finding (< 0.1%) (**Fig. 3.41 a**). Congenital hypoplasia of the gallbladder is also rather rare. If agenesis of the gallbladder is suspected, one should assiduously look for a dystopic gallbladder (e.g., an atypical intrahepatic gallbladder or one hyperextending all the way into the minor pelvis). A completely empty postprandial (or intrahepatic gallbladder) may also be quite hard to visualize (cf. "Nonvisualized Gallbladder," p. 137 ff). A gallbladder completely void of fluid is characterized by homogeneous triple-layering of the wall (**Fig. 3.41 b**).

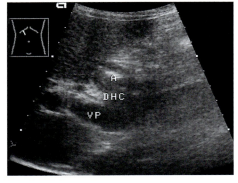

▲ **Fig. 3.41 a** Agenesis of the gallbladder. Previous ultrasound and CT studies diagnosed an atrophic gallbladder; surgery demonstrated agenesis of the gallbladder. A = antrum, DHC = common bile duct, VP = portal vein.

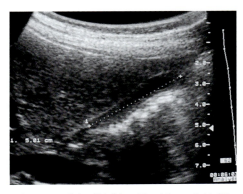

▲ **b** Postprandial gallbladder with minimum fluid. After oral intake the gallbladder may be void of any fluid. This state is characterized by a smooth wall echo with homogeneous triple-layered foldover.

▶ Asymptomatic (Pathological)

The postprandial contracted gallbladder should be differentiated from the asymptomatic cystic duct obstruction with a gallbladder persistently void of any fluid (**Fig. 3.42**).

Gallbladders with low fluid levels and concurrent wall edema are found in severe nonbiliary disorders (**Table 3.1**). They are characterized by a diffuse swelling in the wall, sometimes more pronounced in the fundus, which is hypoechoic or mixed hypoechoic and hyperechoic, and cleanly demarcated from the lumen as well as the outside. If these criteria are demonstrated, the ultrasound study should concentrate on the underlying disease; typical examples are cirrhosis of the liver, right-sided heart failure, acute hepatitis, or severe renal failure. Severe hepatic dysfunction with insufficient secretion of the bile (e.g., in cirrhosis) may decrease the filling volume of the gallbladder and result in wall edema due to hypoalbuminemia (**Fig. 3.43**). Inflammatory lymph nodes along the hepatoduodenal ligament are frequent findings in acute chronic hepatitis. Hypoechoic increases in the wall thickness accompanied by loss of fluid are characteristic for the severe hypoalbuminemia in renal failure or intestinal protein loss as well as for massive chronic cardiac congestion. In these cases hepatomegaly is another regular finding.

Table 3.1 **Gallbladder changes in nonbiliary disorders**

	Right-sided heart failure	*Cirrhosis of the liver*	*Severe malabsorption*	*Acute hepatitis*
Size	Normal or enlarged	More likely small	Normal or enlarged	More likely small
Shape	Normal or little fluid	Normal or little fluid	Smooth or rippled	Ovoid, little fluid
Wall	Smooth hypoechoic wall thickening	Smooth hypoechoic wall thickening, possibly varicose veins	Wall thickening of mixed echogenicity	Smooth hypo- or hyperechoic wall thickening
Surroundings	Signs of cardiac congestion	Ascites	Edema of the intestinal wall	Lymph nodes

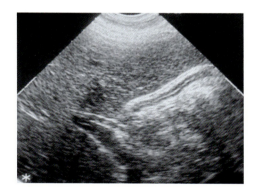

▲ **Fig. 3.42** Completely folded-over gallbladder wall (without calculus); the underlying gallstone obstructing the cystic duct is not depicted in this image.

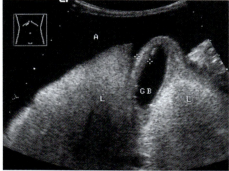

▲ **Fig. 3.43** Gallbladder with little fluid and edema of the wall in cirrhosis of the liver with dysproteinemia. In nonbiliary disorders the hypoechoic increase in wall thickness with decreased fluid level is a typical phenomenon.

▶ Symptomatic (Pathological)

Most fasting gallbladders with low or no fluid levels result from cystic duct obstruction (**Fig. 3.42**).

Inflammatory atrophy of the gallbladder with its lack of fluid is usually caused by chronic cholecystitis, where the shape of the gallbladder is irregular and its wall thickened and inhomogeneous (hyperechoic) (**Figs. 3.44 and 3.45**). During acute exacerbation, hypoechoic areas in the wall may also be visualized. A typical finding would be several, sometimes even encrusted, intraluminal gallstones. In the end the atrophic gallbladder can only be identified by the encrusted calculi within the scar tissue.

This contracted gallbladder with its gallstones is characterized by a crescent-shaped band of echoes without demonstration of the posterior wall. Sometimes even the anterior wall with its scar contraction may hardly be delimited from the gallstone echoes (**Fig. 3.45**). In these patients, differentiation of a possible concurrent gallbladder carcinoma can be problematic. The differential diagnosis should include rare causes such as radiation injuries and traumatic lesions (**Fig. 3.45 a–c**).

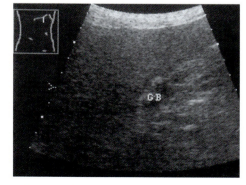

▲ **Fig. 3.44** Inflammatory atrophic gallbladder. Atrophied gallbladder (GB) void of any fluid.

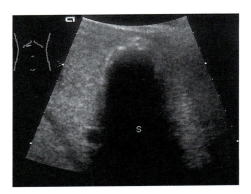

◄ **Fig. 3.45 a** Calculous atrophied gallbladder. The atrophied gallbladder is visualized as a crescent-shaped band of echoes in the hepatic fossa with ill-defined contour of the anterior wall. Usually, the posterior wall cannot be demonstrated due to posterior shadowing (S) of the gallstones.

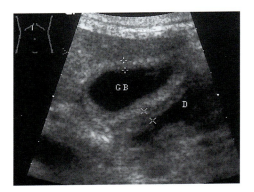
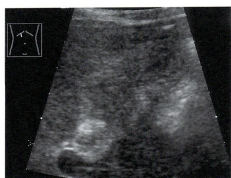
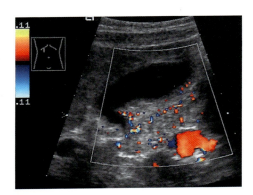

▲ **b and c** Gallbladder with wall thickening and scant fluid.
b Radiogenic wall thickening (cursors) of the gallbladder (GB) and duodenum (D) after radiotherapy for pancreatic head carcinoma.

▲ **c** Traumatic gallbladder contusion: massive wall edema effacing the lumen.

▲ **d** Traumatic wall thickening (with initial obstruction of the lumen) as part of a contusion; sparse vascularization in color-flow Doppler scanning.

Wall Changes

General Hypoechogenicity

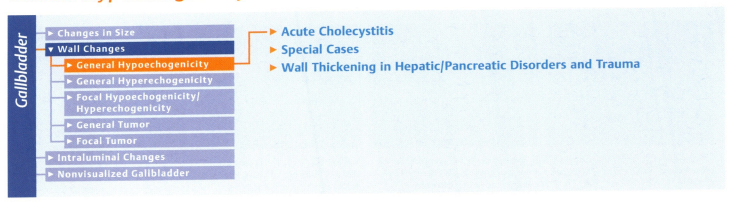

▶ Acute Cholecystitis

Acute and chronic cholecystitis is characterized by uneven thickening of the gallbladder wall with irregular echo pattern. The typical finding in acute cholecystitis is the tensely distended afunctional/dysfunctional gallbladder with its hypoechoic wall that is tender on palpation (positive Murphy's sign). Another sign is the ill-defined intraluminal and extraluminal contour of the wall, accompanied by hypoechoic inflammation of the surrounding tissue (pericholecystitis). Ultrasound morphology of the gallbladder wall spans the spectrum from diffuse hypoechoic thickening with poorly delimited contour of the wall through hypoechoic necrosis all the way to complete destruction of the wall (◧ 3.6a, b; see Table 3.2). Intraluminal hyperechoic or inhomogeneously echogenic material can point the way to the diagnosis of cholecystic empyema.

Advanced and severe courses of acute cholecystitis may result in necrosis of the mucosa and filiform detachment of the tunica mucosa (◧ 3.6d). Usually, these cases present with hyperechoic inhomogeneous necrotic debris within the gallbladder. A pericholecystic film is typical of localized perforation (◧ 3.6c and d). Lacelike structures with hypoechoic necrotic areas are infrequent findings.

Imminent perforation may be preceded by ascites, ulcers of the gallbladder wall, or pericholecystic infiltrates/abscesses (◧ 3.6e). Hypervascularization of the gallbladder wall in color-flow duplex scanning of cholecystitis is by no means mandatory. The histological grading of edematous, phlegmonous, and gangrenous cholecystitis cannot be differentiated all that well by ultrasound.

Special Cases

Emphysematous cholecystitis. The characteristic sign of emphysematous cholecystitis is intraluminal and intramural gas (from infection by gas-producing pathogens) (◻ **3.6f and g**).

Acalculous and xanthogranulomatous cholecystitis. Other special cases are acalculous (◻ **3.6h**) and xanthogranulomatous (◻ **3.6i and j**) cholecystitis. Acalculous cholecystitis is a typical disorder in the immune-compromised patient in the intensive care unit or after chemotherapy. It is characterized by a gallbladder that is tender on palpation, with edema of the wall and possible sludge. In large hydropic gallbladders, ultrasound may only demonstrate slight thickening of the wall despite the presence of phlegmon. Xanthogranulomatous cholecystitis, on the other hand, is characterized by pseudotumorous thickening of the wall with loss of the usual layering. This entity is almost impossible to differentiate from gallbladder carcinoma on the basis of sonographic morphology alone.

Table 3.2 Differentiating cholecystitis

	Acute cholecystitis	Chronic cholecystitis
Size	Large	Normal or atrophied
Shape	Irregular	Round
Echogenicity	Hypoechoic—layered	Hyperechoic
Lumen	Large, calculi	Small or lacking
Wall	Thickened	Thickened

◻ 3.6 Acute Cholecystitis: Complications and Special Cases

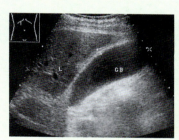

a Acute cholecystitis. Hypoechoic rim around the gallbladder (GB, cursors). L = liver. Positive Murphy's sign.

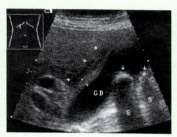

b Acute phlegmonous cholecystitis in cholecystolithiasis (vertical arrows, acoustic shadow S). Laminar wall thickening (cursors) with edema in the gallbladder bed of the liver (horizontal arrows). GB = gallbladder.

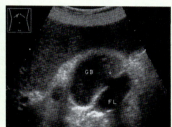

d Perforated gallbladder, gallbladder empyema (GB). Harmonic imaging. The perforation site (arrows) is clearly defined. FL = perivesicular biliary fluid. Upper abdominal longitudinal scan.

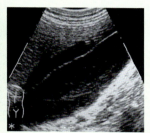

e Perforated gallbladder: phlegmonous gallbladder with filiform desquamation and extensive pericholecystic intraperitoneal fluid (bile).

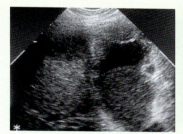

f Empyema of the gallbladder with extensive cholecystitis and pericholecystic abscess.

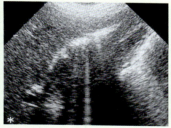

g Emphysematous cholecystitis: extensive intramural gas collection in emphysematous cholecystitis.

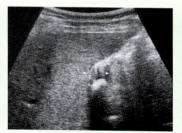

h Emphysematous cholecystitis with mild gas formation: difficult study conditions may render the diagnosis more problematic (image courtesy of Dr. WB Stelzel, Frankfurt, Germany).

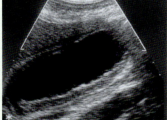

i Acalculous cholecystitis in an ICU patient with total parenteral nutrition: gallbladder tender on palpation, with or without sludge and wall edema.

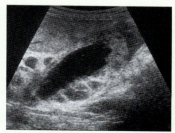

i and j Xanthogranulomatous cholecystitis: rare special case with tumorlike thickening of the gallbladder wall and complete loss of normal wall layering (image courtesy of Dr. WB Stelzel, Frankfurt, Germany).

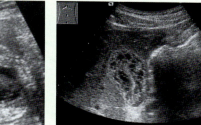

k Intensive complex thickening of the gallbladder wall without fluid in acute hepatitis and AIDS

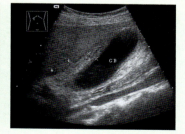

l Concurrent inflammatory wall thickening in an acute episode of chronic pancreatitis; perihepatic fluid film (arrows); surgery did not yield any gallstones.

Wall Thickening in Hepatic/Pancreatic Disorders and Trauma

The differential diagnosis of cholecystic wall changes has to include not only calculous cholecystitis but also wall thickening secondary to acute hepatitis, decompensated cirrhosis of the liver, and acute episodes of (chronic) pancreatitis (**3.6k, l**).

General Hyperechogenicity

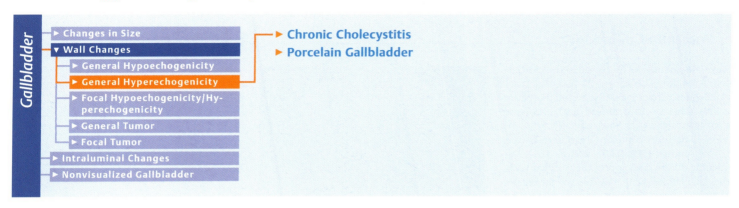

Chronic Cholecystitis

Chronic cholecystitis is accompanied by hyperechoic thickening of the gallbladder wall, spanning the gamut from barely noticeable to pronounced callous thickening. After oral intake these gallbladders present as dysfunctional or even afunctional organs. In the early stages of chronic inflammation the luminal wall displays not only areas of scarred hyperechoic thickening but also acutely inflamed (hypoechoic) lesions of the mucosa. The terminal stage of chronic scarred cholecystitis is characterized by extensive callous (hyperechoic) thickening of the wall with complete loss of layering. The differentiation between acute and chronic cholecystitis is listed in **Table 3.2**.

Mirizzi syndrome. If the inflammatory changes induced by a stone impacted in the neck of the gallbladder spread beyond the border of the gallbladder onto the hepatic portal, leading to obstruction of the CBD, this may result in Mirizzi syndrome (**Fig. 3.46**).

Cholelithic gallbladder perforation. Spontaneous perforation of calculi into the gastrointestinal tract is a rare complication of chronic cholecystitis. Fecal studies have demonstrated spontaneous passage of stones up to 5.7 cm in diameter. Most often the stones perforate from the gallbladder into the duodenum (52%); perforation into the stomach occurs rather infrequently (approx. 3%), while the remainder of the GI tract is affected in 45% of cases. The ultrasound signs of a perforated stone are its atypical anatomical location, gas echoes (pneumobilia) (**Table 3.4**) within the lumen of the gallbladder (may not be present in case of fistulas), demonstration of a fistula, and atrophic gallbladder with visualization of calculi (**Figs. 3.47 and 3.48**).

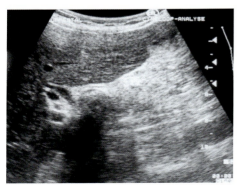

▲ **Fig. 3.46** Mirizzi syndrome: calculus impacted in the neck of the gallbladder, with adjacent inflammation and dilatation of the CBD.

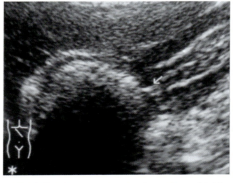

▲ **Fig. 3.47** Gallstone perforation from the gallbladder into the gastric antrum.
a Barrel-shaped gallstone impacted in a fistula (arrow) between gallbladder and gastric antrum.

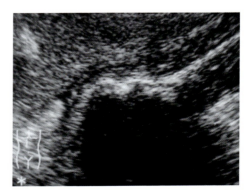

▲ **b** Successful disintegration of the calculus into multiple fragments after extracorporeal shock-wave lithotripsy

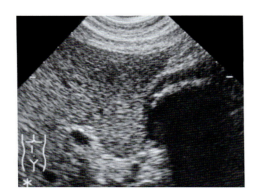
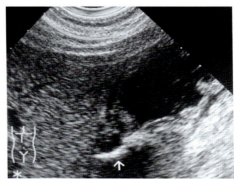

◀◀ **Fig. 3.48** Cholecystoduodenal gallstone perforation.
a Barrel-shaped gallstone impacted in the duodenal bulb after perforation through the gallbladder wall.

◀ **b** Successful shock-wave lithotripsy with spontaneous passage of the fragments, now with demonstration of a wide hyperechoic fistula (arrow) between the atrophied gallbladder and the duodenal bulb (fluid-filled gastric antrum).

▶ Porcelain Gallbladder

Porcelain gallbladder is considered a precancerous condition because in 10–60% of all cases gallbladder carcinoma will develop. Porcelain gallbladder is characterized by intramural shell-like calcification that may affect the entire wall or (more commonly) just parts of it (e.g., the fundus) (**Figs. 3.49 a and b, 3.51**). Depending on the thickness of the calcified layer, the gallbladder wall may be sonolucent. In cases of severe calcification, any ultrasound differentiation of possible malignancy may prove to be infeasible. In the diffuse type there is complete calcification of the gallbladder wall, which may not be penetrated by the ultrasound beam in severe cases. If porcelain gallbladder is suspected, a plain film of the gallbladder should be obtained (**Fig. 3.49 b**).

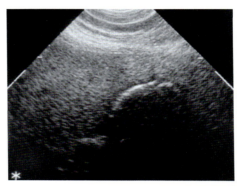

▲ **Fig. 3.49 a** Classic diffuse porcelain gallbladder: visualization of a broad calcified intramural crescent.

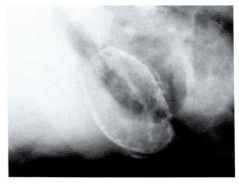

▲ **b** Plain film of the gallbladder: typical radiographic image of diffuse porcelain gallbladder.

Focal Hypoechogenicity/Hyperechogenicity

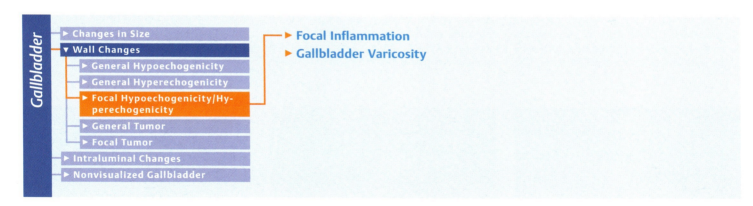

▶ Focal Inflammation

Based on the morphology of the outflow obstruction in gallbladder anomalies, the inflammatory changes of the gallbladder wall may be focal (e.g., inflammation of the fundus in Phrygian cap). The sonographic morphology of focal inflammatory lesions resembles that of the diffuse changes (**Fig. 3.50**). Just as in diffuse calcification, focal calcium deposits are classified as porcelain gallbladders (see above) (**Fig. 3.51**). Cholecystitis in focal porcelain gallbladder may be hard to differentiate.

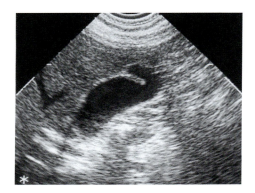
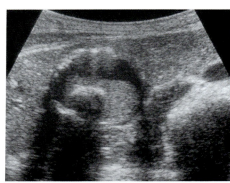

◄◄ **Fig. 3.50** Focal cholecystitis (in Phrygian cap).

◄ **Fig. 3.51** Porcelain gallbladder with sonolucent wall: fine focal calcification of the fundus wall with translucent lumen of the gallbladder and identifiable cholecystolithiasis (with sludge) (image courtesy of Dr. WB Stelzel, Frankfurt, Germany).

▶ Gallbladder Varicosity

When hypoechoic tubular intramural and extramural changes in the gallbladder wall are encountered, the differential diagnosis should include varicosity (**Fig. 3.52 and Fig. 1.99b, p. 44**). It is characteristic of portal hypertension (in prehepatic or posthepatic block). The suspected diagnosis is confirmed by color-flow duplex scanning (**Table 3.3**). This modality is also important in preoperative delineation of vascular anomalies. Its application in the differentiation of a benign polypoid mass (perfusion of the stalk in adenomas) from a malignancy is still experimental (**Table 3.3**).

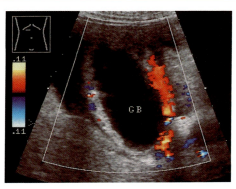
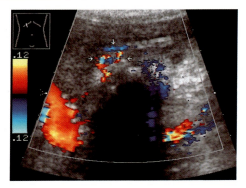

▲ **Fig. 3.52** Thickening of the gallbladder wall.
a Portal venous collaterals in the gallbladder wall.

▲ *b* Thickened gallbladder wall in cholecystolithiasis. Stone shadow, with wall above thickened to 8 mm. Color duplex scan shows aberrant spotlike tumor vessels (arrows). Operative treatment. Histology: carcinoma.

Table 3.3 Color-flow duplex scanning in gallbladder disease

- ▶ Vascular anomalies in the hepatoduodenal ligament before surgery
- ▶ Varicosity of the gallbladder wall
- ▶ Perfusion of the polyp stalk (experimental)
- ▶ Vascularization of tumors (experimental)

General Tumor

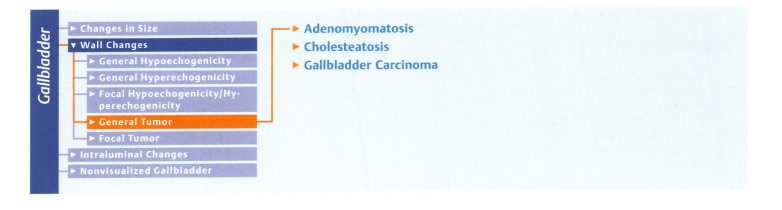

▶ Adenomyomatosis

Adenomyomatosis is a special case of gallbladder cholesteatosis and belongs to the group of hyperplastic cholecystoses. It appears as a hyperechoic tumorous thickening of the wall (generalized or focal), originating from hypertrophied Rokitansky–Aschoff sinuses. This disorder is characterized by coexistent cholesterol deposits (with their typical comet-tail like artifacts) and cystic intramural inclusions (**Fig. 3.53, Table 3.4**).

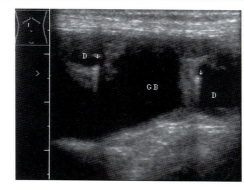

Fig. 3.53 Adenomyomatosis: typical comet-tail pattern (arrows) caused by cholesterol deposits. Wall thickening and large pseudodiverticula (D). GB = gallbladder.

Table 3.4 Comet-tail–like artefacts in gallbladder ultrasound

	Emphysematous cholecystitis	**Cholesteatosis**	**Adenomyomatosis**	**Microliths**	**Pneumobilia**
Size	Large	Normal	Normal or smaller	Normal	Normal
Shape	Round	Normal	Hourglass furrows	Normal	Normal
Lumen	Sludge	Normal	Constricted	Floating (calculi < 5 mm)	Normal
Wall	Hypoechoic wall thickening	Often normal or slightly thickened	Hyperechoic, thickened, cystic inclusions	Normal	Normal
Comet-tail–like artifacts	Intramural or intraluminal gas collections	Intramural, partly few, partly diffuse	Localized, intramural or diffuse	Floating in the lumen	Position-dependent gas collections at the anterior wall

▶ Cholesteatosis

Adenomyomatosis should be differentiated from cholesteatosis (strawberry gallbladder), which is also characterized by numerous comet-tail–like artifacts but mostly without the wall thickening (**Fig. 3.54**).

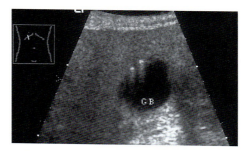

▲ **Fig. 3.54 a** Cholesteatosis ("strawberry gallbladder"): classic intramural hyperechoic "spotted" echoes with comet-tail–like artifacts. GB = gallbladder.

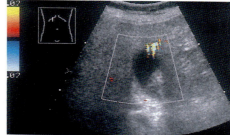

▲ **b** Twinkling artifact in the region of comet-tail artifacts.

▶ Gallbladder Carcinoma

General adenomyomatosis should also be differentiated from diffuse infiltrating gallbladder carcinoma, although the latter completely destroys the regular wall layering (**see Fig. 3.63**). Gallbladder carcinoma lacks the Rokitansky–Aschoff sinuses and intramural comet-tail–like artifacts.

Focal Tumor

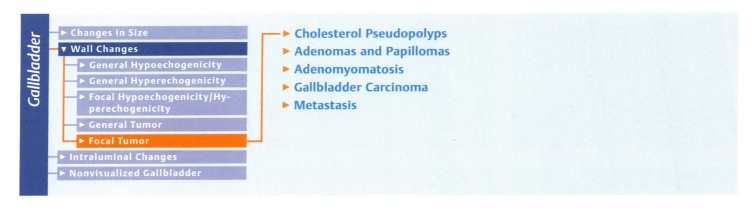

In order of frequency, focal changes in the gallbladder wall are mural polypoid lesions, partial wall thickening, and infiltrating lesions.

▶ Cholesterol Pseudopolyps

Cholesterol pseudopolyps are the most frequently demonstrated. They are hyperplastic polypoid neoplasms, usually hyperechoic, smoothly contoured, round or ovoid. Sometimes they are visualized as small hyperplastic (often hyperechoic) tumors, pendulating from the gallbladder wall, that may display a short stalk (hypoechoic lobulation is rather rare). Usually, their size is less than 6 mm and they are found in multiples (**Figs. 3.55–3.57**). The gallbladder wall always appears normal. Cholesterol polyps measuring more than 1 cm in diameter are the exception and therefore should undergo surgery.

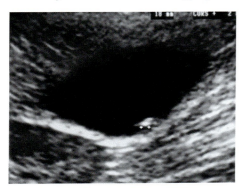

▲ **Fig. 3.55** Cholesterol pseudopolyp: characteristic visualization of a hyperechoic 5 mm cholesterol pseudopolyp at the floor of the gallbladder.

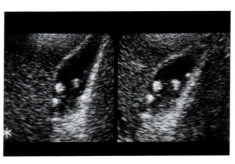

▲ **Fig. 3.56** Cholesterol pseudopolyps. Multiple small sessile hyperechoic polyps of 3–5 mm at the gallbladder wall (some with longer stalks).

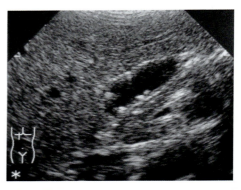

▲ **Fig. 3.57** Characteristic sonographic morphology of five hyperechoic cholesterol pseudopolyps of less than 5 mm diameter.

▶ Adenomas and Papillomas

Adenomas. Compared with the more common cholesterol pseudopolyps (> 1% of the population) adenomas are infrequent findings (**Figs. 3.58–3.60**). Usually, they are hypoechoic sessile structures resting on the intraluminal wall and are frequently found in the neck of the gallbladder. Their size is mostly > 10 mm. Because of the known adenoma → carcinoma sequence they have to undergo surgery.

Papillomas. The differentiation of adenomas from papillomas relies on the fact that papillomas tend to be pedunculated, displaying a lobulated surface. Papillomas tend to be located at the fundus and usually are hypoechoic (**Fig. 3.61, Table 3.5**). All polyps are easily differentiated from calculi by their sessile growth, although sometimes viscous pseudopolypoid sludge may mimic a polyp.

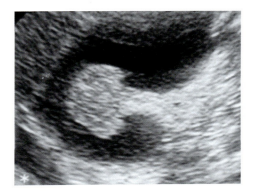

◀ **Fig. 3.58** Pedunculated adenoma of about 2 cm (confirmed histologically) in the body of the gallbladder.

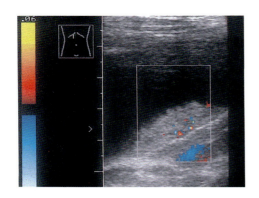 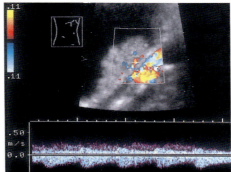

◀◀ **Fig. 3.59 a** Sessile adenoma: sessile adenoma of about 2 cm diameter in the body of the gallbladder.

◀ **b** On spectral analysis, the color-flow signals can definitely be assigned to vessels, ruling out a tumor or sludge.

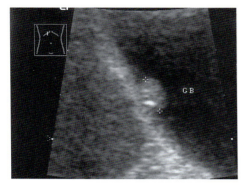 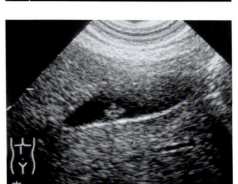 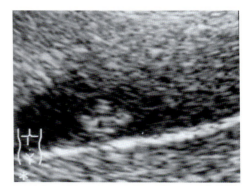

▲ **Fig. 3.60** Polypoid adenoma (cursors). Intact wall, no detectable invasion. GB = gallbladder.

▲ **Fig. 3.61** Papilloma.
a Lobulated papilloma of the body of the gallbladder with a diameter of about 1.2 cm.

▲ **b** Zoomed detail.

Table 3.5 **Focal intraluminal polypoid wall changes**

	Cholesterol pseudopolyp	Adenoma	Papilloma	Carcinoma
Size	Often 2–6 mm and multiple, rarely > 8 mm	Solitary, often > 1 cm	Solitary, > 7 mm	Solitary, > 1–2 cm
Shape	Mostly round, sometimes bizarre, short stalk	Sessile, polypoid, or superficial	Lobulated	Polypoid
Echogenicity	Mostly rather hyperechoic	Usually hyperechoic	Rather more hypoechoic	Hypoechoic, inhomogeneous
Wall	Regular	Normal	Normal	Infiltrated
Location	Varying	Rather more in the neck	Rather more in the fundus	Varying

▶ **Adenomyomatosis**

A good example of partial wall thickening is adenomyomatosis, which may also present as a hyperechoic focal lesion (**Fig. 3.62a**). Combined with the focal cystic inclusions and the classic comet-tail–like artifacts, the focal hypertrophied Aschoff–Rokitansky sinuses will round out the characteristic image in sonographic morphology. In focal adenomyomatosis the gallbladder may undergo segmental constriction (hourglass gallbladder) (**Fig. 3.62b**).

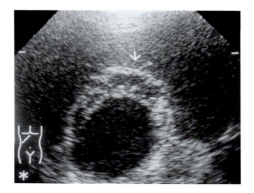 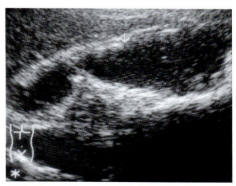

▲ **Fig. 3.62** Adenomyomatosis (focal and segmental).
a Typical adenomyomatosis of the fundus ("fundus adenoma"): hyperechoic wall thickening with hypoechoic inclusions (here no comet-tail–like artifacts).

▲ **b** "Hourglass gallbladder" in adenomyomatosis. In segmental adenomyomatosis the gallbladder displays segmental constriction at the body.

Gallbladder Carcinoma

Every polypoid mass of irregular shape within the lumen of the gallbladder as well as every infiltrating lesion with destruction of the normal wall should be highly suspicious for gallbladder carcinoma. In the early stages (still manageable by surgery), gallbladder carcinoma is clinically quiescent and will typically present in two manifestations: polypoid carcinoma, mostly filling the lumen; or primarily diffuse infiltrating carcinoma, with destruction of the normal texture of the gallbladder wall as well as early invasion of the surrounding tissue (**Fig. 3.63**). The delineation between the mostly hypoechoic infiltrates and the hepatic parenchyma may be ill defined (**Fig. 3.63c and e**). Local lymph node metastasis takes place at an early stage. Histologically, it is a scirrhous adenocarcinoma. Gallstones and chronic cholecystitis play an important role in the carcinogenesis: 2–3% of gallstone carriers will develop a carcinoma of the gallbladder.

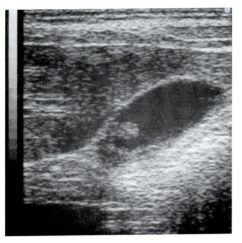
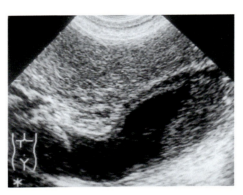
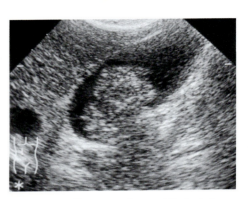

▲ **Fig. 3.63** Gallbladder carcinoma.
a Carcinoma of about 1 cm—with the appearance of a large polyp—in the neck of the gallbladder (image courtesy of Dr. WB Stelzel, Frankfurt, Germany).

▲ *b* Carcinoma of the fundus: hypoechoic adenocarcinoma with segmental infiltration of the fundus and body of the gallbladder.

▲ *c* Polypoid infiltrating carcinoma of the body: hypoechoic carcinoma with impacted gallstone, infiltrating diffusely from the body of the gallbladder into the liver; ill defined delineation between wall and liver parenchyma.

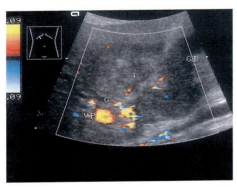
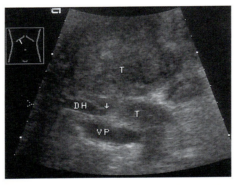
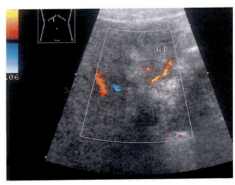

▲ *d* Invasive gallbladder carcinoma (T). Carcinoma infiltrating the liver from the body of the gallbladder, displacing the bile duct (G). Color duplex. VP = portal vein.

▲ *e* Tumor invading the porta hepatis, with cutoff of the hepatic duct (DH, arrow). VP = portal vein.

▲ *f* Differential diagnosis of carcinoma: severe cholecystitis with inflammatory matting (indistinct margins). Echogenic luminal change, presumed infiltration. GB = gallbladder.

Metastasis

Metastases in the wall of the gallbladder and hepatic metastases infiltrating the gallbladder from the liver may mimic primary carcinoma of the gallbladder wall and do not display any characteristic ultrasound morphology (**Fig. 3.64**). Metastasis in the gallbladder wall is a rare finding and cannot be clearly differentiated by sonography from true gallbladder carcinoma.

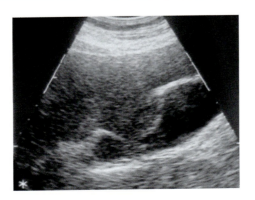

◀ **Fig. 3.64** Metastasis in the gallbladder wall: large hypoechoic metastasis of breast cancer in the gallbladder wall, infiltrating the lumen as well as the liver.

Intraluminal Changes

Hyperechoic

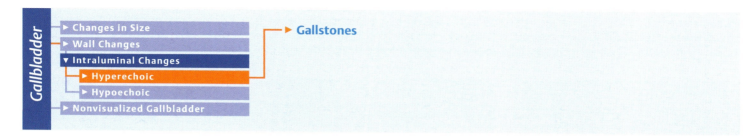

▶ Gallstones

Gallstones are the classic example of mobile changes within the gallbladder. The well-known mnemonic of "the five Fs"—fat, female, fertile, forty, fair—characterizes the segment of the population most at risk for cholecystolithiasis.

The typical gallbladder stones are mobile and differ in their extent of posterior shadowing (depending on the size of the calculus) as well as in their intrinsic pattern (◨ 3.7). The sonographic morphology of the stones depends on their size, shape, and composition. Usually, the gallstones are a mixture of cholesterol, calcium, and bilirubin and are located at the most dependent part of the gallbladder. When looking for calculi it should be remembered that with the patient supine the stones are more likely to be found in the neck of the gallbladder, while in left lateral decubitus position they tend to collect in the region of the fundus/body (◨ 3.7a–c). Fairly large pure cholesterol stones (up to 60 mm) may float in the liquid bile.

Shadowing can be observed in gallstones with a diameter down to about 2–3 mm, depending on the quality of the stone as well the equipment used and the frequency employed. Calculi with a diameter of less than 5 mm are called microliths. From a diameter of 8 mm and upward, subtle differentiation of the gallstones into cholesterol, calcium, and pigmented calculi usually does not present any problem. In microliths with a diameter < 5 mm, assessment of the intrinsic echo pattern may become difficult. Here, additional data such as tabular structure and comet-tail-like artifacts as well as any flotation of the stones (rich in cholesterol) and their size and shape (usually hyperechoic microliths dependent in the gallbladder are of mixed calcium make-up) have to be taken into account (**Table 3.4**). Ultrasound morphology is essential when planning possible lysis or shock-wave lithotripsy.

Differentiating gallstones. The criteria for differentiating gallstones are their intrinsic echo pattern, surface echo, and posterior shadowing (◨ 3.7d–i). Although gallstones are best visualized at the focus of the transducer, the quality and settings of the platform used are eminently important as well. Optimized differentiation of the calculi is possible only if the transmission power matches the situation at hand.

Hypoechoic

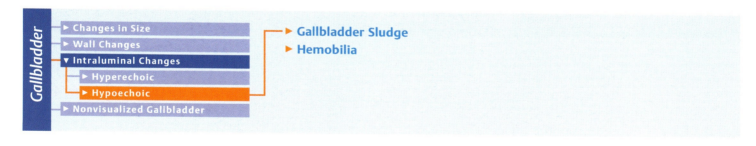

▶ Gallbladder Sludge

Sludge formation in the gallbladder depends on bile concentration, changes in crystallization, and desquamation. The presence of sludge is marked by a hypoechoic layer, or one of mixed echogenicity, at the floor of the gallbladder (no posterior shadowing!), or the gallbladder is filled solid with sluggish floating material. Gallbladder sludge is characterized by its motility upon repositioning of the patient. Depending on make-up and amount, the types of sludge in the gallbladder may be differentiated as shown in **Table 3.6** and ◨ 3.8.

Table 3.6 Types of gallbladder sludge

	Sludge-filled gallbladder	Polypoid sludge	Sludge sedimentation	Floating cholesterol crystals
Size	Gallbladder filled solid	Varying	Varying	Crystalline
Shape	Gallbladder filled solid	Polypoid, dependent on position	Rather dependent on position, often layered	Tabular
Echogenicity	Varying, sometimes hepatized	Varying	Mixed, varying	Hyperechoic, comet-tail–like artefacts
Wall	Normal	Normal	Normal	Normal

3.7 Differentiating Gallstones by Ultrasound

▶ Differentiating calculi in the supine and left lateral decubitus position

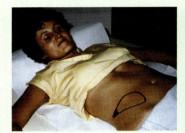
a Supine—the stones are more likely to collect in the neck of the gallbladder.

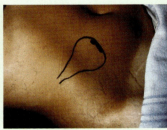
b Left lateral decubitus—the calculi will be located at the fundus/body of the gallbladder.

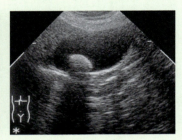
c Typical gallstone with the patient supine: bright echo of the stone, classic posterior shadowing.

▶ Differentiating calculi with a diameter > 8 mm

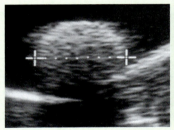
d Cholesterol gallstone: fine crystalline homogeneous intrinsic echo pattern ("through-transmission") with comet-tail–like artifacts, weak surface echo, soft posterior shadowing.

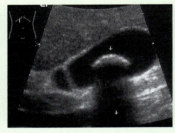
e Calcium stone: shell-like surface echo, pronounced posterior shadowing, inhomogeneous intrinsic echo pattern.

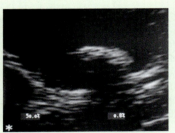
f Mixed pigment gallstone: inhomogeneous intrinsic echo pattern with black voids (pigment), soft surface echo, weak posterior shadowing.

▶ Differentiating calculi with a diameter < 8 mm

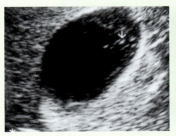
g Cholesterol gallstone: intrinsic echo pattern with tabular structure (with somewhat comet-tail–like artifacts); calculi floating within the lumen of the gallbladder.

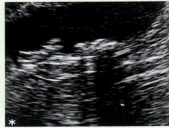
h Mixed calcium stones: rather hyperechoic gallstone dependent in the gallbladder.

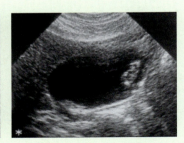
i Mixed pigment gallstone: mixed intrinsic echo pattern (inhomogeneous); stones mostly dependent in the gallbladder.

3.8 Types of Sludge

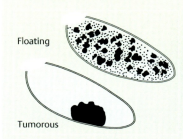
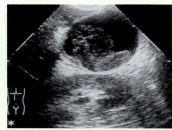
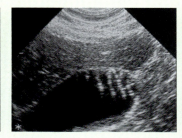
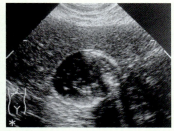

a Sludge may float freely or appear as a "pseudotumor" (modified from Rettenmeier/Seitz[18]).

b Polypoid sludge within the gallbladder.

c Floating sludge: cholesterol tables at the fundus arranged in rouleau fashion.

d Diffuse floating sludge: multiple echoes of different size and echogenicity.

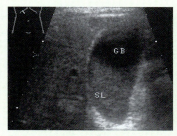
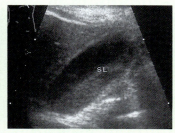
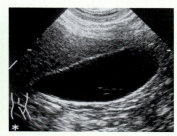

e and f Partially sludge-filled gallbladder

e Pseudotumor, homogeneous sludge.

f Change of shape after a position change excludes a tumor.

g Floating cholesterol crystals.

▶ Hemobilia

Hemobilia is a well-known complication of tumor or, less commonly, inflammatory and traumatic gallbladder lesions. A fresh clot within the gallbladder may mimic hypoechoic sludge. Older traumatic clots adherent to the wall will display as hyperechoic mass (**Fig. 3.65**).

Conclusion

These findings demonstrate the enormous capabilities a subtle ultrasound study can offer in the differential diagnosis of gallbladder disease. Ultrasound is the diagnostic modality of choice in all disorders of the gallbladder, since its resolution is much better than that of all the other modalities. Therefore, sonography is the linchpin in the diagnostic work-up of the gallbladder.

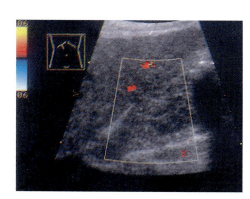
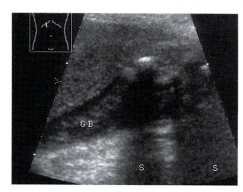

◂◂ **Fig. 3.65** Hemobilia, anticoagulant-related hemorrhage (ERCP).
a Fresh: hyperechoic lumen.

◂ **b** Regression with partially anechoic gallbladder (GB) contents. Cholecystolithiasis. S = shadowing.

Nonvisualized Gallbladder

J. Mueller and L. Greiner

Missing Gallbladder

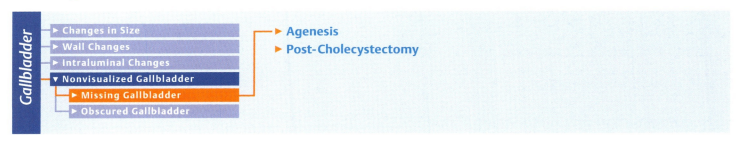

▶ Agenesis

Although agenesis of the gallbladder is a rare anomaly (< 0.1%), it should be of first concern in the differential diagnosis of the nonvisualized gallbladder, because this would raise considerable (also forensic) doubts regarding the proper differential diagnosis and will elucidate the situation quickly. Apparently persistent gallbladders in the immediate postoperative follow-up are not especially infrequent, and indication for surgery, even should it be found during exploration.

▶ Post-Cholecystectomy

In routine studies, nonvisualization of the gallbladder most likely equates with a status post cholecystectomy (**Fig. 3.66**); obtaining a thorough patient history is still a sine qua non for are easily explained as hematoma/seroma (**Fig. 3.67**) which will clear quickly. Only in rare cases do they have to be evacuated by ultrasound guided aspiration.

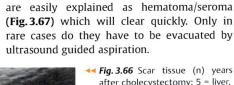

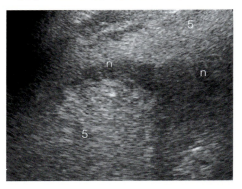
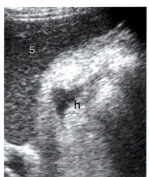
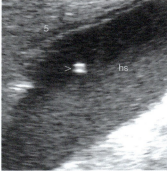

◀◀ **Fig. 3.66** Scar tissue (n) years after cholecystectomy; 5 = liver.

◀ **Fig. 3.67** Status post cholecystectomy. Left: small hematoma (h) a few days after cholecystectomy. Right: hematoseroma (hs) two days post laparoscopic cholecystectomy, ultrasound-guided aspiration (for diagnosis and therapy). > = needle tip artifact; 5 = liver.

Obscured Gallbladder

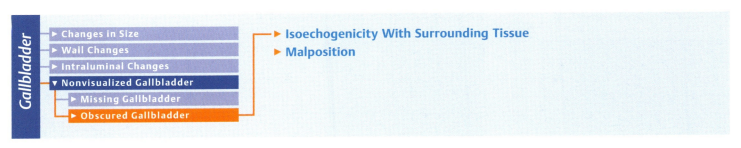

Usually, maximum contraction of the postprandial gallbladder after oral intake does not present any problems, and nor does the gallbladder void of fluid due to lithic obstruction of the cystic duct (**Fig. 3.68**).

If the gallbladder is present but cannot be visualized on ultrasound, this may have to do with the gallbladder itself, its surroundings, or the operator (or a combination of all three). In this case:

▶ the gallbladder cannot be differentiated very well from adjacent structures, e.g., because of unusual content or consumed wall and lumen structure; or

▶ it is outside the "realm of imagination" of the operator, i.e., it is located in unusual ectopic sites.

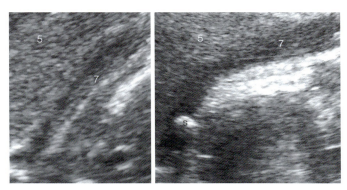

◄ **Fig. 3.68** Left: pronounced postprandial contraction of the gallbladder (7); 5 = liver. Right: gallbladder atrophy (7) in cholelithiasis with calculous obstruction (s).

▶ Isoechogenicity with Surrounding Tissue

Ultrasound may not be able to visualize the gallbladder if it is very small by nature or if it displays maximum volume reduction because of chronic inflammation (**Fig. 3.69**). Somewhat more common is the combination of (calculous atrophic) gallbladder (**Fig. 3.70**) and heavy tympanites (the latter may hinder a study, although any statement to this effect should be taken with a grain of salt).

Most problems in the differential diagnosis result from a gallbladder that is relatively isoechoic with the surrounding tissue and with homogeneous sludge resembling hepatic parenchyma (**Fig. 3.69**), and those gallbladders void of fluid that are being consumed by their own (**Fig. 3.71**) or other malignancy, most commonly HCC (**Fig. 3.72**). This is also true if the gallbladder becomes part of a cystic tumor (e.g., extensive ovarian cancer) or if it cannot be delineated from multicystic processes of the kidneys and/or liver, as well as (much less often) in extreme portal hypertension or cavernous transformation of the portal vein.

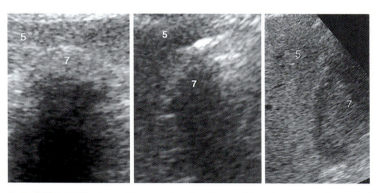

▲ **Fig. 3.69** Left: bile stone with weak echo, almost impossible to demonstrate, in an atrophic gallbladder (7); 5 = liver. Center: small atrophied gallbladder (7); the stone can only be demonstrated indirectly by its shadowing; 5 = liver. Right: "hepatized" gallbladder (7) isoechoic with the liver (5).

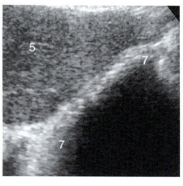

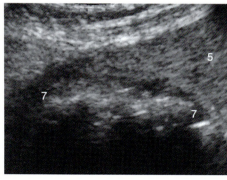

◄◄ **Fig. 3.70** Fluid-filled atrophic gallbladder (7) in cholecystolithiasis and tympanites; 5 = liver.

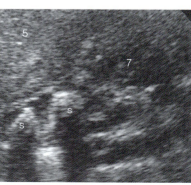

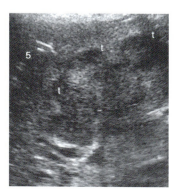

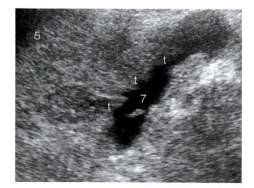

▲ **Fig. 3.71** Left: atrophic calculous gallbladder (7) (stones S) with inflammatory?–malignant? infiltration of the liver (5). Right: gallbladder carcinoma (confirmed by needle aspiration biopsy) with tumor infiltration (t) of the liver (5).

▲ **Fig. 3.72** Tumor infiltration (t) of the gallbladder (7) by hepatocellular carcinoma; liver (5).

▶ Malposition

Malposition of the liver, and thus of the gallbladder, in severe kyphoscoliotic deformity of the chest or paralysis of the right phrenic nerve may limit the accessibility of the gallbladder to ultrasound. Unusual (ectopic) location of the gallbladder is more common than originally thought; in the elderly, the gallbladder may hyperextend all the way into the minor pelvis to be visualized only there. The same holds true for very slim, young patients in left lateral decubitus position: here, the pendulous gallbladder, resembling a clapper, may reach far into the left upper quadrant.

Abnormal locations resulting in poor or even impossible differentiation may be encountered in gallbladders deeply retracted in the portal hilum or in intrahepatic gallbladders, which may then be misdiagnosed as focal liver lesion, particularly so in the case of cholecystolithiasis. Finally, visualization of the gallbladder in a patient with transposition of viscera may also present initial problems.

References

1. Braun, Günther, Schwerk (eds.). Ultraschalldiagnostik. Lehrbuch und Atlas 111-1.1 Biliäres System. Ecomed 1993.
2. Farinon AM et al. Adenomatous polyps of the gallbladder. Adenomas of the gallbladder. HPB Surgery 1991;3:251.
3. Greiner L et al. Biliäre Stoßwellenlithotripsie, Fragmentation und Lyse – ein neues Verfahren. Dtsch Med Wschr 1987;112:1893–6.
4. Hawass ND. False negative sonographic finding in emphysematous cholecystitis. Acta Radiol 1988;29;137.
5. Heyder N et al. Polypoide Läsionen der Gallenblase. Dtsch Med Wschr 1990;115:243–7.
6. Imhof M et al. Sonomorphologie der Streßcholezystitis. Ultraschall in Med 1992;13:96–101.
7. Jakobeit C et al. Probleme der sonographischen Verlaufskontrolle nach ESWL von Gallenblasensteinen. Ultraschall in Klinik und Praxis 1989;Supp.1:20.
8. Jakobeit C, Greiner L et al. Sonographie und biliäre extrakorporale Stoßwellenlithotripsie (ESWL). Ultraschall in Med 1992;13:255–62.
9. Jakobeit C, Greiner L et al. Sonographische Gallensteinmorphologie. Z Gastroenterol 1992;30:594–7.
10. Kubicka S, Manns MP. Das Gallenblasen- und Gallengangskarzinom. Internist (Berlin) 2000;41(9):841–7.
11. Kunisch M et al. Gallenblasenadenokarzinom bei bestehender villöser Adenomatose (Papillomatose) der Gallenblase und des Ductus hepatocholedochus. Rofo Fortschr Geb Röntgenstr Neuen Bildgeb Verfahr 1997;166(5):454–6.
12. Lee KC et al. Mirizzi Syndrom caused by xanthogranulomatous cholecystitis. Report of case. Surg Today 1997;27(8):757–61.
13. Meckler U et al. (eds.). Ultraschall des Abdomen. Diagnostischer Leitfaden. Cologne: Deutscher Ärzteverlag 1998.
14. Meckler U, Wermke W (eds.). Sonographische Differentialdiagnostik: Systematischer Atlas. Cologne: Deutscher Ärzteverlag 1997.
15. Nussie K et al. Adenomyomatose der Gallenblase: Sonographischer Befund. Röntgenpraxis 1998;51(5):155–8.
16. Okabe T et al. Gallbladder-Carcinoma with choledochoduodenal fistula – a case report with surgical treatment. Hepatogastroenterology 1999;46(27):1660–3.
17. Ravo B et al. The Mirizzi syndrome: pre-operative diagnosis by sonography and transhepatic cholangiography. Am J Gastroenterol 1986;81:688.
18. Rettenmaier G, Seitz K (eds.). Sonographische Differentialdiagnostik. Stuttgart: Thieme 2000.
19. Roberts KM, Parsons MA. Xanthogranulomatous cholecystitis: clinico-pathological study of 13 cases. J Clin Pathol 1987;40:412.
20. Sasatomi F et al. Precancerous conditions of Gallbladder-Carcinoma: overview of histopathologic characteristics and molecular genetic findings. J Hepatobiliary Pancreat Surg 2000;7(6):556–67.
21. Schmidt G (eds.). Ultraschall-Kursbuch. 3rd ed. Stuttgart: Thieme 1999.
22. Schölmerich J, Bischoff SC, Manns MP (eds.). Diagnostik in der Gastroenterologie und Hepatologie. Stuttgart: Thieme 1997.
23. Shinizu M et al. Porcelain gallblader: relation between its type by ultrasound and incidence of cancer. J Clin Gastroenterol 1989;11:471.
24. Stelzel WB et al. Perforierte xanthogranulomatöse Cholezystitis. In: Schmitt W, Ottenjann R. (eds.). Der seltene gastroenterologische Fall. Vol 3. Demeter 1990; p. 118–9.
25. Sturm J, Post S. Benigne Erkrankungen der Gallenblase und der Gallenwege. Chirurg 2000;71(12):1530–51.
26. Tsuchiya Y et al. Sonographic diagnosis of gallstones. In: Speranza V, Barbara L, Nyhus LM (eds.). Problems in general surgery. Vol. 8, Nr. 4;541 Philadelphia: Lippincot & Co 1991
27. Weiss A, Weiss H (eds.). Ultraschall in der Inneren Medizin. Edition Medizin 2000.
28. Weiss H et al. Die Schichten der Gallenblasenwand – eine sonographisch-anatomische Vergleichsuntersuchung. Ultraschall Klin Prax 1992;7:142(Abstr.)
29. Wolpers C (eds.). Gallenblasensteine: Ihre Morphogenese und Auswahl zur Litholyse. Karger 1987.

4 Pancreas

Pancreas 143

Diffuse Pancreatic Change — 144

Large Pancreas — 144
- Acute Pancreatitis
- Chronic Pancreatitis
- Tumor Invasion

Small Pancreas — 145
- The Aging Pancreas
- Pancreatic Atrophy
- Post-Pancreatitic Necrosis/Pancreatectomy

Hypoechoic Texture — 147
- Juvenile Pancreas
- Acute Pancreatitis
- Early/Recurrent Chronic Pancreatitis
- Ductal Dilatation

Hyperechoic Texture — 148
- Fibromatosis/Lipomatosis
- Fibrosis in Hemochromatosis/Cystic Fibrosis
- Chronic Pancreatitis

Focal Changes — 152

Anechoic Lesion — 152
- Cysts
- Pseudocysts
- Necrosis
- Vessels/Duct System

Hypoechoic Lesion — 154
- Neuroendocrine Tumors
- Pancreatic Cancer
- Metastasis, Malignant Lymphoma, Inflammatory Lymph Node
- Abscess
- Hemorrhagic/Calcified Cyst/Pseudocyst
- Focal Pancreatitis

Isoechoic Lesion — 158
- Pancreatic Cancer
- Malignant Lymphoma
- Focal Pancreatitis
- Pancreas divisum
- Annular Pancreas

Hyperechoic Lesion — 160
- Calcification/Intraductal Calculus
- Calcified Splenic Artery
- Microcalcification, Calcium Soap
- Intraductal Gas/Stent
- Hemangioma, Lipoma

Irregular Lesion — 163
- Chronic Pancreatitis
- Focal Chronic Pancreatitis
- Pseudocyst
- Cystic Neoplasias: Cystadenoma/Cystadenocarcinoma

Dilatation of the Pancreatic Duct — 164

Marginal/Mild Dilatation — 166
- Bile Duct Disorder
- Acute/Recurrent Pancreatitis, Pancreas Divisum
- Chronic Pancreatitis
- Periampullary Cancer, Cancer of the Pancreatic Head

Marked Dilatation — 167
- Chronic Pancreatitis
- Intraductal Mass
- Pancreatic Cancer

4 Pancreas

G. Schmidt

Anatomy

Size
- Head: 2.5–3 cm
- Body: < 1.8–2 cm
- Tail: 2.5–3 cm

Shape
- Barbell
- Tadpole

The structure of the pancreas shows it to be a composite tubuloalveolar gland. Its size may vary significantly, depending on age and its intrinsic physiological variation in shape; in the elderly the organ becomes smaller and may even atrophy. The variants in shape (barbell and tadpole, **Fig. 4.1**) are characterized by their differences in the size of the pancreatic head and tail. Most of the glands display the dimensions given above.

Microstructure. The enzyme-producing terminal segments of the glands are termed acini ("berries"). The interstice houses blood vessels, fibroblasts, and strands of collagen, and this interstitial connective tissue becomes denser with age. During embryological development, two large ducts (pancreatic duct and duct of Santorini) drain into the duodenum; later the duct of Santorini may degenerate completely, with the pancreatic duct becoming the main drainage. Accessory ducts, termed interlobular excretory ductules, branch off orthogonally. Further branching to the acini within the lobules leads to the so-called intralobular ductules. The lobules of the pancreas are separated from the surrounding tissue not by a firm capsule but by tenuous connective-tissue strands. This explains the blurred outline of the organ in the ultrasound image.

Function. The pancreas is composed of two quite separate types of glandular tissue—the exocrine and the endocrine. The exocrine gland produces the viscous glassy mucus excreted by the acini via excretory ductules into the pancreatic duct. The 0.5–2 million pancreatic islets of Langerhans, diameter 100–200 μm, are cell clusters mainly found in the body and tail of the organ, which constitute the endocrine part of the glandular tissue. They secrete insulin, glucagon, somatostatin, pancreatic polypeptide, and other active peptide hormones and neuropeptides directly into the bloodstream.

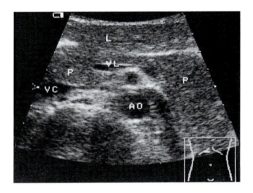
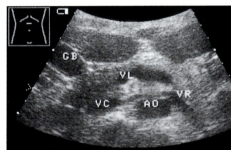

◀◀ **Fig. 4.1** Variant configurations of the pancreas. GB = gallbladder; VR = left renal vein; L = liver; VL = splenic vein; VC = vena cava; AO = aorta.
a Barbell: slender body and prominent head as well as tail of the pancreas (P).

◀ *b* Tadpole: prominent pancreatic head, small body and tail.

Topography

Topographic relationships
- Retroperitoneal location anterior to the upper lumbar spine
- Head — anterior to the inferior vena cava
- Body — transverse in the middle of the upper abdomen anterior to the aorta
- Tail — reaches the hilum of the spleen

Ultrasound landmark structures
- Portal vein confluence and its tributaries
- Inferior vena cava
- Vessels of the celiac axis

The pancreas lies transversely and somewhat obliquely in the retroperitoneum, directly anterior to the spine at the level of the second lumbar vertebra. The head of the pancreas nestles in the posterocaudad concavity of the duodenum; the pancreatic body traverses the spine and courses along the anterior margin of the left kidney, while the tail reaches cephalad into the hilum of the spleen (**Figs. 4.2–4.4**).

Borders. The posterior borders are defined by the spine and the lumbar part of the diaphragm, abdominal aorta, and inferior vena cava, all anterior to the spine. Most of the anterior aspect of the pancreas is covered by the stomach. The omental bursa is formed by the posterior wall of the stomach (up to the lesser curvature) and the anterior aspect of the pancreas. From the border between the head and body of the pancreas to the left, there is the cavity of the omental bursa or lesser sac, which in acute pancreatitis may fill up with exudate. Posterior to the head of the pancreas, the distal segment of the common bile duct and the prepapillary section of the pancreatic duct course together for part of the way to the papilla of Vater, in 75% of cases within a common trough, in the other 25% intrapancreatically.

Blood supply. The origins of the celiac axis and the superior mesenteric artery lie cephalad to the pancreas. Since the celiac axis runs in an anterosuperior direction and the superior mesenteric artery posteroinferior to the pancreas, the organ is caught in a kind of vise. If in pancreatic cancer these vessels are infiltrated, the tumor is no longer amenable to resection. The superior mesenteric artery and vein run in the pancreatic incision across the uncinate process, the latter resting posterior to these vessels.

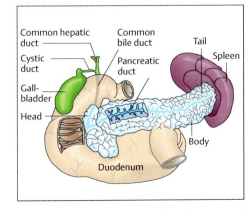

▲ **Fig. 4.2** Schematic diagram of the relationships of the pancreas.

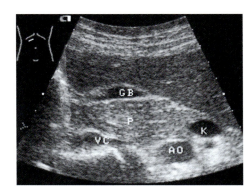 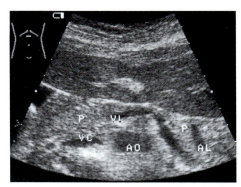 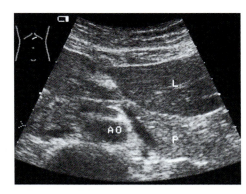

▲ **Fig. 4.3** Ultrasound topography of the pancreas and the relationships with its neighboring organs.
a Oblique right epigastric view: the head of the pancreas (P) is lateral and posterior to the gallbladder (GB), posterior to the right hepatic lobe, and anterior to the vena cava (VC). AO = aorta; K = venous confluens.

▲ **b** Median transverse epigastric view: the median regions of the right and left hepatic lobes are visualized from anterior to posterior; the splenic vein (VL) lies at the inferior border of the pancreas (P), followed by cross-sectional views of the superior mesenteric artery, vena cava (VC), and aorta (AO). AL = splenic artery.

▲ **c** Left oblique epigastric view: demonstration of the entire tail of the pancreas (P) posterior to the left hepatic lobe (L); the splenic artery (AL, **Fig. 4.3b**) meanders through the pancreatic tail.

The splenic vein courses posteroinferior to the pancreas and is completely covered by it, while the splenic artery meanders, partly intrapancreatically and partly retropancreatically, along the superior pancreatic margin toward the hilum of the spleen.

The gastroduodenal artery traverses the anterior part of the pancreatic head, runs anterior to the pars superior duodeni, and branches into the anterior and posterior superior pancreaticoduodenal arteries.

The lymphatics of the pancreatic head drain into the hepatic, pancreaticoduodenal, and superior mesenteric lymph nodes; those of the body and tail of the pancreas drain into the aortic and preaortic nodes. Quite often in malignancy, these lymph nodes harbor metastases and in sonographic staging will become important when considering possible treatment options.

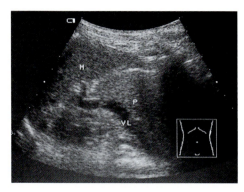

▲ **Fig. 4.4** The tail of the pancreas (P), anterior to the splenic vein (VL), reaches the hilum of the spleen (M); high lateral view.

Diffuse Pancreatic Change

In ultrasonography, diffuse pancreatic change will alter the size and echo texture of the organ.

Large Pancreas

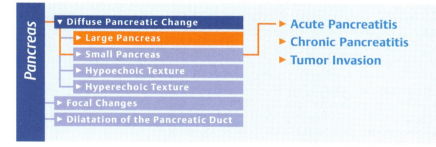

▶ Acute Pancreatitis

Pancreatic edema. Acute pancreatitis will usually lead to diffuse enlargement of the entire pancreas; however, in most cases of concurrent pancreatitis the standard dimensions will not be exceeded. The increase in size is caused by interstitial edema, which in turn decreases the echogenicity. Increased size and hypoechogenicity are the most striking characteristics of mild episodes of acute pancreatitis (**Fig. 4.5**).

Subsiding edema is followed by a return to normal size and echogenicity. However, even after months there may be residual spiculation of the organ contour.

Necrosis of the peripancreatic fat. In severe cases of acute necrotizing pancreatitis, focal masses, such as intrapancreatic and peripancreatic fluid, fatty necrosis, hemorrhage, and exudate, may hamper delineation of the gland, thus resulting in a pseudo-enlargement of the organ (**Fig. 4.6**).

Extensive peripancreatic fatty infiltration in obesity and diabetes may blur the contours of the pancreas by beam scattering and reflection, and therefore may also mimic enlargement of the gland (**Fig. 4.7**).

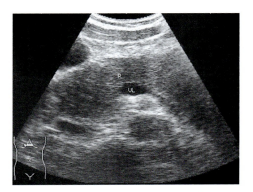
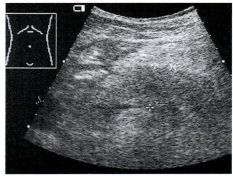
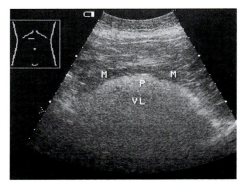

▲ **Fig. 4.5** Acute edematous pancreatitis: diffusely enlarged pancreas (P); blurred hypoechoic texture. VL = splenic vein.

▲ **Fig. 4.6** Acute pancreatitis: apparent enlargement by echogenic peripancreatic areas (fat necrosis, hemorrhagic areas), which indent the posterior stomach wall (cursors). The pancreas (cursors) is of normal size and has a hazy, hypoechoic structure.

▲ **Fig. 4.7** Apparent enlargement of the pancreas (P) because intensive scattering (fibromatosis/lipomatosis, peripancreatic fat) makes delineation by ultrasound impossible; splenic vein (VL) just barely visualized. M = stomach.

▶ Chronic Pancreatitis

It is particularly the early stage and the acute inflammatory episode of chronic pancreatitis that will result in an enlarged pancreas. But in this case texture and contour will tend to undergo mottled, ill-defined, or irregular hyperechoic transformation (**Fig. 4.8**).

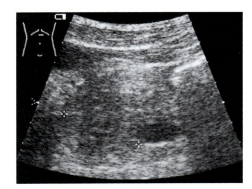

◀ **Fig. 4.8** Recurrent chronic alcohol-associated pancreatitis: distinctive enlargement of the pancreatic body and head; coarse echo pattern due to fibrosis.

▶ Tumor Invasion

In the rather rare case of diffuse carcinoma or in malignant tumor invasion, enlargement of the gland and misdiagnosis may also be encountered (**Fig. 4.9**). The echo pattern may be isoechoic or hypoechoic (**see Fig. 4.36**).

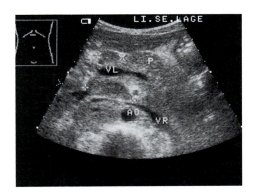

◀ **Fig. 4.9** Confluent intrapancreatic and peripancreatic lymphomas (calipers), resulting in enlargement of the pancreas (P) anterior and posterior to the splenic vein (VL). AO = aorta; VR = renal vein.

Small Pancreas

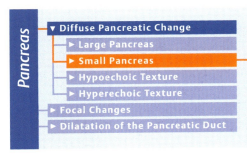

There are no clearly defined dimensional data for the small pancreas, and therefore the assessment of reduced pancreatic size is subjective and depends on the sonographic impression. Nevertheless, a thickness of less than 10mm in the pancreatic head, body, or tail would suggest a smaller than normal size. If the reduced thickness is segmental, it may be simply a physiological variant (**Fig. 4.1**).

▶ The Aging Pancreas

The most common cause of a smaller than normal size of the pancreas is age-dependent atrophy, which is quite common in slim, elderly patients. It affects all parts of the organ evenly. Echogenicity may be normal or increased. Any hypergenicity is due to parenchyma being replaced by fatty and connective tissue (fibrolipomatosis). Problems in differential diagnosis arise if in cachectic patients tubular structures are very closely related, making orientation rather difficult (splenic artery and vein; dilated pancreatic duct/common hepatic artery/renal vein; common bile duct/portal vein/proper hepatic artery). In this case, color-flow Doppler scanning will differentiate the various vessels and facilitate visualization of the narrow pancreatic parenchyma (**Fig. 4.10**).

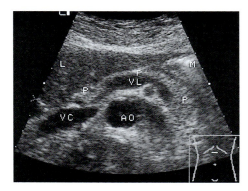

◀ **Fig. 4.10** Pancreas in old age: narrowed pancreas (P), normal texture. VL = splenic vein; AO = aorta; VC = vena cava; L = liver; M = gastric body.

▶ Pancreatic Atrophy

Differentiation of atrophy in chronic pancreatitis from aging pancreas is possible only if there are changes in the texture or in case of ductal dilatation. Pancreatic atrophy is the terminal stage of chronic pancreatitis and may still exhibit the ultrasound criteria of this disease, i.e., calcification and fibrosis. Scarring will often warp the duct and dilate it irregularly, and it may be the only vestige of the gland.

Pancreatic atrophy as a sequel to chronic pancreatitis or in the much more infrequent chronic autoimmune pancreatitis will lead to diabetes mellitus and maldigestion. Newly diagnosed diabetes mellitus or unexplained weight loss may be the only clinical symptoms. Early signs in ultrasound morphology might be localized or diffuse hypoechogenicity without the other signs of chronic pancreatitis[2, 9] (**Fig. 4.11 and Fig. 4.67a–c**).

Hemochromatosis. In atrophy concomitant with advanced hemochromatosis, the fibrosis may lead to diffuse or focal hyperechogenicity of the pancreas (**Fig. 4.12**).

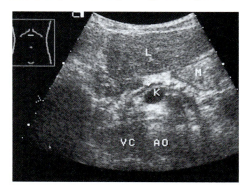

▲ **Fig. 4.11** Atrophy resulting from "burnt out" chronic pancreatitis: only a narrow band of hyperechoic parenchyma and the slightly dilated pancreatic duct are left. K = venous confluence; M = gastric body; L = liver; VC = vena cava; AO = aorta.

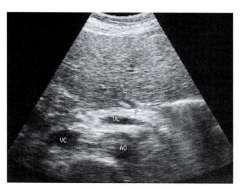

▲ **Fig. 4.12** Fibrosis of the pancreas (P) with diabetes mellitus in hemochromatosis. VL = splenic vein; AO = aorta; VC = vena cava; L = liver.
a Narrow hyperechoic organ.

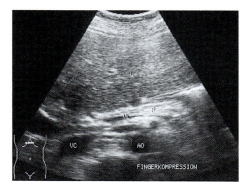

▲ *b* In contrast to lipomatosis, here the pancreas cannot be compressed by the palpating fingers. Fingerkompression = finger compression.

▶ Post-Pancreatitic Necrosis/Pancreatectomy

After necrosis and partial resection of the pancreas as well as after total pancreatectomy it is almost impossible to differentiate sonographically between the peripancreatic fat/connective tissue and the residual pancreatic tissue because they hardly differ in impedance (**Fig. 4.13**). In these cases, differential diagnosis has to fall back on patient history and clinical symptoms.

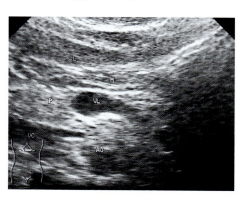

◀ **Fig. 4.13** Three months after necrotizing pancreatitis: while the pancreatic head (P) still appears to be of normal size, the body and tail are missing almost completely. VL = splenic vein; AO = aorta; VC = vena cava; L = liver; M = stomach.

Hypoechoic Texture

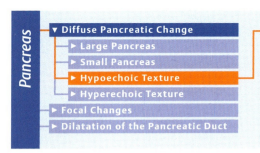

▸ Juvenile Pancreas

Quite often, the juvenile pancreas will be exceptionally hypoechoic and might be mistaken for edematous pancreas in acute pancreatitis, although the "juvenile organ" will demonstrate normal size (**Fig. 4.14**).

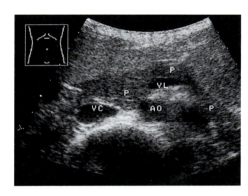

◂ **Fig. 4.14** Juvenile pancreas in a slender female: compared with acute pancreatitis the pancreas (P) is markedly hypoechoic but with unchanged dimensions in all segments. AO = aorta; VC = vena cava; VL = splenic vein.

▸ Acute Pancreatitis

Classification. There are four different international classifications of acute and chronic pancreatitis: the Marseille classification of 1963, the revised Marseille of 1984, the Cambridge classification of 1983 (and of 1984 regarding imaging modalities), and the Marseille–Rome classification of 1988. According to the latter three, the differentiation is only between acute and chronic pancreatitis. In general, the transition from acute to chronic pancreatitis is assumed to be a rare event. The revised Marseille classification of 1984 is listed in the accompanying box.

Ultrasound findings. In a mild episode of acute pancreatitis there is definite ballooning and enlargement of the organ, which is characterized by intensive homogeneous hypoechoic transformation of its texture. These changes correspond to the histological finding of pancreatic edema.

Necrosis of the peripancreatic fat may result in the common ultrasonographic finding of band-shaped hyperechoic peripancreatic masses (**Fig. 4.7**).

Classification of Acute Pancreatitis (Marseille 1984)[8]

Clinical characteristics. Acute onset of abdominal pain, increased blood and/or urine levels of the pancreatic enzymes.

Morphological characteristics
- *Mild form:* necrosis of the peripancreatic fat, interstitial edema.
- *Severe form:* extensive necrosis of the peripancreatic and intrapancreatic fat, necrosis of the parenchymal tissue as well as hemorrhaging; focal or diffuse lesions.

Course. Generally benign course; severe episodes may be fatal; single or recurrent episode; disorder of the exocrine and endocrine pancreas function of varying degree and duration; after elimination of the underlying cause usually complete clinical, functional, and morphological recovery; morphological changes (e.g. scars, pseudocysts) may persist as residual sign of partial recovery.

In addition there also may be fluid-filled spaces around the pancreas, liver, and kidney/spleen, while large exudate tends to be present in the more severe form (**Table 4.1**). Compression-induced dilatation of the pancreatic duct is uncommon and would indicate pancreas divisum or periampullary ductal obstruction (prepapillary gallstone).

On the basis of the ultrasound findings, the differential diagnosis should consider the early stage of chronic or recurrent chronic pancreatitis (**Figs. 4.15 and 4.16**) or even the rarer case of a hypoechoic juvenile pancreas (**Fig. 4.14**).

Table 4.1 Diagnostic ultrasound criteria in acute pancreatitis

Mild pancreatitis	Severe pancreatitis
Enlarged organ (leading sign) Blurred hypoechoic texture Regular size and texture in "concurrent" pancreatitis Heterogeneous texture possible	In addition to the mild form: Focal hypo-/hyperechoic intra- and extra-pancreatic mass (hemorrhage/necrosis/fatty necrosis) Ascites, pleural effusion

▶ Early/Recurrent Chronic Pancreatitis

Chronic pancreatitis is characterized by hyperechoic fibrosis and calcification as well as anechoic/hypoechoic microcysts and macrocysts and ductal dilatation. If all signs are present, the diagnosis is confirmed. In the presence of just one or two criteria, differentiation of chronic pancreatitis from malignancy or other forms of fibrosis, or even acute pancreatitis, becomes difficult. Particularly in alcohol-associated pancreatitis, the texture may become hypoechoic; however, on detailed study it displays the characteristics of chronic pancreatitis, i.e., irregular contour, undulating duct, or interspersed fibrotic regions (**Figs. 4.15 and 4.16**).

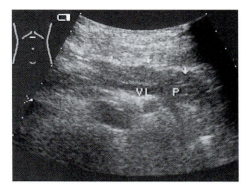

▲ **Fig. 4.15** Early stage of alcohol-associated chronic pancreatitis: hypoechoic pancreas (P), irregular anterior contour (arrows); subsiding acute pancreatitis will demonstrate similar findings. VL = splenic vein.

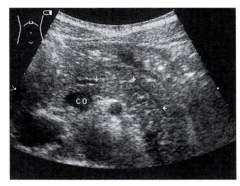

▲ **Fig. 4.16** Hypoechoic pancreas. The diagnosis of chronic pancreatitis is clearly suspected in the presence of sporadically interspersed fibrotic areas and the undulating, barely dilated pancreatic duct (several episodes of inflammation in pancreas divisum). CO = venous confluence.

▶ Ductal Dilatation

Sometimes a "hypoechoic" pancreas is in reality an enormously dilated pancreatic duct which, particularly in the atrophic organ, may constitute almost the entire gland. Detritus, pus, and intraductal calculi produce heterogeneous changes in the texture of the duct that are hard to discriminate from the other pancreatic parenchyma (**Fig. 4.17**).

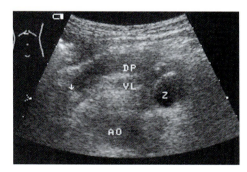

◀ **Fig. 4.17** Misdiagnosis of a hypoechoic pancreas: there is a hypoechoic dilated pancreatic duct (DP); calculi or a protein plug in the pancreatic head (arrow) and the pseudocyst (Z) point the way to the underlying cause (chronic pancreatitis). VL = splenic vein; AO = aorta.

Hyperechoic Texture

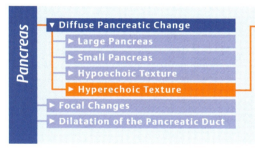

- ▶ Fibromatosis/Lipomatosis
- ▶ Fibrosis in Hemochromatosis/Cystic Fibrosis
- ▶ Chronic Pancreatitis

▶ Fibromatosis/Lipomatosis

Lipomatosis. Very few diffuse changes of the pancreas catch the eye as does pancreatic lipomatosis, and therefore this diagnosis is made without hesitation. Compared with the liver, the pancreas demonstrates normal size and an even, intensively hyperechoic texture. This change is found most often in the overweight non-insulin-dependent diabetic patient.

Fibrolipomatosis. The same holds true for fibrolipomatosis, but here the change is coarser and frequently accompanied by enlargement of the gland. Fibrolipomatosis is more common in the elderly, in whom the loss in parenchyma is made up by fibrosis and fatty tissue (**Fig. 4.18**).

Differentiation. Differentiating siderosis or chronic pancreatitis from pure fibrosis is difficult. It may be aided by checking the build of the organ through palpation: in pure fibrosis there is no compressibility or propagation of the aortic pulse. Usually, the fibrosis results in a significant loss of organ function and will lead to exocrine and endocrine pancreatic insufficiency (**Fig. 4.11**).

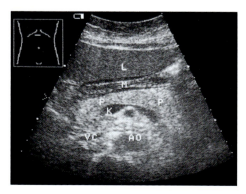

▲ **Fig. 4.18** Fibrolipomatosis of the pancreas (P): hyperechoic, somewhat coarse texture. M = stomach; K = confluence of portal vein; VC = vena cava; AO = aorta; L = liver.

▶ Fibrosis in Hemochromatosis/Cystic Fibrosis

In the more advanced stages, the organ quite often atrophies, thus becoming smaller, and will demonstrate an intensively hyperechoic texture (**Fig. 4.12**). In the early stages, size and texture of the pancreas remain almost normal; as part of hemochromatosis the initial fibrosis may be present without any clear-cut sonographic increase in echogenicity. In cystic fibrosis, there sometimes is additional cystic transformation of the pancreatic texture. Ultrasound cannot differentiate the various causes of pancreatic fibrosis (**Fig. 4.19**).

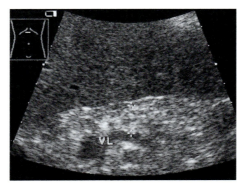 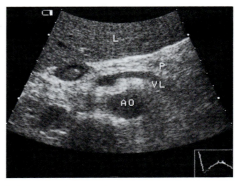

▲ *Fig. 4.19* Fibrosis of the pancreas (calipers, P). VL = splenic vein; AO = aorta; L = liver.
a In chronic alcohol-associated pancreatitis (calipers).

▲ b In hemochromatosis.

▶ Chronic Pancreatitis

Parenchymal changes. Chronic pancreatitis is characterized by fibrotic parenchymal scarring, particularly in the acinar epithelium; with increasing fibrosis, only ectatic excretory ducts, pancreatic islets, obliterated vessels, and some residual parenchyma will remain. In more than 40% of cases this process of fibrosis will be focal within the pancreatic tail or will appear as "groove pancreatitis" or divisum pancreatitis in the head of the pancreas. The frequency of protein deposits and calcification (intraductal calculi) varies, focal necrosis being present in roughly 10% and inflammatory postpancreatitis pseudocysts in 40% of patients. Dilatation of the primary and secondary ducts manifests itself as retention cysts, wich in turn are sequelae to intrapancreatic secretory obstruction and ductal ectasia.

Ultrasound findings. As in siderosis, here too ultrasound can demonstrate the increased echogenicity induced by the fibrosis, but in chronic pancreatitis these fibrotic areas tend to be mottled or cloddy. They may be loosely distributed or bunched together. Additional calcification results in zones of posterior shadowing. Calcifying chronic pancreatitis demonstrates finely or roughly distributed hard echoes. Since the frequent shadowing zones are most often wide, they will conceal the deeper structures such as the retroperitoneal vessels. The pancreas will be difficult to identify because the landmark structures cannot be visualized and the contour of the organ is blurred. Together with the subsequent atrophy, this compounds the fact that ultrasound studies of the pancreas have a sensitivity of only 70–80%[1,4] (**Fig. 4.20**). Pseudocysts and dilatation of the duct tend to result in a more heterogeneous texture (see below).

If all morphological changes are present, chronic pancreatitis is characterized by the following ultrasound criteria (**see Figs. 4.23, 4.25, 4.55**):
▶ Fibrosis
▶ Calcification/Intraductal stones
▶ Microcysts and macrocysts
▶ Ectatic duct
▶ Atrophy in the terminal stage

The majority of all chronic pancreatitis does not exhibit all of the above criteria but rather only fibrosis, dilated ducts, or a combination of two or more of these criteria. In acute episodes the sonographic signs of acute pancreatitis may also be present.

The 1984 Marseille classification[8] of chronic pancreatitis rests on the clinical and morphological aspects.

Imaging modalities play a vital role in the diagnosis of chronic pancreatitis. Ultrasonography and endoscopic retrograde pancreaticography (ERP) are regarded as baseline studies. The guidelines for assessing the severity of chronic pancreatitis also take into account these different imaging modalities (**Table 4.2**).

Classification of Chronic Pancreatitis (Marseille 1984)[8]

Clinical characteristics. Recurrent or persistent abdominal pain; sometimes without pain.

Morphological characteristics
▶ Irregular sclerosis with focal, segmental, or diffuse destruction and permanent loss of exocrine parenchyma of the gland.
▶ Dilatation of varying degree of various ductal segments.
▶ Protein deposits, calcification (intraductal calculi).
▶ Edema, focal necrosis, inflammatory cells, and cysts and pseudocysts are found to a varying degree.
▶ The islets of Langerhans will be affected much later.
▶ The following descriptive morphological terms are used:
1. Chronic pancreatitis with focal necrosis
2. Chronic pancreatitis with segmental or diffuse fibrosis
3. Chronic pancreatitis with or without calcification (calculi)

Course. The irreversible morphological changes will lead to a definite progressive loss of the exocrine and endocrine pancreatic function.

Special case: Obstructive chronic pancreatitis
Morphological characteristics
▶ Dilatation of the ductal tree upstream of the obstruction in a major duct (e.g. tumor or scar).
▶ Diffuse atrophy of the parenchyma and regularly diffuse fibrosis.
▶ Calculi are almost never present.

Course. After the obstruction has been cleared, the morphological and functional changes will usually resolve completely.

Since the different forms of chronic pancreatitis can be differentiated morphologically, and furthermore since there may be focal change, by itself or concomitant with the underlying disease, chronic pancreatitis may be demonstrated in a number of sonographic variants, depending on the predominant histopathological changes. ◻ **4.1** depicts possible sonographic images and variants.

Differentiation. Misdiagnosis may result from pancreatic fibrolipomatosis/lipomatosis due to fatty and fibrotic deposits in elderly obese diabetics, as well as scattering, refraction, and ultrasound absorption by adjacent/superimposed tissue. These factors will blur the margins and texture of the organs and could lead to the mistaken ultrasound diagnosis of chronic pancreatitis (**Table 4.3, Fig. 4.21**).

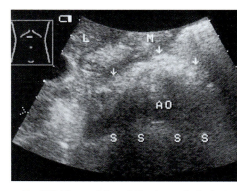
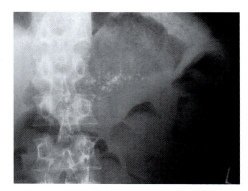
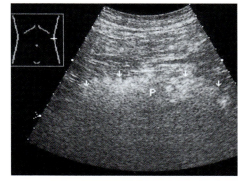

▲ **Fig. 4.20** Micronodular calcification with shadowing (S) in chronic calcifying pancreatitis.
a Sonographic image. M = stomach; AO = aorta; L = liver.

▲ *b* Plain radiographic film.

▲ **Fig. 4.21** Misdiagnosis of chronic pancreatitis (P = pancreas). In this case, ultrasound cannot assess the possible presence of coarse, cloddy fibrosis. CT: normal pancreas (no clinical symptoms). Probably interference by superimposed peripancreatic fat.

Table 4.2 Classification of chronic pancreatitis by imaging modality (Cambridge 1984)[5]

Pancreas/pancreatitis	ERCP	Ultrasound or CT
Normal	Good-quality visualization of the entire gland without pathological signs	
Questionable	< 3 pathological branches	One pathological finding = pancreatic duct 2–4 mm
Mild	> 3 pathological branches	Two pathological findings: cysts < 10 mm irregular duct acute focal pancreatitis parenchymal heterogenicity increased echogenicity of the duct wall irregular contour of head/body
Moderate	All of the above signs plus pathological pancreatitis	All of the above pathological signs
Severe	All of the above signs plus one or more of the following: cyst > 10 mm intraductal voids calculi/pancreatic calcification duct obstruction (stricture) severe dilatation or irregularity of duct adjacent organs affected (demonstrated on ultrasound or CT)	

Table 4.3 Differentiating chronic pancreatitis and fibrolipomatosis

Chronic pancreatitis	Fibrolipomatosis
Hyperechoic, coarse texture	Hyperechoic, fine texture
Inhomogeneities because of – microcysts/macrocysts – parenchymal calcification/intraductal calculi – obstruction/stricture of duct, dilated duct	Homogeneous structure
Increased/decreased size (atrophy)	Normal size
Indurated	No or little induration (palpating finger/propagated aortic pulse)

4.1 Chronic Pancreatitis (CP) on Ultrasound (modified from reference 8)

▶ Chronic pancreatitis with focal necrosis

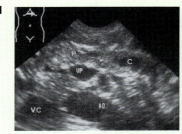
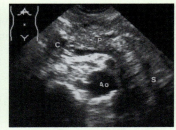
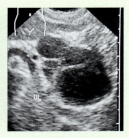

a CP with necrotic episodes, necrosis (C) of the pancreatic tail. VC = vena cava; VP = portal vein; P = pancreas; AO = aorta.

b Six months later: regression accompanied by increased echogenicity and shadowing (S); fresh necrotic area in the head of the pancreas (C). P = pancreas; AO = aorta.

c Months later, another episode of necrosis. VL = splenic vein.

▶ Chronic pancreatitis with segmental or diffuse fibrosis

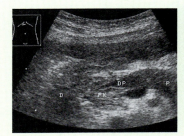
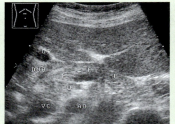
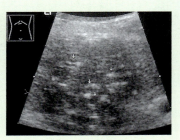

d Fibrosis of the pancreatic head (PK), stenosis of the pancreatic duct (DP); normal body and tail of the pancreas. D = duodenum; P = pancreas.

e Hyperechoic micronodular texture: fibrotic pancreas in cystic fibrosis/hemochromatosis. GB = gallbladder; DUO = duodenum; VC = vena cava; AO = aorta; P = pancreas; U = uncinate process

f Intermittent chronic pancreatitis (pancreas divisum): hyperechoic micronodular fibrosis within the enlarged edematous pancreas. Dilated excretory ducts interspersed in the fibrosis (arrows).

▶ Chronic pancreatitis with calcification/calculi

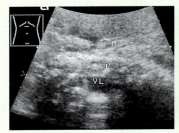
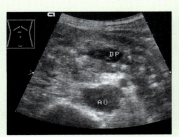
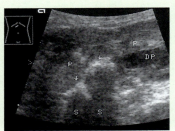

g Chronic pancreatitis: diffuse micronodular calcification with summation shadowing. M = stomach, VL = splenic vein; P = pancreas; L = liver.

h Same patient as in *d* with segmental CP 3½ years later: calcification of the entire pancreas. DP = pancreatic duct; AO = aorta.

i Same patient: oblique right epigastric view: coarse cloddy calcification or intraductal calculi (arrows, shadowing S) along the pancreatic duct in the head. P = pancreas; DP = pancreatic duct.

▶ Obstructive chronic pancreatitis (special variant)

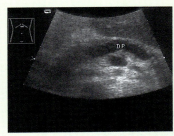
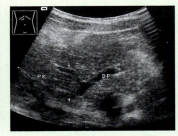
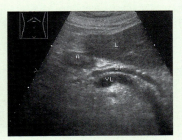

j Chronic obstruction of the pancreatic duct (DP) due to microcystic adenoma, with fibrotic areas in the pancreatic tail and incipient atrophy. Initially interpreted as chronic pancreatitis.

k Pancreas divisum: relative stenosis of the anterior accessory duct of Santorini (downward arrow), filiform stenosis of the posteroinferior duct (upward duct) coursing toward the papilla of Vater. DP = pancreatic duct; PK = pancreatic head.

l Obstruction due to pancreas divisum with loose, echogenic areas of fibrosis and atrophy. A = antrum; L = liver; DP = pancreatic duct; VL = splenic vein.

Focal Changes

Focal changes may display the whole gamut of echogenicity from anechoic to hyperechoic and heterogeneous lesions. They may correspond to anomalies or variants, and may be inflammatory or tumorous. Every so often these focal changes are the result of papillotomy or ductal procedures, which can be confirmed quite easily from the patient's history. Cancer is the most important of these focal changes. It cannot be excluded from diagnostic consideration, unless another origin of the lesion in question has been proven.

Anechoic Lesion

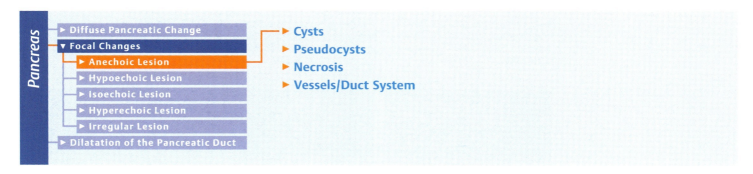

Table 4.4 lists the most important differential diagnoses of the anechoic pancreatic mass.

Table 4.4 Differential diagnosis of the anechoic pancreatic mass

Congenital cyst	Retention cyst	Necrosis	Pseudocyst
Anechoic	Anechoic	Anechoic/hypoechoic	Anechoic/heterogeneous
Round	Round or polygonal	Polycyclic	
Enhancement	< 1 cm together	Mottled or banded	Almost round
Liver/kidney cysts	with: fibrosis, calcification, ductal ectasia	No halo	Echogenic wall

▶ Cysts

Congenital cyst. Congenital cysts may be solitary or multiple, in the latter case accompanied by polycystic kidney disease. Compared with the cysts secondary to inflammation or the frequent cysts in chronic pancreatitis, they are extremely rare and incidental findings.

Retention cyst. Retention cysts are small, come in multiples, and are usually found together with other signs of chronic pancreatitis. They are filled with clear pancreatic secretion.

Hydatid cyst. Intrapancreatic hydatid cyst is a true rarity; as is the case with their hepatic counterparts, these cysts will display a hyperechoic inflammatory wall.

Ultrasound findings. Ultrasound studies of congenital cysts will demonstrate the characteristic criteria of cysts and show them to be anechoic. Retention cysts are also anechoic, often with irregular texture, and frequently hard to differentiate from other anechoic structures such as cross-sectional views of the splenic artery, ectatic pancreatic duct with stricture, dilated prepapillary CBD, and intraparenchymal necrosis (**Figs. 4.22, 4.23**).

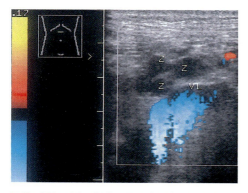

▲ *Fig. 4.22 a* Color duplex: myriad small cysts (C) in the pancreas. VL = splenic vein; red = splenic artery.

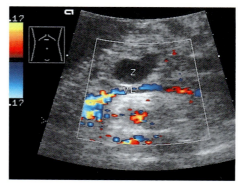

▲ *b* Small pancreatic cyst (Z). Incidental finding in a normal pancreas. Color-flow Doppler.

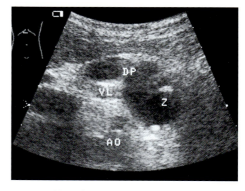

▲ *c* Cyst (Z) in chronic pancreatitis. Ectatic duct (DP), pericystic calcification, fibrosis. AO = aorta; VL = splenic vein.

▶ Pseudocysts

Morphology. Ultrasound morphology differentiates between microcysts of less than 10 mm and macrocysts of more than 10 mm diameter; symptomatic cysts usually have a diameter of more than 60 mm. While in most cases microcysts are simply ectatic sections of the pancreatic duct in chronic pancreatitis, filled with clear juice, and should be properly classified as retention cysts, the larger macrocysts tend to be present in acute pancreatitis or an acute episode of chronic pancreatitis. They are filled with a greenish or brownish cloudy fluid of inflammatory hemorrhagic nature. Pseudocysts will develop in 5–15% of acute pancreatitis and 25% of chronic pancreatitis. Smaller pseudocysts may resolve and vanish. The classification of pancreatic pseudocysts is listed in **Table 4.5**.

Ultrasound findings. Some pseudocysts are extremely large, filling most of the abdomen, and ultrasound may not be able to retrace them to the pancreas with certainty. Anechoic pseudocysts are rare; in most cases, they are filled with hyperechoic irregular intrinsic structures that (in infection, incidence 5%) are rooted in pus and detritus or necrosis and blood clots (**Figs. 4.23–4.25**).

Pathomorphology of Pancreatic Cysts

True cysts
- ▶ *Congenital cysts.* Their wall is made up of simple epithelium, as in liver and kidney cysts, and they are frequently found in conjunction with them.
- ▶ *Retention cysts.* These represent ectatic duct and branch segments and are filled with clear pancreatic juice.
- ▶ *Neoplastic cysts.* These originate from cystadenomas or cystadenocarcinomas; their wall is made up of neoplastic epithelium.

Pseudocysts
- ▶ Pseudocysts are the result of self-digestion of the pancreas in trauma or inflammation.
- ▶ The walls of pseudocysts arise from the reaction of the surrounding tissue to the accumulation of inflammatory fluid.
- ▶ Pseudocysts are most often filled with greenish or hemorrhagic cloudy secretion.

Table 4.5 **Classification of Pancreatic Pseudocysts**

Type I	Pseudocysts in acute necrotizing pancreatitis: usually, no communication with pancreatic duct normal ERCP
Type II	Pseudocysts after an acute episode of chronic pancreatitis: often, communication with pancreatic duct ERCP: irregular duct, no stenosis
Type III	Retention cysts in chronic pancreatitis: internal communication with pancreatic duct ERCP: significant stenoses

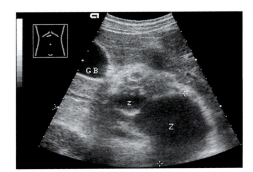

▲ *Fig. 4.23* Microcyst (z) and macrocyst (Z) type II after an acute episode of chronic pancreatitis: anechoic mass in the body and tail of the pancreas. GB = gallbladder.

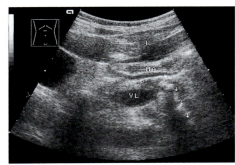

▲ *Fig. 4.24* Same patient as in **Fig. 4.23**. After five months, spontaneous resolution of the pseudocysts; hyperechoic calcification, shadowing (arrows). L = liver; MA = stomach; P = pancreas; VL = splenic vein.

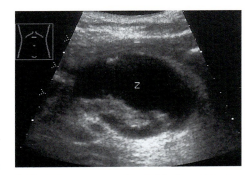

▲ *Fig. 4.25* Incipient pseudocyst (C) after acute pancreatitis: predominantly hypoechoic mass with echogenic sediment. The stomach is displaced anteriorly.

▶ Necrosis

As the term implies, the severe course of acute hemorrhagic necrotizing pancreatitis will produce necrosis within a few days after onset of the disease. Frequently, it is accompanied by collections of peripancreatic fluid, ascites (around spleen, liver, kidney, and in the lower abdomen/Douglas's pouch), and pleural effusion of the left lung (**Fig. 4.26–4.28**).

Ultrasonic differentiation between acute edematous and hemorrhagic necrotizing pancreatitis is based on histopathological criteria; however, in the early stages CT studies might be useful for staging and in obtaining the baseline status when surgery might be an option.

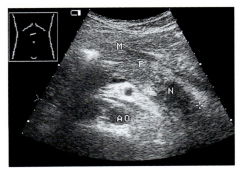

▲ *Fig. 4.26* Necrosis (N, calipers) in the tail of the pancreas (P), acute pancreatitis. M = stomach; AO = aorta.

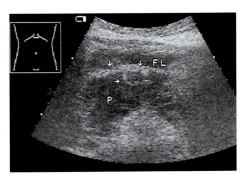

▲ *Fig. 4.27* Acute hemorrhagic necrotizing pancreatitis: extensive edema of the pancreas (P), focal necrosis/bleeding (horizontal arrow), hyperechoic peripancreatic fatty necrosis (arrows), fluid in the lesser sac (FL).

Abscess. Most abscesses arise from infected necrosis; early fine-needle aspiration cytology and culturing of the necroses is necessary in order to decide on possible surgical intervention. Fever and septic temperature are indicative of abscess formation (**Fig. 4.29**).

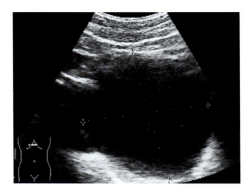

▲ **Fig. 4.28** Extensive anechoic liquid necrosis, severe episode of acute hemorrhagic necrotizing pancreatitis.

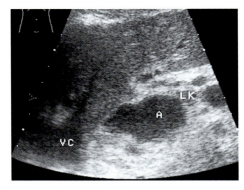

▲ **Fig. 4.29** Peripancreatic abscess after pancreatitis (patient hospitalized because of septic temperatures, no clinical sign of previous pancreatitis): irregularly defined hypoechoic abscess formation (A) below the liver with adjacent inflammatory lymphadenopathy (LK); paracaval (VC) view high in the epigastrium; evacuated by ultrasound-guided fine-needle aspiration.

▶ Vessels/Duct System

Vessels. The splenic and gastroduodenal arteries might be mistaken for microcysts, and the splenic vein for the pancreatic duct (**Figs. 4.30, Fig. 4.31**). Aneurysms of the splenic artery are rare and can be reliably differentiated from cysts by color-flow Doppler scanning.

Ductal cysts. The pancreatic duct has numerous variants. In most patients it is found off-center at the junction between the middle and posterior thirds of the pancreas. It turns caudad in the pancreatic head, and in stenosis of the papilla of Vater it can be traced as a dilated tube running in parallel with the CBD. The cross-sectional view of both ductal systems will visualize them as round cystic structures. Color-flow Doppler scanning identifies them as ducts and not blood vessels.

Dilated segments of the pancreatic duct due to ductal obstruction in chronic pancreatitis may mimic cysts and be easily misdiagnosed (**Fig. 4.32**).

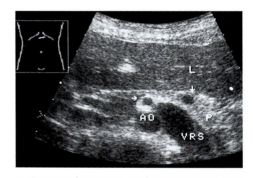

▲ **Fig. 4.30** Splenic artery: anechoic cystic structures in the body and tail of the pancreas (P, arrows). AO = aorta; VRS = left renal vein; L = liver.

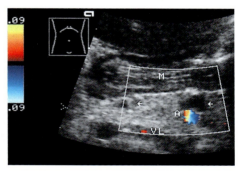

▲ **Fig. 4.31** Microcysts in the pancreas; color-flow Doppler scan: two metastases resolving under chemotherapy, no vascularization. Color-flow Doppler imaging demonstrates the third anechoic mass to be the splenic artery. A = lienal artery; M = stomach; VL = splenic vein.

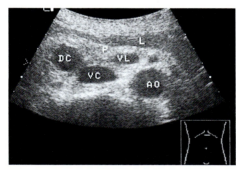

▲ **Fig. 4.32** Significantly dilated prepapillary CBD (DC) within the head of the pancreas (P), in sclerosis of the papilla of Vater. VL = splenic vein; AO = aorta; VC = vena cava; L = liver.

Hypoechoic Lesion

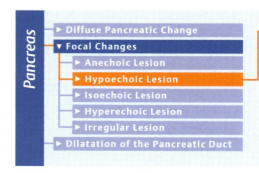

- ▶ **Neuroendocrine Tumors**
- ▶ **Pancreatic Cancer**
- ▶ **Metastasis, Malignant Lymphoma, Inflammatory Lymph Node**
- ▶ **Abscess**
- ▶ **Hemorrhagic/Calcified Cyst/Pseudocyst**
- ▶ **Focal Pancreatitis**

▶ Neuroendocrine Tumors

Neuroendocrine tumors comprise rare intrapancreatic tumors, stemming from the neural crest, with possible endocrine activity. Because the pancreas houses a large number of endocrine cells, endocrine tumors may arise here, particularly insulinoma, a mostly benign tumor while the gastrinoma as a rule can be detected only after it has transformed into malignancy. Even rarer entities are glucagonomas, VIPomas, somatostatinomas, and carcinoid.

Because of their small size (< 2 cm), insulinomas are hardly ever visualized on transcutaneous ultrasound; at best, the clinical diagnosis in the fasting state can only be confirmed by endosonography or intraoperatively.

Ultrasound studies show endocrine tumors to be hypoechoic, round, and smoothly delineated (**Fig. 4.33a**). Endosonography is the most sensitive imaging modality in the diagnosis of neuroendocrine tumors. Endocrine tumors appear as hypoechoic smooth, round structures with increased vascularization; however, further differentiation by ultrasonography is not possible (**Fig. 4.33b**).

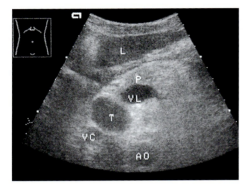
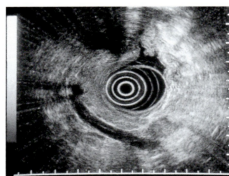

◀◀ *Fig. 4.33 a* Metastasizing neuroendocrine tumor (T) of the head of the pancreas. AO = aorta; L = liver; P = pancreas; VC = vena cava; VL = splenic vein.

◀ *b* Insulinoma in the tail of the pancreas, also visualized is the splenic vein. Endosonography (Dr. N. Heyder, Munic).

▶ Pancreatic Cancer

Pancreatic cancer is a focal, defined solid lesion. The most important criterion of malignancy is its bulging contour; other diagnostic characteristics are tumor spread, cut-off of the pancreatic duct, displacement, invasion, and locoregional as well as distant metastasis (**Fig. 4.34**). Ductal pancreatic cancer arises from the epithelium of the pancreatic duct and therefore will result in a sudden cut-off of the duct and prestenotic dilatation.

Periampullary cancer is a separate and quite different entity because it is an adenocarcinoma of the periampullary mucosa of the papilla of Vater.

Ultrasound findings. As in most other malignancies, the texture of pancreatic cancer is hypoechoic, although assessment of the texture depends on the echogenicity of the pancreas. Since the gland may present as hypoechoic or hyperechoic, depending on the age of the patient, pancreatic cancer will be demonstrated not only as a hypoechoic structure within a hyperechoic pancreas but also as an isoechoic (quite rarely as hyperechoic) lesion within a hypoechoic pancreas of normal texture.

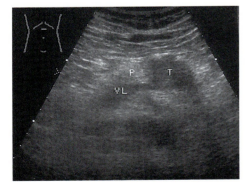
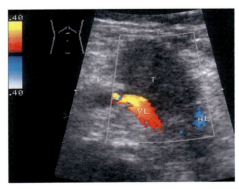

◀◀ *Fig. 4.34* Carcinoma (T) at the junction of the body and tail of the pancreas: elliptical, hypoechoic mass with irregular margins in an echogenic (lipomatous) pancreas (P).
a B-mode image.

◀ *b* Color duplex scan. AL = splenic artery; VL = splenic vein.

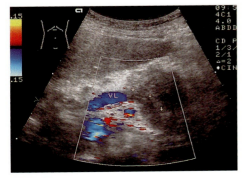
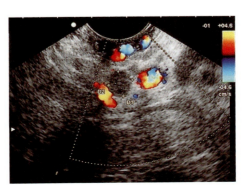

◀◀ *c* Carcinoma at the body/tail of the pancreas with infiltration (arrows) of the splenic vein (VL)

◀ *d* Carcinoma of the pancreas (T), endosonography: multiple lymph nodes, the largest one with cursors. Endosonography is the best imaging modality in the diagnosis of small tumors and operability.

Histological Classification of Pancreatic Cancer

Benign Pancreatic Tumors
- Adenomas, which are quite rare and arise from the acinar or centroacinar cells
- Cystadenomas with cystic and solid parts: cystadenomas are classified into mucinous, macrocystic, and histologically most often already malignant, types and the rather rare microcystic benign cystadenoma
- Mesenchymal tumors (hemangioma, lipoma)
- Endocrine tumors (insulinoma, gastrinoma, VIPoma, and glucagonoma). Insulinoma and gastrinoma are the most common endocrine tumors; rarely do they exceed 1–2 cm and 2–4 cm in diameter, respectively.

Malignant Tumors
- ductal carcinomas; accounting for 80% of pancreatic malignancies, they arise from the epithelium of the duct and originate primarily in the head of the pancreas. They comprise:
  - Tubular adenocarcinoma
  - Mucinous adenocarcinoma
  - Adenosquamous carcinoma
  - Squamous cell carcinoma
  - Pleomorphic giant cell type carcinoma
- Endocrine tumors
- Acinar cell carcinoma.

▶ Metastasis, Malignant Lymphoma, Inflammatory Lymph Node

Differential diagnosis of suspected pancreatic cancer has to consider endocrine tumors, metastasis of, e.g., lung cancer or malignant melanoma, and malignant lymphoma.

Metastases. These appear as smooth round or polygonal structures and are almost impossible to differentiate from primary pancreatic cancer (**Fig. 4.35**).

Lymphoma. The pancreas is permeated by an extensive intrapancreatic and extrapancreatic lymph system, and therefore malignant lymphoma will manifest itself as intrapancreatic as well as extrapancreatic neoplasm. It is seen as a flat or bulky, primarily hypoechoic lesion (**Fig. 4.36**).

Inflammatory lymph node. Sometimes there are inflammatory lymph nodes along the pancreatic margin that may be difficult to separate from the gland. In most cases, confirmation of suspected malignancy has to await fine-needle aspiration biopsy.

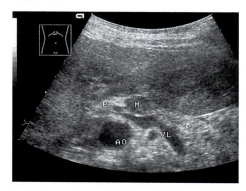
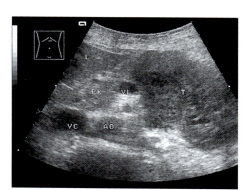

◀◀ **Fig. 4.35** Metastasis (M) of gastric cancer in the pancreatic head. AO = aorta; VL = splenic vein; P = pancreas.

◀ **Fig. 4.36** High-grade non-Hodgkin lymphoma (T) in the body/tail of the pancreas, sole manifestation. Diagnosis confirmed by ultrasound-guided fine-needle aspiration biopsy. PK = head of pancreas; AO = aorta; VC = vena cava; VL = splenic vein.

▶ Abscess

Abscess impresses as an anechoic or, more commonly, hypoechoic mass; frequently, it demonstrates intrinsic structures and may then appear as a hypoechoic inhomogeneous lesion (**Fig. 4.29**).

▶ Hemorrhagic/Calcified Cyst/Pseudocyst

Pancreatic pseudocysts may display a variety of textures, but normally they are anechoic. Bleeding or calcification in the wall will result in a rather hypoechoic mass, even resembling a tumor or abscess (**Fig. 4.37**).

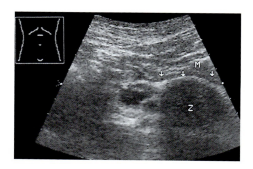

◀ **Fig. 4.37** Pancreatic pseudocyst (Z) with calcification (arrows) at the margin, resembling a hypoechoic (and not anechoic) cystic mass because of the superimposed incomplete shadowing. M = stomach with impression.

▶ Focal Pancreatitis

Focal pancreatitis of the head/tail of the pancreas resembles a tumor, making differentiation from true malignancy difficult. The suspected diagnosis of focal pancreatitis is based on patient history and clinical symptoms, but it should be remembered that pancreatic cancer may also trigger acute pancreatitis. A special form is "groove pancreatitis" (first described by Becker), a focal pancreatitis affecting the head of the pancreas around the intrapancreatic common bile duct. In this case, any increased tumor marker will subside after resolution of the acute symptoms, while in pancreatic cancer the marker will increase steadily. Fine-needle aspiration biopsy will be of differential diagnostic value only if it is positive (**Fig. 4.38, Table 4.6**).

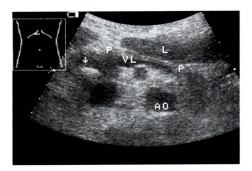
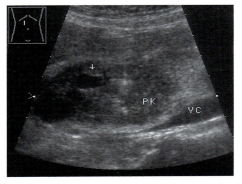
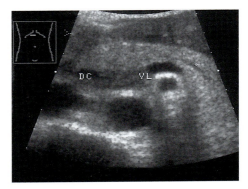
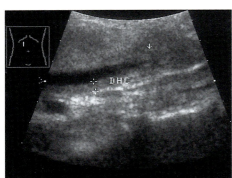

◂◂ *Fig. 4.38 a* Focal pancreatitis in the head of the pancreas (P): hypoechoic, swollen, well-defined head with calcifications, probably intraductal calculus (arrow): the swelling in the pancreatic head is almost impossible to differentiate from cancer. L = liver; AO = aorta; VL = splenic vein.

◂ *b* Acute attack of chronic pancreatitis: hypoechoic swelling of the pancreatic head (PK) with compression of the inferior vena cava (VC). Arrow: dilated pancreatic duct.

◂◂ *c* Focal pancreatitis in the pancreatic head, "groove pancreatitis" with a duct stone, extracted endoscopically. Hypoechoic area in the uncinate process around the common bile duct (DC). VL = splenic vein.

◂ *d* Stenosis of the intrapancreatic common bile duct (arrow); inflammatory wall thickening (calipers).

Table 4.6 Differentiating pancreatic cancer from focal pancreatitis

	Pancreatic cancer	**Focal pancreatitis**
Contour	Bulging (leading sign), small "feet"	Bulging contour (head, tail), smooth/serrated
Texture	Homogeneous to finely mottled irregular (hypoechoic within hyperechoic basic texture, isoechoic within hypoechoic basic texture)	Hypoechoic—homogeneous (acute pancreatitis) Hyperechoic—mottled to irregular (chronic pancreatitis)
Delineation	Blurred to irregular, rarely smooth	Well defined
Pancreatic duct	Prestenotic dilatation common	Rarely dilated
Surroundings	Common: invasion of the duodenum and blood vessels (splenic vein, celiac axis), locoregional metastases, bile duct obstruction, gallbladder with Courvoisier's sign. Rarely: segmental portal hypertension	Rarely: adhesive scarring of posterior gastric wall/duodenum, thrombosis of splenic/portal vein, bile duct obstruction
Color-flow duplex scanning	Almost no intrinsic vascularization, invasion of splenic vein and celiac axis	Normal or marked coloration

Isoechoic Lesion

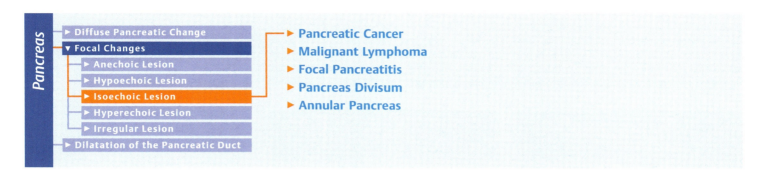

▶ Pancreatic Cancer

If the texture of the pancreas is hypoechoic, as evidenced in slim young patients, the texture of pancreatic cancer will be isoechoic and can only be differentiated by its bulging contour and any secondary signs. Cancers of the pancreatic tail and uncinate process are also hard to detect, and at that only in the special planes of the oblique/transverse epigastric views: on the right for the head and on the left for the tail of the pancreas (**Figs. 4.39 and 4.40**).

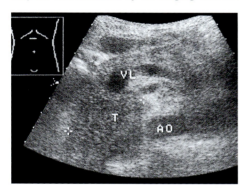
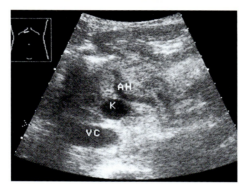

◀◀ **Fig. 4.39** Cancer of the pancreatic head in the uncinate process (T; calipers); isoechoic mass. Direction of spread is posterior, the splenic vein can no longer be demonstrated; color-flow Doppler scanning could help settle the issue of possible invasion into the vena cava. AO = aorta; VL = splenic vein.

◀ **Fig. 4.40** Pancreatic cancer: isoechoic texture of the tumor invading the celiac axis and embracing the hepatic artery (AH); inoperable. K = venous confluence; VC = vena cava.

▶ Malignant Lymphoma

Malignant lymphoma may also be isoechoic with the pancreas, although its characteristic texture is visualized as markedly hypoechoic (**Fig. 4.9**).

▶ Focal Pancreatitis

While in most cases acute focal pancreatitis appears hypoechoic, chronic focal pancreatitis may be isoechoic with the surrounding pancreatic tissue, and therefore can only be differentiated by focal enlargement and a more macronodular texture (**Figs. 4.41 and 4.42**).

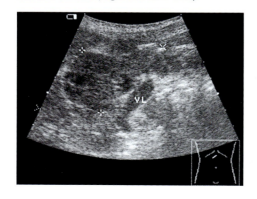
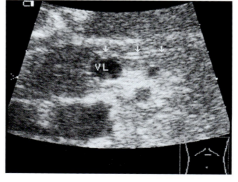

◀◀ **Fig. 4.41** Acute pancreatitis: striking enlargement (calipers) of the pancreatic head with isoechoic texture, tumorlike appearance; slightly inhomogeneous hypoechoic overall pancreatic texture. The bulging tumor cannot be differentiated from a malignant mass. VL = splenic vein.

◀ **Fig. 4.42** Isoechoic enlarged head of the pancreas: chronic focal pancreatitis of the head with significant focal enlargement; slightly irregular diameter of the pancreatic duct (arrows), which is not dilated. VL = splenic vein.

▶ Pancreas divisum

Congenital Anomaly—Pancreas divisum

During embryological development, the smaller, originally ventral anlage and the larger dorsal anlage fuse. The ventral anlage constitutes the inferior parts of the head and uncinate process of the pancreas, as well as the main pancreatic duct, while from the dorsal anlage emanate the remainder of the pancreatic head, the entire body and tail, and the anlage for the accessory duct of Santorini. The latter may sometimes persist after fusion and drains the pancreatic juice to the minor papilla, or it may resolve and drain into the main pancreatic duct to the papilla of Vater.

Fusion anomalies (complete or incomplete pancreas divisum) are quite common. The accessory duct of Santorini will drain most of the pancreatic juice via the minor papilla, while the main pancreatic duct (of Wirsung) drains part of the pancreatic head and the uncinate process and displays either no (complete pancreas divisum) or only a thin (incomplete pancreas divisum) communication with the main duct **(Fig. 4.43)**. The relative stenosis upstream of the minor papilla may cause recurrent episodes of pancreatitis.

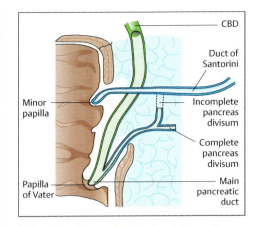

▲ **Fig. 4.43** Schematic drawing of complete and incomplete pancreas divisum.

Pancreas divisum is characterized by a strikingly enlarged head of the pancreas with normal texture, segmental ductal dilatation in the pancreatic body, and the demonstration of two distinct ductal systems in the pancreatic head **(Fig. 4.43–4.45)**.

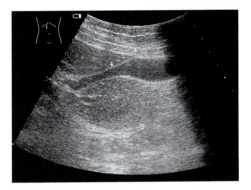
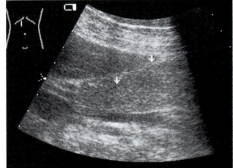

◀◀ **Fig. 4.44** Enlarged head of the pancreas.
 a Impressing the posterior wall of the gallbladder (arrow).

◀ **b** Impressing the vena cava (arrows). CT study suspected malignancy. Ultrasound diagnosis: probably pancreas divisum. ERCP: pancreas divisum.

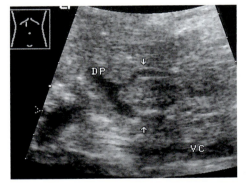
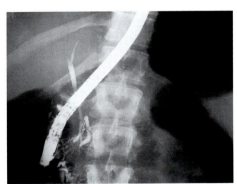

◀◀ **Fig. 4.45** Pancreas divisum, recurrent pancreatitis.
 a Longitudinal ultrasound view demonstrating two pancreatic ducts (arrows). The ventral duct is seen to possess a narrow communication with the main pancreatic duct (DP); the larger posterior duct is the accessory duct of Santorini. VC = vena cava.

◀ **b** ERCP through the papilla of Vater, with visualization of the CBD and rudiments of the main pancreatic duct.

▶ Annular Pancreas

Annular pancreas is another example of an isoechoic focal lesion with changes in size and shape; only in rare instances is it completely annular. In most patients it is completely or incompletely annular around the pancreatic head, which envelops the descending duodenum and may result in stenosis.

In ultrasonography there is definite compression of the descending duodenum by the enlarged head of the pancreas, which is missing its usual border with the duodenum and extends further to the right, posterior and lateral to the duodenum (◻ **4.2**).

4.2 Annular Pancreas

▶ Annular pancreas: at the head the pancreas presents as a complete or incomplete ring around the descending duodenum and may lead to stenosis.

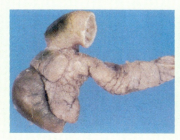 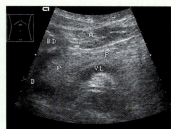 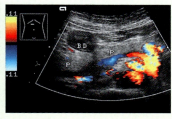

a Pathological specimen (from: Riede and Stolte, General and Special Pathology, Thieme Verlag).

b Pancreatic tissue (P), unusually far to the right; the descending duodenum (D) is stenosed by the formation of the pancreas. A = antrum, BD = duodenal bulb. GB = gallbladder; U = uncinate process; VC = vena cava; AO = aorta

c Transverse epigastric view. The pancreas (P) continues rather strikingly to the right (arrows) posterior to the dilated (prestenotic) duodenum (BD). VL = splenic vein.

L = liver
M = stomach
P = pancreas
VL = splenic vein

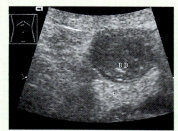 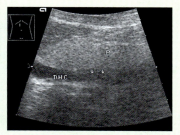

d and e Direct demonstration of the ring formation posterior to the duodenal bulb in a view shifted somewhat compared with *b* and *c*. The CBD is also stenosed upstream of the papilla (incidental clinical finding of cholestasis; the pancreas was demonstrated first in the CT study).

DP = pancreatic duct
S = shadowing
AO = aorta

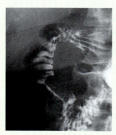 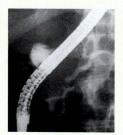

f and g Hypotone duodenogram and ERCP: stenosis of the descending duodenum. In the ERC distal stenosis (not demonstrated here) of the CBD of intermittent character and pancreatic duct enveloping the contrasted duodenum.

Hyperechoic Lesion

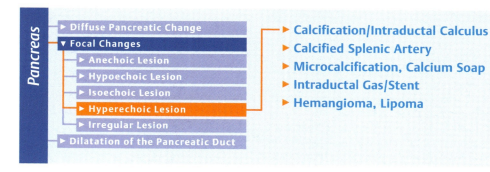

▶ Calcification/Intraductal Calculus

The most striking, and in addition pathognomonic, criteria for chronic pancreatitis are calcification and intraductal calculi. They are made of calcium carbonate precipitates and are located in the main pancreatic duct (intraductal calculi) and the branching ductules ("parenchymal calcification"). They appear as intensively hyperechoic structures with posterior shadowing (**Fig. 4.46, Table 4.7**).

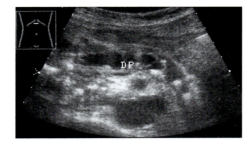

◀ **Fig. 4.46** Chronic calcifying pancreatitis with pancreatic duct stones (DP), and calcified areas in the parenchyma.

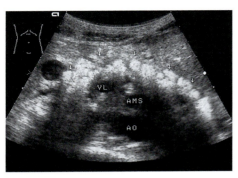
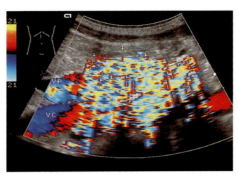
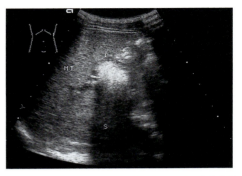

▲ **Fig. 4.47 a–c** Chronic calcifying pancreatitis.
a Brightness picture: coarse diffuse echogenic structure with multiple posterior shadowing and summation shadowing. VL = splenic vein; AMS = superior mesenteric vein; AO = aorta.

▲ *b* Color Doppler "twinkling artifact" with confetti phenomena. VP = portal vein; VC = vena cava.

▲ *c* Trans-splenic section. Calcification (arrows) in the tail of the pancreas, shadowing (S). MI = spleen.

Table 4.7 Diagnostic criteria for calcification/intraductal calculi

Parenchymal calcification	Intraductal calculi
Individual or multiple intensive echoes with posterior shadowing; broad irregular band of echoes	Intensive echoes with posterior shadowing, individual or loosely strung along the duct
Summation shadowing with nonvisualization of the structures behind	Dilatation of the prestenotic duct due to calculi
No landmark structure because of thrombosis or warping of the splenic vein, celiac axis, aorta, and vena cava!	

▶ Calcified Splenic Artery

Diffuse calcification of the splenic artery presents as a similar structure (**Fig. 4.48**).

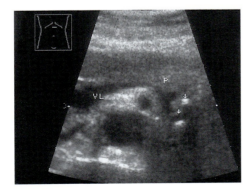

◀ **Fig. 4.48** Echogenic calcified mottling (arrows): calcified splenic artery. VL = splenic vein; P = pancreas.

▶ Microcalcification, Calcium Soap

Microcalcification can be found in chronic pancreatitis, in pancreatic cancer, and as sclerosis in arterial walls. Calcium soap as part of acute pancreatitis will appear as focal echogenic peripancreatic mottling/bands (**Fig. 4.49, 4.50** and **Fig. 4.24**).

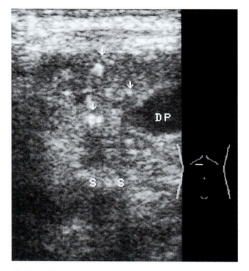

▲ **Fig. 4.49** Echogenic microcalcification with shadowing (S) in pancreatic cancer; cut-off of the pancreatic duct (DP).

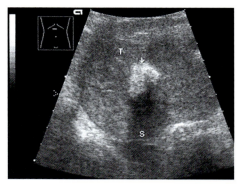

▲ **Fig. 4.50** Microcalcification and macrocalcification (arrows, shadowing S) in advanced pancreatic cancer (T).

▶ Intraductal Gas/Stent

After endoscopic intervention at the papilla or pancreatic duct, gas (after papillotomy) or stents may be evidenced as echogenic foreign bodies within the duct (**Fig. 4.51–4.53**). Usually, their differential diagnosis becomes self-evident from the patient's history.

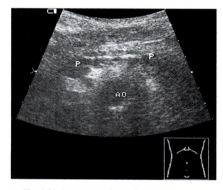

▲ **Fig. 4.51** Pancreatic duct after ERCP; in serial views the gas (arrows) beads around the duct on repositioning of the patient. P = pancreas; AO = aorta.

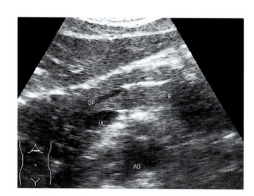

▲ **Fig. 4.52** Echogenic stent in the pancreatic duct (arrow; DP). P = pancreas; VL = splenic vein; AO = aorta.

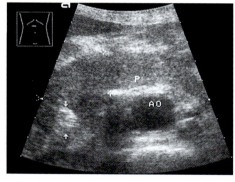

▲ **Fig. 4.53** Diffuse pancreatic cancer in the head/body of the pancreas (P) (calipers 20 mm); CBD stent (arrows) in place. AO = aorta;.

▶ Hemangioma, Lipoma

Hemangioma and lipoma will both be visualized as round, intensively hyperechoic lesions that cannot be differentiated by ultrasound. Both are rare entities within the pancreas. Their sonographic characteristics are those of typical hepatic hemangiomas (**Fig. 4.54**).

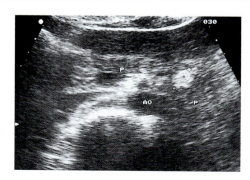

◀ **Fig. 4.54** Hyperechoic, smoothly delineated, ovoid lesion at the junction of the pancreatic body and tail: hemangioma (calipers differential diagnosis lipoma;). P = pancreas; AO = aorta.

Irregular Lesion

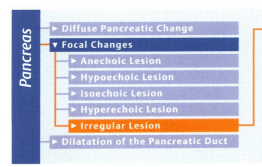

▶ Chronic Pancreatitis

If several or all of the criteria are present, quite often chronic pancreatitis will resemble a "lively" picture, where the individual criteria (cyst, fibrosis, calcification, dilated duct) can only be discerned with difficulty or not at all (**Fig. 4.55**).

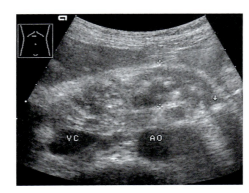

◀ **Fig. 4.55** Chronic pancreatitis: without the splenic vein as landmark structure (here thrombosed/obliterated), the pancreas is almost impossible to delineate (calipers); the "lively" image is due to ductal ectasia (arrow), here, with calculus, fibrosis, calcification, and microcysts. VC = vena cava; AO = aorta.

▶ Focal Chronic Pancreatitis

Here, too, the texture is heterogeneous, but because of the fibrosis and/or calcification it is micronodular to macronodular. Differential diagnosis has to consider pancreatic cancer (**Fig. 4.56**).

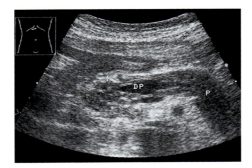

◀ **Fig. 4.56** Mottled hypoechoic/hyperechoic texture of the pancreatic head (P): focal chronic pancreatitis in the head, cut-off of the pancreatic duct (DP) (caution: cancer!)

▶ Pseudocyst

The retention cyst in chronic pancreatitis is anechoic, while the inflammatory pseudocyst in acute pancreatitis is characterized by detritus, hemorrhage, and pus collections, constituting the "lively" ultrasound image of this lesion with its hypoechoic as well as hyperechoic areas (**Fig. 4.57**).

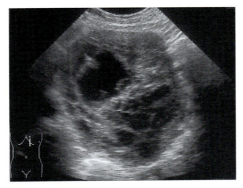 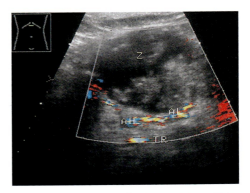

▲ **Fig. 4.57 a** Large, symptomatic pancreatic pseudocyst: complex masses in the left upper abdomen. Initial symptoms were caused by mass effects from the cyst.

▲ **b** Incipient pseudocyst (Z) after acute pancreatitis: complex mass displacing the hepatic artery (AH) and splenic artery (AL). Color duplex. TR = celiac axis.

▶ Cystic Neoplasias: Cystadenoma/Cystadenocarcinoma

Cystic neoplasias of the pancreas are rare. Ductal carcinomas comprise approximately 80% of all malignant neoplasms of the pancreas, and some 90% of those are ductal adenocarcinomas. Variants are intraductal papillary mucinous neoplasia and mucinous cystic neoplasia. The most common differential diagnosis of pseudocyst is versus neoplasms with a cystic appearance (IPMN, MCN and SPN[3]) because the gross appearance of the latter neoplasms may be similar to that of pseudocysts. Histologically and cytologically, however, pseudocysts differ from the cystic neoplasms in that they lack any epithelial lining but display hemorrhagic debris and inflammatory cells. Moreover, pseudocysts contain pancreatic enzymes, such as amylase and lipase, and lack elevated levels of CEA and CA 19–9.

▶ Mucinous Cystic Neoplasms (MCN)

MCNs of the pancreas affect women almost exclusively, do not communicate with the ductal system, and may be unilocular or multilocular.

More than 90% of MCNs occur in the body and tail of the pancreas, where they form large round cystic tumors showing a unilocular or multilocular appearance and diameters between 2 and 35 cm (**Fig. 4.58**).

▶ Serous Cystic Neoplasms: Serous Microcystic Adenoma (SMA)

Most common are SMAs, which make up 60% of all SCNs. They present as single, well-circumscribed, slightly bosselated round tumors, with diameters ranging from 1 to 25 cm.

About two thirds of the SMAs occur in the body-tail region and almost all in elderly women. They are usually found incidentally. Ultrasound shows numerous small (honeycomb-like) cysts up to two cm. The tumor occurs predominantly in the head of the pancreas, where it may obstruct the common bile duct and more often the pancreatic duct (**Fig. 4.59**).

▶ Intraductal Papillary-Mucinous Neoplasms

IPMNs are characterized by intraductal proliferation of mucin-producing cells, wich are arranged in papillary patterns. In many IPMNs hypersecretion of mucin leads to a cystic dilatation of the involved ducts. In a few IPMNs, focal or diffuse intraductal papillary growth causes duct dilatation (**Fig. 4.60a**).

▶ Ductal Adenocarcinoma and Variants with Cystic Features

DACs and variants thereof showing cystic features are relatively frequent among cystic tumors and account for 10%[3] (**Fig. 4.60b**).

▶ Solid Pseudopapillary Neoplasms (SPN)

SPNs are round tumors (diameters ranging from 3 to 18 cm) which are found in any region of the pancreas or loosely attached to it.

Table 4.8 is a summary list of the differential diagnoses of diffuse and focal changes in the texture and size of the pancreas.

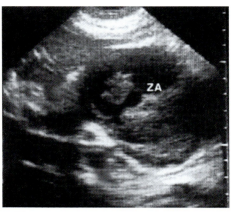

▲ *Fig. 4.58* Macrocystic cystadenoma (ZA) (confirmed by histology): anechoic (cystic) and hyperechoic (solid) regions of the tumors; longitudinal and transverse epigastric view.

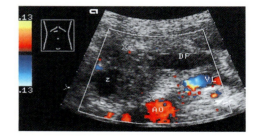

◀◀ *Fig. 4.59 a* Microcystic cystadenoma of the pancreas (calipers), confirmed by histology: hypoechoic microcystic tumor with a larger cyst (Z); cut-off of the pancreatic duct (DP). After two year follow-up there has so far been no change of this finding in a rather old female patient. AO = aorta; VL = splenic vein.

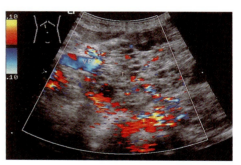

◀ *b* Microcystic cystadenoma: large tumor (T) of the head of the pancreas with microcysts and spot-like vascularization. VP = portal vein.

Dilatation of the Pancreatic Duct

Under good conditions ultrasound will demonstrate the normal pancreatic duct in the body of the pancreas as a narrow anechoic ligamentous structure with delicate, smooth, echogenic margins. If it appears marked or dilated, it may be traced all the way to the papilla of Vater (**Fig. 4.60**).

In dilatation of the pancreatic duct, appropriate views (oblique or sagittal epigastric) will help identify and differentiate the nature of the obstruction. A ductal diameter of 2 mm or less is considered normal. The marginal diameter of 2–4 mm is much more common; its assessment can be difficult, in which case additional diagnostic measures are called for to settle the issue. The widely dilated duct is found in chronic pancreatitis, cancer, and metastasis. **Table 4.9** lists possible causes.

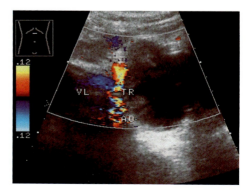

▲ *Fig. 4.60 a* Malignant pancreatic pseudocyst. The celiac axis (TR) and splenic vein (VL) have been infiltrated by a papillary bile-duct carcinoma invading the pancreas, forming a malignant pseudocyst. AO = aorta.

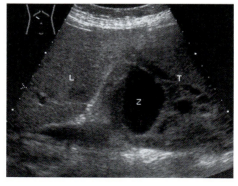

▲ *b* Intraductal Papillary-Nucinous Neoplasm (?), identified histologically as mucinous ductal carcinoma. Ultrasound shows a small, solid, cystic tumor with smooth margins and moderately large echo-free areas (C) displacing, but not infiltrating, the portal vein. The disease took a relatively benign two-year course.

Table 4.8 Differential diagnosis of textural and ductal changes

Structural change

Diffuse	Focal
	Anechoic lesion – pancreatic cysts/pseudocysts – renal/splenic cyst – splenic artery – gastroduodenal artery – arterial aneurysm – pancreatic duct – dilated prepapillary CBD
Hypoechoic structure – juvenile pancreas – acute pancreatitis – cancer with diffuse spread – autoimmune chronic pancreatitis	Hypoechoic lesion – pancreatic cancer – necrosis/hemorrhage – hemorrhagic pancreatic cyst/pseudocyst – abscess – focal acute pancreatitis of the head/tail – metastasis of cancer – metastasis of lymphoma – peripancreatic inflammatory lymph node
Hyperechoic texture – pancreas in the elderly – pancreatic lipomatosis/fibrolipomatosis – pancreatic fibrosis in hemochromatosis/cystic fibrosis – chronic pancreatitis (with fibrosis/calcification)	Hyperechoic/echodense lesion – intraparenchymal calcification – intraductal calculus of the pancreatic duct – stented pancreatic duct – intraductal gas bubbles – calcified splenic artery – calcified tumor
Irregular/heterogeneous structure – pseudocystic transformation of the pancreas – acute pancreatitis – chronic pancreatitis	Irregular/heterogeneous lesion – pancreatic pseudocyst – cystadenoma – pancreatic cancer – focal chronic pancreatitis

Size change

Diffuse	Focal
Enlarged – juvenile pancreas – acute pancreatitis – pancreatic edema – diffuse cancer – pancreas divisum	Variant shapes – bar-bell – tadpole Pancreatitis – pancreatitis of the head – pancreatitis of the tail
Reduced – pancreas in the elderly – atrophic pancreas (terminal stage of chronic pancreatitis) – status post necrotizing pancreatitis – status post surgery – advanced pancreatitis fibrosis (hemochromatosis)	Pancreatic cancer Enlarged head in pancreas divisum and annular pancreas

Table 4.9 Causes of pancreatic duct dilatation

Ductal diameter marginal (2–4 mm) Smooth	Ductal diameter > 4 mm Smooth	Ductal diameter > 4 mm Convoluted
Postprandial cholelithiasis	Pancreatic cancer Periampullary cancer	Chronic pancreatitis Atrophy in chronic pancreatitis
Pancreas divisum	Chronic pancreatitis Obstructive chronic pancreatitis	

Marginal/Mild Dilatation

- Diffuse Pancreatic Change
- Focal Change
- Dilatation of the Pancreatic Duct
  - Marginal/Mild Dilatation
  - Marked Dilatation

▶ Bile Duct Disorder
▶ Acute/Recurrent Pancreatitis, Pancreas Divisum
▶ Chronic Pancreatitis
▶ Periampullary Cancer, Cancer of the Pancreatic Head

▶ Bile Duct Disorder

Marginal diameters of 2–3 mm occur as a postprandial functional response, but often they are based on a disease of the biliary system. In the case of somewhat blurred ducts, it is well worth the effort to take a look at the gallbladder and to trace the CBD all the way to the papilla of Vater. In many cases, ductal dilatation is nothing more than postcholecystectomy, often preceded by recurrent colics (with accompanying pancreatitis?). The underlying cause would have to be increased intraductal pressure (**Fig. 4.61**).

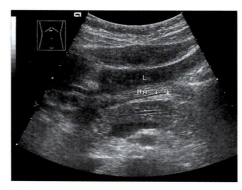
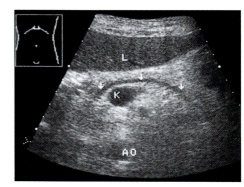

▲ **Fig. 4.61** Pancreatic duct of marginal diameter.
a Postprandial: marked pancreatic duct (calipers) of normal diameter in postcholecystectomy; echogenic peripancreatic bandlike mass (arrows): fatty necrosis after biliary pancreatitis? MA = stomach; L = liver.

▲ *b* Dilated pancreatic duct (arrows) in postcholecystectomy. K = venous confluence; AO = aorta; L = liver.

▶ Acute/Recurrent Pancreatitis, Pancreas Divisum

Here, ductal dilatation is infrequent since this is counteracted by the edema. However, if there is edema the differential diagnosis should include biliary pancreatitis and obstruction of the pancreatic duct (**Figs. 4.62 and 4.63**).

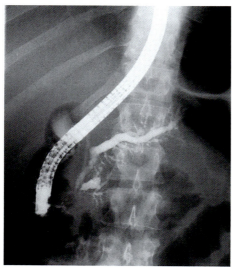
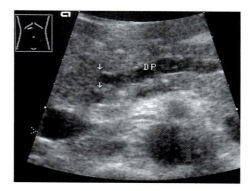
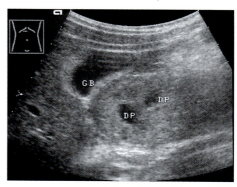

▲ **Fig. 4.62** Pancreas divisum: prominently dilated stubby pancreatic duct terminating in a cul de sac; dilated accessory duct (of Santorini), which has taken over as primary drain via the minor papilla (see **Fig. 4.45**, p. 159, years later; filling via the major and minor papilla).

▲ **Fig. 4.63** Pancreas divisum. GB = gallbladder; DP = pancreatic duct.
a Longitudinal section through the accessory duct of Santorini; two duct systems are evident in the head of the pancreas (arrows).

▲ *b* Shifted view: oblique section through both ducts (accessory and main pancreatic duct) which are visualized as being dilated. GB = gallbladder; DP = pancreatic duct.

▶ Chronic Pancreatitis

Dilatation of the pancreatic duct in chronic pancreatitis tends to be more marked rather than marginal. The obstruction may be caused by intraductal calculi, prepapillary gallstones, protein plugs, and in a few rare cases a slowly growing malignancy. The fibrosis of the adjacent tissue can result in a tortuous duct with variations in its diameter, beaded irregularities, and twisting, mostly in an advanced state (**Fig. 4.64**).

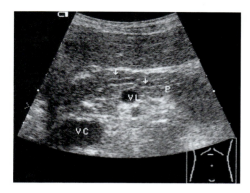

◀ **Fig. 4.64** Dilated undulating pancreatic duct (arrows) in chronic pancreatitis (P). This appearance of the duct is characteristic of chronic pancreatitis and not ductal obstruction. VL = splenic vein; VC = vena cava.

▶ Periampullary Cancer, Cancer of the Pancreatic Head

Here, dilatation of the pancreatic duct is normal and in the advanced stage quite marked. Cancer of the tail of the pancreas will not result in ductal dilatation, while cancer of the uncinate process will sometimes do so. Cancer in the head of the pancreas is usually accompanied by dilatation of the CBD (**Fig. 4.65**).

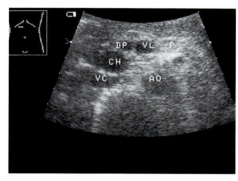

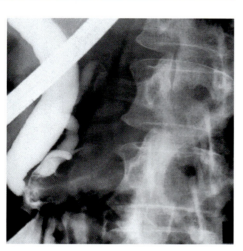

▲ **Fig. 4.65** Dilated prepapillary ducts.
a Transverse epigastric view: cross-sectional view of the pancreatic duct (DP) and CBD (CH) (double-duct sign); periampullary ductal cancer of the pancreas. The carcinoma could not be demonstrated on ultrasound or CT scanning. AO = aorta; VC = vena cava; VL = splenic vein; P = pancreas.

▲ **b** ERCP film with tumorous void in the pancreatic duct.

Marked Dilatation

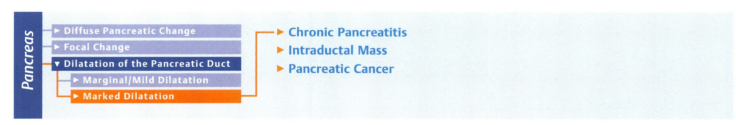

▶ Chronic Pancreatitis

According to the Marseille Classification, calculous obstruction with dilatation of the pancreatic duct is classified as obstructive chronic pancreatitis. The calculus will be visualized when following the duct sonographically to the papilla of Vater. One treatment option is ultrasound guided lithotripsy (**Fig. 4.66**).

Prominent dilatation of the pancreatic duct with no obstruction delineated on ultrasound or endoscopy is also seen in the rare patient with chronic autoimmune pancreatitis. In these cases, it is of vital importance that possible malignancy be ruled out for certain (**Fig. 4.67**).

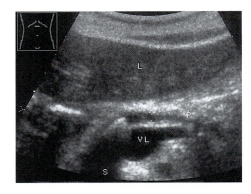
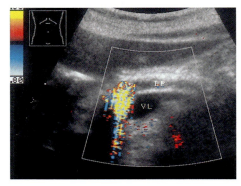

▸▸ *Fig. 4.66* Dilated pancreatic duct (DP) in chronic obstructive pancreatitis. L = liver; VL = splenic vein.
a Site of the obstruction (gallstone; acoustic shadow S) at the junction of the head and body. Subsequent prestenotic dilatation of the duct. Patient presented clinically with diabetes mellitus.

◂ *b* Color duplex: the "twinkling artifact" aids in stone detection (as with renal stones). VL = splenic vein; DP = pancreatic duct.

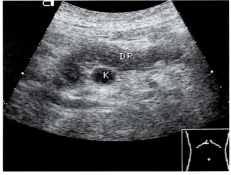
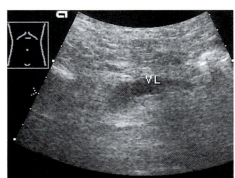
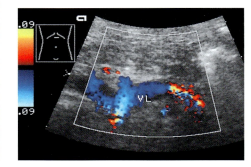

▴ *Fig. 4.67* Chronic pancreatitis. Clinical symptoms: diabetes and weight loss. VL = splenic vein; K = venous confluence.
a Prominent undulating dilated duct (DP). ERCP: no obstruction, no branches whatsoever.

▴ *b* Same patient after one year: additional loss of the pancreatic duct. Without knowledge of the previous findings and the clinical symptoms, the diagnosis of CP would have been missed. VL = splenic vein.

▴ *c* Color-flow Doppler scan: no dilatation of the duct evident, atrophy of the pancreas, no history of pancreatitis, probably primary autoimmune chronic pancreatitis.

▸ Intraductal Mass

By far the most common causes of intraductal mass are echogenic calculi with posterior shadowing, followed by sediments and pus, while protein plugs are infrequent findings (**Fig. 4.68**).

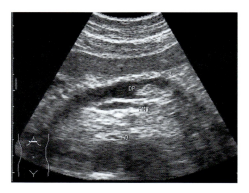

◂ *Fig. 4.68* Chronic (autoimmune?) pancreatitis, ectatic duct with protein plug (DP, arrow); ERCP: wide open papilla of Vater; biopsy and cytology negative three years after these procedures periampullary carcinoma. Surgery confirmed the protein plug. AMS = superior mesenteric artery; AO = aorta.

▸ Pancreatic Cancer

Dilatation of the pancreatic duct without discernible cause of the obstruction has to raise a high degree of suspicion of malignancy unless another cause can be confirmed (calculus, fibrosis, pseudocyst, twisted duct, ductal stricture). Ultrasound will demonstrate the duct all the way to the tumor. In the selective enlargement, the ductal cut-off will be either ovoid, convex, or tapering.

Concurrent dilatation of the CBD is indicative of a malignancy in the vicinity of the papilla (periampullary cancer) and is termed "double duct sign". ERCP with brush cytology and ductal biopsy or CT study will help with the final diagnosis; fine-needle aspiration biopsy should be reserved for uncertain findings and inoperable cases because of the risk of implantation of tumor cells along the needle track.

In 5 to 10%[3] of patients, pancreatic cancer will coexist with chronic pancreatitis. The cumulative risk of pancreatic cancer in chronic pancreatitis is 1.8% after 10 years, and 4% after 20 years. Therefore, chronic pancreatitis is considered a precancer. When the symptoms persist, cancer cannot be ruled out and the issue has to be settled by surgery (**Figs. 4.69–4.71**).

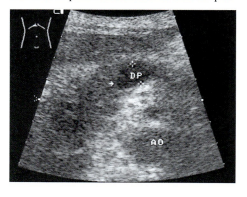

◂ *Fig. 4.69* Pancreatic duct (DP) with prestenotic dilatation and ductal cut-off without direct visualization of the tumor; but, together with the cut-off (arrow), the diffuse ill-defined enlarged head of the pancreas suggests the malignancy. AO = aorta.

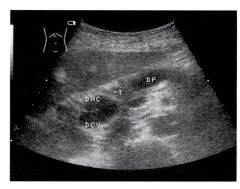 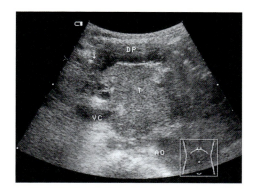 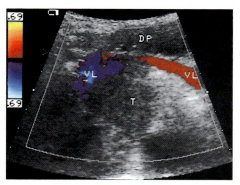

▲ **Fig. 4.70** Small cancer (T) of the pancreatic head; duct (DP) with prestenotic dilatation; dilated CBD (DHC) and cystic duct (DCY).

▲ **Fig. 4.71** Cancer (T) of the uncinate process. AO = aorta; VC = venous confluens; VL = splenic vein.
a With invasion of the pancreatic duct (arrow, DP).

▲ *b* Color-flow Doppler scan: invasion of the splenic vein. The invasive spread confirms malignancy and rules out surgery as an option.

Table 4.10 summarizes the differential diagnosis of the pancreatic duct with prestenotic dilatation.

Table 4.10 Differential diagnosis of the pancreatic duct with prestenotic dilatation

Intraductal calculus	Hard echo due to calculus, posterior shadowing Frequently in the head/body of the pancreas
Pancreatic cancer	Hypoechoic (isoechoic) tumor mass downstream of the stenosis Tapered or convex cut-off of the duct (on selective enlargement)
Metastasis/lymphoma	Impossible to differentiate from pancreatic cancer by ultrasound morphology alone (ultrasound-guided fine-needle aspiration biopsy)
Periampullary cancer (pancreas/CBD)	Concurrent dilatation of the pancreatic duct and CBD Usually, no direct visualization of the tumor possible
Pancreas divisum	Ductal cut-off in the head/body without definite cause Conspicuously enlarged head of the pancreas Demonstration of two ductal systems in the pancreatic head

References

1. Bosseckert H. Diagnosestandards bei chronischer Pankreatitis (CP) – Bildgebende Verfahren. Verh Dtsch Ges Verdau.- u. Stoffwechselkr. 1991;26:53.
2. Etemad B, Whitcomb DC. Chronic Pancreatitis: Diagnosis, Classification and New Genetic Developments. Gastroenterology 2001; 120: 682–707.
3. Klöppel G, Kosmahl, M. Cystic Lesions and Neoplasms of the Pancreas. Pancreatology, Basel 2001.
4. Lankisch PG, Löhr-Happe A, Otto J, Creutzfeldt W. Natural course in chronic panreatitis. Pain, exocrine pancreatic insufficiency and prognosis of the disease. Digestion 1992;54:148–55.
5. Lankisch PG, Staritz M, Freise J. Sicherheit bei der Diagnostik der chronischen Pankreatitis. Z Gastroenterol 1990;28:253.
6. Löser CH, Fölsch UR. Diagnostik der chronischen Pankreatitis. Dtsch Med Wschr 1996;121:243–7.
7. Lowenfels AB, Maisonneuve P, Cavallini G et al. International Pancreatitis Study Group. Pancreatitis and the risk of pancreatic cancer. N Engl J Med 1993;328:1433–7.
8. Sarner M, Cotten PB. Classification of pancreatitis. Cambridge 1983. Gut 1984;25:756–9.
9. Singer MV, Gyr K, Sarles H. Revidierte Klassifikation der Pankreatitis – Marseille 1984. Inn Med 1985;12:242–5.
10. Taniguchi T, Seko S, Azuma K, Tamegai M, Nishida O, Inone F, Okamoto M, Mizumoto T, Kobayashi H. Autoimmune Pancreatitis detected as a mass in the tail of the Pancreas. Am J Gastroenterol 1995; 90:1834–7.

5 Spleen

Spleen 173

▼ Nonfocal Changes of the Spleen — 176
▼ Diffuse Parenchymal Changes — 176
- Malignant Invasion
- Benign Nonhomogeneity

▼ Large Spleen — 177
- Infection
- Congestive Splenomegaly
- Systemic Hematological Malignancy

▼ Small Spleen — 180
- Variants, "Aged Spleen"
- Functional Hyposplenism/Asplenia

▼ Focal Changes — 182
▼ Anechoic Mass — 182
- Dysontogenetic Cysts
- Pseudocysts
- Infective Cysts

▼ Hypoechoic Mass — 184
- Invasive Lymphoma
- Splenic Infarction
- Splenic Abscess
- Splenic Trauma
- Splenic Metastasis

▼ Hyperechoic Mass — 193
- Hemangioma
- Hamartoma
- Lymphoma and Myeloproliferative Disorders

▼ Splenic Calcification — 195
- Focal Calcification
- Diffuse Calcification
- Vascular Calcification

5 Spleen

C. Goerg

The spleen appears about the fifth week of embryonic development as a localized thickening of the coelomic epithelium of the dorsal mesogastrium near its cranial end. Its characteristic shape is evident even during initial development, and the early lobulated appearance of the fetal spleen will resolve until birth. The spleen fulfills numerous functions:

- **Hematopoiesis**: normally only during fetal life
- **Immune function**: antibody and lymphocyte production
- **Erythrocyte storage**: in the human spleen not nearly as marked as in other species
- **Phagocytosis**: removal of old and pathological blood cells, immune complexes, and particulate matter in the bloodstream.

The arterial hemodynamics of the spleen must be viewed within the context of the other splanchnic organs. On the venous side it is regarded as part of the portal venous system.

Anatomy

Size
- Length along the maximum cephalocaudal diameter ≤ 11 cm
- Thickness from hilum to surface (cortex) ≤ 5 cm

Shape
- Crescent/coffee bean configuration, highly variable

Size. Intercostal scanning will provide the most reliable measurements of splenic dimensions. In this view the largest distance between the two poles should be determined (maximum length). The thickness is determined orthogonal to the maximum length by measuring from the hilum to the apex of the splenic convexity (**Fig. 5.1**). Additional measurement of the width for computation of the splenic volume by the ellipsoid method has not become part of routine clinical practice.

Normal dimensions of the adult spleen are a maximum length ≤ 11 cm and a thickness ≤ 5 cm. The severity of any splenomegaly depends on the size of the spleen:
- Mild to moderate: ≥ 5 cm × 11 cm
- Marked: ≥ 6 cm × 16 cm
- Extreme: ≥ 8 cm × 20 cm

Any splenic dimensions above these normal values have to result in the presumed diagnosis of an enlarged spleen. Depending on the patient's age (juvenile) and physique, a slightly longer and thinner (asthenic) or shorter and plumpish (pyknic) spleen can be regarded as normal. During childhood the spleen tends to be smaller.

Shape. The shape of the spleen is that of a half-moon or crescent/coffee bean but is highly variable and depends on the plane of the ultrasound view. The diaphragmatic surface is convex and smooth, while the concave visceral surface presents gastric, renal, pancreatic, and colic impressions.

Vestiges of the complex embryological development of the splenic anlage in the dorsal mesogastrium may also be found as notches and septa in the diaphragmatic surface (**Fig. 5.2**). Complete congenital cleft with separate hilar blood supply may be demonstrated in rare cases (**Fig. 5.3**).

Sometimes branches of the vasculature penetrate the visceral surface at various points. In a few patients, blood vessels terminating on the diaphragmatic aspect will also be seen. Usually, the splenic vein has a diameter < 0.5 cm and runs straight from the hilum of the spleen. Varicosities and kinking along the course of these vessels have been visualized.

Ultrasound texture. Comparison of the healthy liver and spleen in the same patient demonstrates a slightly diminished echogenicity of the spleen, but the organ is significantly more echogenic than the kidney.

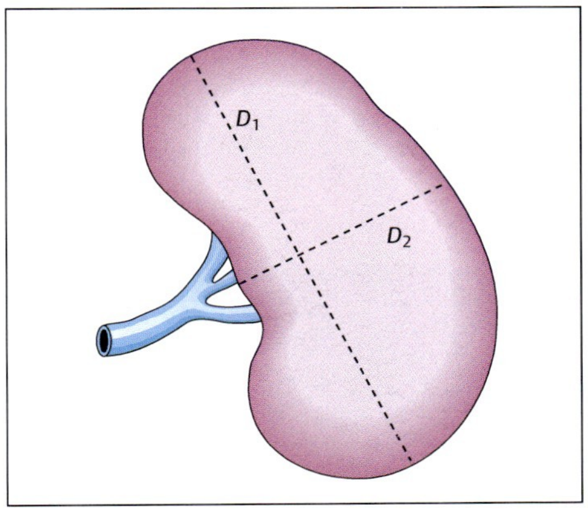

▲ **Fig. 5.1** Sonographic illustration of the splenic hilum with assessment of length (D_1) and thickness (D_2).

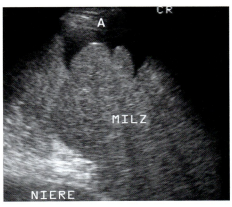

▲ **Fig. 5.2** Splenic septa at the diaphragmatic aspect may become evident in the presence of ascites (A). Milz = spleen; Niere = kidney.

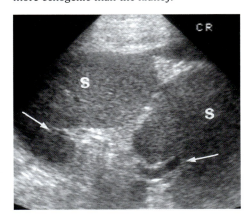

▲ **Fig. 5.3** Congenital cleft of the spleen (S) with demonstration of separate hilar blood supply (arrows).

Topography

The spleen is situated principally in the left hypochondric region of the abdomen and is an almost completely intraperitoneal organ. Its convex diaphragmatic aspect is in wide relation with the abdominal surface of the diaphragm (**Fig. 5.5**). Posterior and lateral protection is by the 9th to 12th ribs, and the organ is covered by the costophrenic recess, which may extend down as far as the inferior border of the organ. The longitudinal axis of the spleen roughly parallels the course of the 10th rib. The anteromedial aspect of the concave gastric surface is in relation with the posterior wall of the gastric body, while the inferior renal surface abuts the superior pole of the left kidney

(**Fig. 5.6**). The anteroinferior aspect of the spleen is in close relation with the left colic flexure (**Fig. 5.4**).

Apart from the hilum, the spleen is almost entirely surrounded by peritoneum. It remains connected with the stomach by a peritoneal fold, the so-called gastrosplenic ligament (**Fig. 5.7**). Visualization of the splenorenal ligament depends on the extent of fusion with the dorsal peritoneum. Sometimes the gastrosplenic ligament may become evident in patients with ascites. In the presence of an enlarged left hepatic lobe the liver may be in contact with the diaphragmatic aspect of the spleen and cover it like a cap (**Fig. 5.8**).

Blood vessels. The splenic artery originates at the celiac axis and then runs straight along the superior margin of the pancreas. On arriving near the spleen it follows a rather tortuous course and close to the hilum it divides into several branches. There are only infrequent variants of its origin at the celiac axis. The segmental branches of the splenic artery are terminal arteries resulting in separate splenic segments. The spleen is tied into the systemic circulation via the splenic artery, and into the portal circulation via the splenic vein (◻ **5.1 d and e**). The trunk of the splenic vein (sometimes located up to 6 cm from the actual splenic hilum) commences from several tributaries issuing from the stomach and spleen, courses posterior to the tail and body of the pancreas, and unites with the superior mesenteric vein to form the portal vein.

Vascular appearance. On color-flow Doppler scanning, the vascular appearance is dominated primarily by the spokelike course of the segmental arteries and veins, which run in fan-like fashion to and from the splenic hilum, respectively (◻ **5.1 a and b**). The arterial blood is supplied by the splenic artery (◻ **5.1 c**) and only rarely via accessory arteries in the gastrosplenic ligament. The trunk of the splenic vein is a landmark structure in ultrasound studies for locating the tail of the pancreas (◻ **5.1 f and g**). Quite frequently it is possible to visualize the area of the pancreatic tail by insonation through the spleen from the patient's left side ("ultrasound window"); this might be possible, even if the tail of the pancreas cannot be demonstrated from anterior because of intestinal gas (◻ **5.1 h and i**).

Relations (Fig. 5.4)
▶ Diaphragmatic surface with the left dome of the diaphragm
▶ Gastric surface with the posterior gastric wall
▶ Renal surface with the upper pole of the left kidney
▶ Pancreatic tail touching the hilum of the spleen

Ultrasound landmark structure
▶ Hilar blood vessels of the spleen

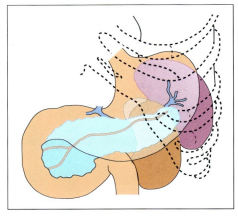

▲ *Fig. 5.4* Anatomical relations of the spleen, pancreas, stomach, and kidney.

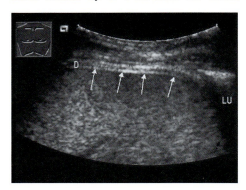

▲ *Fig. 5.5* Left lateral intercostal view. D = diaphragm.
a Visualization of the anterior crus of the diaphragm. LU = lung.

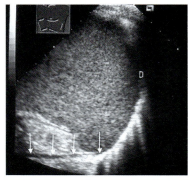

▲ *b* Dome of the diaphragm and the posterior crus of the diaphragm (arrows).

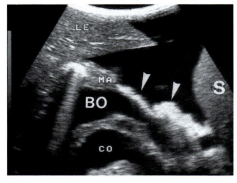

▲ *Fig. 5.7* Transverse left hypochondric view visualizing the gastrosplenic ligament (arrows) due to the presence of intraperitoneal fluid. The ligament is anterior of the lesser sac (BO). CO = venous confluence; S = spleen; LE = liver; MA = stomach.

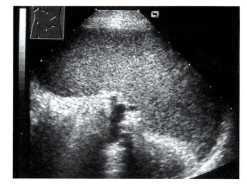

▲ *Fig. 5.6* Splenic dimensions.
a Maximum length (polar diameter).

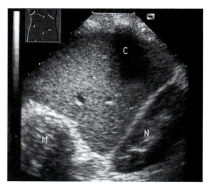

▲ *b* Transverse view visualizing the posterior renal and anterior gastric aspects. N = kidney; M = stomach; C = posterior shadowing of the rib.

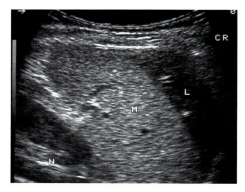

▲ *Fig. 5.8* In hepatomegaly the liver (L) may cap the spleen (M). N = kidney.

5.1 Blood Supply of the Spleen

▶ Parenchymal vessels

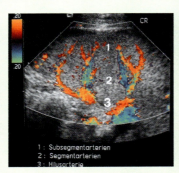 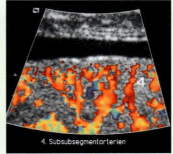

a 1: subsegmental arteries
2: segmental arteries
3: hilar artery

b 4: subsegmental arteries

a and b Vessels of the splenic parenchyma on color-flow Doppler imaging.

▶ Splenic artery

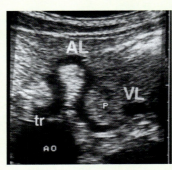 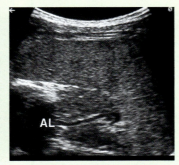

c Quite often the splenic artery (AL) displays a tortuous course. VL = splenic vein; AO = aorta; tr = celiac axis; P = pancreas.

d The splenic artery (AL) courses through the pancreas.

▶ Splenic vein

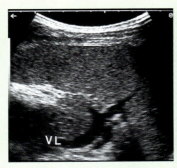 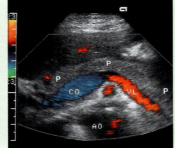

e In the vicinity of the splenic hilum the splenic vein (VL) will be visualized posterior to the pancreas.

f and g Color-flow Doppler imaging: splenic vein (VL) at the central hypochondric region and the hilum of the spleen. P = pancreas; CO = venous confluence; AO = aorta; AL = splenic artery; S = spleen.

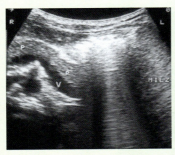 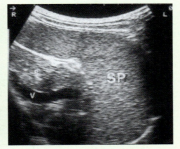

h Landmark structure: splenic vein (V). Quite often the pancreatic tail cannot be visualized because of the gastric gas. P = pancreas; Milz = spleen.

i The region of the pancreatic tail (P) may be assessed by insonation through the spleen. P = pancreas; V = splenic vein; SP = spleen.

Nonfocal Changes of the Spleen

Diffuse Parenchymal Changes

Diffuse nonhomogeneity of the splenic texture is rare, especially when compared with textural nonhomogeneity of the liver. Definite diagnosis is based on history, clinical picture, sonographic follow-up, and possibly ultrasound-guided fine-needle aspiration biopsy[2].

The sonographic appearance is characterized by a "subjectively" inhomogeneous splenic parenchyma without definite delineation of individual focal masses (compared with healthy hepatic parenchyma, the tissue of the healthy spleen appears somewhat "more homogeneous"). However, the transition to focal micronodular splenic disorder is fluent.

▶ Malignant Invasion

Diffuse splenic change as a sign of malignant invasion is frequently found in low-grade lymphomas (**Fig. 5.9**), in Hodgkin disease (**Fig. 5.10**), and rarely as diffuse splenic invasion by a solid tumor (**Fig. 5.11**).

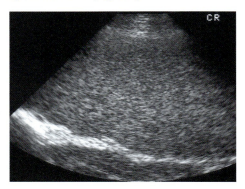

▲ *Fig. 5.9* Splenomegaly with coarse splenic parenchyma in malignant lymphoma. This finding is compatible with splenic invasion.

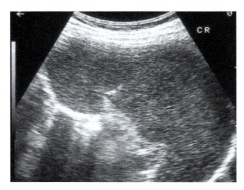

▲ *Fig. 5.10* Diffuse textural nonhomogeneity compatible with splenic invasion in Hodgkin disease.

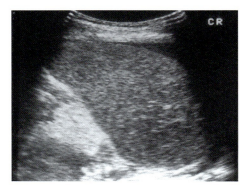

▲ *Fig. 5.11* Coarse splenic parenchyma in metastasizing breast cancer. This finding is suspicious for splenic metastasis.

▶ Benign Nonhomogeneity

Diffuse nonhomogeneity may be demonstrated in some cases of:
- ▶ Collagen disease (e.g., rheumatoid arthritis, lupus erythematosus, polyarteritis nodosa)
- ▶ Benign granulomatous disease (**Fig. 5.12**) (e.g., tuberculosis, Wegener granulomatosis, sarcoidosis)
- ▶ Bacterial infection
- ▶ Amyloidosis (**Fig. 5.13**)
- ▶ Obstruction of the splenic artery
- ▶ Thorotrast exposure (**Fig 5.14**)
- ▶ Portal hypertension (**Fig. 5.15**)
- ▶ Incidental finding in "healthy" patients (**Fig. 5.16**)

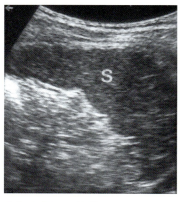
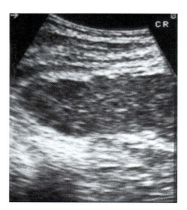

▲ *Fig. 5.12a and b* Diffuse textural nonhomogeneity of the spleen (S) with undulating surface in Wegener disease. This finding is compatible with granulomatous invasion.

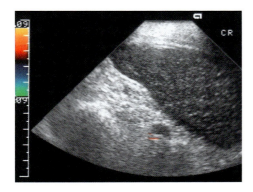
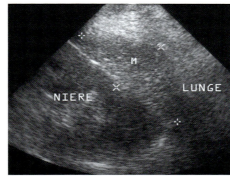
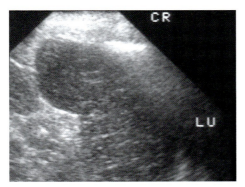
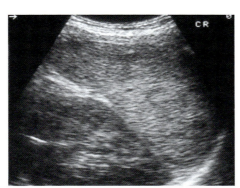

◄◄ **Fig. 5.13** Coarse splenic parenchyma in amyloidosis. Color-flow Doppler scanning cannot demonstrate any flow signals. This finding is indicative of functional hyposplenism.

◄ **Fig. 5.14** Small spleen with increased echogenicity in known thorotrast exposure. M = spleen. Niere = kidney; Lunge = lung.

◄◄ **Fig. 5.15** Coarse splenic parenchyma in long-term portal hypertension and hepatic cirrhosis. This finding is compatible with splenic fibrosis. LU = lung.

◄ **Fig. 5.16** Textural nonhomogeneity of the spleen in a patient without obvious clinical pathological findings. The etiology remains uncertain.

Large Spleen

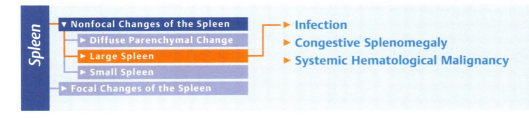

Differential diagnosis of splenomegaly covers an extremely wide range of possibilities (**Table 5.1**). From experience, any ultrasound study of the spleen is not by itself sufficient for pinpointing the definite cause of splenomegaly.

Severity. Although the size of the spleen may vary rather widely between patients with the same disease, assessing the dimensions of the organ may yield some differential diagnostic clues.

Mild to moderate splenomegaly is encountered, e.g., in infections and granulomatous disease (**Fig. 5.17**), portal hypertension (**Figs. 5.20 and 5.21**), and acute leukemia.

Severe splenomegaly is typical of, e.g., malignant lymphoma, hemolytic anemia (**Fig. 5.18**), storage disease, infectious mononucleosis (**Fig. 5.19**), and leishmaniasis.

Extreme splenomegaly is seen in myelofibrosis, in terminal chronic myelocytic leukemia (**Fig. 5.23**), and also in advanced low-grade malignant lymphomas (**Fig. 5.24**). In some cases ultrasound may not be able to ascertain the exact size of the spleen.

◄ **Fig. 5.17a and b** Hepatosplenomegaly in sarcoidosis. Hepatic involvement was confirmed by histology.

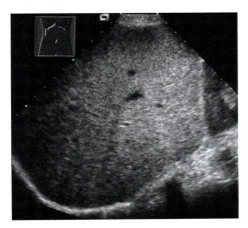
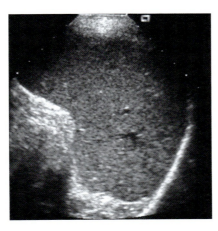

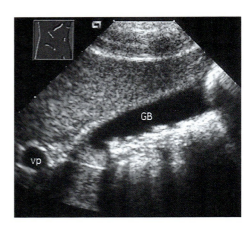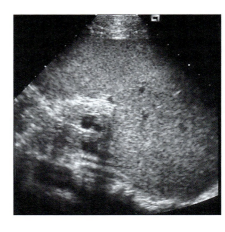

Fig. 5.18 A 40-year-old patient with spherocytosis.
a Frequently there are bilirubin gallstones in the gallbladder (GB) due to the chronic hemolysis.

b Splenomegaly. GB = gallbladder; VP = portal vein.

Table 5.1 Possible causes of splenomegaly

Acute and chronic systemic infection
Infectious mononucleosis, chickenpox, hepatitis, AIDS, sepsis, endocarditis, typhus, tuberculosis, malaria, toxoplasmosis, leishmaniasis, candidiasis

Disorders of the portal circulation
Hepatic cirrhosis, thrombosis of the portal and splenic veins, AV fistula of the spleen

Hemolytic disorders
Pernicious anemia, spherocytosis, thalassemia, sickle-cell anemia

Malignant systemic disease
Leukemia, myeloproliferative disorders, myelodysplastic syndrome, non-Hodgkin lymphoma, Hodgkin lymphoma, malignant histiocytosis, systemic mastocytosis

Immune disorders
Collagen disease, idiopathic thrombocytopenic purpura, Evans syndrome

Other
Amyloidosis, Wegener disease, sarcoidosis, hemochromatosis, lipidosis

▶ Infection

In viral or bacterial infections, moderate splenomegaly will sometimes display a slightly inhomogeneous splenic parenchyma without definite delineation of focal masses. In a few patients, infectious mononucleosis may be accompanied by extreme splenomegaly (**Fig. 5.19**). Complete resolution of this state may take months. Spontaneous splenic hemorrhage or rupture after inadequate incidental trauma has been reported in a rare few cases, mostly in spleens with rapidly enlarged volume.

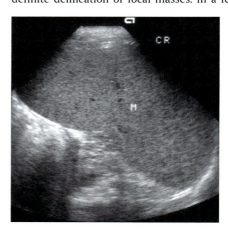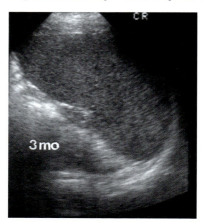

Fig. 5.19 Infectious mononucleosis.
a Marked splenomegaly (M).

b The splenic enlargement resolved over time (3 months).

▶ Congestive Splenomegaly

Hepatic cirrhosis and portal hypertension. Splenomegaly will be observed in 50–75% of patients with cirrhosis of the liver and portal hypertension **(Figs. 5.20 and 5.21)**. The causes are:
- ▶ Passive congestion (diminished portal venous outflow)
- ▶ Hypercirculation (increased splanchnic inflow)
- ▶ Intrinsic splenic factors (e.g., autoimmune processes)

This is counteracted by hemodynamically important portosystemic shunts, the extent of which may vary significantly from patient to patient. A regular-sized spleen does not rule out portal hypertension.

Splenic vein thrombosis. In thrombosis of the splenic vein, splenomegaly will be observed in approximately 60% of patients. A regular-sized spleen does not rule out splenic vein thrombosis. Ultrasound will visualize thrombosis of the splenic vein as a homogeneously echogenic mass of varying severity within the lumen of the vessel **(Fig. 5.22)**. Color-flow Doppler imaging will demonstrate the lack of flow as well as the collateral circulation and thus confirm the preliminary diagnosis.

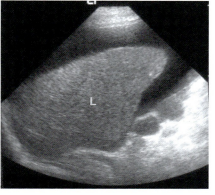
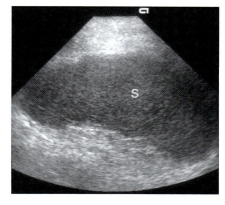

◂◂ **Fig. 5.20** Cirrhosis of the liver.
 a Hepatic cirrhosis (L) and ascites confirmed by histology.

◂ *b* Congestive splenomegaly (S).

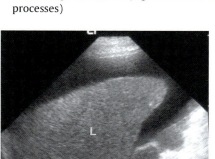
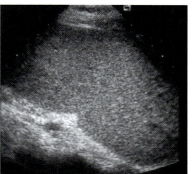

◂◂ **Fig. 5.21** Congenital hypoplasia of the portal vein.
 a Hypoplasia of the portal vein and esophageal varices.

◂ *b* Congestive splenomegaly.

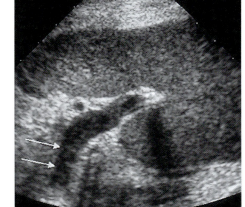
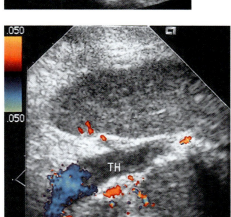

◂◂ **Fig. 5.22** Partial thrombosis (TH) of the splenic vein.
 a Color-flow Doppler image.

◂ *b* Mild splenomegaly.

▶ Systemic Hematological Malignancy

Myeloproliferative disorder. Splenomegaly is regarded as the principal diagnostic sign in myeloproliferative disorders, particularly in myelofibrosis and chronic myelocytic leukemia (CML) **(Fig. 5.23)**. It is found in approximately 70% of CML cases at the time of primary diagnosis, and after several years frequently results in an extremely large spleen. The number of circulating blast cells and the size of the spleen are decisive prognostic parameters.

High-grade lymphoma. In high-grade lymphoma, the size of the spleen is unreliable regarding possible splenic involvement. Despite the fact that increasing splenic size will raise the probability of invasion by the lymphoma, a normal-sized spleen does not rule out possible involvement of the spleen[1].

Low-grade lymphoma. In low-grade lymphoma, particularly in chronic lymphocytic leukemia (CLL) **(Fig. 5.24)**, hairy cell leukemia, and also immunocytoma, splenomegaly will point toward a highly probable invasion of the spleen, even if the sonographic echo pattern of the organ is homogeneous. This has to do with the fact that these entities are characterized by a leukemic course. Demonstration of splenomegaly is of prognostic significance, particularly in CLL.

Hodgkin disease. Use of splenic size as the sole criterion for possible involvement of the spleen has been abandoned. Approximately one-third of all affected spleens are normal sized. In contrast to almost all non-Hodgkin lymphomas, in Hodgkin disease the correlation between splenic size and extent of organ involvement is only tenuous.

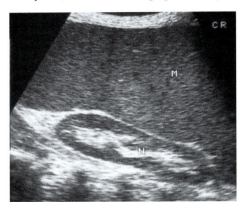

▲ *Fig. 5.23* Extreme splenomegaly (M) in myeloproliferative disorder.

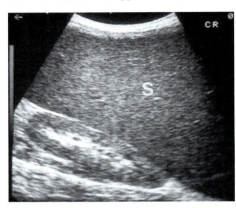

▲ *Fig. 5.24* Hepatosplenomegaly (S) in CLL.
a Ultrasound does not yield accurate dimensions of the spleen.

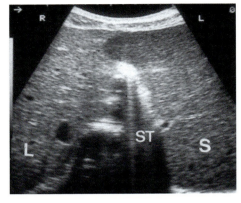

▲ *b* Both organs may touch in the upper abdomen (ST = stomach). L = liver.

Small Spleen

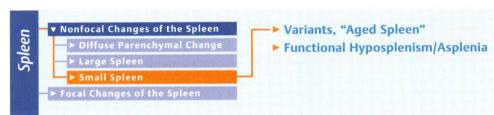

▶ Variants, "Aged Spleen"

Sonographic determination of a longitudinal diameter < 11 cm and a thickness < 5 cm should be recorded and documented as a "small" spleen **(Fig. 5.25)**.

To date, this finding has been regarded as a variant and certainly does not seem to be of any clinical consequence in most cases. Splenic size varies with the type of patient, but the volume of the organ also decreases with age. On color-flow Doppler scanning, these spleens will be visualized with a normal fanlike vasculature of the parenchyma. At present, it is unknown whether this age-dependent decrease in splenic size has any functional significance.

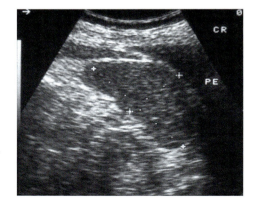

◀ *Fig. 5.25* Small spleen in a 75-year-old patient, possibly corresponding to an "aged spleen." PE = pleural exudation.

▶ Functional Hyposplenism/Asplenia

In recent years functional autosplenectomy syndromes have increasingly been reported in sickle-cell anemia (◻ **5.2a**), after extensive splenic trauma and septic disease, in autoimmune disease (◻ **5.2b and c**), as part of thorotrast exposure of the spleen, and particularly on the heels of allogeneic bone marrow transplantation as a complication of chronic GVHD (graft-versus-host disease) (◻ **5.2d–f**) **(Table 5.2)**.

Apart from the clinical symptoms, the principal sonographic sign of functional splenic changes is the diminishing size of the spleen (◻ **5.2g–i**). The findings in color-flow Doppler scanning vary. Although in some cases there is no vascularization whatsoever, most organs will demonstrate a rarefied vascular bed. However, sonographic confirmation of splenic blood flow cannot rule out functional asplenia. This requires additional functional studies of the spleen (technetium-99m [^{99m}Tc] sulfur colloid labeling, platelet count, demonstration of Howell–Jolly bodies).

Table 5.2 Possible causes of functional hyposplenism/asplenia

Vascular	Parenchymal

▸ Obstruction of the large blood vessels
  – embolic splenic infarction
  – torsion of the splenic pedicle
  – complete splenic vein thrombosis
▸ Obstruction of the smaller blood vessels
  – sickle-cell anemia
  – vasculitis
  – sepsis with DIC
  – thorotrast exposure
	▸ Bone marrow transplantation
	▸ Amyloidosis
	▸ Thyrotoxicosis
	▸ Post radiotherapy/chemotherapy
	▸ Autoimmune disorders
	  – celiac disease
	  – Crohn disease
	  – ulcerative colitis
	  – collagen disease
	▸ Malignant invasion

5.2 Functional Asplenia

▸ Sickle–cell anemia, amyloidosis

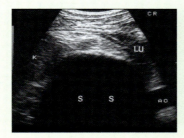
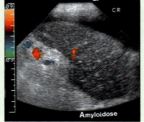

a Small hyperechoic spleen with hypoechoic mass and crescent-shaped calcification with posterior shadowing (S) in homozygous sickle-cell anemia. Splenic scarring as sequelae of recurrent splenic infarction, suspected functional asplenia. LU = lung; K = kidney; AO = aorta.

b and c Color-flow Doppler scanning of a small inhomogeneous spleen with spurious flow signals in amyloidosis; suspected functional hyposplenism.

▸ Bone–marrow transplantation (GVHD)

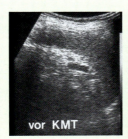
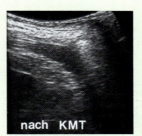
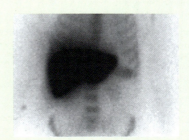

d–f Acute leukaemia.
d Normal-sized spleen before bone marrow transplantation.

e Shrunken spleen after allogeneic bone marrow transplantation in severe GVHD.

f Colloid-labeled scintiscan: the spleen is barely visible, indicating functional hyposplenism.

▸ Sepsis, ulcerative colitis, radiotherapy

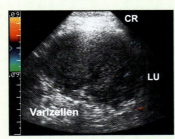
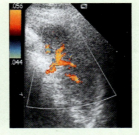
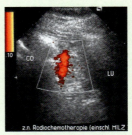

g Small spleen with lack of flow signals in sepsis and diffuse splenic hemorrhage one year earlier; suspected functional hyposplenism. LU = lung; Varizellen = chicken pox.

h Small spleen with normal flow signals in chronic ulcerative colitis.

i Small spleen with marked hilar flow signals in malignant lymphoma and post radiotherapy of the spleen; suspected functional hyposplenism. LU = lung; CO = venous confluence.

Focal Changes

Focal changes of the spleen are rare. Ultrasound detects them in approximately 0.2% of cases. They are characterized sonographically similarly to hepatic masses, i.e., according to echogenicity, size, shape, delineation, and number. Compared with hepatic masses, the nosological assessment of a focal splenic mass is often difficult and becomes possible only when taking into account the history and clinical symptoms of the patient as well as the sonographic follow-up. In case of doubt, the diagnosis is confirmed by definite cytology/histology via ultrasound-guided fine-needle aspiration cytology/biopsy.

The differential diagnostic consideration in the sections below adheres to the morphological typing. This is somewhat fraught with problems since, for instance, splenic cysts may be demonstrated as being anechoic, hypoechoic, or also hyperechoic. Therefore, an additional classification according to the frequency of diagnosis has been introduced.

Anechoic Mass

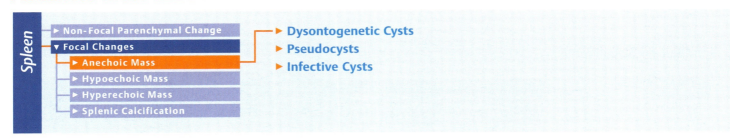

Splenic cysts are rare benign lesions with an incidence of less than 0.1%. They are differentiated by their origin as being infective (hydatid disease) or noninfective. The latter group breaks down into "true" cysts (dysontogenetic, epidermoid, and dermoid cysts) and pseudocysts (not lined with epithelium).

▶ Dysontogenetic Cysts

True splenic cysts are characterized by an epithelial lining and are congenital in origin. On ultrasound, they appear as round, smooth, anechoic lesions, well-defined from the surrounding splenic texture, with signs of distal acoustic enhancement. Sometimes echogenic septation, internal echoes, sedimentation phenomena, sequestered tissue, and calcification of the wall may be observed. The contents of the cyst may be watery clear or dark brown owing to hemorrhage. In other cases the lumen of the (pseudo-)cyst is filled with pulpy material. On ultrasound, the fluid within the cysts is at times visualized with a floating, moving hyperechoic mass ("snowstorm"), corresponding to cell conglomerates, sequestered tissue, or crystals (◻ 5.3). This may complicate differentiation from a solid mass. There are no certain sonographic signs ruling out pseudocysts. Fifty-two patients with noninfective splenic cysts (24 true cysts and 28 pseudocysts) did not show any significant difference regarding size, intrinsic echogenicity, or contents of the cyst. Only calcification of the wall appeared to be more frequent in pseudocysts.

◻ 5.3 Splenic Cysts

▶ Different ultrasound appearance of splenic cysts

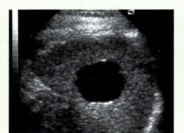
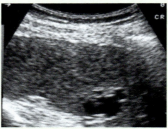
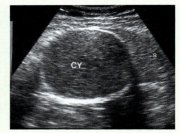

a Central anechoic, smoothly delineated round mass within the spleen, with posterior acoustic enhancement, compatible with splenic cyst.

b Anechoic splenic cysts of irregular margin and with small septa.

c Hyperechoic splenic cyst (cy) with signs of intramural calcification.

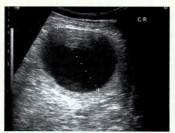
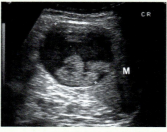

d and e Anechoic splenic cyst (*d*). Follow-up demonstrates intrinsic sedimentation phenomena as in old hemorrhage (*e*). M = spleen.

f Large cyst (C) with signs of intramural calcification. S = spleen.

▶ Pseudocysts

By definition, pseudocysts are not lined with epithelium. Almost without exception they are solitary lesions and, as such, sequelae to liquefactive, hemorrhagic, or encapsulating processes after pancreatitis, splenic trauma (◻ 5.4b and c), infarction (◻ 5.4a), and metastasis (◻ 5.4d). Since splenic trauma and infarction are somewhat common, the percentage of secondary cysts (approx. 80%) is not only far larger than that of primary cysts (approx. 20%), but also larger than for other parenchymal organs (e.g., the liver).

General treatment of splenic cysts depends on the clinical symptoms, which in turn are a function of the size of the cyst. Cysts with a diameter < 5 cm should be followed up. Large lesions occupying the spleen are mostly treated by surgery, even today when conservative procedures are increasingly preferred. Ultrasound-guided catheter drainage with sclerosing agents is becoming a more viable option. Rupture and carcinoma of splenic cysts have been reported in a few rare cases.

Table 5.3 Differential diagnosis of anechoic splenic masses

Frequent	Rare
▶ Dysontogenetic splenic cyst	▶ Abscess
▶ Pseudocyst	▶ Hemorrhage
▶ Infective splenic cyst	▶ Infarction
	▶ Metastasis
	▶ Pseudoaneurysm
	▶ Lymphangioma
	▶ Hemangioma
	▶ Hamartoma

Table 5.3 lists other rare anechoic splenic masses (◻ 5.4e–k).

◻ 5.4 Pseudocysts and Other Anechoic Masses

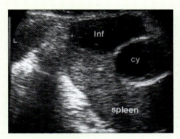
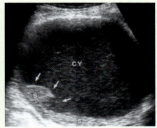
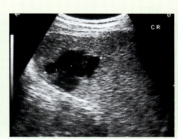
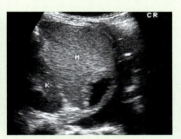

a–d Pseudocysts.
a Central anechoic cyst (Cy) with calcified wall. Triangular hypoechoic structure at the margin as in splenic infarction (Inf).

b Large old posttraumatic splenic cyst (CY). The splenic parenchyma is lacerated (arrows). S = spleen.

c Central anechoic splenic mass after bicycle accident, compatible with splenic hemorrhage.

d Echogenic mass within the spleen, with central anechoic liquefaction, in cancer of the floor of the mouth, compatible with colliquated splenic metastasis. M = spleen; K = Kidney.

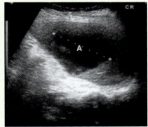

e and f Anechoic splenic abscess (A) (e); after needle evacuation hyperechoic air is seen (f).

g and h Anechoic intrasplenic mass in hepatic cirrhosis, with demonstration of arterial flow. Intrasplenic pseudoaneurysm; the patient underwent splenectomy. C = cyst–like mass; M = spleen.

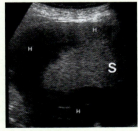
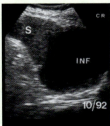
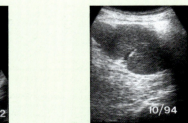

i Anechoic encasement of the spleen (S) in malignant lymphoma, compatible with spontaneous subcapsular hemorrhage (H).

j to l Somewhat older anechoic splenic infarction (INF) in endocarditis of the aortic valve; follow-up demonstrated spontaneous resolution. S = spleen.

▶ Infective Cysts

Infective cysts are rare and are encountered in less than 2% of all patients infected with hydatid disease. In most cases the infective agent is *Echinococcus cysticus* or *E. granulosus*.

Most cysts are visualized as anechoic lesions with a double wall (pericyst and endocyst). In rare cases they may demonstrate daughter cysts. In exceptional cases these secondary cysts may be very small and numerous; and, because of the large number of wall echoes (**Fig. 5.26**), the sonographic appearance of such a hydatid cyst may resemble that of a hyperechoic lesion. Intracystic membranes, hydatid sand (scolicial sedimentation), and calcification have been reported. In general, the ultrasound appearance of infective splenic cysts is quite characteristic, although sometimes they are hard to differentiate from incidental splenic cysts. When there is doubt, the diagnosis has to be confirmed by laboratory work-up.

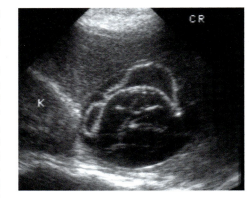

◀ **Fig. 5.26** Anechoic mass with festoonlike structures corresponding to a hydatid cyst. K = Kidney,

Hypoechoic Mass

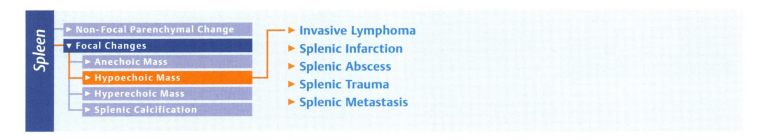

Table 5.4 lists the most important hypoechoic splenic masses.

Table 5.4 Differential diagnosis of hypoechoic splenic masses

Frequent	Rare
▶ Invasive lymphoma	▶ Metastasis
▶ Infarction	▶ Tuberculosis
▶ Abscess	▶ Sarcoidosis
▶ Splenic trauma	▶ Collagen disease
	▶ Amyloidosis
	▶ Histoplasmosis
	▶ Leukemic infiltrate
	▶ Microabscess
	▶ Peliosis
	▶ Cyst

▶ Invasive Lymphoma

Splenic involvement may generally be diagnosed sonographically by the presence of splenomegaly (primarily in low-grade lymphoma) or the demonstration of hypoechoic focal or diffuse textural lesions of the splenic parenchyma. However, splenic involvement cannot be ruled out for certain even if the spleen is of normal size and homogeneous texture.

Ultrasound differentiates between five different patterns of invasion (**Fig. 5.27**), with the micronodular and macronodular invasion as well as the bulky formation corresponding to focal parenchymal lesions.

Diffuse splenic involvement. As in all parenchymal organs, the greatest difficulty ultrasound faces is with diffuse splenic involvement, and this is the main reason for the poor sensitivity (albeit for all imaging modalities) in diagnosing possible invasion of the spleen. Compared with the adjacent liver, a normal spleen will appear to be somewhat more homogeneous. The (subjective or operator-dependent) assessment of the splenic texture should be based on the liver as an in-vivo reference (◨ 5.5a–c).

Focal parenchymal lesions. The value of ultrasonography in the detection of focal parenchymal lesions is well known, having a sensitivity of more than 90% and a specificity of 96%. Since the general incidence of focal splenic destruction is low, hypoechoic splenic masses in pa-

5.5 Invasion by Lymphoma

▶ Diffuse invasion

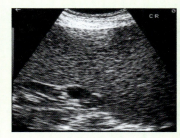
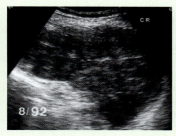

a Diffuse splenic invasion in malignant lymphoma.

b and c Diffuse hypoechoic invasion of the entire spleen in Hodgkin disease. Resolved under therapy (**c**).

▶ Focal (micronodular and macronodular) lesions

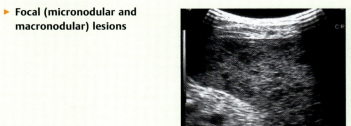
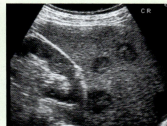
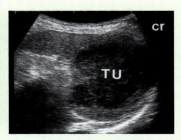

d Micronodular splenic invasion in Hodgkin disease. The hypoechoic masses resolved under chemotherapy.

e Micronodular hypoechoic splenic masses in malignant lymphoma.

f Macronodular hypoechoic splenic mass (TU) in malignant lymphoma.

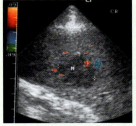
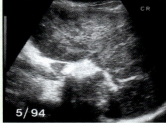

g Hypoechoic mass within the spleen; splenectomy confirmed primary lymphoma of the spleen.

h and i Large complex masses within the spleen, with hyperechoic as well as hypoechoic areas, in Hodgkin disease. Resolved under therapy (**i**).

▶ Perisplenic invasion

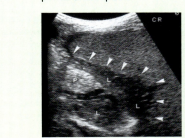
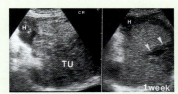
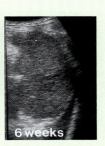

j Perisplenic invasion (L) originating at the hilum in malignant lymphoma.

k and l Extensive invasion (TU) of the spleen in malignant lymphoma; subcapsular hemorrhage (H). Under therapy, demarcation of the intrasplenic lesion (arrows) with resolution.

▶ Perivascular invasion

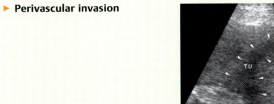
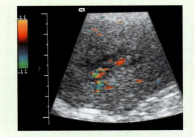

m and n Perivascular invasion (TU) at the splenic hilum in Hodgkin disease (arrowheads); resolved under therapy (**n**). S = spleen.

o Perivascular invasion in malignant lymphoma.

tients with lymphoma have to be regarded as neoplastic with a high degree of certainty (5.5d–g).

Frequently, large lesions will display an inhomogeneous echo texture (5.5h and i) with hyperechoic areas. Calcification is rare and will occur mostly after treatment.

Corresponding with the macroscopic findings, low-grade non-Hodgkin lymphoma as well as Hodgkin lymphoma tend toward diffuse or micronodular invasion, while high-grade non-Hodgkin lymphoma will lead to larger masses.

Perisplenic invasion. Perisplenic invasion by lymphoma is extremely rare; it may originate at the hilum and spread in caplike fashion (5.5j). Perisplenic invasion is also possible by the lymphoma spreading from the thorax through the diaphragm into the capsule of the spleen. In individual cases this may result in complications such as hemorrhage, rupture (5.5k and l), and infarction of the spleen.

Hypoechoic perivascular structural transformation. Hypoechoic perivascular structural transformation of the hilar vessels of the spleen is a rare entity in patients with malignant lymphoma. The etiology is unknown and it resolves under chemotherapy. Similar changes have been reported in the liver as hypoechoic structural lesions encompassing the portal vein ("periportal cuffing"). They have also been observed in systemic hematological malignancy as well as in benign disorders. Apart from invasion by the lymphoma, perivascular edema by lymphatic obstruction has also been suggested as one possible explanation (5.5m–o).

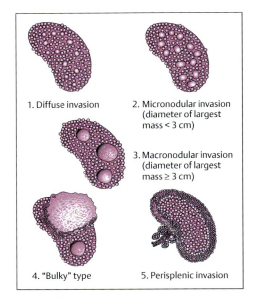

▲ **Fig. 5.27** Schematic illustration of the different sonographic patterns of splenic invasion in malignant lymphoma.

▶ Splenic Infarction

Splenic infarction is relatively common. It is the result of embolic or thrombotic obstruction of branches of the splenic artery.

Clinical symptoms. The clinical picture is unremarkable and is characterized by:
▶ Lack of any symptoms
▶ Diffuse abdominal pain, or
▶ Left upper quadrant pain

Because of the textural difference with regular parenchyma, splenic infarction and its complications may be visualized by ultrasound (**Fig. 5.28**).

Acute splenic infarction. Ultrasound shows acute splenic infarction as more or less hypoechoic lesions of the parenchymal texture, differing in size and extending to the splenic margin (5.6a). If the ultrasound beam parallels the longitudinal axis of the infarct, it may be possible to visualize the typical pyramid or wedge shaped defect, with its base pointing toward the surface and the apex toward the hilum (5.6a and b). In these cases, the characteristic shape alone is sufficient to differentiate between splenic infarction and the similar sonographic morphology of splenic abscess or neoplastic splenic invasion.

Color-flow Doppler imaging will delineate infarction from regular splenic parenchyma by the lack of flow signals in the former.

The wide spectrum of sonographic visualization in splenic infarction reported in the literature is partly due to the lack of methods (primarily because of the unspecific clinical picture) for determining the age of the infarction in retrospect.

Chronic recurrent infarction. It is chronic (recurrent) infarction (5.6c) in particular, typical in homozygous sickle-cell anemia, for example, that displays calcification and focal hypoechoic as well as hyperechoic masses with increasing atrophy of the organ, corresponding to autosplenectomy (5.6d). In color-flow Doppler scanning of the scarred spleen, circulation in the organ is markedly reduced.

Causes of Splenic Infarction

Thromboembolism. Depending on the patients studied, thromboembolism is the cause of splenic infarction in up to 70% of cases. It complicates various cardiovascular diseases (arteriosclerosis, myocardial infarction with intramural thrombus, atrial fibrillation, bacterial endocarditis, cardiac catheterization, but also in microangiopathy syndromes).
There have been reports of septic emboli in AIDS patients without any underlying cardiac disease.

Myeloproliferative and lymphoproliferative disorders. The pathogenetic mechanism of splenic infarction in myeloproliferative and lymphoproliferative disease is certainly multifactorial. Apart from congestion due to invasion by malignancy and/or extramedullary hematopoiesis (primarily in myeloproliferative disorders), the mismatch between the increased oxygen consumption incurred by the enlarged organ and the decreased oxygen supply in anemia plays a certain role.

Total splenic infarction. Infarction of the entire spleen may be the result of acute splenic vein thrombosis in the wandering spleen, torsion of the vascular pedicle, acute sequestration in homozygous childhood sickle-cell anemia, septic disorders, disseminated intravascular coagulation (DIC), or as part of pancreatitis (5.6g–i). The sonographic image is charac-

Sickle-cell anemia. In homozygous sickle-cell anemia, oxygen deficiency and/or acidosis will lead to abnormal crystallization of hemoglobin with subsequent erythrocyte adhesion and manifestation of splenic infarction. This complication is less common, but still possible, in carriers (heterozygous sickle-cell anemia).

Thrombophilia. Congenital or acquired thrombophilia (e.g., congenital protein C or S deficiency, lupus anticoagulant, erythropoietin therapy) is an infrequent cause of splenic infarction.

Partial splenic dearterialization. Some children with thalassemia major undergo therapeutic partial dearterialization of the splenic artery with subsequent splenic infarction. In myeloproliferative disorder, hypersplenism may be palliated by embolization of branches of the splenic artery.

terized by hypoechoic inhomogeneous transformation of the entire splenic texture.

Healing phase. Increasing echogenicity and shrinking size of the infarct characterize the healing phase. Sometimes local textural inhomogeneity or calcification will remain as a scar. In 80% of cases the infarction will heal without any complication (◨ **5.6e and f**).

Complications. Twenty percent of patients will suffer complications, including:
▸ Increasing liquefaction of the infarct (◨ **5.7a–c**)
▸ Development of subcapsular hemorrhage (◨ **5.7d–f**),
▸ Flow phenomena identifiable on color-flow Doppler scanning as indication of pseudoaneurysm or arteriovenous fistula (◨ **5.7g–i**)
▸ Demonstration of free intraperitoneal fluid (blood) (◨ **5.7j and k**)

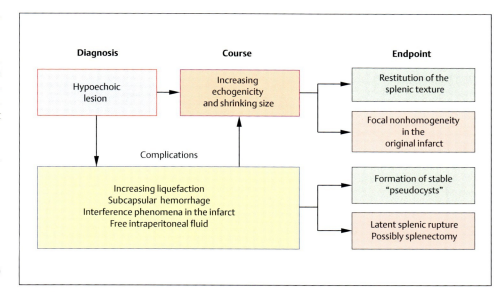

▲ **Fig. 5.28** Sonographic visualization and complications of splenic infarction.

◨ 5.6 Acute and Chronic Recurrent Splenic Infarction

▸ **Fresh and old infarctions**

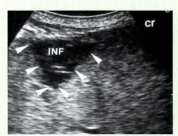

a and *b* Wedge-shaped splenic infarct (INF); in a slightly different view mimicking a round mass (*b*).

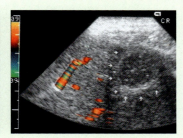

c Old complex splenic infarct as residual scar; hyperechoic delineation (arrows) of the margin.

▸ **Follow-ups**

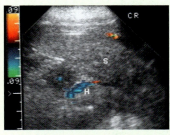

d Small echogenic spleen lacking any vascular flow signals; chronic recurrent infarction in homozygous sickle-cell anemia. H = hematoma; S = spleen.

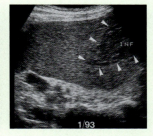

e and *f* Course of splenic infarction (INF).
e Hypoechoic appearance during the acute stage.

f Later, increasing echogenicity of the infarct.

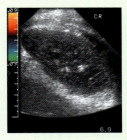

g–i Acute pancreatitis.
g Formation of a hypoechoic perisplenic abscess (A). SP = spleen; E = pleural exudation.

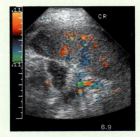

h During the course, transient hypoechoic transformation of the spleen, lacking flow signals because of splenic artery obstruction.

i Two days later, revascularization is evident.

▶ Splenic Abscess

Macroabscess. Most of these are pyogenic. On ultrasound, a macroabscess is visualized as a smooth or irregularly shaped, primarily hypoechoic lesion that is delineated from the normal parenchymal texture. However, as for hepatic abscess, there is a wide spectrum of ultrasound morphology of these splenic abscesses, which can be traced back to the difference in the number of acoustically relevant echo boundaries. These morphologies include:
- ▶ Completely anechoic abscess resembling a cyst with posterior acoustic enhancement
- ▶ Hypoechoic abscess with different degree of textural echo pattern (◻ 5.8a–c)
- ▶ Markedly hyperechoic abscess, sometimes gaseous, with or without posterior acoustic enhancement (**Fig. 5.29**)

Pathogenesis

One of the explanations for the rather low incidence of splenic abscess is the high degree of phagocytosis in the spleen. Hematogenous bacterial spread accounts for approximately 75% of all abscess formation, bacterial endocarditis being the most common cause (possibly via infected splenic infarct).
Superinfection of hematoma in splenic hemorrhage or a liquefying infarct accounts for only 15% of cases.

Other predisposing factors are diabetes, immunosuppression, and neoplastic disease cancer of the stomach, colon, and pancreas. These cancers tend to invade the spleen, with secondary infection after the original organ is perforated.
A distinction has to be made between macroabscesses and microabscesses.

◻ 5.7 Complications of Splenic Infarction

▶ **Liquefaction of the infarct**

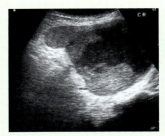 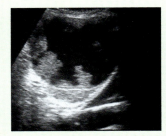 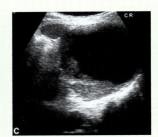

a–c Large liquefying splenic infarct with pseudocyst formation in endocarditis.

▶ **Subcapsular hemorrhage**

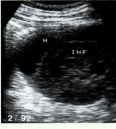 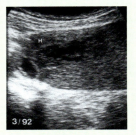 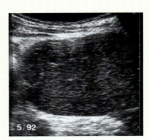

d–f Apart from a splenic infarct (INF) there is a subcapsular hematoma (H) with subsequent resolution.

▶ **Pseudoaneurysm and AV fistula**

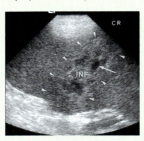 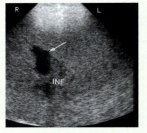 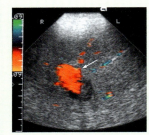

g–i Complex transformation of splenic tissue with small anechoic area (arrow). There are arterial flow signals compatible with intrasplenic pseudoaneurysm (arrow). INF = infarct.

▶ **Free intraperitoneal fluid**

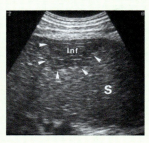 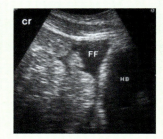

j and k Wedge-shaped splenic infarct (inf) with tenuous intraperitoneal fluid (FF) posterior to the urinary bladder (HB). Fine-needle aspiration confirmed the presence of blood within the peritoneal cavity. S = spleen.

Differentiating splenic abscess from other focal masses (hematoma, infarct, cyst, tumor) by ultrasound criteria for contour and texture alone, not taking into account any clinical parameters, is fraught with problems. Since splenic abscess has a mortality of up to 100% if left untreated, a tentative diagnosis should be confirmed by ultrasound-guided fine-needle aspiration (3–4 Fr) with bacteriological and cytological work-up (◾ **5.8d–f**). If it is an abscess, the diagnostic procedure can be expanded to definitive treatment in terms of quantitative evacuation; an abscess of less than 8–10 cm across may be aspirated repeatedly, while catheter drainage is recommended for abscess diameters > 8–10 cm (◾ **5.8g–i**). Splenectomy should be reserved for very special cases. Since the parenchymal trauma carries with it the risk of potential hemorrhage, any interventional procedures in splenic abscess should involve close cooperation with the surgeons at an early stage.

Microabscess. Microabscesses within the spleen, or liver, are uncommon and are seen primarily in immunocompromised patients. The prevalence is about 26% of all splenic abscesses. The most important etiology is that of chronic disseminated candidiasis, manifested as hepatosplenic candidiasis; microabscess as part of bacterial infection, such as miliary tuberculosis or infection with *Pneumocystis carinii*, is infrequent (**Fig. 5.30**).

Establishing a prognosis in candida abscess is impossible unless the clinical picture is considered. It is not possible to differentiate a hypoechoic mass from micronodular invasion, as in malignant lymphoma or leukemia, by sonographic morphology alone. The diagnosis is confirmed by clinical parameters, following up the antimycotic treatment by ultrasound, and sometimes even ultrasound-guided fine-needle aspiration biopsy; because of the concurrent antimycotic therapy, cytohistology mostly demonstrates the presence of necrosis and granulation. Frequently, calcification will be seen as residual scar after splenic microabscess.

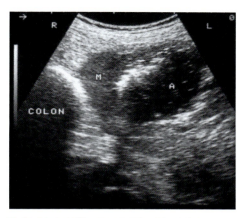
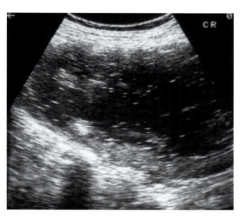

▲ **Fig. 5.29a and b** Large complex splenic abscess (A) with intralesional gas. M = spleen.

◾ 5.8 Treatment of Splenic Abscess

▶ **Repeated aspiration**

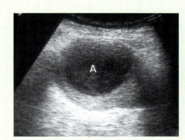
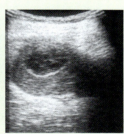

a Hypoechoic splenic abscess (A); 80 ml

b and c Resolution four weeks later after two aspiration cycles.

▶ **Abscess drainage without catheter**

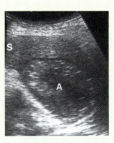
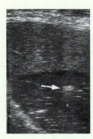
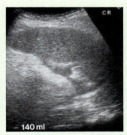

d Complex splenic abscess (A) within the hilum. S = spleen.

e In ultrasound-guided fine-needle aspiration of the abscess the echo of the tip of the needle is seen within the mass (arrow).

f Complete evacuation of the material.

▶ **Catheter drainage of abscess**

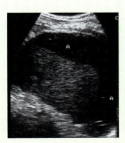
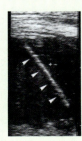
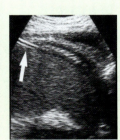

g Large abscess (A) capping the spleen.

h Puncture and placement of the guidewire.

i The catheter is placed by Seldinger technique and the abscess is drained.

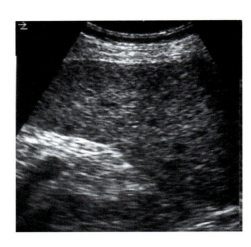 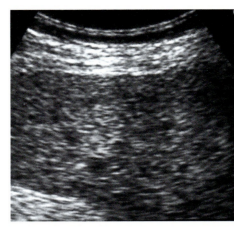

▲ *Fig. 5.30a and b* Diffuse micronodular splenic invasion in a patient with systemic hematological malignancy, in complete remission, with septic temperature; highly indicative of splenic candidiasis.

▶ Splenic Trauma

Sonographic findings. Ultrasound can visualize the following alterations indicative of splenic trauma.
- **Hematoperitoneum**: free intraperitoneal, perisplenic, perihepatic fluid and/or fluid in the rectovesical pouch or Douglas's space in primary splenic rupture with hemorrhage into the peritoneal cavity.
- **Subcapsular splenic rupture**: liquid zones (anechoic, isoechoic, or hyperechoic!) between the parenchyma and capsule of the spleen.
- **Organ injury**: destruction of the parenchymal texture, with visualization of textural nonhomogeneity or splenic laceration of varying severity as direct indication of tissue lesions and/or hemorrhage.

Subcapsular splenic rupture. External trauma leading to subcapsular splenic rupture (5.9a–f) frequently results in the hemorrhage between parenchyma and capsule capping the organ, primarily along the convex diaphragmatic surface; this can produce a double contour on ultrasound examination. Subcapsular hemorrhage around the splenic hilum is less common.

As in the posttraumatic subcapsular hemorrhage of the liver, it has to be pointed out that the acute subcapsular splenic hemorrhage may also be distinctly hyperechoic and could easily be overlooked on cursory examination. Sometimes an enlarged left hepatic lobe may mimic a subcapsular mass.

Organ injury. A careful ultrasound study will be able to successfully demonstrate most cases of organ injury, although sometimes short-term follow-up will become necessary. Injuries to the spleen are recognized by:
- Irregularly defined hypoechoic, isoechoic, as well as hyperechoic lesions of the usually homogeneous parenchymal texture (5.9g–l)
- Destruction of the splenic contour (5.9m–o)

Treatment. In traumatic and nontraumatic splenic rupture, the current regimen calls for preservation of the spleen, if at all possible. This depends on the extent of the injury, for which there are several grading systems. These are founded on ultrasound studies and have become quite useful as additional parameters in the decision how to tailor treatment. However, imaging modalities cannot be the sole foundation on which to rest the decision against surgery. The clinical picture and laboratory work-up still play the primary role here. Repeated short-term (possibly even hourly) follow-up ultrasound studies have proved to be very useful.

Ultrasound Grading System in Splenic Trauma

▶ **Grade 1**
Subcapsular hematoma, thickness < 3 cm, and/or intraparenchymal lesion < 3 cm diameter, splenic capsule unbroken.
▶ **Grade 2**
Subcapsular hematoma, thickness ≥ 3 cm, and/or intraparenchymal lesion > 3 cm diameter, splenic capsule unbroken.
▶ **Grade 3**
Splenic fragmentation, avascular spleen, or flow phenomena (arteriovenous pseudoaneurysms) in liquefied intraparenchymal areas.

A retrospective study of 30 patients with splenic rupture demonstrated that "watchful waiting" was justified in grade 1 patients ($n = 6$), while surgery became necessary in all grade 3 trauma cases ($n = 8$). Patients with grade 2 splenic trauma ($n = 16$) had to undergo surgery in 62% of cases ($n = 9$).

▶ Splenic Metastasis

Splenic metastasis is detected in approximately 7% of autopsies. Metastasis in the spleen is far less common than in the liver, the hypothesis being that the spleen is equipped with a special immunological microenvironment.

Ultrasound appearance. Classification of splenic metastasis is along the same lines as in the liver, the splenic parenchyma being the in-vivo reference. The metastases can be classified as being anechoic, hypoechoic, isoechoic, hyperechoic, and complex. The most common sonographic types demonstrated in the spleen are hypoechoic metastases. Larger metastases may exhibit central colliquation.

All metastases may present with or without a halo, which can be regarded as typical of, but not specific to, hepatic and splenic malignancy (5.10a–d).

Metastasis in direct extension. Splenic metastasis may also arise by direct extension of pancreatic, colonic, and gastric cancer (5.11). In rare cases, malignancies of the lung or diaphragm may break through and invade the spleen in continuity. Also peritoneal metastasis may encase and invade the spleen.

Complications. Complications may be localized perforation, abscess, splenic hemorrhage, and rupture (5.10e–i). Calcification of splenic metastasis has also been reported as well as tumor-induced splenic vein thrombosis.

5.9 Splenic Trauma

► Subcapsular hematoma

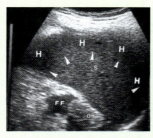 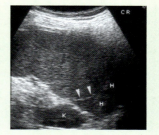 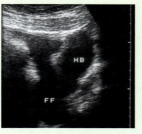

a–c Almost isoechoic subcapsular hematoma (H) in mononucleosis. Free fluid (FF) in Douglas's space. HB = bladder; K = kidney; S = spleen.

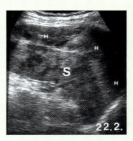 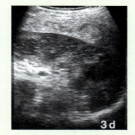 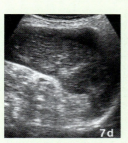

d–f Subcapsular hematoma (H) in chickenpox sepsis. During the course, changing echogenicity of the hematoma with resolution. S = spleen.

► Intraparenchymal splenic trauma

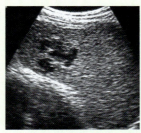 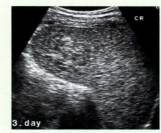 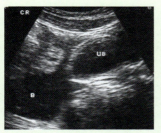

g–i Intraparenchymal splenic trauma with increasing echogenicity over time. In addition, free fluid (probably blood: B) in Douglas's space. UB = urinary bladder.

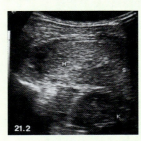 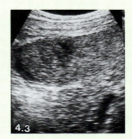 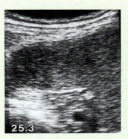

j–l Intraparenchymal, irregularly defined echogenic defect after blunt abdominal trauma, resolving eventually. H = hematoma; S = spleen.

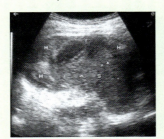 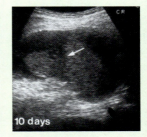 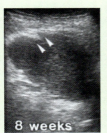

m–o Large complex subcapsular splenic hemorrhage (H) with demarcation of a parenchymal laceration (arrow); eventually resolved but with scarring. S = spleen.

5.10 Splenic Metastasis

▶ Anechoic/complex

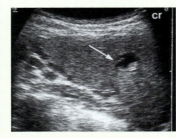 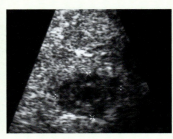 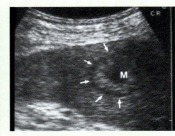

a Splenic metastasis.

b Hypoechoic splenic mass with central liquefaction in colon cancer: splenic metastasis.

c Hyperechoic splenic mass (M) with hypoechoic margin ("halo") and central liquefaction in colon cancer: splenic metastasis.

▶ Echogenic

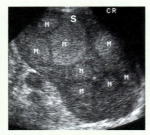 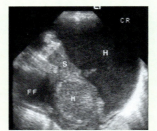 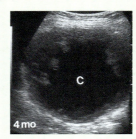

d Splenic metastasis (M).

e and f Splenic metastasis (M) in ENT malignancy. Large intrasplenic hematoma (H); at the same time a large amount of free intraperitoneal fluid (FF) can be demonstrated. The weak, emaciated patient refused surgery. UB = urinary bladder; S = spleen.

▶ Hemorrhagic areas

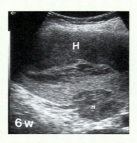 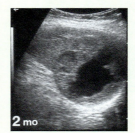 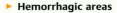

g–i Malignant melanoma. Slowly resolving splenic metastasis (M) and subcapsular hematoma (H); in addition, formation of a liquefied splenic metastasis.

5.11 Splenic Metastasis in Direct Extension

▶ Pancreas, stomach

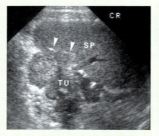 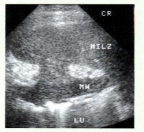 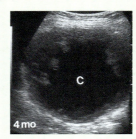

a Cancer of the pancreatic tail (TU) invading the spleen (SP) in direct extension.

b and c Gastric cancer (TU) invading the spleen (Milz). The blood supply of the tumor (arrow) can be demonstrated. LU = lumen; MW = stomach wall.

▶ Colon, ovary

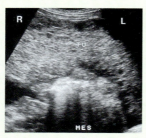 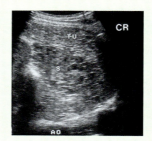 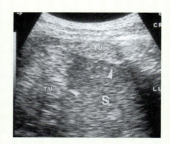

d–f Mucinous cancer of the colon. *d* Tumor (TU) invasion of the greater omentum (MES).

e Perisplenic and splenic invasion by the tumor (TU). S = spleen; AO = aorta.

f Hyperechoic perisplenic invasion by the tumor (TU) in ovarian cancer with peritoneal metastasis. S = spleen.

Hyperechoic Mass

Spleen — Focal Changes ▸ Hyperechoic Mass
- Non-Focal Parenchymal Change
- Focal Changes
  - Anechoic Mass
  - Hypoechoic Mass
  - **Hyperechoic Mass** → Hemangioma, Hamartoma, Lymphoma and Myeloproliferative Disorders
  - Splenic Calcification

Table 5.5 lists the differential diagnosis of hyperechoic splenic masses and their incidence.

Benign solid hyperechoic splenic tumor is usually diagnosed as an incidental finding in abdominal ultrasound studies. It is extremely rare, the most common being hemangiomas and hamartomas.

The main advantage of ultrasound and other tomographic imaging modalities is their ability to differentiate these entities from primarily malignant splenic tumors, splenic metastases, or infiltrates in malignant lymphoma, and from other hyperechoic intrasplenic masses. Only rarely is ultrasound alone able to do that.

Table 5.5 Differential diagnosis of hyperechoic splenic mass

Frequent	Rare
▸ Hemangioma	▸ Lymphoma infiltrate
▸ Hamartoma	▸ Hemorrhage
	▸ Abscess
	▸ Metastasis
	▸ Hemangiosarcoma
	▸ Extramedullary hematopoiesis
	▸ Gaucher disease
	▸ Niemann–Pick disease
	▸ Peliosis
	▸ Spherocytosis
	▸ Schistosomiasis
	▸ Littoral cell angioma

▸ Hemangioma

Hemangiomas are the most common benign tumors of the spleen. Their incidence in autopsy studies ranges from 0.03% to 14%. They are mostly asymptomatic and are diagnosed as incidental findings. Their size varies from just a few millimeters to 15 cm. This predominantly cavernous and rarely capillary tumor arises from the sinus epithelium. Hemangiomas may be solitary or come in multiples and are seen as part of a generalized angiomatosis. Isolated splenic hemangiomatosis is a rare entity and is usually detected as incidental finding after splenectomy. Splenic hemangiomas will grow slowly; rupture is the most common complication, with an incidence of up to 25%.

5.12 Splenic Hemangioma

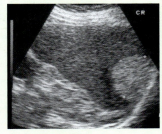
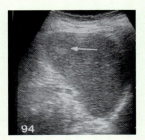
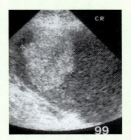
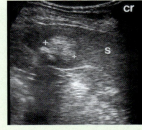

a Hyperechoic splenic mass compatible with hemangioma.

b and *c* Growing hyperechoic splenic mass; splenectomy confirmed the diagnosis of a cavernous hemangioma.

d Hyperechoic calcified splenic mass corresponding to hemangioma. S = spleen.

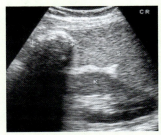
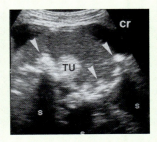

e Calcified splenic mass; these phenomena are more frequent in hemangiomas.

f Multiple hyperechoic splenic masses, compatible with hemangioma; in addition, marked intrasplenic calcification. TU = tumor; S = spleen.

Ultrasound appearance. Ultrasound can differentiate between two separate types:
- A primarily smooth, homogeneous, hyperechoic and mostly round lesion (◨ **5.12a–c**)
- A complex lesion with hypoechoic, partly anechoic, areas and sometimes also calcification with posterior shadowing (◨ **5.12d–f**).

In terms of anatomical pathology, this corresponds to a homogeneous vascular pattern or liquid areas (partly hemorrhagic, partly filled with serous fluid).

Cystic hemangioma is a rare variant.

▶ Hamartoma

Hamartomas (splenomas or nodular hypersplenism) are regarded as infrequent congenital neoplasias of the spleen. Most often they will be solitary and are diagnosed as an incidental finding. Anatomical pathology shows them to be made up of normal splenic parenchyma. Their size ranges from several centimeters to more than fist-sized masses, but they rarely cause any symptoms (**Fig. 5.31**).

Ultrasound appearance. Ultrasound visualizes hamartomas as smoothly delineated tumors weakly contrasted against the splenic parenchyma, with a primarily homogeneous textural echo pattern, good through-transmission of the ultrasound waves, and mild posterior enhancement. Their echogenicity is probably due to the density of breaks in acoustic impedance at the walls of their numerous microscopic fissured cavities. On color-flow Doppler scanning this mass will present as "silent tumor."

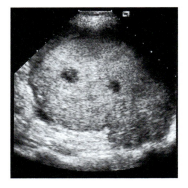
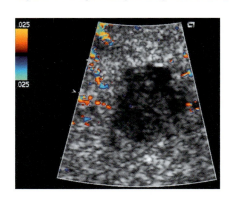

◀ **Fig. 5.31a and b** Large hyperechoic splenic mass with hypoechoic central areas. Splenectomy confirmed a splenoma.

▶ Lymphoma and Myeloproliferative Disorders

Hyperechoic lesions may be identified as lymphoma infiltrates in just a few cases (< 10%) (**Fig. 5.32**). They are primarily seen in chronic lymphocytic leukemia (CLL) and marked splenomegaly. Hyperechoic masses are also found in some patients with extramedullary splenic hematopoiesis in myeloproliferative disorders (**Fig. 5.33**).

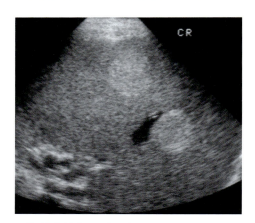
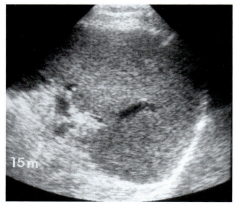
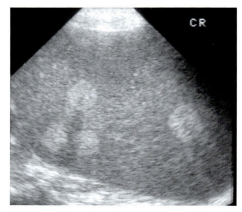

▲ **Fig. 5.32** Malignant lymphoma.
a Multiple hyperechoic masses. The pathological morphology of this finding remains unclear.

▲ **b** These masses resolved under chemotherapy, indicating that they might have been lymphoma infiltrates.

▲ **Fig. 5.33** Multiple hyperechoic masses in a patient with myeloproliferative disorder. The pathological morphology of this finding remains unclear, possibly corresponding to extramedullary hematopoiesis.

Splenic Calcification

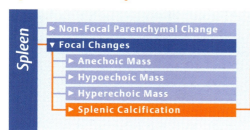

Table **5.6** summarizes the differential diagnosis of splenic calcification.

On ultrasound calcification of the splenic parenchyma presents as solitary or multiple hyperechoic structures, characterized by total or partial posterior shadowing.

Definitive correlation with certain diseases, based only on the ultrasound findings, is impossible in most cases. Since they do not require any treatment, the etiology of these mostly incidental findings remains unclear.

Table 5.6 Differential diagnosis of splenic calcification

Frequent	Rare

▶ Metainfective "starry sky"
 ▶ Calcified cyst
 ▶ Vascular calcification
	▶ Splenic calcification
	 ▶ Calcified metastasis
	 ▶ Calcified hemangioma
	 ▶ Scarring after
	  – abscess
	  – lymphoma
	  – trauma
	  – infarction

▶ Focal Calcification

Focal calcification will be seen as residual scarring after infarction, hematoma, abscess, or invasive lymphoma, or as part of a metabolic disorder (e.g., chronic renal insufficiency) (**Fig. 5.34**). Calcification of metastases (e.g., medullary thyroid carcinoma) is rare. Splenic cysts may exhibit intramural calcification. In larger hemangiomas, hemorrhage may lead to calcification as well. Sometimes recurrent splenic infarction will leave substantial splenic scarring. Such a spleen will rarely be visualized as just a calcareous crescent, but this would be characteristic in homozygous sickle-cell anemia. Calcified lymph nodes at the splenic hilum will sometimes be seen as sequelae of tuberculosis.

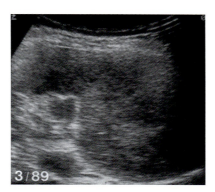

▲ **Fig. 5.34** Malignant lymphoma.
a Splenic involvement.

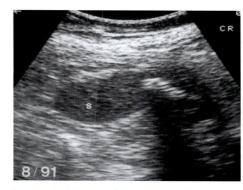

▲ *b* Focal calcification of the spleen (S) after treatment as residual scarring.

▶ Diffuse Calcification

Diffusely distributed fine reflectors in the spleen will produce a pattern resembling a "starry sky" (**Fig. 5.35**). Quite often it is visualized as metainfective scarring and may be associated with calcification of other abdominal organs (e.g., in tuberculosis, systemic histoplasmosis, brucellosis, sarcoidosis, aspergillosis, candidosis, lupus erythematosus, pneumocystis infection, and also amyloidosis).

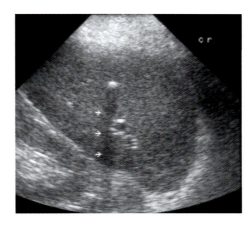

◀ **Fig. 5.35** Multiple small calcifications in an elderly patient with miliary tuberculosis in her youth.

▶ Vascular Calcification

This should be differentiated from the vascular calcification of the arteries and veins (phleboliths), which is primarily seen at the splenic hilum but also as diffuse calcification within the parenchyma. The etiology remains unclear. It has been reported in a few patients with general vascular sclerosis, renal insufficiency, and long-standing portal hypertension (**Fig. 5.36**).

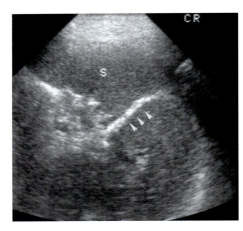

◀ **Fig. 5.36** Vascular calcification in chronic renal insufficiency. S = spleen.

References
1. Falk S. Maligne Lymphome in der Milz. Stuttgart: Fischer 1991.
2. Görg C, Schwerk WB. Milzsonographie. In: Braun B, Günther R, Schwerk WB (eds.). Ultraschalldiagnostik – Lehrbuch und Atlas. Landsberg: ECO med 2000.
3. Neiman RS, Orazi A. Disorders of the spleen. 2nd ed. Philadelphia: W. B. Saunders 1999.

6 Lymph Nodes

Lymph Nodes 199

- **Peripheral Lymph Nodes** — 207
  - **Head/Neck** — 207
    - Inflammatory Lymph Nodes
    - Metastases
    - Malignant Lymphoma
    - Other Structures
  - **Extremities (Axilla, Groin)** — 210
    - Inflammatory Lymph Nodes
    - Metastases
    - Malignant Lymphoma
    - Other Structures

- **Abdominal Lymph Nodes** — 212
  - **Hepatic Portal** — 212
    - Inflammatory Lymph Nodes
    - Metastases
    - Malignant Lymphoma
    - Other Structures
  - **Splenic Hilum** — 215
    - Inflammatory Lymph Nodes
    - Metastases
    - Malignant Lymphoma
    - Other Structures
  - **Mesentery (Celiac, Upper and Lower Mesenteric Station)** — 216
    - Inflammatory Lymph Nodes
    - Metastases
    - Malignant Lymphoma
    - Other Structures
  - **Retroperitoneum (Para-Aortic, Paracaval, Aortointercaval, and Iliac Station)** — 219
    - Inflammatory Lymph Nodes
    - Metastases
    - Malignant Lymphoma
    - Other Structures

6 Lymph Nodes

C. Goerg

Together with the spleen and the mucosa-associated lymphoid tissue [MALT], lymph nodes form the essential barrier of the secondary immune system. The usual lymph node diameter varies between 0.2 cm and 2.5 cm and depends on the functional state of the lymph node as well as the age of the patient. Lymph nodes are in connection with the lymphatics.

Assessment of possible lymph node malignancy is based primarily on the clinical picture (history, workplace, and age of patient, location of lymph node in question, palpation of finding, experience of examining physician) and only secondarily on the ultrasound findings. A definite diagnosis has to await confirmation by histology. Sonographic follow-up has proved to be invaluable in terms of assessing possible malignancy as well as documenting the response to therapy. The diagnostic armamentarium for the follow-up and detection of recurrence, particularly in diseases of the peripheral lymph nodes, has gained immeasurably by the addition of ultrasound.

A summary of possible differential diagnosis in pathological lymph nodes is listed in **Table 6.1**.

Table 6.1 Differential diagnosis in lymphadenopathy (modified from reference 2)

Infectious disease
- Viral infection
  Infectious mononucleosis (EBV), cytomegalic inclusion disease, infectious hepatitis, AIDS, rubella, human herpesvirus 3 (varicella-zoster)
- Bacterial infection
  Streptococci, staphylococci, salmonellae, *Tropheryma whippelii* (Whipple disease), *Francisella tularensis* (tularemia)
- Mycotic infection
  Histoplasmosis, coccidioidomycosis, blastomycosis
- Chlamydial infection
  Lymphogranuloma venereum, cat-scratch disease, trachoma
- Mycobacterial infection
  Toxoplasmosis, trypanosomosis, microfilariae
- Spirochetosis
  Syphilis, leptospirosis

Malignancy
- Hodgkin disease, non-Hodgkin lymphoma, chronic lymphocytic leukemia, acute lymphocytic leukemia
- Myelogenous leukemia (chloromas = extramedullary manifestation of myelogenous leukosis): acute myelogenous leukemia, blast crisis in chronic myelogenous leukemia
- Metastasis of epithelial or mesenchymal tumors

Immunological disease
- Rheumatoid arthritis
- Systemic lupus erythematosus
- Dermatomyositis
- Allergic reaction to drugs such as phenytoin, hydralazine, allopurinol

Other
Sarcoidosis
Lipid storage disease (Gaucher disease, Niemann–Pick disease)

Anatomy

The trabeculae extend from the capsule, composed of connective tissue and a few elastic fibrils, into the substance of the lymph node and result in a radial configuration. From the outside to the inside, the cortical substance is made up of the cortex, the paracortex, and the medulla where the immune response takes place. The hilum is rich in connective tissue and houses the afferent and efferent lymphatics and blood vessels.

Topography

Overall, the normal patient harbors approximately 1000 lymph nodes. The lymphatic system in mammals may be grouped into five large regions, and the lymph of each drains into a major lymphatic trunk:
1 Head/neck
2 Axilla (including ipsilateral arm, mammary gland, and thoracic wall)
3 Groin (including ipsilateral leg and abdominal wall)
4 Intra-abdominal and pelvic organs
5 Intrathoracic organs

Each of these major drainage regions is subdivided into several lymphatic subregions, the names of which are primarily taken from the adjacent blood vessels. For didactic as well as differential diagnostic reasons, the lymph nodes should be classified as peripheral or nonperipheral. Mediastinal and pulmonary lymph nodes will be excluded from this discussion since transcutaneous sonography cannot visualize them by conventional means.

Peripheral lymph nodes include the following regions:
- Head/neck
- Axilla/groin

Lymph node regions of the head/neck (Fig. 6.1)

- I   Submental, submandibular
- II Lymph nodes draining into the upper third of the jugular vein
- III Lymph nodes draining into the middle third of the jugular vein
- IV Lymph nodes draining into the lower third of the jugular vein (including the supraclavicular lymph nodes)
- V   Nuchal

Relations
- Cervical lymph nodes along the jugular vein and carotid artery
- Submandibular lymph nodes along the muscles of the root of the tongue
- Nuchal lymph nodes posterior to the sternocleidomastoid muscle

Landmark structure in ultrasound
- Jugular vein
- Carotid artery
- Subclavian artery and vein

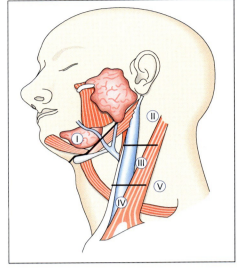

▲ **Fig. 6.1** Topography of the lymph nodes in the head and neck.

Regions of the axillary lymph nodes (Fig. 6.2)
- I   Lymph nodes of the lower axillary region
- II Lymph nodes of the central axillary region
- III Lymph nodes of the upper axillary region (including the infraclavicular lymph nodes)

Relations
- Lymph nodes along the axillary vessels
- Lymph nodes anterior, along, and posterior to the pectoralis major muscle

Landmark structure in ultrasound
- Axillary vessels
- Pectoralis major muscle

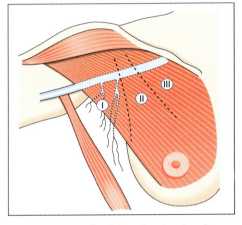

▲ **Fig. 6.2** Topography of the axillary lymph nodes.

Nonperipheral lymph nodes. The abdominal (nonperipheral) lymph nodes comprise the following regions (**Fig. 6.3**):
- Intraperitoneal (splanchnic) lymph nodes (hepatic hilum, splenic hilum, mesentery)
- Retroperitoneal (parietal) lymph nodes (para-aortic, iliac)

Regions of the intraperitoneal lymph nodes
- I   Lymph nodes at the hepatic hilum
- II Lymph nodes at the splenic hilum
- III Mesenteric lymph nodes

Regions of the retroperitoneal lymph nodes
- I Para-aortic/paracaval lymph nodes
- II Iliac lymph nodes

Usually, only enlarged lymph nodes will be visualized for certain, but normal lymph nodes can be detected down to a size of just 2–3 mm (**Fig. 6.4**). Lymph nodes of the head and neck measuring more than 10 mm across are considered as being pathologically enlarged. Quite often a central hyperechoic ovoid hilum can be differentiated from a peripheral hypoechoic concentric cortex (**Fig. 6.5**).

The sonographic parameters for lymph node assessment are listed in **Table 6.2**.

Relations
- Intraperitoneal along the blood vessels leading to liver and spleen
- Along the mesenteric blood vessels
- Along the retroperitoneal iliac blood vessels

Landmark structures for ultrasound
- Arteries and veins

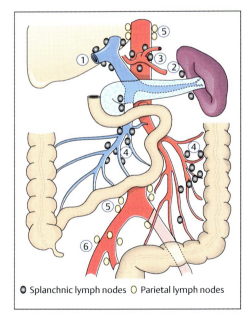

▲ **Fig. 6.3** Topography of the abdominal lymph nodes.
1 = hepatic portal
2 = hilum of spleen
3 = celiac group
4 = upper and lower mesenteric group
5 = para-aortic group
6 = iliac group

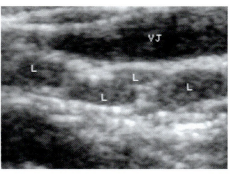

▲ **Fig. 6.4** Demonstration of an 8-mm-long enlarged lymph node (L) of homogeneous echogenicity in an otherwise asymptomatic patient. The lymphadenopathy was considered as being reactive. VJ = jugular vein.

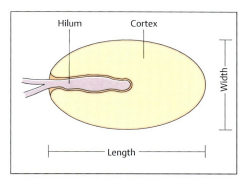

▲ **Fig. 6.5** Schematic illustration of a lymph node.

Table 6.2 Sonographic parameters for lymph node assessment

Location
Region involved
Pattern of involvement

Morphology
Size
Shape
Delineation from adjacent tissue

Structural parameters
Hilar sign
Echogenicity
Homogeneity

Vascularization
Concentration of blood vessels
Pattern of vascularization
Flow parameters

Normal lymph node morphology
- Size <1 cm
- Discernible hilum
- Cortex and hilum distinctly different
- Ellipsoid shape (length : width ≥ 2)

Location. The location alone of a lymph node may point the way to the etiology (supraclavicular sentinel, or Virchow's, node in gastric cancer, painful inguinal lymphadenopathy in erysipelas (alarm-bell sign), unilateral axillary lymphadenopathy in breast cancer). (■ 6.1 a–d).

■ 6.1 Location and Morphology of Abnormal Lymph Nodes

▶ **Location**

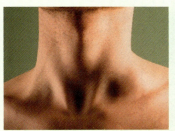 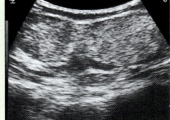

a and b A 29-year-old patient with lymph node in left supraclavicular fossa ("Virchow's sentinel node"). Ultrasound demonstrates two large hyperechoic lymph node metastases caked together (gastroscopy confirmed the suspected diagnosis of gastric cancer). This localization signals malignancy.

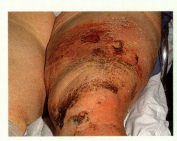 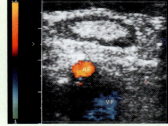

c and d A 51-year-old patient with erysipelas. Enlarged lymph node in the left groin with wide hyperechoic hilum and thin hypoechoic parenchymal border; reactive lymphadenopathy.

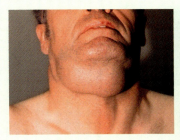 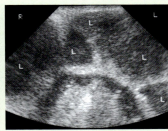

e and f Chronic lymphocytic leukemia.
e A 63-year-old patient with submandibular tumor formation.

f Ultrasound demonstrates large lymph nodes (L) invaded by tumor and caked together.

6.1 Location and Morphology of Abnormal Lymph Nodes

▶ Morphological criteria: Size, shape, delimitation

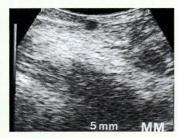
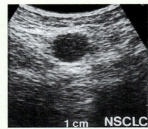
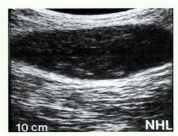

g–i Lymph nodes of different size invaded by tumor.
g Small lymph node metastasis in the left groin in malignant melanoma.

h Lymph node metastasis of the lower jugular region in lung cancer.

i Malignant lymphoma invading an inguinal lymph node.

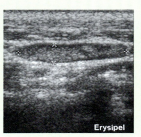
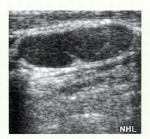
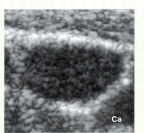

j–l Peripheral lymph nodes of different shape.
j Elongated hypoechoic reactive lymph node in erysipelas.

k Ovoid hypoechoic lymph node invaded by malignant lymphoma.

l Round hypoechoic lymph node invaded by carcinoma.

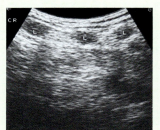
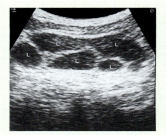
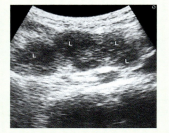

m Multiple round hypoechoic tumor-infiltrated well defined lymph nodes (L) in lung cancer.

n Multiple ill-defined lymph nodes (L) invaded by malignant lymphoma.

o Multiple lymphomas caked together in Hodgkin disease.

One important criterion for assessing possible malignancy is the pattern of involvement, i.e., whether this is localized or generally spread.

The relation with the blood vessels is of particular importance in ENT since it could spell the difference between surgery and inoperability. If ultrasound demonstrates contact between the tumor and the vascular wall over a distance of more than 3.5 cm or more than half the circumference, invasion of the vessel no longer amenable to resection is indicated.[3]

Morphology. Apart from the size (◻ 6.1e–j), morphological assessment has to consider the shape of the lymph nodes as well (◻ 6.1k–n). The parameter commonly used is the ratio of length (*L*) to width (*W*); a *L/W* ratio > 2 is more indicative of reactive changes, while a *L/W* ratio < 2 suggests malignancy (**Fig. 6.5**). The information gained by palpation can be supplemented by ultrasound because of its ability to differentiate between a well-defined lymph node and festoonlike lymphadenopathy or lymphomas caked together like potatoes in a bag (◻ 6.1 o–p).

Structural parameters. Regarding the structural parameters, the importance of any hilar sign (present or missing) is generally accepted, and it supposedly is indicative of malignant lymphadenopathy (◻ 6.2a and b).

When assessing the echogenicity of any lymph node, this should always be based on an "in vivo" reference, usually the adjacent tissue (◻ 6.2c–e). It has been stated that hypoechoic nodes would be typical for invasion by malignant lymphoma, while hyperechoic parenchyma seems to be more common in cancer metastasis and lymph nodes with chronic inflammation or regression scars.[1]

The normal parenchyma is homogeneous but may be clustered with anechoic (◻ 6.2g and h), hypoechoic (◻ 6.2f and i) as well as hyperechoic (◻ 6.2m, n) masses. Anechoic lesions are seen in granulomatous or suppurating inflammation corresponding with necrosis, but also in cancer metastases where the lesions would correspond with colliquation. Hypoechoic lesions may be indicative of beginning malignant lymph node invasion. Hyperechoic regions in lymph nodes are seen in low-grade malignant lymphoma and could correspond with regressive changes. Calcification may represent lymph node scarring. However, sometimes lymph node metastases tend to calcify as well (e.g., medullary thyroid carcinoma) (◻ 6.2j–l).

Vascularization. Color-flow Doppler scanning can demonstrate lymph node vascularization only indirectly by the presence or absence of flow phenomena.

The afferent and efferent hilar vessels in a normal-sized lymph node can be visualized by color-flow Doppler imaging. Depending on the state of the lymph node, the cortical region will display a spokelike or increased parenchymal vascularization with a markedly hilar aspect

6.2 Structural Parameters of Abnormal Lymph Nodes

▶ Hilar sign, echogenicity, homogeneity

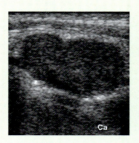 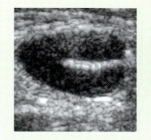 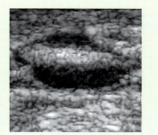

a and b Peripheral lymph nodes with different levels of the hilar sign.
a Lymph node with malignant invasion and no or just a faint hilar sign.

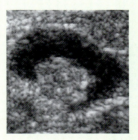 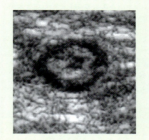 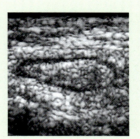

b Enlarged reactive lymph node with mild to marked hilar sign.

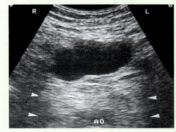 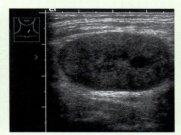 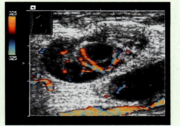

c–e Enlarged lymph nodes displaying different levels of echogenicity.
c Hypoechoic to "anechoic" mesenteric lymph node invaded by malignant lymphoma.

d Hypoechoic cervical lymph node metastasis in ovarian cancer.

e Structural inhomogenicity of a lymphoma infiltration in a groin lymph node with hyper- and hypoechoic parts at chronic lymphocytic leukemia (regressive changes).

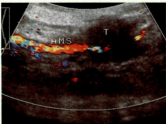 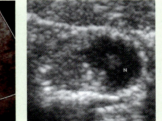 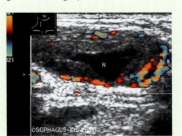

f Marked structural nonhomogeneities in a tuberculous axillary lymph node (LK) with hyperechoic and hypoechoic elements (foci of liquefaction found at surgery).

g Colliquation of an enlarged cervical lymph node (N) in bacterial lymphadenitis.

h Lymph node (N) with liquefied center invaded by cancer of the esophagus.

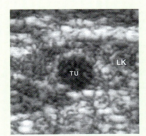 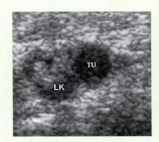 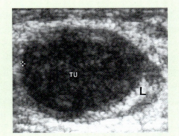

i Enlarged lymph node (LK) with focal hypoechoic lesions. In all three cases beginning lymph node metastasis in malignant melanoma. The hypoechoic regions correspond with the malignant tissue (TU).

6.2 Structural Parameters of Abnormal Lymph Nodes

▶ **Peripheral lymph nodes with calcification**

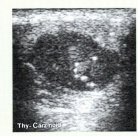
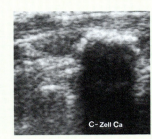
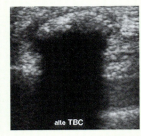

j–l Different forms of lymph node calcification.
j Cervical lymph node metastasis with mild calcification in carcinoid of thymus.

k Large plaquelike calcification in medullary thyroid carcinoma.

l Calcified cervical lymph node as end stage of tuberculous lymphadenitis.

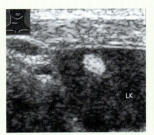
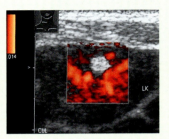

m CLL. Focal hyperechoic masses in an enlarged lymph node (LK) invaded by lymphoma. The pathomorphological substrate of the hyperechoic lesion remains unclear.

n Color-flow Doppler scanning shows a hypervascularisation of the lymph node.

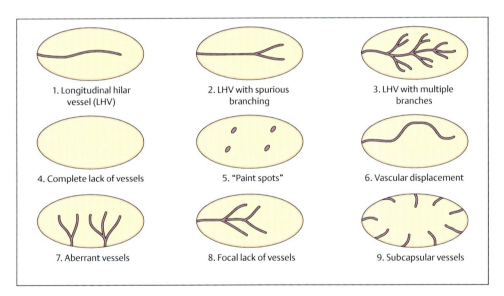

◀ **Fig. 6.6** Schematic illustration of various vascular patterns in peripheral lymph nodes on color-flow Doppler scanning (from reference 5).

(◨ 6.3a–f). Semiquantitative assessment of the concentration of blood vessels differentiates between increased vascularization (◨ 6.3g and h), and a focal decrease or lack of flow phenomena in the lymph node. "Increased vascularization" is said to be indicative of reactive lymphadenopathy in acute inflammation (◨ 6.3i and j), but it is also seen in malignant lymphoma. A focal lack of flow phenomena in lymph nodes has frequently been observed in metastasis.[4] In addition, this lack of flow signals is also quite common post therapy (◨ 6.3k and l).

Apart from the intranodal vascular bed visualized on ultrasound in peripheral lymph nodes, vascular displacement, aberrant vessels, focal lack of vessels, subcapsular vessels, and so called "paint spots" all point more toward malignant lymphadenopathy (**Fig. 6.6,** ◨ **6.3m and n**).[5] Enlarged reactive lymph nodes tend to be characterized by more horizontal hilar or longitudinal parenchymal vessels as well as treelike branching.

Flow parameters, such as the resistance indices measured in the lymph node arteries (resistance index, RI; pulsatility index, PI), seem to offer some benefit in the differential diagnosis of enlarged lymph nodes. A large resistance index (RI > 85) is considered indicative of a lymph node invaded by metastasis.

Abdominal lymph nodes. Compared with the peripheral lymph nodes, sonographic parameters of the vascularization in abdominal lymph nodes are difficult to obtain. Because of the location away from the probe, B-mode imaging yields less detailed sonographic resolution of the parenchymal structures; this implies that any differential diagnosis has to rely primarily on location and morphology, while structural parameters are relegated to a minor role. The

6.3 Vascularization in Abnormal Lymph Nodes

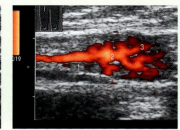
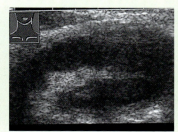
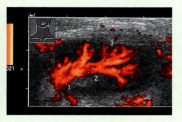

a and b Reactive lymph node enlargement.
a Small ovoid hypoechoic lymph node, diameter approximately 15 mm.

b On color-flow Doppler scanning hilar flow signal (1) and regular intraparenchymal vascular branches (2, 3).

c and d Reactive lymph node enlargement (resolved during follow-up).
c Enlarged lymph node in the upper jugular region, hilar sign present.

d Color-flow Doppler scanning demonstrates increased vascularization.
1 = hilar vessel, 2 = longitudinal vessel, 3 = intraparenchymal vascular branches.

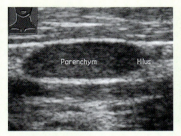
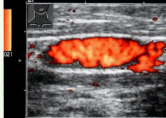
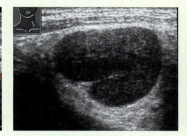
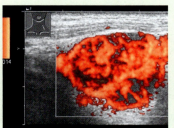

e and f Infectious mononucleosis confirmed by serology. Enlarged lymph node.

f Color-flow Doppler scanning demonstrates hypervascularization in reactive lymph node enlargement.

g and h Cancer of the prostate.
g Lymph node metastasis.

h Hypervascularization on color-flow Doppler scanning.

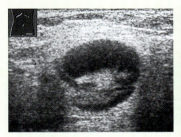
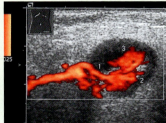
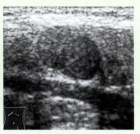
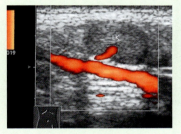

i and j Reactive lymph node enlargement in autoimmune vasculitis.
i Lymph node enlargement.

j On color-flow Doppler scanning marked vascularization with demonstration of hilar (1), longitudinal (2), and peripheral vessels (3).

k and l Hodgkin disease.
k Persistent lymph node enlargement after chemotherapy.

l On color-flow Doppler scanning no flow signals within the lymph node parenchyma. The nodular enlargement was regarded as being reactive.

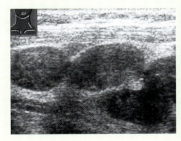
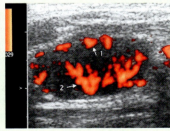

m and n Gastric cancer.
m Lymph nodes invaded by tumor.

n On color-flow Doppler scanning subcapsular (1) and aberrant (2) vessels.

criteria above for the diagnosis of possible malignancy in peripheral lymph nodes have been confirmed far better than for abdominal lymph nodes, since their sonographic pattern of involvement and the ultrasound visualization differ substantially from those of the peripheral lymph nodes. The one important factor in abdominal lymph nodes is their size. In most cases it becomes impossible to demonstrate the hilum, and thus in many patients selective visualization of the cortex is also not feasible.

Ultrasound distinguishes four basic patterns in the invasion of abdominal lymph nodes (**Fig. 6.7**). The diffuse speckled micronodular invasion (primarily of the mesenteric lymph nodes) is quite different from the focal enlargement of lymph nodes (micronodular and macronodular). The "bulky" formation is characterized by its large mass of tumor, which may represent confluent lymphomas, or excessive growth of individual lymph nodes (**Fig. 6.8**).

Ultrasound studies of abdominal lymph nodes labor under the following disadvantages:
▶ Only enlarged lymph nodes will be detected.
▶ Specificity is rather low in lumbar and iliac lymph nodes.
▶ Intestinal gas can limit the usefulness of the study.
▶ Misdiagnosis is possible in solitary lymphomas.
▶ It requires substantial experience of the operator in terms of technique and assessment.

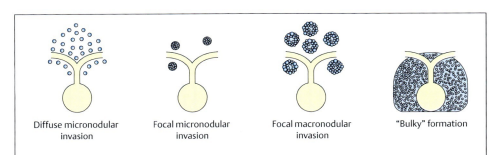

◀ *Fig. 6.7* Schematic illustration of the different patterns of invasion in abdominal lymph nodes around the celiac axis.

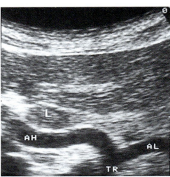 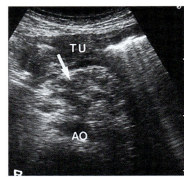
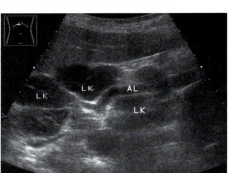 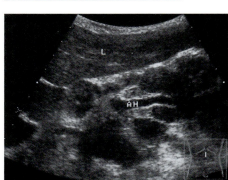

◀ *Fig. 6.8* Different patterns of invasion in abdominal lymph nodes (L) around the celiac axis.
a Individual enlarged lymph nodes in hepatitis. AH = hepatic artery; AL = splenic artery; TR = celiac axis.

◀◀ **b** Plaquelike micronodular lymph node metastasis in gastric cancer (TU). AO = aorta.

◀◀ **c** Low-grade non-Hodgkin lymphoma, celiac lymph nodes. Scan shows hypoechoic lymph node tumors (LK) displacing the splenic artery (AL) and hepatic artery.

◀ **d** High-grade non-Hodgkin lymphoma. Multiple lymph node metastases in the upper abdomen. AH = hepatic artery; L = liver.

Staging in Abdominal Lymph Node Involvement

Solid gastrointestinal tumors. Ultrasound cannot differentiate reliably between lymph nodes with metastatic invasion and those with benign lymphadenopathy. Frequently the lymph nodes are located within the drainage region of the tumor. Lymph node involvement has great prognostic significance in tumor staging (TNM system). When removing the tumor and the regional lymph nodes, the number of metastatic lymph nodes and their distance from the primary tumor are of additional prognostic importance **(Fig. 6.9)**. In most cases, exact staging is possible only after pathological work-up since the mesenteric and parietal lymph nodes are superimposed on each other and thus defy precise demonstration. Endosonography is the imaging modality of choice when staging gastrointestinal tumors (except in the large and small intestines). In solid tumors the primary pattern of lymph node invasion is diffuse and micronodular as well as focal lymphadenopathy (micro and macro). "Bulky" formations are infrequent findings.

Malignant lymphoma. In the staging of malignant lymphoma, possible involvement of the abdominal lymph nodes carries with it far-reaching therapeutic consequences. If ultrasound cannot resolve the issue, additional CT studies are warranted. In patients with Hodgkin disease, staging laparotomy becomes necessary in only a few cases and is performed only if it results in consequences for the treatment regimen. The sonographic image of abdominal lymph node involvement in malignant lymphoma covers a broad spectrum. Focal lymphadenopathy is most prevalent, with the lymphomas being well defined or confluent. Extremely "bulky" formations with concomitant displacement phenomena are not especially rare. If there is concurrent lymphoma, involvement of parenchymal organs of the GI tract with an invasion pattern characteristic of lymphoma ultrasound will often be the first measure to raise the suspected diagnosis of malignant lymphoma.
In localized, primarily gastrointestinal lymphomas, any additional splanchnic (regional) lymph node involvement implies stage II$_{E1}$, while parietal (nonregional) involvement would indicate stage II$_{E2}$ according to Musshoff. Sometimes this situation is difficult to differentiate from primary lymph node involvement with organ involvement by direct extension.

Low-grade and high-grade non-Hodgkin lymphoma (NHL). While the most common manifestation of low-grade NHL is systemic lymphadenopathy (the clinical symptoms frequently being rather mild), high-grade NHLs often manifest themselves by their enlarged lymph nodes in localized anatomical regions, but also by "bulky" formation. The diagnosis has to be confirmed by histology (also needed for subtyping of the lymphoma). Ultrasound-guided fine-needle aspiration biopsy will be able to distinguish benign lymphadenopathy from cancer metastasis or malignant lymphoma; however, typing of malignant lymphoma usually requires substantially more material, which often can only be obtained by laparotomy (unless there are peripheral lymph nodes easily accessible for excision).

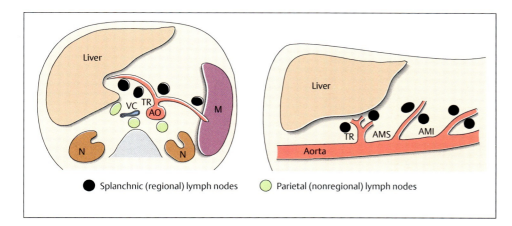

Fig. 6.9 Schematic illustration of the splanchnic and parietal lymph nodes. TR = celiac axis; VC = vena cava; N = kidney; M = stomach; AO = aorta; AMS = superior mesenteric artery; AMI = inferior mesenteric artery.

Peripheral Lymph Nodes

Head/Neck

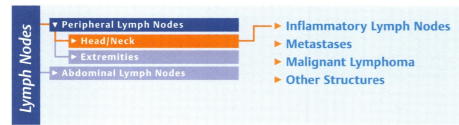

▶ Inflammatory Lymph Nodes

About 300 of the about 1000 lymph nodes in the human body are located in the cervical region. Depending on the age during childhood/adolescence, more than 80% of all enlarged lymph nodes are reactive in nature. Posterocervical nuchal lymph nodes tend to be benign, while the lymph nodes of the supraclavicular fossa often are malignant.

Acute inflammatory lymphadenopathy (▣ 6.3c and d) has to be differentiated from the chronic inflammatory (regressive) lymph node enlargement (▣ 6.4). Usually, acutely inflamed lymph nodes are small (< 1.5 cm), the hilar sign is present, and the ratio of length to width (L/W) is greater than 2; they are not caked together and mostly display a homogeneous parenchyma (note: liquefying suppurating lymph node). Acute lymphadenitis is characterized by homogeneous hyperperfusion (▣ 6.3e and f), but low-level perfusion, or even lack of it, does not rule out reactive lymph node enlargement (**Fig. 6.10**). It has been suggested that on color-flow Doppler scanning of the vascular supply of the lymph nodes, horizontal hilar vessels, longitudinal branches, and homogeneous vascular branching are indicative of reactive lymphadenopathy (▣ 6.3i and j).

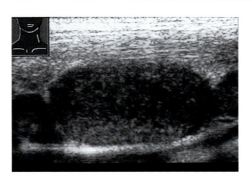

▲ *Fig. 6.10* A 13-year-old girl with fever and cervical lymphadenopathy.
a Enlarged homogeneous hypoechoic lymph node.

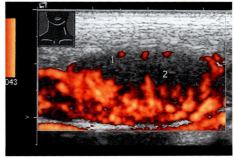

▲ *b* Subcapsular vessels (1) and a focal lack of blood vessels (2) on color-flow Doppler imaging. The initial findings raised a high suspicion of malignancy, while the follow-up indicated reactive lymphadenopathy.

In regressive lymph nodes, parenchymal calcification is possible (▣ 6.2j–l). On color-flow Doppler imaging, chronic inflammatory lymph nodes are characterized by a lack of flow.

▶ Metastases

In metastasis, size is not a typical parameter and usually the hilar sign is missing (▣ 6.3g and h). This type of lymph node tends to be round and hyperechoic (▣ 6.1a and b). Sometimes invasive growth can be demonstrated, necrosis is possible, and calcification of the parenchyma has also been observed (▣ 6.2j–l). The concentration of blood vessels varies on color-flow Doppler scanning. The vascular supply of the lymph nodes has been said to indicate malignancy if color-flow Doppler imaging visualizes vascular displacement, aberrant vessels, and regions lacking any vascularization, and capsular vessels (▣ 6.3m and n). Metastases exhibiting rapid growth have been shown to display a pathological vascularization with corkscrew-like vessels (**Fig. 6.11**). It is important to determine before surgery whether the metastatic cervical lymph nodes can be delineated from the large blood vessels of the neck or whether there is vascular

6.4 Lymph Nodes in Hodgkin's Disease

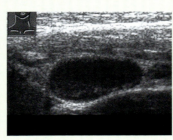
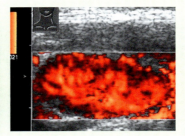

a and *b* **A 32-year-old patient with Hodgkin disease four years previously, presenting with an acutely enlarged lymph node.**
a Homogeneous hypoechoic lymph node.

b Hypervascularization on color-flow Doppler scanning. Follow-up indicated reactive lymphadenopathy.

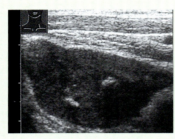

c and *d* **A 33-year-old patient with Hodgkin disease.**
c Persistently enlarged lymph node.

d Lack of any flow signals on color-flow Doppler scanning. Follow-up indicated reactive lymphadenopathy.

▶ **Follow-up studies post treatment**

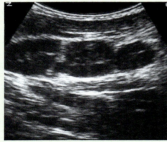
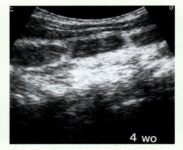
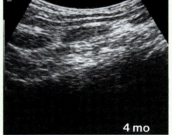

e–g A 22-year-old patient with Hodgkin disease and enlarged cervical lymph nodes that resolved under treatment. Scarred enlarged lymph nodes may be demonstrated for years.

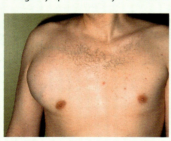
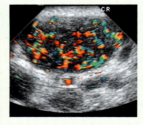

h–j **Chronic lymphocytic leukemia.**
h A 25-year-old patient with a large tumor in the right axilla.

i and *j* Intensified vascularization on color-flow Doppler scanning before therapy; after chemotherapy no more flow signals are detected (further resolution during follow-up).

invasion. Contact between tumor and vessel wall over a distance of more than 3.5 cm, or over more than half the circumference, suggests vascular invasion (**Fig. 6.12**).

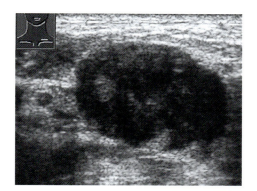
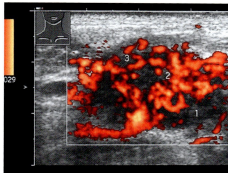

Fig. 6.11 A 72-year-old patient with malignant lymphoma and cervical lymph node metastasis.
a Hypoechoic lymph node.

b Corkscrew-like neovascularization. 1 = focal lack of vessels; 2 = aberrant vessels; 3 = subcapsular vessels.

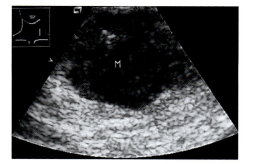
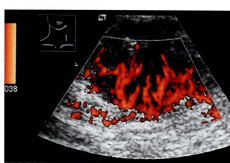

c Hypoechoic lymph node. M = metastasis.

d Marked neovascularization in metastases with rapid clinical growth.

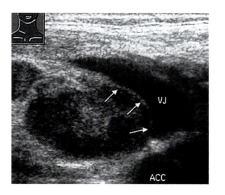
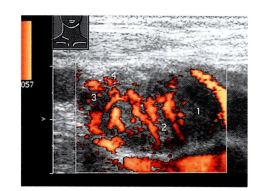

Fig. 6.12 Lymph node invaded by an ENT tumor.
a The lymph node covers the vessel wall over more than one-quarter of the circumference. ACC = common carotid artery; VJ = jugular vein.

b Color-flow Doppler imaging demonstrates a lack of blood vessels (1), aberrant vessels (2), "paint spots (3)" and subcapsular vessels (4).

▶ Malignant Lymphoma

In many cases the lymph nodes will be visualized as being large, hypoechoic, and in multiples. The normal ratio of length to width is < 2. Their texture is mostly homogeneous and they are clustered like grapes or in festoonlike fashion. Color-flow Doppler scanning will show them to be characterized by a homogeneous increase in the vascular images (**6.4a and b**). Not only will they decrease in size during treatment but the flow phenomena observed on color-flow Doppler scanning will also diminish (**6.1h–m**, **6.4c–j**). Sometimes the end stage will be an echogenic lymph node, varying in size, with hyperechoic capsule and no discernible flow signals.

▶ Other Structures

- **Head/neck.** Tumor of the parotid gland, lymphangiomatosis, abscess, hemorrhage, carotid artery aneurysm, branchial cyst (**Figs. 6.13 and 6.14**), parathyroid adenoma
- **Supraclavicular.** Pancoast tumor, bone tumor, abscess.

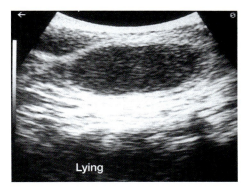
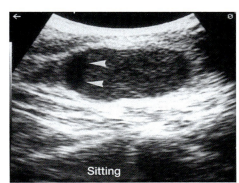

Fig. 6.13a and b Formation in the right lateral neck with sedimentation phenomena, compatible with a branchial cyst.

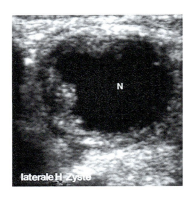
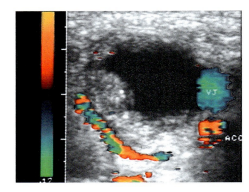

◀ **Fig. 6.14 a and b** Formation in the right lateral neck with liquefied center (N). The diagnosis of a branchial cyst was made only after surgery. ACC = common carotid artery; VJ = jugular vein.

Extremities (Axilla, Groin)

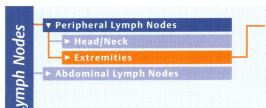

Enlargement of locoregional lymph nodes is observed particularly in injuries of the extremities. If axillary lymph nodes are enlarged, the possibility of involvement of the breast has to be kept in mind.

▶ Inflammatory Lymph Nodes

Sometimes reactive lymph nodes can become rather large (**Figs. 6.15 and 6.16**); in most cases the hilar sign is present and marked (**Fig. 6.17**). In a few patients, the cortex of the lymph nodes may be nothing more than a delicate hypoechoic border. Vascularization may be rarefied or marked. Complete healing will leave constant regressive hyperechoic lymph nodes. Reactive regressive lymph nodes in the groin are almost mandatory.

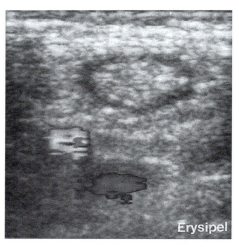
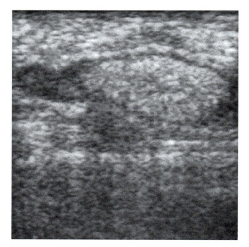
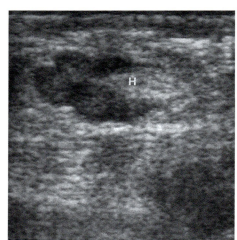

▲ **Fig. 6.15 a–c** Reactive inguinal lymph nodes in erysipelas displaying different levels of hypoechoic parenchyma. H = hilum.

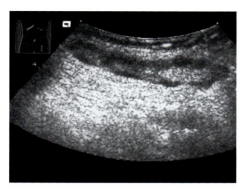
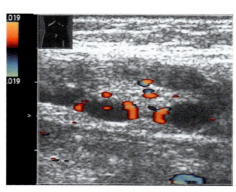
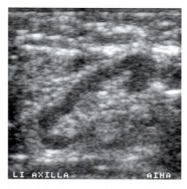

▲ **Fig. 6.16 a and b** A 42-year-old patient with known Hodgkin disease, now presenting with lymphadenopathy in the left groin; elongated lymph node with hilar sign and markedly inhomogeneous texture of the parenchyma. Histology confirmed reactive lymphadenopathy.

▲ **Fig. 6.17** A 33-year-old patient with autoimmune hemolytic anemia and sarcoidosis. Large lymph node with hilar sign present in the left axilla. Follow-up indicated reactive lymphadenopathy.

▶ Metastases

Metastases are much more common in the axilla than in the groin (**Fig. 6.18–6.22**). In breast cancer they are mostly homogenous and hypoechoic (**Fig. 6.18**) and their sizes differ widely. Very small lymph node metastases are frequently found in malignant melanoma (**Fig. 6.22**); in vascular invasion, compression syndrome is a not uncommon finding.

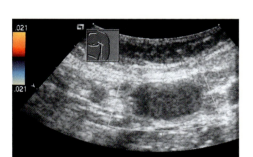
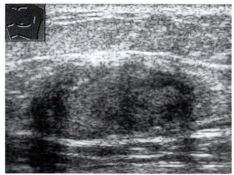
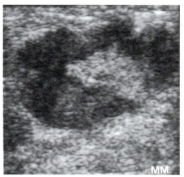

▲ **Fig. 6.18** Homogeneous hypoechoic lymph node in breast cancer. After two cycles of adriamycin plus cyclophosphamide, no more flow signal was observed; this was interpreted as positive response to treatment. Histological work-up of the lymph node did not yield any remaining vital tumor tissue.

▲ **Fig. 6.19** Lymph node invaded by neuroendocrine cancer.

▲ **Fig. 6.20** Lymph node in the left axilla invaded by malignant melanoma; the hilar sign is still present.

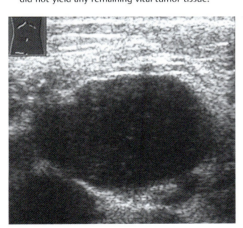
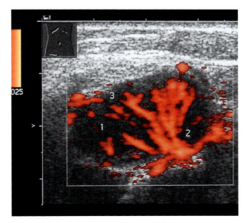
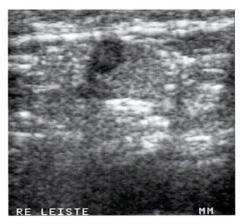

▲ **Fig. 6.21 a** Large hypoechoic lymph node invaded by cancer of the rectum.

▲ **b** Abnormal flow pattern on color-flow Doppler scanning. 1 = focal lack of vessels; 2 = aberrant vessels; 3 = subcapsular vessels.

▲ **Fig. 6.22** Hyperechoic metastasis of malignant melanoma in an inguinal lymph node. re Leiste = right grein.

▶ Malignant Lymphoma

The picture is similar to that of the head/neck region (**Fig. 6.23**). Here, too, impaired venous or lymphatic drainage due to lymphomas can often be expected (**Fig. 6.24**). Invasive growth into the soft tissue has been observed, particularly in T-cell lymphoma of the groin. In these cases, the lymphoma may be visualized as being hyperechoic and ill defined to the adjacent soft tissues.

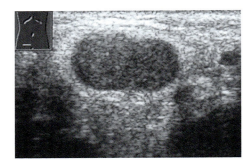
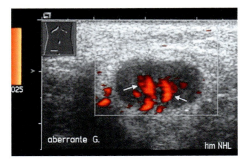

◀ **Fig. 6.23** Lymph node with pathological vascular pattern in malignant lymphoma.

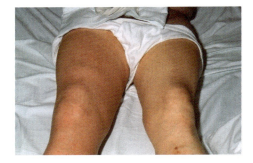
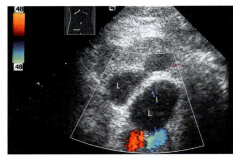

◀ **Fig. 6.24** A 55-year-old patient with swollen right leg. Ultrasound showed multiple abnormally large lymph nodes (L) without any sign of deep venous thrombosis. Needle biopsy confirmed the diagnosis of Hodgkin disease. The swollen leg was explained by impaired lymphatic drainage.

▶ Other Structures

- ▶ **Axilla**. Scar, postoperative fibrosis, seroma, thrombosis of the axillary vein, cellulitis, panniculitis, abscess, myositis.
- ▶ **Groin**. Undescended testis, inguinal hernia, varicosity, lymphocele, hematoma, abscess, false aneurysm (**Fig. 6.25**).

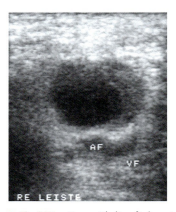
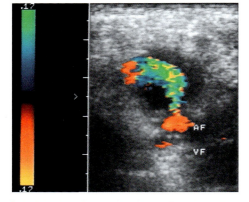

▲ **Fig. 6.25 a** Mass with liquefied center in the right groin. AF = femoral artery; VF = femoral vein.

▲ **b** Color-flow Doppler imaging confirmed the diagnosis of a false aneurysm.

Abdominal Lymph Nodes

Hepatic Portal

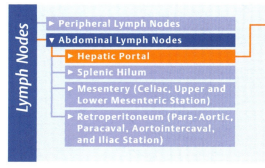

▶ Inflammatory Lymph Nodes

Enlarged inflammatory lymph nodes at the hepatic portal are quite common and can easily be demonstrated on ultrasound. Most of these lymph nodes are small (< 2 cm), ovoid or elongated, and likely echogenic. They are almost always found in acute hepatitis (A, B, C), concomitant hepatitis (EBV, chickenpox, HIV, etc.), autoimmune hepatitis, primary biliary cirrhosis, primary sclerosing cholangitis, and bacterial cholangitis (◻ 6.5).

▶ Metastases

There are no definite ultrasound criteria for ruling out possible malignancy. Enlarged lymph nodes in primary tumors of the liver will be diagnosed as definite metastasis or reactive lymphadenitis only after surgery; however, it can be stated that the probability of malignant invasion will increase with increasing size of the lymph node (**Fig. 6.26**).

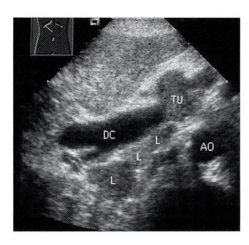
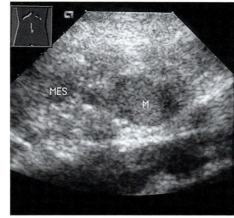

◀ **Fig. 6.26 a and b** Enlarged lymph node (L) in pancreatic cancer (TU). Only histology can confirm possible lymph node metastasis. AO = aorta; DC = common hepatic duct; M = mesenteric lymph node; MES = mesentery.

◻ 6.5 Enlarged Reactive Lymph Nodes at the Hepatic Portal

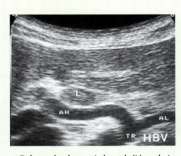
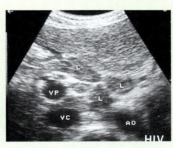
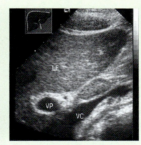
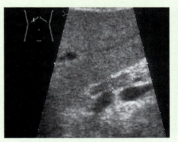

a Enlarged echogenic lymph (L) node in hepatitis. AH = hepatic artery; AL = splenic artery; TR = celiac axis.

b Enlarged lymph node (L) in an HIV-positive patient. AO = aorta; VC = vena cava; VP = portal vein.

c and d Mononucleosis.
c Echogenic lymph node at the hepatic portal. LE = liver; VC = vena cava; VP = portal vein.

d Enlarged lymph node (cursors) with subtle hilar signs.

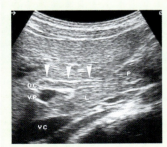
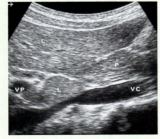

e and f Enlarged reactive lymph node (L) in primary sclerosing cholangitis. DC = common bile duct; P = pancreas; VC = vena cava; VP = portal vein.

Abdominal Lymph Nodes

▶ Malignant Lymphoma

Involvement of the hepatic portal is observed particularly in systemic low-grade lymphoma. Different patterns of invasion have been noted (**Fig. 6.7**). Hypoechoic perivascular transformation of the portal vein and its intrahepatic branches close to the hilum (so-called "periportal cuffing") has to be differentiated from actual lymphoma involving the hepatic portal. Periportal cuffing is more likely to be found in impaired lymphatic drainage (**Fig. 6.27**).

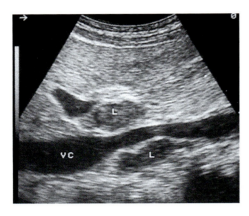
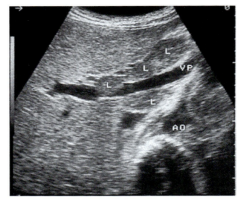

◀◀ *Fig. 6.27* Different invasion patterns in lymph nodes (L) of the hepatic portal in malignant melanoma. L = lymph node; VC = vena cava; VP = portal vein; AO = aorta.

a Individual lymph nodes in high-grade lymphoma.

◀ *b* Multiple lymph nodes in lymphocytic lymphoma (LC).

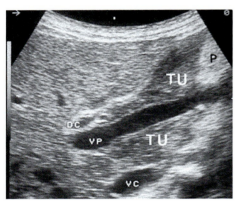
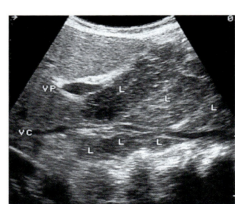

◀◀ *c* Extensive lymph nodes (TU) in lymphocytic lymphoma.

◀ *d* Large "bulky" tumor transformation in lymphocytic lymphoma. DC = common bile duct; VP = portal vein; VC = vena cava; P = pancreas.

▶ Other Structures

▶ Hematoma at the hepatic portal, abscess
▶ Cavernous transformation of the portal vein, thrombosis of the portal vein, varicosities in portal hypertension, aneurysm of the hepatic artery (**Fig. 6.28**).

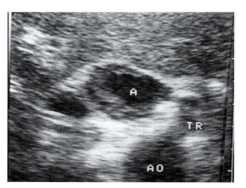
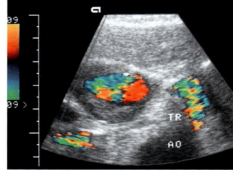

▲ *Fig. 6.28 a* Hypoechoic mass with anechoic center (A). TR = celiac axis; AO = aorta.

▲ *b* Color-flow Doppler scanning confirms the tentative diagnosis of hepatic artery aneurysm.

Splenic Hilum

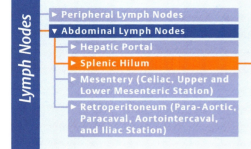

▶ Inflammatory Lymph Nodes

Enlargement of the lymph nodes of the splenic hilum is somewhat infrequent but is visualized quite well by insonation through the spleen. Reactive lymphadenitis of lymph nodes at the splenic hilum is almost never seen.

▶ Metastases

Metastases have been demonstrated in adenocarcinoma of the pancreatic tail, neuroendocrine tumors of the pancreas, gastric cancer, and less frequently in peritoneal metastasis. The principal misgivings about assessment of possible malignancy apply here as well. Possible invasion of the tumor into the spleen can be demonstrated on ultrasound (**Fig. 6.29**).

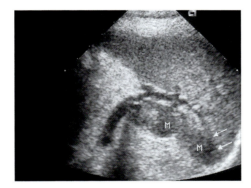

◀ **Fig. 6.29** Lymph node metastasis at the splenic hilum in ovarian cancer. M = stomach.

▶ Malignant Lymphoma

It is particularly the low-grade lymphomas that display involvement of the splenic hilum as part of systemic disease (**Fig. 6.30**).

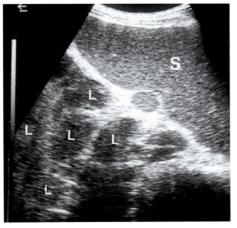 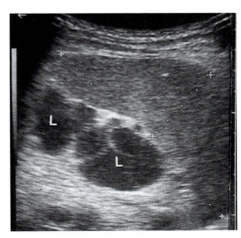

▲ **Fig. 6.30** Different invasion patterns visualized in lymph nodes (L) of the splenic hilum in malignant lymphoma. S = spleen.
a Individual lymph nodes in chronic lymphocytic leukemia (CLL).

▲ *b* Numerous confluent lymph nodes in CLL.

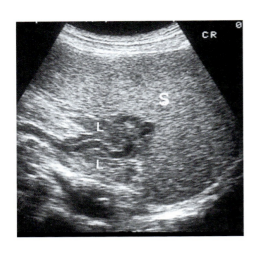
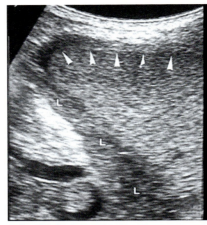

◂◂ **Fig. 6.27**
  c Extensive lymph node (L) invasion in mantle cell lymphoma.

◂ d Perisplenic invasion by follicular center lymphoma.

▶ **Other Structures**

- Accessory spleen (**Fig. 6.31**), abscess
- Pancreatic mass (tumor, cyst, necrosis) (**Fig. 6.32**)
- Adrenal mass (metastasis, pheochromocytoma, incidentaloma)
- Vascular process (splenic varicosity, thrombosis of the splenic vein, splenic artery aneurysm)

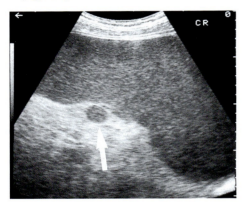
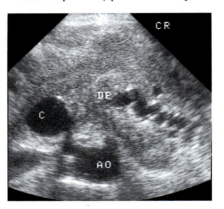
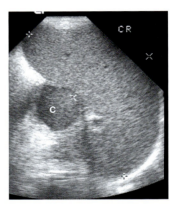

▲ **Fig. 6.31** Small accessory spleen (arrow) at the splenic hilum in CLL.

▲ **Fig. 6.32 a** Signs of chronic pancreatitis with enlarged pancreatic duct (DP) and anechoic pseudocyst (C) at the head of the pancreas. AO = aorta.

▲ **b** Echogenic pseudocyst (C) at the splenic hilum in the same patient.

Mesentery (Celiac, Upper and Lower Mesenteric Station)

Lymph Nodes
- ▶ Peripheral Lymph Nodes
- ▼ Abdominal Lymph Nodes
  - ▶ Hepatic Portal
  - ▶ Splenic Hilum
  - ▶ **Mesentery (Celiac, Upper and Lower Mesenteric Station)**
  - ▶ Retroperitoneum (Para-Aortic, Paracaval, Aortointercaval, and Iliac Station)

- ▶ Inflammatory Lymph Nodes
- ▶ Metastases
- ▶ Malignant Lymphoma
- ▶ Other Structures

Although sometimes the mesenteric lymph node stations are difficult to visualize (**Fig. 6.33** and **Fig. 6.34**), they play an important role in clinical practice.

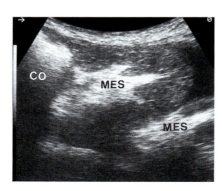

◂ **Fig. 6.33** Usually the mesentery (MES) of the individual hypoechoic loop of the small intestines will be visualized as being homogeneously hyperechoic. CO = colon.

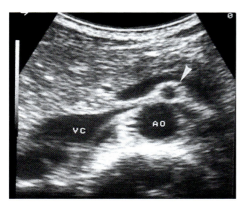 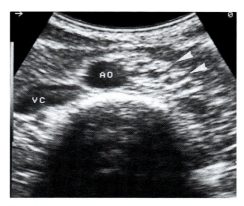 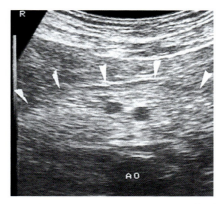

▲ **Fig. 6.34** Transverse section of the mesentery. AO = aorta; VC = vena cava.
a The mesentery, inferior to the splenic vein at the pancreas, displays a hyperechoic texture.

▲ *b* Once the mesenteric vessels have branched off the aorta, they rest within this hyperechoic mesentery.

▲ *c* Mesenteric lipomatosis is characterized by homogeneous echogenic thickening of the mesentery.

▶ Inflammatory Lymph Nodes

Most of these lymph nodes are situated in the mesenteric fat along the unpaired branches of the aorta (celiac axis, superior and inferior mesenteric artery). Since the majority of these lymph nodes are small, the mesentery displays a "dirty" pattern. In some cases the diameter of an enlarged lymph node may be several centimeters. One important differential diagnosis of acute appendicitis, particularly during childhood, is mesenteric lymphadenitis, which can be assessed as such once ultrasound has demonstrated or excluded other local inflammation (nonspecific gastroenteritis, Crohn disease, ulcerative colitis, yersiniosis, ileocolitis, appendicitis) (▣ **6.6a–e**).

▣ 6.6 Enlargement of the Mesenteric Lymph Nodes

▶ Size, shape, and structure are not criteria for benignancy or malignancy

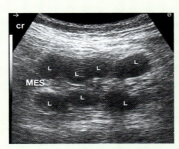 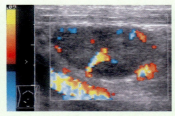 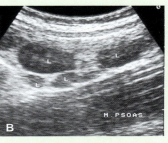

a and *b* Marked reactive lymphadenitis (L) along the mesenteric vessels in mesenteric lymphadenitis.
MES = mesentery
a Longitudinal view.

b Color duplex: central vessel and peripheral vascularity; no aberrant vessels as with a nodal metastasis.

c Enlarged individual lymph nodes (L).

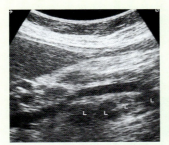 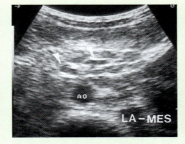 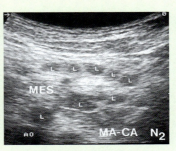

d In the epigastric longitudinal view, numerous lymph nodes (L) along the mesenteric vein; definite diagnosis: reactive lymphadenitis in tuberculosis.

e and *f* Differential diagnosis of "dirty" mesenteric invasion; assessment regarding possible malignancy based on the sonographic morphology alone is impossible. AO = aorta; MES = mesentery
e Enlarged lymph nodes in mesenteric lymphadenitis.

f Enlarged lymph nodes (L) in gastric cancer.

▶ Metastases

Enlarged mesenteric lymph nodes are a frequent finding in ultrasound studies of abdominal cancer (carcinoma of the stomach, pancreas, esophagus, colon, etc.). The definitive diagnosis of malignancy is a prerogative of the pathologist (postoperatively) (■ 6.6f).

▶ Malignant Lymphoma

Possible involvement of the mesenteric lymph nodes is seen in all the various lymphomas. The sonographic morphology is rather diverse and may lead to problems in the differential diagnosis (■ 6.7). In case of primary involvement of the abdominal lymph nodes, the diagnosis is confirmed by ultrasound-guided needle biopsy; however, sometimes the issue can only be resolved by laparotomy.

■ 6.7 Malignant Lymphomas in Mesenteric Lymph Nodes

▶ Nodular, confluent, extended

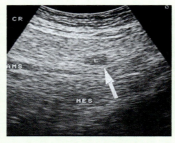
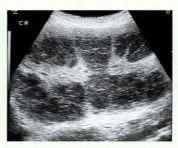
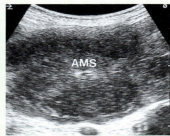

a–c Different nodular patterns of invasion in malignant lymphoma.
a Small solitary lymph node (L) in CLL. AMS = superior mesenteric artery; MES = mesentery.

b Numerous confluent lymph nodes in CLL.

c Extended tumor formation encasing the superior mesenteric artery (AMS) in mantle cell lymphoma

▶ Atypical patterns

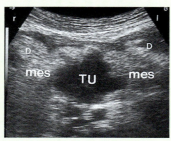
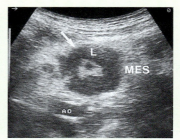
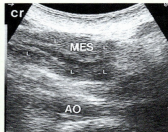

d–f Atypical pattern of mesenteric involvement in malignant lymphoma: extremely difficult diagnosis in case of sole mesenteric involvement.
d Cross-sectional view: hypoechoic mesenteric tumor formation in high grade lymphoma. D = intestine; mes = mesentery; TU = tumor.

e Cross sectional view with annular hypoechoic tumor formation around the mesenteric artery in follicular center lymphoma. AO = aorta; L = liver; MES = mesentery.

f Longitudinal epigastric view with extended, partly nodular, ill defined tumor formation in CLL. AO = aorta; L = liver; MES = mesentery.

▶ Small confluent nodes, bulky formation

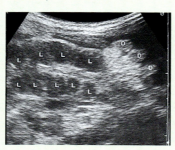
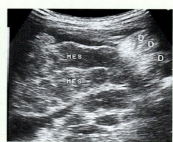
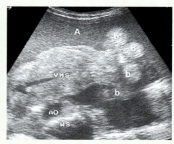

g–i Patterns of mesenteric invasion in malignant lymphoma and ascites.
g Micronodular confluent lymph nodes (L) in high grade T-cell lymphoma. D = intestine.

h Extended sheets of lymphomas in lymphoblastic lymphoma (LB-NHL). D = intestine; MES = mesentery.

i Homogeneous hyperechoic tumor formation invading all of the mesenteric root in Hodgkin disease. A = ascites; AO = aorta; b = bowels; VMS = superior mesenteric vein; WS = vertebral column.

Other Structures

The differential diagnosis of an isolated mesenteric mass covers a whole gamut of possibilities, including:
- Intestinal loop, mesenteric cyst (**Fig. 6.35**), necrosis in pancreatitis, abscess
- Mesenteric varicosities in portal hypertension, thrombosis of the mesenteric vessels, mesenteric artery aneurysms, hematoma
- Inflammatory pseudotumor (**Fig. 6.36**), lipoma, primary mesenchymal tumor

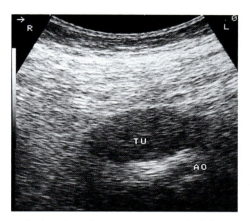

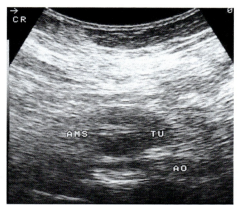

▲ **Fig. 6.35** Transverse epigastric view with anechoic mesenteric mass corresponding with a cyst (C). AO = aorta; L = liver; MA = stomach; MES = mesentery.

▲ **Fig. 6.36** Hypoechoic mesenteric mass (TU); histology confirmed an inflammatory pseudotumor. AO = aorta.
a Transverse epigastric view.

▲ **b** Longitudinal view. AMS = superior mesenteric artery.

Retroperitoneum (Para-Aortic, Paracaval, Aortointercaval, and Iliac Station)

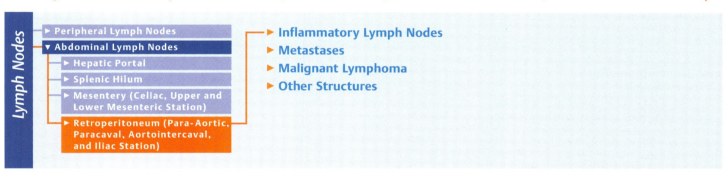

In ultrasound studies gas shadowing frequently makes it quite difficult to visualize the retroperitoneal lymph nodes.

Inflammatory Lymph Nodes

Para-aortic lymph nodes with reactive enlargement are rare. In the iliac region they may be demonstrated in the presence of local inflammation (appendicitis, diverticulitis, adnexitis) (**Figs. 6.37 and 6.38**).

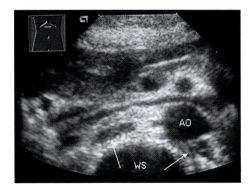

◀ **Fig. 6.37** Transverse epigastric view with reactive enlargement of the para-aortic lymph nodes in lupus erythematosus. AO = aorta; WS = spine.

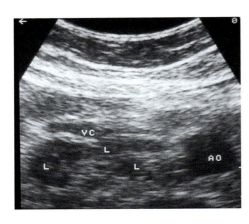 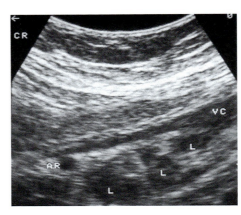

Fig. 6.38 Enlarged inflammatory lymph nodes (L) in tuberculosis. AO = aorta; AR = renal artery; VC = vena cava.
a Cross-sectional view.
b Longitudinal view.

▶ Metastases

Enlarged para-aortic lymph nodes are malignant unless proven otherwise. They are seen in, e.g., cancer of the kidney, testis, esophagus, prostate, colon, and rectum. Their sonographic pattern of invasion cannot be distinguished from malignant lymphoma. Despite the principal uncertainty in the assessment of possible malignancy if there is nonregional (parietal) lymphadenopathy in cancer of the stomach, pancreas, gallbladder, or liver, because of the location alone (para-aortic, aortointercaval, paracaval) it has to be regarded as metastasis with a frequently unfavorable prognosis (**6.8**).

▶ Malignant Lymphoma

Quite often as part of a systemic lymphoma the retroperitoneum will be invaded by lymphoma masses. The sonographic patterns of invasion are rather varied. As in all other lymph node stations, here too there is "bulky" disease, as well as micronodular and macronodular and diffuse involvement. Isolated retroperitoneal manifestation of lymphoma is rare but possible (**6.9**).

▶ Other Structures

Particularly in local retroperitoneal tumor formations, the differential diagnosis covers a wide spectrum of possibilities.
- **Para–aortic region**. Crura of diaphragm, horizontal part of the duodenum, horseshoe kidney, hematoma, abscess, aortic aneurysm, retroperitoneal fibrosis, necrosis in pancreatitis, lymphocele, primarily retroperitoneal tumors (**6.10a–d**).
- **Iliac region**. Ovary, undescended testis, lymphocele, hematoma, abscess (**6.10e–h**).

6.8 Retroperitoneal Lymph Node Metastasis

▶ Varying patterns of involvement of para-aortic lymph nodes

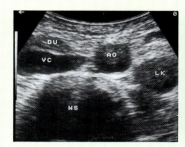 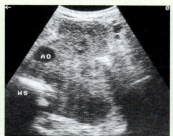 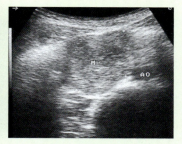

a–c Different patterns of invasion of para-aortic lymph nodes in cancer (cross-sectional view).
a Individual hypoechoic lymph nodes (LK) in cancer of the colon. AO = aorta; DU = intestine; WS = spine; VC = vena cava.

b Large para-aortic hyperechoic tumor formation encasing the aorta (AO) in esophageal cancer. WS = spine.

c Large para-aortic lymph node to the right of the aorta (AO) in testicular cancer. M = metastasis.

▶ Multiple, confluent lymph node metastases

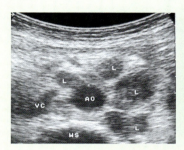 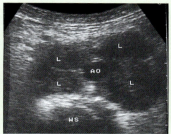 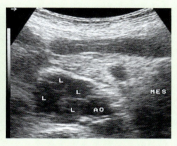

d Numerous para-aortic lymph nodes (L) in malignant melanoma. AO = aorta; VC = vena cava; WS = spine.

e Marked hypoechoic lymph node (L) metastasis in cancer of the bladder. Cross-sectional view. AO = aorta; WS = spine.

f Transverse epigastric view with isolated lymph node metastasis (L) in ovarian cancer. The mesentery (MES) is not involved. AO = aorta.

6.9 Para-aortic and Iliac Lymph Node Metastasis in Malignant Melanoma

▶ Varying patterns of involvement of para-aortic lymph nodes

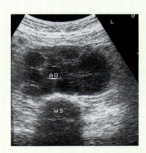 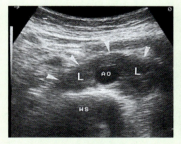 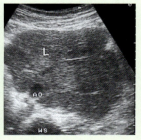

a–c Different patterns of invasion in para-aortic lymph nodes.
a Confluent lymphomas encasing the aorta in centroblastic lymphoma. AO = aorta; WS = spine.

b Extended tumor formation (arrowheads) in low-grade lymphoma (L). AO = aorta; WS = spine.

c "Bulky" tumor formation (L) in CLL. AO = aorta; WS = spine.

▶ Varying infiltration patterns of iliac nodes

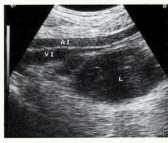 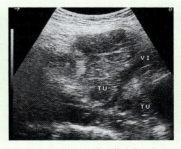 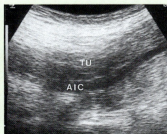

d–f Different patterns of invasion in iliac lymph nodes.
d Large solitary hypoechoic tumor formation (L) in Hodgkin disease. AI = iliac artery; VI = iliac vein.

e Large complexes of well-defined lymphoma masses (TU) in high-grade lymphoma. VI = iliac vein.

f Large, faint, ill-defined hypoechoic tumor formation (TU) in high-grade lymphoma. AIC = common iliac artery.

6.10 Differential Diagnosis in Enlarged Para-aortic and Parailiac Lymph Nodes

▶ Para-aortic masses

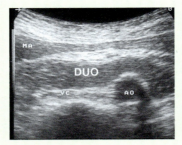
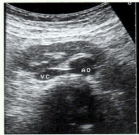

***a–d* Para-aortic.**
a Transverse epigastric view with duodenum (DUO). AO = aorta; MA = stomach; VC = vena cava.

b Transverse epigastric view with visualization of the parenchymal bridge in a horseshoe kidney. AO = aorta; VC = vena cava.

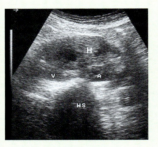
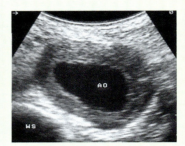

c Transverse view of the lower abdomen with retroperitoneal hematoma (H). A = iliac artery; V = iliac vein; WS = spine.

d Transverse view of the lower abdomen with partially thrombosed aortic aneurysm. AO = aorta; WS = spine.

▶ Parailiac masses

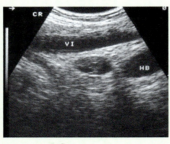
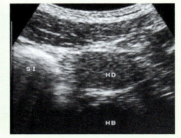

***e–h* Parailiac.**
e Parietal view on the right with the ovary. HB = urinary bladder; VI = iliac vein.

f Transverse view of the lower abdomen with the inguinal ligament. HB = urinary bladder; HD = testicle; SI = sigma.

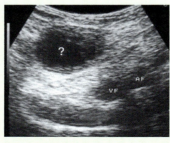
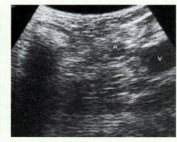

g Transverse view of the right groin with a varicosity (?). AF = femoral artery; VF = femoral vein.

h Transverse view of the right groin with an inguinal hernia. A = iliac artery; V = iliac vein.

References

1. Ahuja et al. The use of sonography in differentiating cervical lymphomatous lymph nodes from cervical metastatic lymph nodes. Clin Radiol 1996;51:186.
2. Fischer et al. Lymphknotenvergrößerung. Internist 1994;35:301.
3. Gritzmann et al. Invasion of the carotid artery and jugular vein by lymph node metastases: Detection with sonography. Am J Radiol 1990;154:411.
4. Tschammler et al. Dignitätsbeurteilung vergrößerter Lymphknoten durch qualitative und semiquantitative Auswertung der Lymphknotenperfusion mit der farbkodierten Duplexsonographie. Fortschritte Röntgenstr 1991;154:414.
5. Tschammler et al. Lymphadenopathie: Differentiation of benign from malignant disease - Color Doppler US assessment of intranodal angioarchitexture. Radiology 1998;208:117.

7 Gastrointestinal Tract

Gastrointestinal Tract 225

Stomach — 229

▼ Focal Wall Changes — 229
- Gastric Polyps
- Stromal Tumor
- Carcinoma
- Lymphoma
- Gastric Varices
- Ulceration
- Diverticula, Mucosal Folds
- Hypertrophic Pyloric Stenosis

▼ Extended Wall Changes — 232
- Carcinoma/Scirrhus
- Lymphoma
- Gastritis
- Congestion, Edema
- Peritoneal Carcinomatosis

▼ Dilated Lumen — 233
- Physiological Dilatation
- Inflammation
- Gastric Outlet Obstruction
- Functional Disorder

▼ Narrowed Lumen — 234
- Impression
- Compression
- Tumor
- Postoperative Status

Small/Large Intestine — 235

▼ Focal Wall Changes — 236
- Carcinoma
- Lymphoma
- Hematoma
- Polyp
- Intussusception
- Gallstone/Bezoar
- Diverticula
- Diverticulitis
- Appendix
- Appendicitis
- Hernia

▼ Extended Wall Changes — 241
- Enteritis
- Sprue
- Crohn Disease
- Ulcerative Colitis
- Amyloidosis
- Ischemia
- Pseudomembranous (Antibiotic-associated) Enterocolitis
- Hypertrophy
- Tumor
- Lymphoma

▼ Dilated Lumen — 245
- Physiological Dilatation
- Prepping for the Study
- Inflammation
- Ileus
- Coprostasis
- Tumor
- Foreign Body

▼ Narrowed Lumen — 247
- Tumor Stenosis
- "Starvation Gut"
- Ischemia
- Atrophy

7 Gastrointestinal Tract

M. Brandt

In humans the food is ingested, transported, and stored by the gastrointestinal (GI) tract, which may be subdivided into four major sections: esophagus, stomach, small intestine, and large intestine.

The esophagus propels food taken up in the mouth into the stomach, where it is mixed, ground down, digested, and stored. The ingesta are then passed into the small intestine, where they undergo selective absorption. The residual indigestible parts of our food become thickened in the large intestine and are stored there until evacuation.

In addition, the gastrointestinal tract plays an important role as defensive barrier, and its Peyer's patches and lymphocytes comprise the most extensive immune system in the human body.

Successful realization of these functions is based on a common wall structure of the gastrointestinal tube: the innermost mucous membrane secretes and absorbs; the submucous layer in the middle with its blood vessels, lymphatics and nerves and the majority of the enteric lymphatic organ lets the outer tela muscularis slide with respect to the mucous membrane. This muscular coat is characterized by longitudinal and circular muscle fibers arranged in different fashions in the various parts of the gastrointestinal tract; their peristaltic contraction mixes and propels the intestinal contents as well as controlling this transport by means of special sphincter organs.

Anatomy and Topography (Fig. 7.1)

Esophagus
- Wall thickness 3–4 mm
- Length 40 cm
- Transitory transport of the ingesta

Stomach
- Wall thickness 5–7 mm
- Length 20 cm
- Capacity: fasting 50 ml; postprandial up to 2000 ml

Duodenum
- Wall thickness 3–4 mm
- Length 30 cm
- Transitory transport of the chyme

Jejunum and Ileum
- Wall thickness 3–4 mm
- Total length 150 cm
- Transitory transport of the chyme

Colon
- Wall thickness 2–3 mm
- Length 120 cm
- Scybala/air

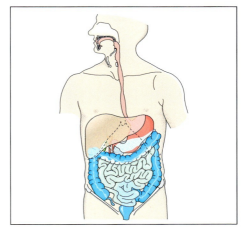

▲ **Fig 7.1** Topographical anatomy of the intestinal tract.

Esophagus. The esophagus is a muscular tube about 40 cm long connecting the pharynx to the stomach and is located in the posterior mediastinum. Its distal segment is anterior to and parallels the aorta. It penetrates the diaphragm through the so-called esophageal hiatus (hiatus oesophagei) terminating at the esophagocardiac transition zone.

Stomach. The stomach is one of the intraperitoneal organs and is situated in the left upper quadrant. This hook- or comma-shaped hollow organ runs from the cephalad left to the caudad right and has a length of approximately 20 cm. Under fasting conditions it contains about 50 ml of fluid, but will expand physiologically up to a maximum capacity of 2 liters.

The stomach is subdivided into cardia, fundus/fornix, body, and pyloric antrum. The cardiac opening of the stomach is situated anterior to the aorta at the level of the esophageal hiatus; its anterior aspect is covered by the inferior surface of the left hepatic lobe. The fundus/fornix of the stomach with its round dome fills the space in the left upper quadrant, the superior border of which is formed by the diaphragm, while the left fundic aspect is in contact with the spleen. The distal part of the stomach comprises the body and the pyloric antrum, which are defined on the anterior aspect by the left hepatic lobe. The muscular opening into the duodenum is the pyloric orifice, which is in direct contact with the head of the pancreas.

Small intestine. The small intestine is subdivided into the duodenum, which is about 30 cm long, and the jejunum plus ileum, which altogether measure approximately 1.5 m. The duodenum is only partially covered by peritoneum, its shape resembling an arc (slightly larger than a semicircle) that encloses the head of the pancreas. The superior duodenal segment crosses the structures of the hepatic portal, i.e., common bile duct, portal vein, and hepatic artery, while the gallbladder is anterolateral to it. The descending duodenal segment parallels the posterolateral vena cava and borders the right kidney. The inferior duodenal segment, situated about two fingerbreadths inferior to the mesenteric root and caudad of the pancreas, crosses anterior to the vena cava and the aorta. Cross-sectional views of the superior mesenteric artery and vein can be demonstrated anterior to the intestine. The retroperitoneal duodenum continues as intraperitoneal organ at the level of the mesenteric root slightly left of the aorta.

The jejunum and ileum are attached to the posterior abdominal wall by the fan-shaped folds of the peritoneum known as the mesentery proper; most of the coils of the small intestine are found in the left upper (jejunum) and lower (ileum) quadrant. The jejunum and ileum account for most of the intraperitoneal space. The terminal ileum ascends from the pelvis over the right psoas major muscle, the iliac vessels paralleling its medial margin, at the level of McBurney's point and ends in the right iliac fossa by opening into the medial side of the cecum at the ileocecal (Bauhin's) valve.

Colon. The colon is about 120 cm long and runs along the margins of the intraperitoneal cavity. In a clockwise direction (from the subject's point of view) it is subdivided into cecum, ascending, transverse, descending, and sigmoid colon, and the rectum.

The cecum is situated anterior to the psoas major muscle in the right lower quadrant. The ascending colon parallels the right lateral abdominal wall and its superior segment is anterior to the inferolateral part of the right kidney. The hepatic flexure comprises the terminal part of the ascending colon and the commencement of the transverse colon; usually, the convex part of this flexure hugs the gallbladder and the lower right margin of the liver, but as a variant it may dome up far superior and may even be situated between the lower right thoracic wall and the right hepatic lobe. The transverse colon touches the anterior abdominal wall and traverses the upper abdomen from right to left; elongated variants may have a drooping center section reaching all the way into the pelvis. The splenic flexure connects the transverse and descending colon, its convex aspect being inferior to the spleen. The proximal part of the descending colon is anterior and lateral to the left kidney. The S-shaped sigmoid colon forms a loop that, depending on its length, frames the roof of the urinary bladder more or less markedly. The rectum descends into the pelvis posterior to the bladder and terminates at the anus.

Ultrasound Morphology

With enough training and experience the sonographer will be able to identify and demonstrate most regions of the gastrointestinal tract (◻ 7.1).

Esophagus. The proximal part of the cervical esophagus posterior to the left lobe of the thyroid lends itself to sonographic study **(Fig. 14.5, p. 418)**; although for all practical purposes the thoracic segment is beyond the reach of transcutaneous ultrasound, ultrasonography can demonstrate the distal esophagus at the level of the gastric cardia.

Stomach and duodenum. With appropriate techniques all of the stomach and duodenum are accessible to sonographic study.

Jejunum and ileum. In the fasting state the individual loops of the jejunum cannot be differentiated, while their mesenteric attachment and the Kerckring's folds characterize the postprandial fluid-filled loops. Later, the postprandial ileum loops in the lower abdomen will also be fluid-filled and display vivid peristalsis.

Colon. Usually, the ileocecum and colon can be visualized reasonably well and, taking into account the anatomical relations, the topography of these parts of the gastrointestinal tract can be identified for certain. Sometimes an elongated sigmoid colon or drooping transverse colon may interfere and be the reason for misclassification. Almost always the colon will appear as a tube filled with a varying amount of feces and lacking peristalsis.

Gut signature. The morphological criterion to look for in the ultrasound study of the gastrointestinal tract is the so-called gut signature. At any place of the gut this cross-sectional view will demonstrate the GI tube as an annular structure, while the longitudinal view depicts it as a tubular structure. Assessment of the intestinal wall and differentiation of its characteristic layered structure becomes possible only with high-frequency probes (5, 7 or 7.5 MHz) **(Table 7.1)**.

Gut signature criteria. Detection of a gut signature calls for analysis of its ultrasound morphology, lumen, and peristalsis as well as of the surroundings and the intestinal segments upstream and downstream. Only all of these criteria together will permit typing and assessment with a clear-cut diagnosis in many cases. The criteria to be considered are listed below.

▶ **Location/relation**. Specifying the position of a gut signature offers the first chance of defining the anatomical relations. It is impor-

Gut Signature

The normal "gut signature" is known as the "cockade," a term whose origins date back to Old French and refer to a rosette-shaped badge. In ultrasound, the "gut signature" and its pathological variant the "target sign" have come to denote the round cross-sectional view of the intestinal wall with its different layers. Although it has also been used to describe the longitudinal view of the gastrointestinal tube, it is reserved exclusively for the GI tract and should not be applied to other rosette-shaped structures, such as hepatic metastasis, which are given their own terms (e.g., "halo" or "bull's-eye" sign).

Thus, in the cross-sectional view the gut signature/target sign refers to the annular image of the layered intestinal wall and its center, while in the longitudinal view it refers to the parallel arrangement of adjacent intestinal segments with the lumen in between.

Physiological gut signature. A so-called physiological gut signature refers to a lumen that is normal for this segment, a wall structure with characteristic layering, well-defined wall thickness, and normal peristalsis.

Pathological gut signature. A so-called pathological gut signature is characterized by changes in the normal appearance of lumen, wall thickness, and/or peristalsis/pliability **(Table 7.2)**. Pathological wall changes may be circular or eccentric and focal, or they may be continuous or discontinuous along the longitudinal axis. Intussusception will be seen on ultrasound as the "target/doughnut sign" (cross-sectional view) or "pseudokidney sign" (longitudinal view). Adjacent target signs fixed in space are characteristic of a conglomerate.

Table 7.1 Layers of the intestinal wall

Sonographic layer	Histological layer
Entrance echo—innermost hyperechoic layer	Mucosal surface
Innermost hypoechoic layer	Mucosa
Central hyperechoic layer	Submucosa
Outermost hypoechoic layer	Muscularis propria
Outermost hyperechoic layer—entrance/exit echo	Serosal surface

Table 7.2 Criteria of the pathological gut signature

Wall thickness	> 4 mm Circumferential thickening Off-center appearance
Wall layering	Pronounced Interrupted Missing
Peristalsis	Rigid wall Lack of pliability Lack of peristalsis
Lumen	Constricted Distended
Vascularity	Missing Enhanced

7.1 Visualization of the Gastrointestinal Tract

▶ Stomach and duodenum: physiological gut signature

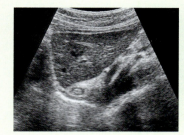

a Typical gut signature of the esophagocardiac junction anterior to the aorta at the esophageal hiatus.

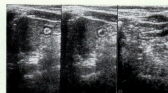

b Gut signature of the antrum: longitudinal (contraction [left] and beginning [center] dilatation) and cross-sectional view.

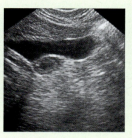

c Normal gut signature of the superior part of the duodenum indenting the gallbladder, longitudinal and cross-sectional view.

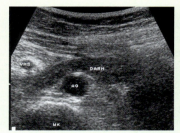

d Normal gut signature of the inferior part of the duodenum where it crosses the aorta (AO). VMS = superior mesenteric vein; WK = spine; Darm = intestine.

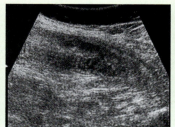

e Jejunum, slightly fluid-enhanced, after oral fluid intake; note the clearly delineated Kerckring's folds.

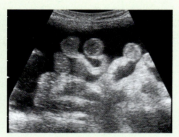

f Loops of the small intestine at their mesenteric attachment, floating in ascites of cardiac origin.

▶ The differential diagnosis of fluid-filled intestinal loops has to rely on peristalsis

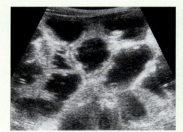

g Chronic ileus in obstructing tumor of the hepatic flexure, exhibiting distended intestinal loops and abnormally sluggish and ineffective peristaltic movement.

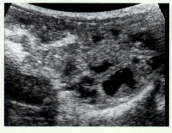

h Sprue with so-called "tumbler phenomenon."

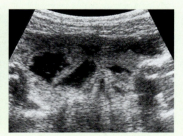

i Mechanical ileus (adhesions) with focal fixation of the intestinal loops, resulting in impaired peristalsis.

▶ Colon

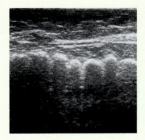

j Haustra in a colon displaying meteorism and scybala.

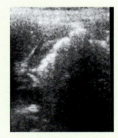

k Haustra of the hepatic flexure indenting the gallbladder may mimic gallstones.

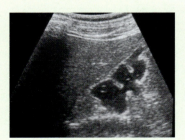

l Haustra after a saline enema.

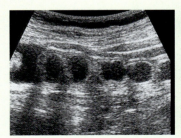

m Descending colon post enema.

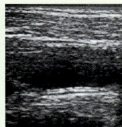

n Hydrocolonic sonography demonstrating the intestinal wall of the descending colon.

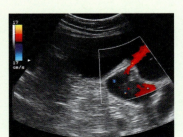

o Hydrocolonic sonography demonstrating the ileocolic valve and an ileocecal jet of fluid.

tant to recognize whether the pathology exhibits a fixed location or is mobile.
- **Echogenicity**. Basically, the echogenicity of the gut signature may be normal, hypoechoic, or hyperechoic; since one is dealing with a layered anatomical structure, this criterion has to be applied to the predominant elements of the wall or should reflect the possible loss of layering.
- **Wall thickness**. Numerous standard dimensions have been listed for the wall thickness (see above). Measurement of the wall thickness has to account for the degree of filling and the functional state (contraction/dilatation) of the intestines, and it also has to specify whether the wall is thickened or thinned out or whether its outline is interrupted or ill defined.
- **Wall layering**. The wall may display a normal layered structure or it may be markedly layered, may demonstrate thickening of just one particular layer, may present with layer defects, or may have lost its layered makeup altogether.
- **Shape/texture of the gut signature**. The cross-sectional view of the gut signature may be round or ovoid, or it may be characterized by asymmetrical changes; one characteristic pathological sign is the so-called target or bull's-eye sign.
- **Extent**. In terms of length, the short focal or extended lesions have to be differentiated from the diffuse changes in the intestinal wall.
- **Internal delineation**. Assessment of the luminal surface of the bowel wall will be able to differentiate between normal as well as pathological Kerckring's folds and haustra (preserved or lost) and also focal polypoid/tumorous changes, ulcers, and other surface irregularities.
- **External delineation**. The outside of the gastrointestinal tube may be smooth or irregular; it may exhibit pod-like extensions or invade other structures.
- **Changes in the surroundings**. The surroundings of the gut signature may be absolutely normal or there may be free air or fluid; ultrasound may be able to visualize focal reactions in the surrounding tissue, e.g., hyperechoic pannus, abscess and fistula formation, as well as lymphadenopathy.
- **Lumen**. Assessment of the lumen has to account for the functional state/degree of contraction; it may be normal, distended, or reduced/narrowed.
- **Stenosis**. A stenosis is a circumscribed functionally narrowed lumen of the bowel with prestenotic distension and poststenotic narrowing of the intestinal tube; usually, a pathological gut signature or "target sign" will be seen at the stenosis itself.
- **Contents**. Within the lumen of the gut there may be anechoic fluid, echogenic chyme/ingesta, hyperechoic feces/scybala, air, and foreign bodies.
- **Peristalsis**. Assessment of the peristalsis differentiates between physiological contraction/distension on the one hand and normal, missing, increased, impaired, or pathological peristalsis (pendulating peristalsis) on the other.
- **Texture/pliability**. Normal intestinal loops are compliant; lack of pliability suggests invasive inflammatory or malignant changes.
- **Painfulness**. A normal gut signature is not painful; if localized pain can be triggered at a focal change in the intestinal wall, this indicates either an inflammatory or a functional disorder (e.g., irritable bowel syndrome).
- **Vascularity**. The intestinal wall and its surrounding tissues may be hypervascular or avascular, or the vascularity may be normal.
- **Changes in intestinal segments upstream**. Upstream of a focal lesion one may find characteristic changes in the intestinal lumen (e.g., distension in the presence of ileus), peristalsis, and texture (e.g., thickening of the muscularis propria in case of hypertrophy).
- **Changes in intestinal segments downstream.** In case of mechanical ileus, a typical sign downstream is the so-called "starvation gut."
- **Changes observed over time**. The quality and/or quantity of one or more of the observed criteria may become more or less pronounced.
- **Changes in other organs**. Additional findings in other organs may help immensely in the correct interpretation of intestinal sonographic observations (e.g., gallbladder, biliary tree, and liver in case of gallstone ileus; assessment of the flow signals in the superior and inferior mesenteric artery in ischemic and inflammatory bowel disease).

Peristalsis

Peristalsis comprises a wave of contraction, followed by immediate relaxation, passing along the longitudinal axis of the intestinal tube; under physiological conditions it may be visualized sonographically at the stomach and small intestine. Next to a segment actively contracting and displaying a thickened intestinal wall with narrowing of the lumen, the segments upstream and downstream will undergo concurrent relaxation of the intestinal wall musculature with thinning of the wall, dilatation, and widening of the lumen.

Stomach. Gastric peristalsis is best seen around the antrum and is characterized by rhythmic contractions with a frequency of 2–4 times per minute and a period of 2–20 s. The dilatation phases with discernible passage of chyme subsequent to swallowing are best observed at the esophagogastric junction.

Small intestine. Under fasting conditions, the empty small intestine (the Latin word "jejunus" means empty, dry, barren) is hard to visualize sonographically and thus its peristaltic movement remains hidden. Under physiological conditions the postprandial peristalsis usually appears as a steady and orderly alternation of muscular contraction and dilatation propelling chyme and fluid in a directed fashion.
In inflammatory disorders the lumen of the small intestine will still be filled with some fluid even when fasting; by itself this demonstration of intraluminal fluid (e.g., within the duodenum in case of pancreatitis or cholecystitis) may be enough to suggest the underlying inflammation. Depending on the severity of the inflammation, the peristalsis may be vigorous, increased or even turbulent (e.g., the so-called "tumbler phenomenon" in sprue). Disturbed peristalsis with pathological contractions, mandatory pathological distension of the lumen, and conspicuously uncoordinated movement of the intestinal wall and intraluminal chyme/fluid are characteristic of ileus (see below).

Large intestine. Under physiological conditions, ultrasonography cannot visualize peristaltic activity in the large intestine. However, the characteristically impaired peristalsis in the presence of ileus does become evident on ultrasound.

Stomach

Although the stomach is not part of a routine transabdominal ultrasound study, except for some special cases, it quite often produces typical findings, which have to be interpreted correctly. This calls not only for a systematic analysis of the above criteria but also for the use of a 5 MHz probe, which will improve the diagnostic interpretation (differentiation of the wall layers).

Assessment of any sonographic findings at the stomach has to consider somewhat precisely the time of the patient's last ingestion. Interpretation may be facilitated and improved by oral fluid intake (with an antifoaming agent added). Specific sonomorphological analysis of the gastric wall requires endoscopic/bioptic and endosonographic procedures.

Focal Wall Changes

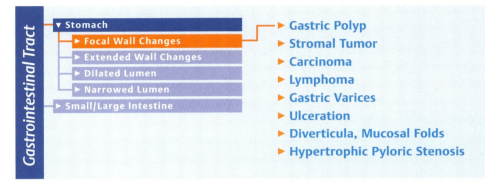

▶ Gastric Polyps

Polypoid changes of the gastric wall are purely incidental findings and are best visualized with the stomach containing only very little fluid (**Fig. 7.2**). The polyp will appear as a sessile focal mass protruding into the gastric lumen and presenting as an atypical (off-center) pathological gut signature. Polyps arise from certain layers of the gastric wall, most often the mucosa and submucosa, but may also involve the deeper layers of the wall. A more precise analysis of the wall layers would require the use of high-frequency probes or even endoscopic/endosonographic procedures. In larger polyps, color-flow Doppler imaging may be able to demonstrate the intravascular blood flow. Polyps do not affect the outer delineation of the gastric gut signature. Being subjected to the peristaltic movement of the stomach wall, the sessile polyp will be moving passively and thus can be better differentiated from the mucosal folds. Since ultrasound cannot distinguish between benign and malignant polyps, it is impossible to differentiate a benign polyp from gastric adenocarcinoma type I.

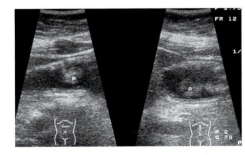

▲ **Fig. 7.2** Gastric polyp (P). Demonstration of a sessile polypoid gastric tumor awash in fluid/secretions. Left: transverse plane. Right: longitudinal plane.

▶ Stromal Tumor

These most frequent benign fibroid tumors (e.g., leiomyoma), with their smooth margins, are found in the layered wall of the stomach, quite often relate to one of the central layers, and are well vascularized. They exhibit interstitial growth and may become as large as several centimeters. Although these firm, elastic tumors display a somewhat varied echogenicity, they are mostly hypoechoic (**Fig. 7.3**). The following stromal tumors may be found in the stomach:
- Leiomyoma
- Leiomyoblastoma
- Neurinoma
- Neurofibroma

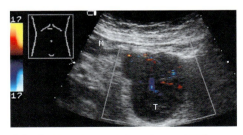

▲ **Fig. 7.3** Gastrointestinal stromal tumor (GIST).
a Hypoechoic tumor (T) with extramural spread and vascularity. M = stomach.

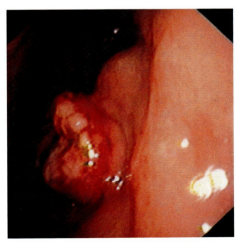

▲ *b* Endoscopic view; the biopsies were negative.

▶ Carcinoma

Focal adenocarcinoma may arise anywhere within the stomach (**Table 7.3**). Frequently, sonography will demonstrate a pathological concentric gut signature limited to the gastric antrum or cardia, while focal pathological atypical (off-center) gut signatures are more common in the corpus and rare in the fundus of the stomach. The typical lesion is visualized as a pathological thickening of the gastric wall with loss of the usual layering. Quite often the lesion is poorly delineated at the gastric lumen, and in case of concentric tumors it is not uncommon to encounter a stenotic lumen; in such cases there will be retention of food proximal to the stenosis. The immediate vicinity of the tumor shows a characteristic loss of peristalsis, while the pathological gut signature is hard and not compliant. The surface of the tumor may either be smooth or irregular. In advanced gastric carcinoma, there may be free fluid as well as lymphadenopathy around the pancreas, the hepatic portal, and/or the celiac axis (**Figs. 7.4, 7.5**).

Table 7.3 **The sites of gastric adenocarcinoma**

Site	Frequency (%)
Antrum	50–80
Corpus/fundus	20–30
Cardia	10–20

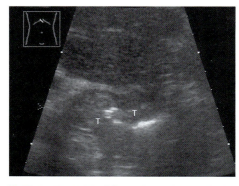

▲ **Fig. 7.4** Carcinoma of the gastric cardia (T) impinging on the fornix. Irregular, abnormal target sign (compare with ▣ 7.1a).

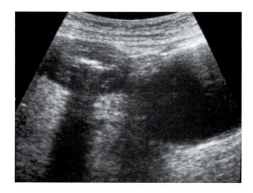
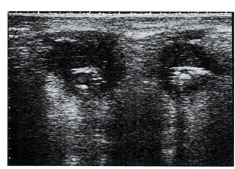
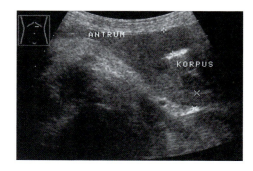
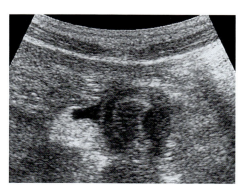

◂◂ **Fig. 7.5** Gastric carcinoma.
 a Thickened ovoid pathological gut signature of the gastric antrum in the longitudinal plane, right next to an abdominal aortic aneurysm.

◂ **b** Pathological gut signature with loss of wall layering, irregular and clearly thickened wall, ill defined outer margin, and narrowed lumen.

◂◂ **c** Carcinoma of the gastric body (signet-ring carcinoma). The stomach wall is markedly thickened to 14 mm (cursors) and shows intense, hypoechoic structural transformation with loss of the normal layered pattern.

◂ **d** Irregular thickened pathological gut signature of the gastric antrum; the free fluid present in the perigastric space indicates local metastasis (in addition there is ascites in Morrisons pouch as well as hepatic metastasis)

▶ Lymphoma

Gastric lymphoma may be visible on ultrasound as a focal hypoechoic mass involving the wall of the stomach, with clearly evident hypervascularity and loss of its typical layered appearance (**see Fig. 7.11**).

▶ Gastric Varices

Varices of the gastric wall are quite common in portal hypertension; owing to their tortuous course, sectional views of these varices will appear as small anechoic/hypoechoic cystoid structures on the outside of the gastric wall (**Fig. 7.6**). At the gastric fundus and cardia, as well as at the distal esophagus, they may protrude transmurally into the lumen of the stomach as esophageal or fundic varices. Color-flow Doppler scanning will demonstrate a ribbon-like hepatofugal portovenous blood flow.

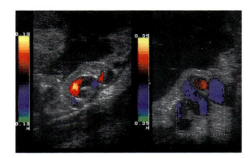

◀ **Fig. 7.6** Gastric varices. Endosonography demonstrating varices in the gastric wall in portal hypertension.

▶ Ulceration

The majority of gastric ulcers are far too small to be visualized on transabdominal ultrasound. At the ulceration, the gastric wall is thinned out and has lost its layered appearance; trapped air or food particles will often be seen within the cavity of the ulcer, resulting in a coarse echo. Peristalsis will spare the area of the lesion. The liver, pancreas, or greater omentum may wall off any possible penetration, and in other cases there may be free fluid, while free air can sometimes be demonstrated in frank perforation (**Figs. 7.7 and 7.8**).

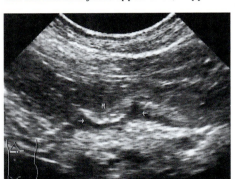
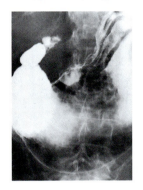

◀◀ **Fig. 7.7** Benign gastric ulcer.
   a Craterlike benign gastric ulcer (M; arrows) after fluid ingestion. Note the rigid wall thickening along the lesser curvature (beam directed obliquely upward from the greater to lesser curvature).

◀ *b* Double-contrast radiograph of the stomach demonstrates a benign ulcer in the lesser curvature.

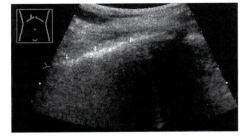
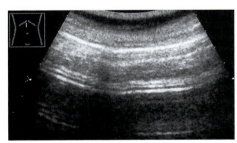

◀◀ **Fig. 7.8** Free air caused by an intra-abdominal perforation.
   a Perforated diverticulum: grainy, hyperechoic air bubbles between the parietal and visceral peritoneum of the hepatic surface with a reverberation artifact.

◀ *b* Complete sound reflection from copious free intra-abdominal air. Perforated ulcer.

▶ Diverticula, Mucosal Folds

Diverticulum-like sacculation in the gastric wall is rare; when looking at all wall layers there will be focal excavation of the lumen.

Transverse sections through rugal hypertrophy at the gastric body may mimic focal polypoid wall lesions.

▶ Hypertrophic Pyloric Stenosis

Hypertrophic pyloric stenosis (**Fig. 7.9**) is a relatively common condition affecting the newborn—recurrent projectile vomiting is almost pathognomonic. On ultrasonography, the pylorus appears as a circumscribed lengthy circular thickening of the muscle, the total pyloric diameter being > 12 mm and the pyloric canal being compressed (so-called "cervix sign"); at the same time the stomach will display marked fluid retention.

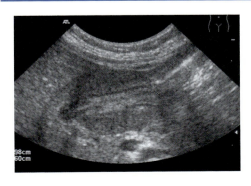

◀ **Fig. 7.9** Hypertrophic pyloric stenosis. So-called cervix sign with marked circumscribed thickening of the lamina propria mucosae and tight pyloric canal, accompanied by gastric distension and fluid retention (with the kind permission of Dr. R. Kardorff, Wesel, Germany).

Extended Wall Changes

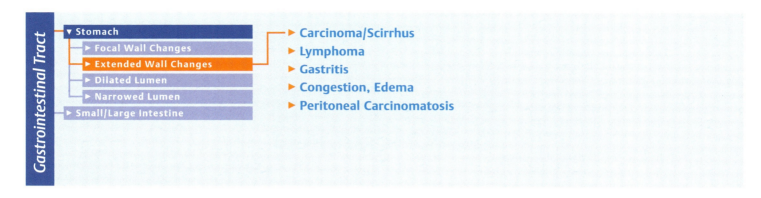

▶ Carcinoma/Scirrhus

Scirrhous carcinoma is characterized by diffuse extensive invasion of the gastric wall by the tumor, resulting in a narrowed lumen and loss of the layered wall architecture. Owing to the intramural spread of the carcinoma, the inner and outer margins of the gastric wall are still smoothly defined irrespective of a possible wall thickness of several centimeters. The region of the tumor will be void of any peristaltic movement, and the pathological gut signature will demonstrate a coarse texture and lack any pliability (**Figs. 7.10 and 7.17**).

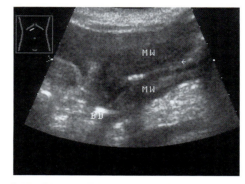 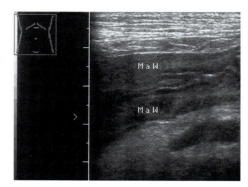

▲ **Fig. 7.10 a, b** Scirrhous carcinoma. Oblong abnormal target sign produced by a scirrhous signet-ring cell carcinoma of the stomach. MW, MaW = gastric wall.

▶ Lymphoma

Diffuse invasion of the gastric wall by lymphoma may lead to clearly recognizable irregular and noncompliant hypoechoic thickening of the wall, with easily visualized hypervascularity and loss of its layered architecture (**Fig. 7.11**).

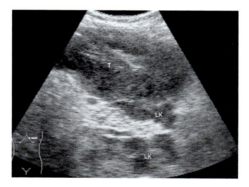

◀ **Fig. 7.11** Gastric lymphoma: diffuse tumor invasion of the gastric wall (T) with lymph node metastasis (LK).

▶ Gastritis

The different types of gastritis (*Helicobacter pylori* infection, long-term therapy with proton pump inhibitors), as well as Ménétrier disease, display a markedly pronounced emphasis of the layering and rugal coarsening (**Fig. 7.12**).

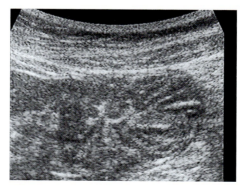 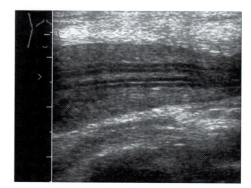

▲ **Fig. 7.12 a** Marked corporic rugae, fasting state.

▲ **b** Hypertrophic antral folds in gastritis, with normal wall layers.

▶ Congestion, Edema

Congestion. In cardiac congestion, the outer layers of the gastric wall will undergo a marked hypoechoic thickening; other signs of the cardiac congestion will always be present as well (distended hepatic veins, engorged vena cava, possibly ascites, and pleural effusion).

Edema. Concomitant inflammatory reaction of the gastric wall as part of pancreatitis could result in a more pronounced appearance of the layering as well as discrete extended thickening of the gastric wall. Owing to the concurrent paralytic ileus, there is no peristalsis and the pliability of the wall is diminished by the inflammatory invasion.

▶ Peritoneal Carcinomatosis

As part of diffuse peritoneal carcinomatosis the gastric wall may undergo appositional thickening from the outside, and it is quite typical of these cases that marked ascites can frequently be demonstrated (**see Fig. 7.16**).

Dilated Lumen

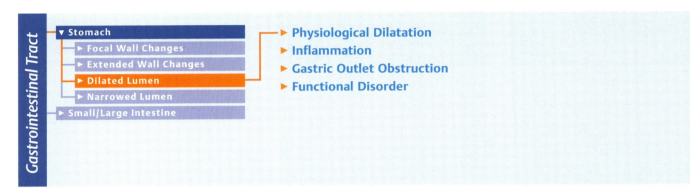

Being a storage organ, the stomach may hold up to 2000 ml of food even under physiological conditions. Conditioning and disease/disorders can increase this volume beyond 3000 ml. In the fasting state (6 hours, at most 12 hours, after the last ingestion) under physiological conditions the stomach will empty completely; with the patient in the supine position the small residual secretion of about 50 ml can be demonstrated at the gastric fundus. The echogenicity of the gastric contents depends on the type of food ingested.

▶ Physiological Dilatation

The postprandial chyme can be visualized at the gastric fundus with the patient in the supine position (**Fig. 7.13**). Peristaltic activity will mix it and then transport it to the gastric outlet, where it is portioned through the pylorus into the duodenum. Here, the chyme becomes visible only because of the peristalsis and can then be demonstrated within the lumen along its brief passage through the duodenum.

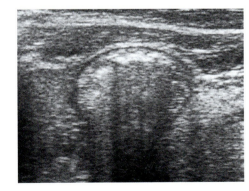

◀ **Fig. 7.13** Postprandial lumen of the stomach, markedly dilated by ingesta; thinned out, dilated gastric wall.

▶ Inflammation

When dealing with inflammation near the duodenal C (pancreatitis, cholecystitis, complicated ulcer, ileus) one can always demonstrate fluid within the duodenal lumen (indirect sign), the latter displaying a markedly pathological and diminished peristalsis with sloshing of the fluid. At the same time, the gastric lumen will contain an increased amount of food particles and fluid. Because of the lack of peristalsis, the solid particles will settle in layers beneath the fluid and gas and can be churned by deliberate palpation or by repositioning the patient.

▶ Gastric Outlet Obstruction

Gastric outlet stenosis or obstruction by the duodenum will result in a markedly ectatic stomach, retaining the food and fluid previously ingested as well as the increased amount of gastric juice produced (**Fig. 7.14b**)

▶ Functional Disorder

Functional disorders of gastric emptying are encountered in ileus and diabetic gastroparesis (**Fig. 7.14**); here, it is primarily the retention of fluid characterized by fine echoes.

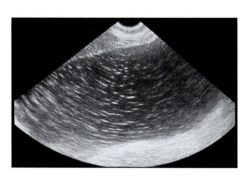
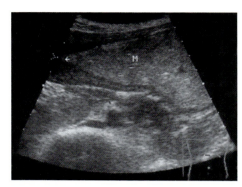
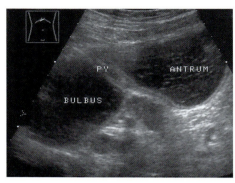

▲ **Fig. 7.14 a** Pathological dilatation of the stomach in diabetic gastroparesis (in this case more than 3000 ml of hematinic fasting secretion was drained).

▲ **b** Gastric lumen narrowed by scirrhous carcinoma of the antrum with antral stenosis (arrow) and ensuing massive dilatation of the stomach (M).

▲ **c** Abnormal dilatation of the antrum and duodenal bulb, indicating a postbulbar location of the stenosis (here, duodenal carcinoma with locoregional metastasis; hypoechoic retrogastric and retrobulbar masses).

Narrowed Lumen

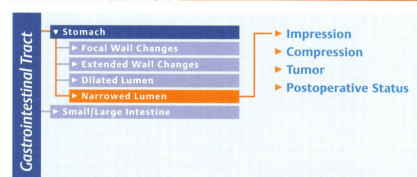

In fasting, peristaltic movement of the antrum will result in concentric contraction of the gastric wall with complete loss of the lumen; depending on the degree of prefilling, this narrowing of the lumen may be incomplete.

▶ Impression

Impression of the stomach from the outside may result in eccentric narrowing of the gastric lumen, the primary such cause being masses in adjacent organs, e.g., hepatic (**Fig. 7.15**) or pancreatic cysts, but also the gallbladder.

Fig. 7.15 a Anterior impression of the stomach by a liver ▶ cyst.

b Posterior indentation of the stomach (MA) by an ▶▶ area of pancreatic necrosis (N).

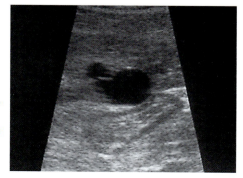
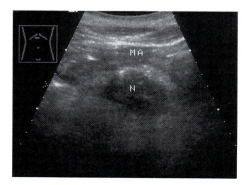

▶ Compression

Compression of the gastric lumen from the outside is seen in massive ascites (e.g., in peritoneal carcinomatosis; **Fig. 7.16**) and severe pancreatitis with retroperitoneal edema and ascites.

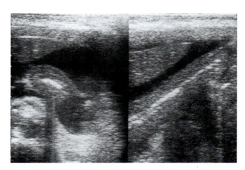

▲ **Fig. 7.16 a** Gastric compression by ascites in a gynecological tumor with peritoneal carcinomatosis, the stomach lacking any dilatability.

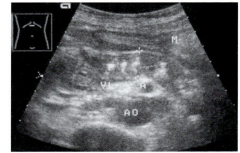

▲ **b** Gastric compression (M) by chronic calcifying pancreatitis (calipers). AO = aorta; A = antrum; VL = splenic vein.

▶ Tumor

Focal circular tumors of the gastric antrum, body, and cardia as well as scirrhous carcinoma (**Fig. 7.17**) will lead to significant narrowing of the lumen, accompanied by dilatation of those segments of the stomach and/or esophagus upstream.

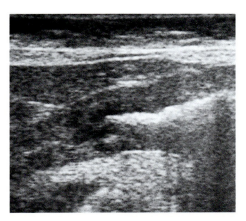

▲ **Fig. 7.17 a** Narrowing of the gastric lumen by an oblong scirrhous carcinoma of the antrum, upper abdominal transverse scan.

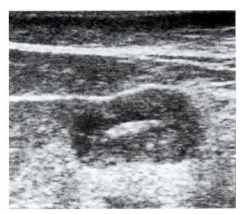

▲ **b** Longitudinal scan showing the antrum in transverse section: target sign.

▶ Postoperative Status

Depending on the degree of resection in stomach operations, the lumen of the gastric stump may be markedly smaller.

Small/Large Intestine

Small intestine. Ultrasonographic assessment of the jejunum and ileum is successful only if certain conditions are met. When differentiating sonographic findings of the small intestine, it is vital to know the time of the last ingestion. In a fasting patient these segments of the small intestine do not display a filled lumen, and unless there are pathological findings, such as ascites or inflammatory or neoplastic changes, this "empty intestine" is masked from diagnostic ultrasonography. The only section of the small bowel regularly identified during ultrasound scanning is the terminal ileum where it crosses anterior to the psoas muscle and where it terminates at the colon (ileocecal valve). Visualization and assessment of the jejunal and ileal loops can be facilitated and improved by examining the patient postprandially or after oral intake of fluid (with antifoaming agent added). Apart from a systematic analysis based on the above criteria, assessment profits from the 5 MHz probe since this allows better differentiation of the wall layers. In the visualization and assessment of peristaltic activity, no other abdominal organ, except the small bowel, has to rely so heavily on real-time scanning. Wall thickening in the setting of inflammatory bowel disease can be detected with an accuracy of 90.5% (sensitivity 90.3%, specificity 88.4%).

Colon. The large bowel frames the abdominal cavity. It is always filled to a varying degree by feces, scybala, and gas, thus being more of a hindrance for abdominal ultrasound scanning than offering easy access for diagnostic sonography. The physiological peristaltic movement of the colon cannot be visualized. The wall, lumen, and peristalsis can only be identified in large-bowel pathology or when employing special examination techniques (retrograde saline lavage, hydrocolonic sonography).

Focal Wall Changes

- Stomach
- ▼ Small/Large Intestine
  - Focal Wall Changes
  - Extended Wall Changes
  - Dilated Lumen
  - Narrowed Lumen

▶ Carcinoma
▶ Lymphoma
▶ Hematoma
▶ Polyp
▶ Intussusception
▶ Gallstone/Bezoar
▶ Diverticula
▶ Diverticulitis
▶ Appendix
▶ Appendicitis
▶ Hernia

Focal wall changes at the small and large intestine always present as a localized finding at the intestinal loop itself. However, there will usually be characteristic reactions and changes in the vicinity of this target sign as well, particularly in those intestinal segments upstream of the lesion.

▶ Carcinoma

Focal adenocarcinoma is a common pathological finding in the large bowel, while it is a rare entity in the small intestine (**Figs. 7.18–7.20**). Ultrasonography will demonstrate a typical concentric or atypical off-center target sign with loss of the normal wall layers. Irregular delineation at the luminal surface is not uncommon, and in concentric malignancies quite often the lumen will be narrowed. This stenosis may result in dilatation of the intestinal segments upstream, finally leading to full-blown ileus. The area around the neoplasm is characterized by a lack of peristaltic movement. The texture of the target sign is coarse, lacks pliability, and sometimes may be painful, signifying peritonitis.

The tumor may present a smooth or irregular surface, and in advanced stages free fluid and localized lymphadenopathy around the tumor may be demonstrated. Presently, there are no clear-cut color-flow Doppler criteria characteristics of intestinal malignancy.

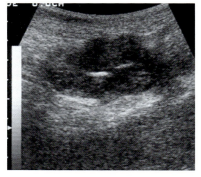

▲ **Fig. 7.18** Cancer of the small intestine.

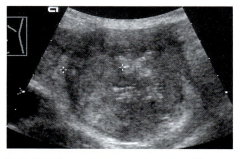

▲ **Fig. 7.19** Cancer of the ascending colon with target sign due to tumor-induced concentric swelling of the wall.

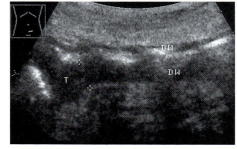

▲ **Fig. 7.20** Tumor (T, cursors) has invaded a long segment of the sigmoid colon, growing into and along the bowel wall (DW). Harmonic imaging.

▶ Lymphoma

Lymphoma of the small and large bowel presents as a focal hypoechoic mass in the intestinal wall with loss of the normal layered architecture (**Fig. 7.21**). One often encounters bizarre neoplasms with luminal stenosis, which are difficult to delineate from the adjacent tissue and frequently are hypervascular.

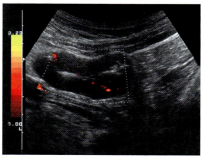

▲ **Fig. 7.21 a** NHL of the jejunum.

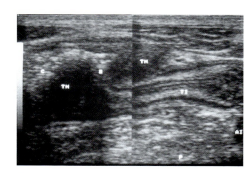

▲ **b** Lymphoma at the ileocecal valve in AIDS.

▶ Hematoma

Sometimes coumarin anticoagulant therapy will be complicated by bleeding into the intestinal wall, leading to circular hypoechoic thickening of the wall or a focal hypoechoic mass, with subsequent narrowing of the lumen and loss of peristalsis (**Fig. 7.22**).

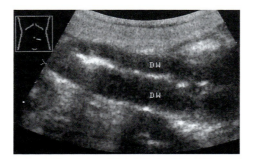

◀ **Fig. 7.22** Bleeding into the small bowel wall (DW) in a patient on anticoagulant medication has produced a thickened wall with a homogeneous, very hypoechoic structure ("garden hose" appearance).

▶ Polyp

Polypoid changes of the intestinal wall are purely incidental findings best visualized when the lumen of the bowel contains only a trace of fluid (**Fig. 7.23**). Such a polyp will appear as a focal sessile protrusion into the intestinal lumen characterized by an atypical pathological gut signature. In larger polypoid lesions, color-flow Doppler scanning may demonstrate the presence of vessels, thus permitting these neoplasms to be differentiated from scybala. Polyps do not alter the outer margin of the intestinal wall. During peristaltic movement of the bowel, such a sessile polyp may be localized, but sometimes large polyps can induce intussusception.

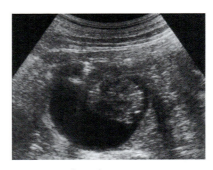

▲ **Fig. 7.23** Colon polyp.

▶ Intussusception

In intussusception one part of the intestine prolapses along the longitudinal axis into an immediately adjoining part. Intussusception of early childhood, where the abnormal mobility of various intestinal segments will lead to the well-known enteric (**Fig. 7.24**) and ileocecal intussusception, has a different etiology from that in adults. In the latter case, there will always be a lead point triggering and leading the way for the prolapse. Such lead points include polyps (**Figs. 7.25 and 7.26**), large mural lymph nodes, and tumors; in addition, intussusception may also arise in small bowel affected by Crohn disease.

Intussusception will present intermittently as a multilayered pathological gut signature or target sign (**Fig. 7.27**). Edema and inflammation produce marked thickening, thus emphasizing the various layers of the wall, the outermost hypoechoic layer (muscularis propria) of the intussusceptum being especially thick. The intussusceptum can be identified by its own peristalsis, and in adults a tumorous lesion (polyp, tumor, lymph node) will provide the lead point. When bowel loops are invaginated, the patient suffers from massive localized pain and tenderness.

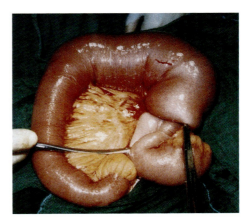

▲ **Fig. 7.24** Enteric intussusception.

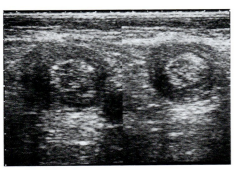

▲ **Fig. 7.25** Cross-sectional view of an intussusception. Left: through the apex. Right: through the neck of the polyp.

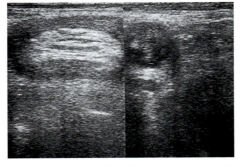

▲ **Fig. 7.26** Intussusception. Left: longitudinal view with muscular hypertrophy in the thickened outer and delicate invaginated inner gut signature. Right: cross-sectional view of a polyp as the leading point.

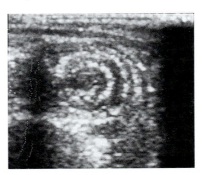

▲ **Fig. 7.27** So-called target sign (layered pathological gut signature) in intussusception.

▶ Gallstone/Bezoar

Large foreign objects may impact in the small bowel, thus producing localized reaction and even triggering mechanical ileus. The most common such object is a large gallstone that has perforated the gallbladder into the duodenum (**Fig. 7.28**). If it obstructs the lumen of the small intestine it will be visualized as a ball-shaped, inhomogeneous hyperechoic mass with posterior shadowing. There is very little localized tenderness and the findings and symptoms of the mechanical ileus dominate the picture. In addition, unequivocally pathological findings can be demonstrated at the gallbladder and possibly the biliary tree (pneumobilia).

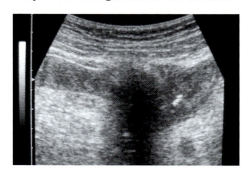

▲ **Fig. 7.28** Gallstone ileus.
a Ultrasound image.

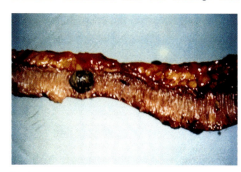

▲ **b** Surgical specimen.

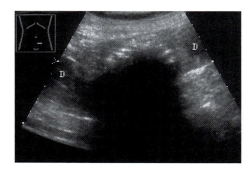

▲ **c** Differential diagnosis: bezoar, distinguished from a gallstone by its irregular surface. D = intestine.

▶ Diverticula

Besides the typical clinical findings, ultrasound has become the most important method for the diagnosis of diverticulitis, providing a sensitivity of 98.1% and a diagnostic accuracy of 97.7%.

Diverticula of the sigmoid colon are echogenic because of the gas or feces they contain; sometimes the outer hypoechoic layer of the intestinal wall (muscularis propria) becomes more pronounced owing to the concurrent muscular hypertrophy.

At times, periampullary duodenal diverticula (**Fig. 7.29**) may be recognized by the alternating presence of air and fluid within the lumen. However, Meckel's diverticulum may only be visualized in the presence of pathological changes.

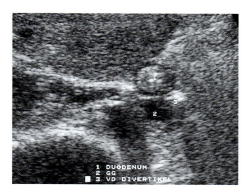

◀ **Fig. 7.29** Visualization of a periampullary duodenal diverticulum filled with air.

▶ Diverticulitis

Inflammation of a diverticulum will always result in localized tenderness. The diverticulum itself displays marked distension; the diverticular wall will appear as edematous hypoechoic crescent-shaped halo around the lumen which, when filled with feces, will be hyperechoic or hypoechoic in the presence of fluid.

Apart from this typical local finding, diverticulitis will demonstrate two other characteristic findings: particularly proximal of the diverticulum, the intestinal loop shows extended muscular hypertrophy of the wall and thickening of the outermost hypoechoic layer, as well as edema with pronounced layering of the wall and marked narrowing of varying degree of the gut lumen. There will be significant inflammatory hypervascularity at the diverticulum, which is surrounded by a localized massive reaction of the adjacent tissue: its being walled off by the greater omentum may result in a hyperechoic halo several centimeters thick. Complications are heralded by peridiverticular fluid, local collection of gas, abscess formation and fistulization (◻ **7.2**).

Diverticulosis/Diverticulitis

True diverticula are sacculations of the intestinal wall involving all layers and resulting in localized outpouching, e.g., duodenal diverticula (**Fig. 7.29**), Meckel's diverticulum, diverticula of the ascending colon. However, false diverticula, also known as pseudodiverticula, are by far more frequent: here, gaps (defects) in the muscularis propria lead to localized sacculation of mucosa and submucosa (e.g., sigmoid diverticula). Local findings always comprise hyperplasia of the muscularis propria, and the musculature of the surrounding intestinal wall becomes hypertrophied.

The formation of numerous pseudodiverticula in the sigmoid colon (diverticulosis) is seen as sequela of local pressure increases within the intestinal lumen, which in turn arises from nutrition low in dietary fiber. In addition, focal weakening of the bowel wall around the afferent and efferent vessels is also considered a causative factor. Feces impacted and inspissated in the extruded diverticular sac induce local pressure erosion of the mucosa, chronic inflammatory granulation (diverticulitis), and also possibly abscess formation and perforation (◻ **7.2**). Apart from muscular hypertrophy of the intestinal wall (particularly of the proximal segments), recurrent and chronic inflammation with edema and narrowing of the lumen will finally result in cicatricial contraction of the chronically inflamed bowel segment.

7.2 Acute Sigmoid Diverticulitis

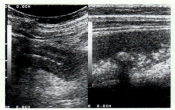

a Left: Extensive edematous pathological gut signature in the left lower quadrant with muscular hypertrophy of the intestinal wall and narrowed lumen. Right: Edematous wall of the sigmoid colon with stool-filled diverticulum and hypoechoic halo.

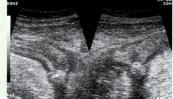

b Accentuated edematous intestinal wall. Diverticulum filled with feces; marked reaction of the adjacent tissue with hyperechoic halo.

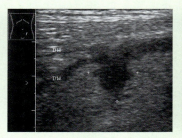

c Edematous diverticulum (arrows) with hyperechoic panniculitis.

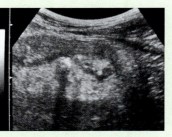

d Walled off perforation with localized collection of free air and free fluid.

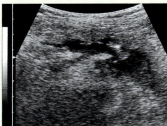

e Perforation with demonstration of free fluid and abscess formation.

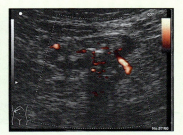

f Demonstration of inflammatory hypervascularity.

▶ Appendix

High-resolution probes can visualize a normal appendix in approximately 40% of cases; a gut signature displaying normal architecture will be seen at the cecum, terminating blindly and lacking in peristalsis, with a maximum diameter > 6 mm (**Fig. 7.30**).

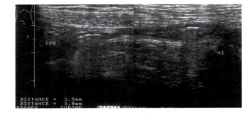

◀ **Fig. 7.30** View of the appendix from the cecum (COE) to its blind end over the iliac artery (AI). Inflammatory wall thickening at that site is consistent with appendicitis (surgery).

▶ Appendicitis

Acute appendicitis can be diagnosed sonographically with a positive predictive value of 95.7% and a sensitivity of 88.5%. Thus, the diagnostic accuracy of ultrasound is only marginally below that of bolus CT (sensitivity 96%, positive predictive value 95–96%). Inflammation of the appendix is characterized by enlargement, dilatation, and thickening, initially with demonstration of edema and accentuated layering of the wall; quite often fecaliths will be seen within the lumen. Appendicitis is always accompanied by localized tenderness (**Fig. 7.31**). Advanced stages will destroy the layered structure of the wall and produce a hyperechoic echo, local accumulation of fluid, and abscess formation (**Table 7.4, Figs. 7.32–7.34**). In such an advanced stage of the inflammation, the appendix itself is almost impossible to identify, and frequently localized lymphadenopathy will be evident.

Table 7.5 summarizes the differential diagnosis of appendicitis by ultrasound (**Fig. 7.35**).

Table 7.4 Sonographic signs in acute appendicitis

- ▶ Swelling of the appendix
- ▶ Thickening of the wall
- ▶ Fluid-filled lumen
- ▶ Tenderness
- ▶ Fecalith
- ▶ Hyperechoic omental cap
- ▶ Free fluid
- ▶ Perityphlitis
- ▶ Loss of peristalsis

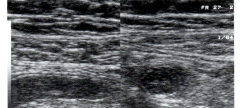

▲ **Fig. 7.31** Acute appendicitis. Pathologically distended and thickened appendix with local tenderness.

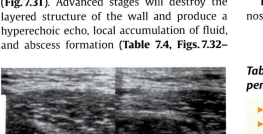

▲ **Fig. 7.32** Acute appendicitis. Thick pathological gut signature with pronounced wall layering and hyperechoic halo.

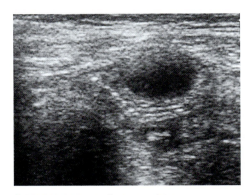

▲ *Fig. 7.33* Acute purulent appendicitis.

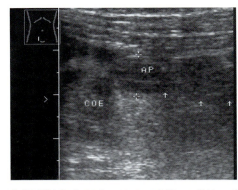

▲ *Fig. 7.34* Perforated acute appendicitis: partial loss of delineation of the appendix (AP) and thickening of the cecal wall (COE). Arrows: swelling. The patient also had fluid around the liver and an atonic, congested gallbladder (not shown).

◄ *Fig. 7.35* Purulent salpingitis.

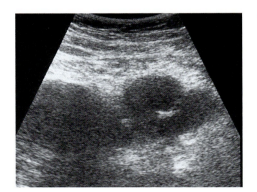

Table 7.5 Differential diagnosis of acute appendicitis by ultrasound

Bowel	► Enteritis
	► Terminal ileitis
	► Intussusception
	► Diverticulitis
	► Tumor
Adnexa and ovary	► Adnexitis
	► Tubo-ovarian abscess (Fig. 7.35)
	► Ectopic pregnancy
	► Hemorrhagic cyst
	► Torsion of ovarian tumor
Psoas muscle	► Hematoma of the psoas muscle
Ureter	► Stenotic ureteral origin
	► Ureterolith
Lymph node	► Mesenteric lymphadenitis
Vessels	► Thrombosis
	► Arterial dissection
	► Aneurysm
Other	► Cholecystitis
	► Pancreatitis
	► Perforated gastric ulcer

► Hernia

Hernias are defects in the abdominal wall. Ultrasound can identify the location (inguinal, femoral, umbilical, incisional, spigelian, epigastric) and size of the fascial defect as well as the contents. Demonstration of an edematous gut signature with accentuated wall architecture in the hernial sac proves that bowel is involved in the herniation; in these cases, stasis and even mechanical ileus may be present in the more proximal intestinal segments (**Fig. 7.36**).

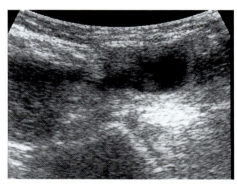

▲ *Fig. 7.36 a* Inguinal hernia on the left with incarcerated intestinal loop and mechanical ileus.

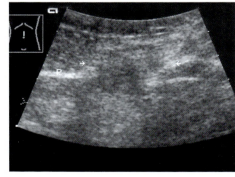

▲ *b* Incisional hernia (arrows); interrupted peritoneal contour (P).

Extended Wall Changes

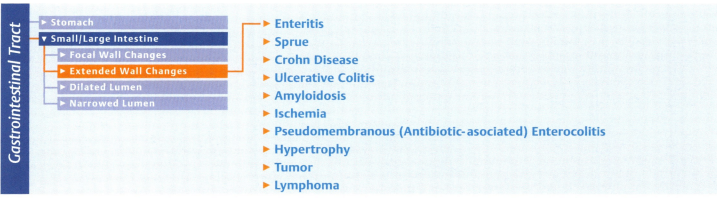

Extended changes in the jejunal, ileal, and colonic wall are primarily due to acute infection or chronic inflammation, while toxic, allergic, ischemic, invasive, and functional causes are much less common. Differential diagnosis has to rule out extended malignant wall changes.

▶ Enteritis

The continuous, extended edematous thickening of the mucosa in enteritis is seen primarily in the ileum but also in the jejunum and colon. There is markedly accentuated wall layering, with the mucosa and/or submucosa being particularly thick, resulting in a narrowed lumen of the bowel. In acute enteritis the intestinal lumen always contains some fluid, even in the fasting state, and this finding is present even before the clinical symptom of diarrhea (**Figs. 7.37–7.41**).

In the small intestine the folds of Kerckring may be pronounced, while in the colon the haustra and folds may intertwine in gyrose fashion. One characteristic sign in the small bowel is vigorous peristalsis that propagates in an orderly antegrade way and does not exhibit any tendency to pendulate. In acute enteritis the colon, too, will demonstrate peristaltic activity. Color-flow Doppler scanning may visualize inflammatory hypervascularity in the intestinal wall that, at least in its initial stages, seems to correlate with the severity of the inflammation. Outside the bowel, ascites may be present, signifying the inflammatory peritoneal reaction, as well as enlarged mesenteric lymphadenopathy.

In severe necrotizing inflammation the peristaltic activity and the inflammatory hypervascularity will subside again. There will be diffuse tenderness along the diseased bowel segment, and the intestinal wall will be characterized by indistinct wall layering; the appearance of gas bubbles has to be regarded as a particularly ominous sign. These gas bubbles will be carried along the venous system of the mesentery and are the cause of portovenous gas embolism in the liver.

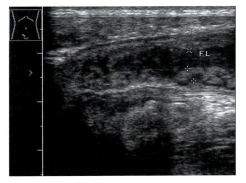

▲ **Fig. 7.37** Infectious enteritis, probably yersiniosis (patient presented clinically with suspected appendicitis). Scan shows "gyral" wall thickening with an accentuated layered structure (cursors) and intraluminal fluid (FL).

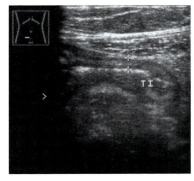

▲ **Fig. 7.38** Microbial invasive enterocolitis (*Campylobacter jejuni*). Scan demonstrates the thickened, layered wall of the terminal ileum (TI, cursors).

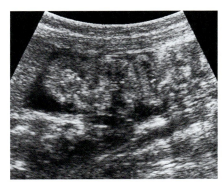

▲ **Fig. 7.39** Enterocolitis with free peritoneal fluid.

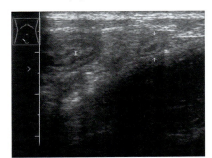

▲ **Fig. 7.40** Acute ileitis with appendicitis, each shown in transverse section: layered wall thickening of the terminal ileum (I) and appendix (arrows; histologically confirmed at operation).

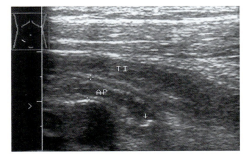

▲ **Fig. 7.41 a and b** Similar appearance as in **Fig. 7.40**, with longitudinal sections of the terminal ileum (TI) and appendix (AP; cursors 4.5 mm). These findings, along with the mesenteric lymph nodes (L in **b**), are suggestive of yersiniosis. Acute appendicitis also requires differentiation from mesenteric lymphadenitis, which may occur in the absence of ileitis and can cause significant lymph node enlargement. D = intestine.

▶ Sprue

Being a special case of enteric reaction, celiac disease is characterized by edema with hypoechoic thickening of the intestinal wall and marked distension of the fluid-filled lumen. The hyperperistaltic loops of the small bowel spin around each other, giving rise to the term "tumbler phenomenon" (**Fig. 7.42**).

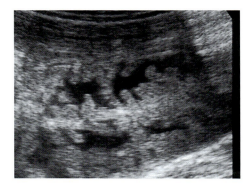
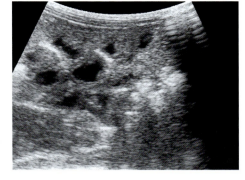

▲ *Fig. 7.42 a and b* Sprue.

▶ Crohn Disease

Crohn disease is a chronic inflammatory bowel disease occurring anywhere in the gastrointestinal tract, with discontinuous extended involvement of individual bowel segments, the primary location being the terminal ileum and colon. In addition to the segmental pattern of the typical pathological changes demonstrated by ultrasound, the type and severity of the most frequent transmural inflammation and its complications, with their wildly mixed and constantly alternating pattern, are characteristic of Crohn disease (**7.3**).

Type of wall change. In Crohn disease various types of change in the intestinal wall can be seen, depending on the transmural severity of the inflammation.

▶ On the one hand, the layering of the wall becomes more pronounced and thickened,

7.3 Crohn Disease

▶ **Accentuated wall, inflammatory hypervascularity**

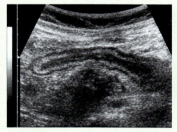
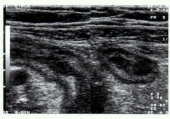
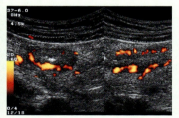

a–d Involving the terminal ileum.
a Terminal ileitis.

b Accentuated layering of the intestinal wall in the terminal ileum.

c Terminal ileitis with inflammatory hypervascularity.

▶ **Colon involvement**

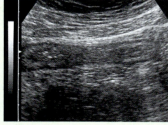
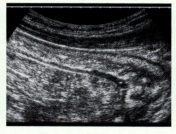
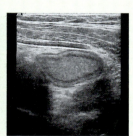

d Crohn colitis.

e Accentuated wall of the descending and sigmoid colon.

f Crohn colitis.

▶ **Complications**

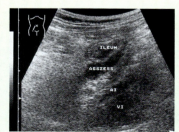
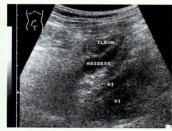
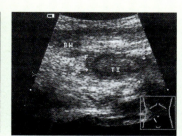

g Crohn colitis, hyperactive phase: hypoechoic swelling of the wall (DW) with loss of all layering. AI = iliac artery; VI = iliac vein.

h–i Complications.
h Accentuated wall of the terminal ileum post appendectomy with abscess formation. AI = iliac artery; VI = iliac vein.

i Crohn disease of the terminal ileum (TI) with a hazy, thickened wall and "mesenteritis" (arrows with echogenic "omental cap"). Fistulous tract (F) leads from the wall-thickened loop of ileum into the abdominal wall (BW). Confirmed at operation.

the intestinal lumen is narrowed, and, because of the impaired peristalsis (inflammatory rigidity), the segment involved may act as functional stenosis.
- On the other hand, the intestinal wall may display a complete loss of normal layering, and diffuse and irregular hypoechoic thickening or hyperechoic widening, which may also result in aperistaltic narrowing of the lumen.

There is a gradual transition from one type of wall change to the other.

Complications. Complications of Crohn disease can be expected to arise from the functional and/or organic stenosis (colicky pain upstream of the stenotic segment, signs of mechanical ileus in the proximal bowel loops) as well as the local inflammation. Apart from local tenderness, color-flow Doppler scanning will reveal inflammatory hypervascularity in the intestinal wall and its vicinity. There will be hyperechoic panniculitis and inflammatory reaction of the greater omentum (hyperechoic halo) as well as complications such as formation of abscesses, fistulas, and conglomerates comprising several loops of bowel.

Sensitivity and specificity in the diagnosis of inflammatory bowel disease are reported between 90.3% and 95%[1, 2]; in detecting strictures a sensitivity and specificity of 100% and 91%, respectively, and in the diagnosis of fistulas 87% and 90%, respectively with a bowel wall thickening of at least 3 mm[3]. Power Doppler has a high accuracy in the detection of disease acitivity[4].

▶ Ulcerative Colitis

Ulcerative colitis is a continuous chronic inflammation of the distal left or even the entire colon. It manifests as an extended homogeneous slight thickening of the colonic wall with clearly identifiable wall layers and a tight lumen. There is neither peristaltic activity nor clear-cut hypervascularity or concurrent reaction of the adjacent tissue. On physical examination, extended diffuse tenderness may be triggered along the pathological gut signature (**Fig. 7.43**).

It seems possible to discriminate severe and moderately extend and activity with a specificity, sensitivity, and diagnostic accuracy of 96%, 90.3%, and 92.9%, respectively[5].

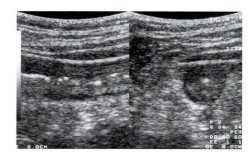
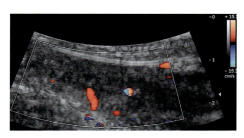

▲ **c** There is no hypervascularity.

▲ **Fig. 7.43** Ulcerative colitis.
a and b Thickened wall of the bowel with tight lumen.

▶ Amyloidosis

Amyloid deposits in the wall of the bowel are a rare finding: they are seen as hyperechoic, homogeneous thickening of the entire intestinal wall with filiform stenosis of the lumen (**Fig. 7.44**), and there is no peristalsis.

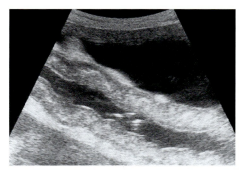
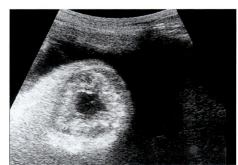

▲ **Fig. 7.44** Amyloidosis.
a Hyperechoic homogeneous thickening of the entire intestinal wall.

▲ **b** Amyloidosis. Filiform narrowing of the lumen.

▶ Ischemia

In acute ischemia there will be edematous swelling of the bowel wall and, while initially the layering of the wall persists, eventually it will end in hypoechoic thickening and narrowing of the lumen. The lack of vascularization (especially since the diseases to be considered in the differential diagnosis tend to be hypervascular) raises the suspicion of a circulation disorder (**Fig. 7.45**).

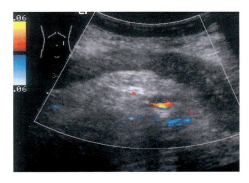

▲ **Fig. 7.45 a–c** Ischemic colitis on the left side.
a Descending colon wall shows hypoechoic swelling that starts abruptly in the distal transverse colon. Color duplex shows no evidence of vascularity.

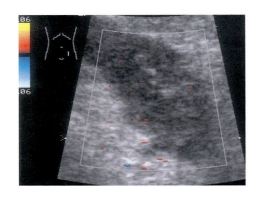
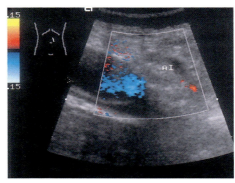

◂◂ **b** Close-up view, caudal end: no vascularity.

◂ **c** Occlusion of the inferior iliac artery (AI) with slight evidence of retrograde flow (red).

▶ Pseudomembranous (Antibiotic-associated) Enterocolitis

This type of colitis is characterized by a marked hypoechoic hypervascular swelling of the intestinal wall (**Fig. 7.46**).

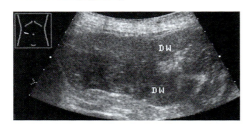

▲ **Fig. 7.46 a–c** Pseudomembranous (antibiotic-associated) pancolitis. The inflammatory wall swelling is most pronounced in the ascending colon and diminishes toward the sigmoid colon.
a Ascending colon: massive, tumorlike wall swelling with loss of the normal layered pattern (DW).

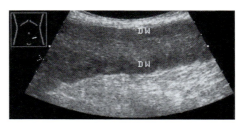

▲ **b** Sigmoid colon: hypoechoic wall swelling with a faint layered pattern (DW)

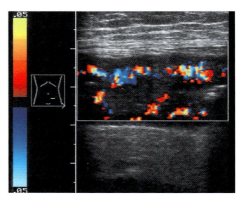

▲ **c** Marked swelling of the intestinal wall, intensive hyporeflectivity, pronounced vascularization.

▶ Hypertrophy

The musculature of the intestinal wall upstream of a stenosis or a functionally stenosed bowel segment will become hypertrophic because of increased activity and will display widening of the outermost hypoechoic layer (muscularis propria) despite the dilated lumen. Typical such examples are the wall of the descending colon and sigmoid in stenotic sigmoid diverticulitis and the prestenotic bowel segments in Crohn disease.

▶ Tumor

Extended tumor growth may mimic diffuse changes in the wall of the bowel and has to be differentiated especially from Crohn disease as well as ischemia; however, these present the typical characteristics of a focal tumor lesion (**Fig. 7.20**). The musculature of the intestinal wall upstream of a stenosis or a functionally stenosed bowel segment will become hypertrophic because of increased activity and will display widening of the outermost hypoechoic layer (muscularis propria) despite the dilated lumen.

▶ Lymphoma

Lymphoma may lead to extended diffuse involvement of the bowel wall.

Dilated Lumen

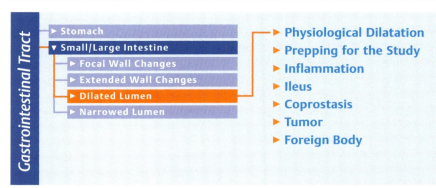

Small intestine. Under physiological conditions no chyme can be demonstrated in the small intestine (hence its name "intestinum jejunum": empty intestine). Oral intake of food and fluid will result, after some delay (temporary retention of the ingesta in the stomach), in a dilated lumen of the small bowel. Demonstration of fluid within the intestinal lumen in the fasting patient has to be regarded as pathological; further differentiation should include the size of the lumen, peristaltic activity, and the wall changes.

Large intestine. Because of its storage function, the large bowel is always full of scybala and air and therefore the sonographic assessment of its diameter is irrelevant. In pathological conditions or when particular types of bowel preparation are employed, fluid or sonolucent chyme can be visualized in the lumen, in which case the diameter of the lumen, particularly any change in lumen diameter, can be assessed during the sonographic study.

▶ Physiological Dilatation

Fluid can be demonstrated in the small intestine within just a few minutes after oral intake; the lumen becomes fluid-filled in segmental fashion, waves of contraction alternating with distension of the intestinal loops and propelling the column of ingesta forward. The loops of small bowel display a normal wall texture. In those jejunal segments filled with fluid, the Kerckring's folds will be visualized as fine corrugations, while at the ileum the intraluminal surface will be smooth. Even a distended lumen will not have a diameter exceeding 15–20 mm, and during contraction the bowel will be wrung dry; here, the loops of the small bowel will evidence a thick muscular layer. The fine film of remaining fluid permits excellent delineation of the mucosa as well.

▶ Prepping for the Study

Specific loading by oral fluid uptake for sonographic Sellink studies or rectal enemas for hydrocolonic sonography (HCS) permit assessment of changes in the lumen and of focal and extended changes in the intestinal wall, detection and localization of circumscribed obstructions and stenosis, and especially assessment of the peristalsis.

▶ Inflammation

In a fasting patient suffering from enteritis, the intestinal lumen will exhibit some fluid, but here the dilatation is less than after oral intake and rarely goes beyond a luminal diameter of 10 mm (**Fig. 7.47**). The primary aspect is edematous thickening of the intestinal wall of varying degree, accompanied by vigorous or even swirling hyperperistalsis characterized by constant alternation between contraction and dilation without any rest in these phases. During their peristaltic movements the loops of the small bowel constantly change their location. Other findings in enteritis may be the signs of peritonism (free intra-abdominal fluid) as well as regional lymphadenopathy.

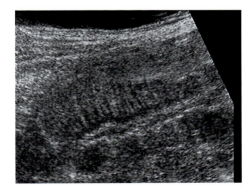

◀ **Fig. 7.47** Enteritis with a thin film of fluid covering the folds of Kerckring in the jejunum.

▶ Ileus

The leading sonographic sign of ileus is distension of the bowel. In the small intestine this dilatation of the lumen may be several centimeters. The lumen is filled with fluid (in the small bowel) or echogenic chyme (in the large bowel and in chronic ileus). Because of the constant filling of the lumen, the intestinal wall can be assessed quite well at the intraluminal surface. The Kerckring's folds in the small bowel appear rigid, giving rise to the so-called "piano key phenomenon," and in the large intestine the haustra are easily identifiable. Despite the dilatation, with increasing duration and severity of the damage the intestinal wall itself may appear thickened and full of edema (■ 7.4).

Peristalsis. The most important sonographic criterion in the differential diagnosis of ileus is assessment of the peristaltic movement. The early stages of mechanical ileus will demonstrate vigorous peristaltic activity of the wall, which, however, is ineffective and only results in incomplete contraction. The intraluminal column of fluid exhibits pendulating peristalsis, while during the later stages the unsuccessful peristalsis of the intestinal wall will cease completely. The intraluminal fluid will slosh back and forth gently and finally will simply stop moving. This stage of the mechanical ileus can no longer be differentiated from paralytic ileus, with the same rigidly distended lumen, thickened wall, and signs of peritonism (free fluid). The possible causes of mechanical ileus are summarized in **Table 7.6**.

Table 7.6 The causes of mechanical ileus

- Adhesions
- Tumor
- Hernia
- Inflammatory stenosis (Crohn disease)
- Intussusception
- Volvulus and torsion
- Gallstone
- Foreign body

The Various Types of Ileus

Ultrasound may be able to diagnose ileus six hours before it shows up on regular radiographic films.

All types of ileus. All types of ileus are characterized by significant distension of the lumen, signs of wall thickening (edema, hypertrophy), and finally signs of peritonitis with demonstration of an increasing amount of free fluid between the bowel loops. The typical air–fluid interfaces have a sonographic counterpart: with the patient supine, the air-filled intestinal loops will block imaging with the probe on the anterior abdominal wall, while a study with the probe on the lateral abdominal wall will demonstrate quite well the intestinal loops, distended by the fluid/chyme, and their peristalsis, thus permitting better differentiation of the ileus.

Mechanical ileus. Initially this will demonstrate hyperperistalsis in those intestinal segments upstream of the obstruction, which itself can quite often be visualized sonographically, but the chyme/fluid will no longer be propelled in a directed fashion. In addition to antegrade "squirty" movements, more and more retropulsion (backward sloshing) becomes evident as well as pendulating motion of the intraluminal fluid. During the late stages of mechanical ileus this hyperperistalsis will disappear completely, the intestinal wall will be seen to initiate some ineffective efforts of contraction, and the intraluminal column of fluid sloshes back and forth gently until it finally rests. Downstream of the mechanical obstruction the bowel will be contracted, demonstrating a collapsed lumen and lacking any obvious peristaltic activity (so-called starvation gut).

Paralytic ileus. This type of ileus is characterized by luminal distension, thickening of the wall, and the signs of peritonism (free fluid). The intestinal wall does not exhibit any peristaltic activity and the intraluminal column of fluid is static; this situation cannot be differentiated from advanced mechanical ileus, unless it is possible to visualize the cause underlying the mechanical obstruction.

■ 7.4 Ileus

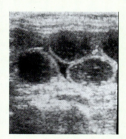

a Ileus with peritonism and rigid distended ileal loops.

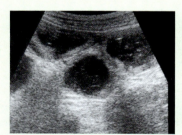

b Chronic ileus.

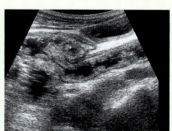

c Ileocecum in chronic ileus (stenotic tumor of the hepatic flexure).

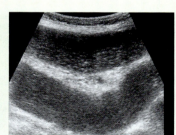

d Chronic ileus in incarcerated inguinal hernia (**Fig. 7.36**).

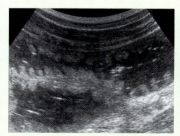

e Chronic ileus of the small bowel with distended lumen and edematous thickened Kerckring's folds.

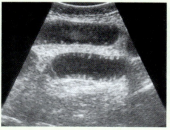

f Rigid Kerckring's folds displaying the so-called piano key phenomenon.

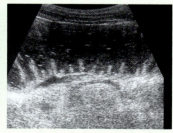

g In addition, free fluid signifying peritonism.

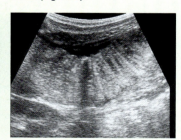

h Free fluid in peritonism and intramural gas in the jejunal wall.

▶ Coprostasis

The colon filled with gas or feces can be identified by its prominent arching haustra, which would be a perfectly normal finding, intensified however in coprostasis. In the irritable bowel syndrome, local tenderness may often be elicited along the course of the colon.

▶ Tumor

A large polypoid tumor may fill the lumen completely. It may be identified by indirect signs (e.g., as cause of mechanical ileus) or the visualization of tumor vessels in the polypoid mass may facilitate the differentiation of tumor from feces. A possible complication is the tumor acting as the leading point in intussusception.

▶ Foreign Body

It is the rare exception for foreign bodies to be identified and located as such; quite often, it is possible only if they are sufficiently large to produce complete obstruction with subsequent mechanical ileus.

Narrowed Lumen

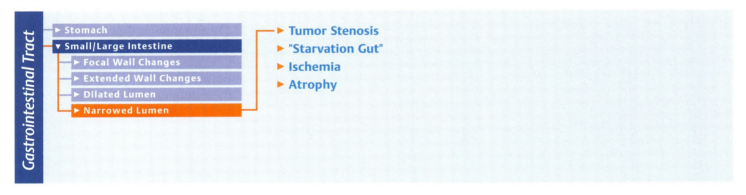

The lumen may be narrowed by changes in the bowel wall (tumor, inflammation, invasion) or by external effects (adhesions, tumor, hernia).

▶ Tumor Stenosis

Carcinomas that grow primarily in circular fashion, but also off-center, as well as lymphomas can narrow the lumen until there is a filiform stenosis, and finally a complete stoppage with the full-blown clinical picture of mechanical ileus (**Fig. 7.48**). Apart from the pathological gut signature of the tumor, ultrasonography can demonstrate the distended intestinal loops proximal of the obstruction, while downstream there is the poststenotic "starvation gut" (see below).

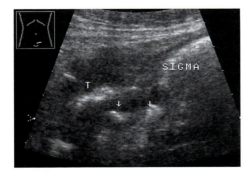

◀ **Fig. 7.48** Sigmoid carcinoma. Solid, hypoechoic tumor mass (T). Prestenotic dilatation of the sigmoid colon, markedly overdistended with gas (echogenic zone with an acoustic shadow obscuring the posterior wall). Arrows = diverticulum.

▶ "Starvation Gut"

Compared with the distended intestinal loops proximal to the obstruction, in mechanical ileus the bowel segment distal to the obstruction will be contracted and empty.

▶ Ischemia

In chronic ischemia there is extended hyperechoic thickening of the intestinal wall with a markedly narrowed lumen.

▶ Atrophy

Bypassed intestinal loops demonstrate a constricted lumen.

References
1. Schwerk WB BK, Raith M. A prospective evaluation of high-resolution sonography in the diagnosis of inflammatory bowel disease. Eur J Gastroenterol Hepatol 1992;4:173–182
2. Solvig J, Eckberg O, Lindgren S, et al. Ultrasound examination of the small bowel: Comparison with enteroclysis in patients with Crohn's disease. Abdom Imaging 1995;20;323–326
3. Gasche C, Moser G, Turetschek K, Schober E, Moeschl P, Oberhuber G. Gut 1999;44:112–117
4. Neye H, Voderholzer W, Rickes S, Weber J, Wermke W, Lochs H. Evaluation of criteria for the activity of Crohn's disease by power Doppler sonography. Digestive Diseases 2004;22:67–72
5. Arienti V, Campieri M, Boriani L, et al. Management of severe ulcerative colitis with the help of high-resolution ultrasonography. Am J Gastroenterol 1996;91(10):2163–9

8 Peritoneal Cavity

Peritoneal Cavity 251

Diffuse Changes 254

Anechoic Structure 256
- Cirrhosis of the Liver
- Heart Failure
- Peritonitis
- Hypoalbuminemia
- Peritoneal Carcinomatosis
- Hemoperitoneum

Hypoechoic Structure 258
- Pancreatitis
- Cirrhosis of the Liver with SBP (Spontaneous Bacterial Peritonitis)
- Peritoneal Carcinomatosis
- Purulent Peritonitis
- Tuberculosis
- Choleperitoneum
- Hemoperitoneum
- GI Tract Perforation
- Chyloperitoneum

Hyperechoic Structure 261
- Pneumoperitoneum

Localized Changes 262

Anechoic Structure 263
- Septated Ascites
- Intra-abdominal Abscess

Hypoechoic Structure 264
- Abscess
- Bilioma
- Hematoma
- Necrosis after Pancreatitis

Hyperechoic Structure 265
- Localized Perforation
- Gas Abscess

Wall Structures 266

Smooth Margin 266
- Right-Sided Heart Failure
- Cirrhosis
- Peritoneal Carcinomatosis

Irregular Margin 267
- Pancreatitis
- Peritonitis
- Peritoneal Carcinomatosis

Differentiating Intra- and Extra-luminal GI Tract Fluid 269

Intragastric Processes 269
- Gastric Outlet Obstruction

Intraintestinal Processes 270
- Duodenal Stenosis
- Small Bowel Obstruction
- Large Bowel Obstruction

8 Peritoneal Cavity

D. Nuernberg

Anatomy

Definition
▶ Capillary space between the parietal and visceral peritoneum

Synonyms
▶ Peritoneal cavity
▶ Greater peritoneal cavity
▶ Intraperitoneal space
▶ Abdominal cavity
▶ Intra-abdominal space

The abdominal organs (viscera) are invested by a thin serous membrane, the so-called visceral peritoneum, while its continuation lining the abdominal wall (parietes) is known as the parietal peritoneum. The peritoneum continuously transudes serous fluid, thus enabling the organs, lined by the visceral peritoneum, to glide over each other. Since the peritoneum reabsorbs this peritoneal fluid constantly, the imaging modalities will not be able to demonstrate any significant amount of fluid. Thus, the peritoneal cavity usually exists as a "peritoneal gap" and is that space that can be visualized sonographically only in pathological conditions. A true space or cavity exists only if fluid or another substrate collects in the gap between the visceral and parietal peritoneum (intraperitoneal position).

Intraperitoneal fluid may stem from hypersecretion or impaired absorption, e.g., when there is inflammation (peritonitis). This intraperitoneal fluid may also arise from injuries of fluid-filled organs, e.g., bleeding (hemoperitoneum) or perforation of the bile system (choleperitoneum) or the gastrointestinal (GI) tract. Another reason for these fluid collections may be pressure changes in the venous system (right-sided heart failure, portal hypertension). The peritoneal cavity may contain not only collections of fluid but also gas and solid matter.

Topography

If an organ is completely invested by peritoneum it is called 'intraperitoneal' (e.g., stomach, spleen, liver, small intestine, transverse and sigmoid colon, ovaries). Retroperitoneal organs are the kidneys, adrenal glands, aorta, and vena cava. If only the anterior part of an organ is invested by peritoneum and otherwise it is directly fixed to the posterior abdominal wall, it is also regarded as being retroperitoneal (e.g., pancreas, descending part of the duodenum).

The reflections of the peritoneum divide it into different abdominal compartments. **Figures 8.1–8.4** illustrate this concept. The significance of these compartments becomes evident when the question arises whether there is diffuse fluid within the peritoneal cavity or if it only involves certain subspaces (e.g., in "trapped" ascites).

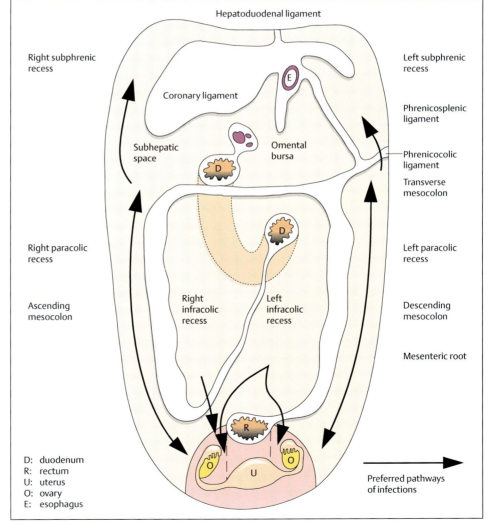

▲ **Fig. 8.1** Peritoneal reflections and the recesses thus created (based on reference 2).

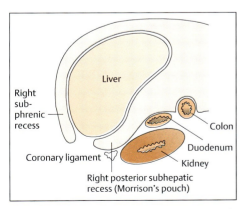

▲ **Fig. 8.2** Delineation and correlation of the longitudinal recesses on the right (based on reference 2).

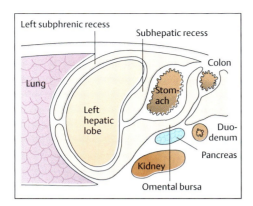

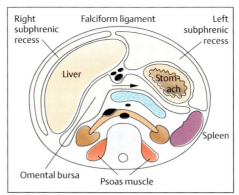

Fig. 8.3 Delineation and correlation of the longitudinal recesses in the midclavicular line (based on reference 2).

Fig. 8.4 Delineation and correlation of the transverse recesses (based on reference 2).

Ultrasound Morphology

The peritoneum itself cannot be demonstrated by ultrasound since it does not exhibit a large enough impedance gradient. However, in ultrasound studies of the viscera it seems to be an integral part of their boundary layers, e.g., the hepatic surfaces, the boundary layer between the liver and the right kidney, the splenic surfaces, and the inner lining of the abdominal wall, and therefore appears as a hyperechoic band investing the capsule of the organ. When the visceral relations change (for instance, between liver and right kidney) the "gliding" motion of the peritoneum becomes quite evident (**Fig. 8.5**).

Visualization of the peritoneal *space* implies the presence of pathology! But there is always an exception to the rule: in menstruating young females a scant amount of free fluid can be demonstrated in Douglas's pouch. The same is true in patients after abdominal surgery.

Ultrasonography of the Peritoneal Cavity

- Sonographic accessibility
- Preferred localization for fluid and/or gas collections
- Classification as to intraperitoneal, extraperitoneal, and retroperitoneal location
- Retroperitoneal space

Fluid collections. Fluid collections are seen as anechoic/hypoechoic structures between the abdominal viscera. Owing to gravity, fluid will always collect in the dependent areas, i.e., while recumbent in the posterior parts of the body and while upright in the lower abdomen (**Fig. 8.6**).

Preferred localizations for fluid (anechoic/hypoechoic) collections are (◻ 8.1 a–f):
- Perihepatic right
- Perihepatic left
- Subhepatic right (between the right lobe of the liver and the right kidney = Morrison's pouch)
- Subphrenic
- Perisplenic
- Omental bursa
- Douglas's pouch, perivesical
- Between the bowel loops (characteristic for ascites)
- Pericolic ("paracolic gutter")
- Below the abdominal wall (knee-elbow position).

Gas collections. The accumulation of free intra-abdominal gas may result in the formation of hyperechoic structures. Physics dictates that gas will rise, and therefore it will be found in locations different from those for fluid, i.e., in the more superior regions such as the subphrenic recess (**Fig. 8.7**, see ◻ 8.1 g–i).

Knowledge of these preferred localizations helps to identify substrates and recesses: *when the patient is repositioned, fluids will gravitate to the more dependent parts of the abdominal cavity while gases will rise.*

Extraperitoneal and intraperitoneal location. Determination whether a formation is intraperitoneal, extraperitoneal, or retroperitoneal may be quite difficult. Visualization of the organ surfaces is the most decisive factor in this correlation; in the case of fluid collections in the gastrointestinal tract, precise correlation requires demonstration of the stomach or bowel wall. Differential diagnosis becomes especially problematic when the fluid or gas does not relocate upon patient repositioning. This repositioning does not produce any significant alterations in extraperitoneal and retroperitoneal formations.

Differentiating intraluminal air within the GI tract from hyperechoic intra-abdominal structures (gas collections) can become rather difficult (◻ 8.2a and b).

Retroperitoneal space. Here too this space as such may only be demonstrated by the organs it contains or by collections of foreign structures such as fluid, gas, or solid tissue. The retroperitoneal space is delineated by correlating it with the retroperitoneal organs, e.g., the kidneys, large vessels, or pancreas (◻ 8.2 c–h).

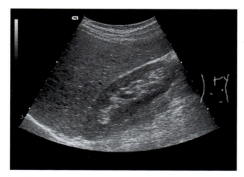

▲ *Fig. 8.5* The hyperechoic boundary between the right hepatic lobe and the right kidney (Morrison's pouch) is formed by the surfaces of these two viscera and the investing peritoneum.

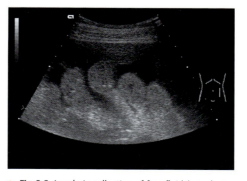

▲ *Fig. 8.6* Anechoic collection of free fluid (e.g., hepatogenous ascites) within the peritoneal cavity, characterized by the bowel loops floating in the fluid.

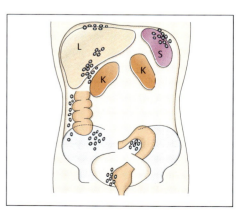

▲ *Fig. 8.7* Gas collection as sequela of GI tract perforation (based on reference 1). L = liver; K = kidney; S = spleen.

8.1 Gas and Fluid Collections within the Peritoneal Cavity

▶ **Fluid collections**

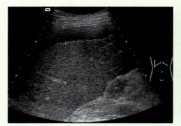

a Perihepatic: anechoic film anterior and lateral to the right hepatic lobe. Ascites due to alcoholic cirrhosis. The amount of ascites may be guessed by the thickness of the film.

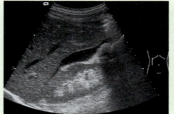

b Morrison's pouch: already there is a small amount of free fluid in the hepatorenal recess, seen as anechoic gap between the liver and kidney. Malignant ascites in ovarian cancer.

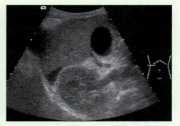

c Subhepatic: free fluid below the liver in the right transverse plane; ascites (transudate) in right cardiac failure. The hyperechoic delineation anterior to the kidney corresponds with the peritoneum plus the renal capsule.

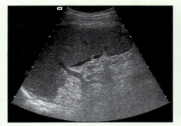

d Perisplenic: anechoic film around the spleen, particularly at the hilum. In the presence of just a minute amount of fluid only hypoechoic organ surfaces will be visualized.

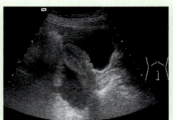

e Douglas's pouch: in the lesser pelvis even minute amounts of fluid can be demonstrated. In this longitudinal plane the uterus is bathed by the fluid.

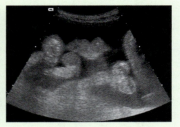

f Interenteric: in the presence of large amounts of free intra-abdominal fluid the bowel loops float in the fluid and weave around like underwater plants ("sea anemone phenomenon").

▶ **Gas collections**

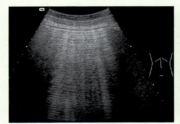

g Hyperechoic intra-abdominal mass caused by free air. Note the characteristic reverberations.

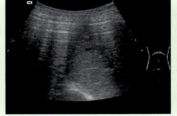

h Characteristic image of the hyperechoic gas collection anterior to the left hepatic lobe in the transverse plane, with the patient supine. The left hepatic lobe can be seen between the "curtain" of free air.

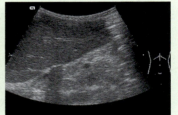

i Gas collection inferior to the left hepatic lobe; visible in the longitudinal plane and posterior to the left hepatic lobe in the area around the perforation (duodenal ulcer).

8.2 Correlation of Extraperitoneal or Intraperitoneal Location

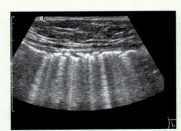

a Intraluminal air within the GI tract. Compared with the free air anterior to the reverberation artifacts, the multi-layered bowel wall is demonstrated.

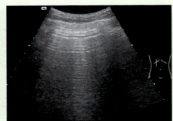

b In a free perforation, repositioning the patient will not yield any changes and the wall of the GI tract will not be visualized.

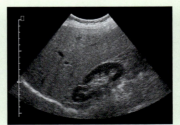

c The cardinal structures of the retroperitoneal space are its viscera, e.g., the kidneys.

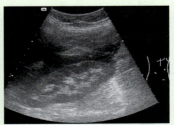

d Intraperitoneal and retroperitoneal hypoechoic masses anterior to and around the right kidney in status post rupture of the bile duct, with bile leaking into the peritoneal cavity and the retroperitoneal space.

8.2 Correlation of Extraperitoneal or Intraperitoneal Location

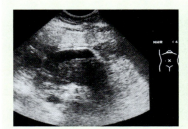 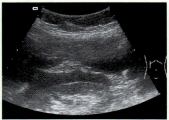 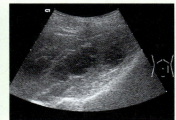 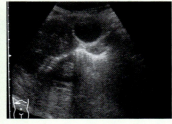

e Peripancreatic hypoechoic mass; fluid collection anterior to the head of the pancreas in acute hemorrhagic pancreatitis.

f Hypoechoic film enveloping the right kidney in retroperitoneal bile collection due to a lesion during endoscopy of the bile duct.

g Inhomogeneous hypoechoic retroperitoneal mass on the left, particularly in the left psoas muscle: hematoma in coumarin anticoagulant overdosage.

h Hyperechoic band anterior to the right kidney and posterior to the gallbladder and duodenum: pneumoperitoneum due to retroperitoneal perforation during ERCP.

Diffuse Changes

Diffuse intra-abdominal formations may either be anechoic, hypoechoic (echogenic!), or hyperechoic (**Table 8.1**). Patient repositioning will alter the sonographic image of this diffuse distribution, an almost pathognomonic characteristic. The formation will change its location and can be visualized in different compartments.

Amount. The bigger the collection, the better this effect will be noted. In anechoic substrates (fluid) a small volume of 5–10 ml can already be demonstrated, particularly within Morrison's pouch. Between the bowel loops (preferred localization of ascites) and within Douglas's pouch very small amounts may also become visible. An amount of about 700–1000 ml is required to become clinically detectable! When the collection is large (several hundred milliliters, or liters), if not all compartments then at least several compartments will be involved. The "floating" loops of the small intestine in the anechoic fluid are particularly impressive (so-called "sea anemone phenomenon," **Fig. 8.9**).

Determination of the volume involved can be fraught with problems. Some authors rely on the width of the right perihepatic film with the patient supine (1 cm = approx. 1 liter; 2 cm = 1.5 liter; 3 cm = 2 liters) (**Fig. 8.10**). When the patient is sitting or standing, the fluid will gravitate into Douglas's pouch and the amount can be approximated by the ellipsoid method: $0.5 \times h \times w \times l$ (**Fig. 8.11**). Rule-of-thumb approximation is more practicable than exactness in the form x milliliters, x hundred milliliters, or x liters. Follow-up studies by one and the same sonographer have proved to be rather helpful and may sometimes determine the course of treatment.

Table 8.1 **The echogenicity of diffusely distributed substrates**

Echogenicity	Substrate	Contents	Translucency
Anechoic	Fluid	Transudate Exudates Blood (early phase)	Good translucency; surroundings can be assessed
Hypoechoic (echogenic)	Fluid	Exudate Blood (late phase) Bile Pus Chyle	Good translucency; surroundings can be assessed
Hyperechoic	Gas	Gas/air (pus + gas)	No translucency; reverberation artifacts; severely curtailed assessment of the surroundings

Origin. The origin of peritoneal fluid collections (ascites) may be quite varied (**Table 8.2**). The rate at which a particular type of ascites is observed depends on the profession of the sonographer and the patient population studied. In gastroenterology ascites tends to be hepatogenic in origin; in oncology malignant ascites prevails; while in gynecology ascites may be due to ovarian cancer or ectopic pregnancy, and hemoperitoneum will be most common in the surgical emergency room. The makeup

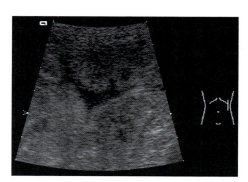

▲ **Fig. 8.8** Minute fluid collection between the bowel loops (several milliliters) resembling an obtuse angle.

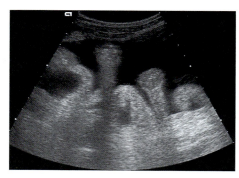

▲ **Fig. 8.9** "Sea anemone phenomenon": in the case of large amounts of diffusely distributed free fluid the bowel loops will float unencumbered in the fluid.

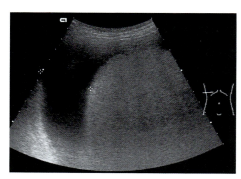

▲ **Fig. 8.10** When "guesstimating" the amount of free fluid, the distance between the surface of the liver and the lateral abdominal wall is a good marker.

Table 8.2 Origin of intra-abdominal fluid collections (by organ)

Hepatogenic/portal	Cirrhosis, portal vein thrombosis, Budd-Chiari syndrome
Peritoneal	Peritoneal carcinomatosis, peritonitis
Cardiac	Right-sided heart failure
Pancreatogenous	Acute/chronic pancreatitis
Ovarian	Ectopic pregnancy, ovarian cancer
Vascular	Portal hypertension, ruptured vessel
Chylous	Lymphatic aplasia

Table 8.3 Type of ascites by origin and its rate

Cirrhosis	30–50%
Malignancy	30–50%
Cardiac origin	10–15%
Other origins	10%

of a patient population with ascites seen in a regular hospital is listed in **Table 8.3**.

The most important parameters for the differential diagnosis of intra-abdominal fluid are patient history, clinical signs, distribution of the fluid in the ultrasound study, sonographic morphology, and finally ultrasound-guided fine-needle paracentesis (**Fig. 8.12**).

Figure 8.13 illustrates an algorithm for the differential diagnosis in ascites, based on diagnostic paracentesis.

The differential diagnosis of fluid collections within the peritoneal cavity is quite varied; an overview is listed in **Table 8.4**.

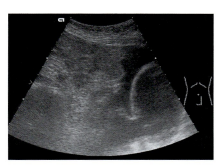

▲ **Fig. 8.11** The amount of free fluid in the lesser pelvis (Douglas's pouch) may also be "guesstimated" when viewed in the longitudinal plane. Since this is a dependant region of the body, even minute amounts of fluid can be detected here.

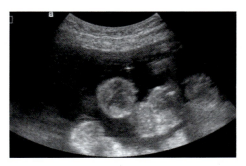

▲ **Fig. 8.12** Ultrasound-guided fine-needle paracentesis in the differential diagnosis of ascites. The tip of the needle is visible as a small echogenic structure anterior to the bowel loops. Ultrasound guidance will help avoid injuries to intra-abdominal structures.

Ultrasound-guided Fine-needle Paracentesis

Quite often the clinical data and the patient's history, supplemented by ultrasound morphology and the pattern of distribution, are not enough to confirm the precise type of ascites. Ultrasound-guided fine-needle paracentesis is an efficient and proven method with few potential complications that can help ascertain the final diagnosis. For diagnostic purposes it uses needles of up to 3Fr (1 mm diameter), while bigger needles are employed in therapeutic procedures.

Ultrasound targeting. Ultrasound targeting helps to avoid injury to vascular structures on the inside of the abdominal wall (e.g., internal Medusa's head) as well as dry aspiration due to the tip of the needle adhering to tissue. Furthermore, it permits atypical needle insertion sites in the left lower quadrant (inverse McBurney's point). While any site may be selected, the distance to the target should be as short as possible and also should avoid any obstacles, such as the bowel, omentum, etc.

Laboratory studies. If fluid can be aspirated, thus confirming the suspected ultrasound diagnosis of "free fluid," it first undergoes gross examination; this will allow the ascites to be classified as transudate/exudate, blood, bile, pus, urine, or chyle. Then the liquid substrate is subjected to additional cytological, bacteriological, and other laboratory studies.

While one aspiration would be enough for the laboratory panel, in the case of peritoneal carcinomatosis cytology sometimes requires several aspirations and work-ups. The sensitivity depends directly on the number of aspirations. If a malignant fluid collection is suspected clinically and the cytology is negative, the fine-needle aspiration has to be repeated. For differential diagnosis, the following laboratory parameters are cardinal findings:

Protein	↑ in exudate
Amylase, lipase	↑ in pancreatogenous ascites
Hemoglobin	↑ in status post bleeding
Granulocytes	↑ in peritonitis
Cholesterol	↑ in malignant ascites
Tumor cells	↑ in malignant ascites
Bacteria	↑ in peritonitis

Table 8.4 Differential diagnosis of intraperitoneal fluid (based on reference 7)

Transudate (anechoic)	Exudate (anechoic or echogenic)	Hemorrhage	Postoperative, posttraumatic (echogenic)
Cirrhosis of the liver	Peritoneal carcinomatosis	Trauma	Hematoma
Budd–Chiari syndrome	Peritonitis	Iatrogenic	Seroma
Right-sided heart failure	Pancreatitis	Ectopic pregnancy	Biloma
Inferior vena cava syndrome	Tuberculosis	Coagulation disorder	Urinoma
Nephrotic syndrome	Peritoneal dialysis	Ruptured abdominal aortic aneurysm	Chyme
Mesenteric venous thrombosis	Mesothelioma		Contents of a cyst
Hypoalbuminemia			Lymphocele (chyliform ascites)

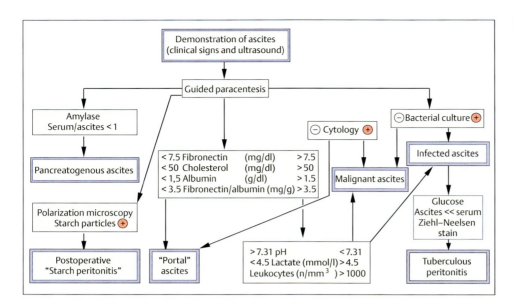

◀ **Fig. 8.13** Algorithm for differentiating ascites by diagnostic paracentesis (based on reference 9)

Anechoic Structure

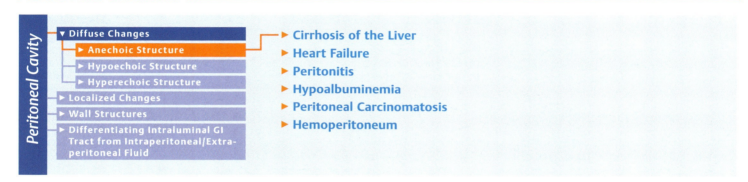

Transudate. Most anechoic intra-abdominal masses are transudates. There are no fine particles floating in the fluid, no strands of fibrin, and no irregularities in the wall, examples being cirrhosis of the liver, heart failure, and peritoneal carcinomatosis. During its early phase, acute hemorrhage after blunt abdominal trauma may also appear as anechoic fluid!

▶ Cirrhosis of the Liver

In most cases ascites in cirrhosis with hepatic failure is anechoic (**Fig. 8.14**). When the patient is being repositioned it will shift location and may be demonstrated in all compartments. The underlying disease can be diagnosed quite easily based on the organ changes in the liver: altered shape, outline, size, intrahepatic vascular pattern, and the extrahepatic signs of portal hypertension, splenomegaly, and portovenous shunts (collaterals) (see ▣ **2.2, p. 56,** and ▣ **2.7, p. 73**). The irregular surface of the liver and the splenomegaly are the easiest and most reliable signs to detect.

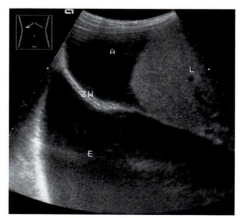
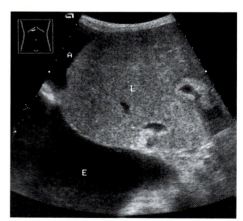

▲ **Fig. 8.14** Diffuse collection of anechoic fluid in alcoholic cirrhosis of the liver.
a Transverse view high up in the upper right quadrant: ascites (A) and pleural effusion (E); the abdominal and thoracic cavity are separated by the echogenic diaphragm (ZW). L = liver.

▲ **b** Coarsely structured hepatic parenchyma, changes in the vascular pattern, rounded margin.

▶ Heart Failure

Transudate in decompensated right-sided heart failure is a late symptom and appears after or concomitant with pleural effusion (right > left). Apart from the general clinical signs, ultrasound will demonstrate a markedly wide and rigid inferior vena cava and wide hepatic veins (with pronounced starlike junction) as definite signs firming up the suspected diagnosis **(Fig. 8.15)**.

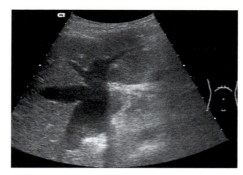

▲ *Fig. 8.15* Right-sided heart failure.
a The wide and rigid inferior vena cava and the wide hepatic veins are characteristic for right ventricular failure.

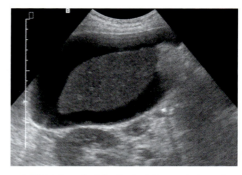

▲ ***b*** Right hepatic lobe bathed in anechoic ascites (transudate) in decompensated right-sided heart failure.

▶ Peritonitis

Inflammation and infection in the peritoneal cavity mostly result in exudates, and thus in echogenic ascites with strands of fibrin and septation. If there is only a small amount of hypersecretion, e.g., in viral infection with polyserositis, the ascites may also be anechoic **(Fig. 8.16)**. Markedly purulent peritonitis is characterized by echogenic contents, adhesions, and bowel loops that no longer glide unencumbered. In "spontaneous bacterial peritonitis" (SBP) complicating decompensated cirrhosis of the liver, there will often be fine echoes within the fluid.

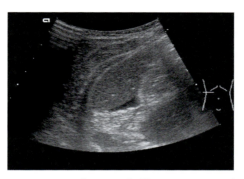

▲ *Fig. 8.16 a* Small amount of subhepatic ascites in viral polyserositis (accompanied by pleural and pericardial effusion = multicavity effusion).

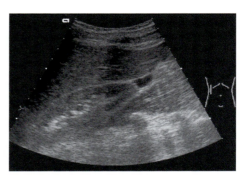

▲ ***b*** Small 'angle of ascites' between the right hepatic lobe and the inferior pole of the right kidney in concomitant viral peritonitis.

▶ Hypoalbuminemia

Irrespective of its origin, protein deficiency with a markedly low level of plasma albumin may result in the production of a hypoechoic transudate. In these cases the wall of the gallbladder is thicker than normal (> 3 mm). Apart from this observation, the liver appears unchanged and there are no wide veins. Laboratory studies will yield further diagnostic clues.

▶ Peritoneal Carcinomatosis

The malignant ascites in peritoneal carcinomatosis may also be anechoic **(Figs. 8.17 and 8.18)**, but internal echoes within the fluid are much more common. In anechoic ascites, the lack of any signs for cirrhosis of the liver or portal hypertension on the one hand and the demonstration of a possible primary tumor or metastases on the other will lead one to suspect the malignant origin. A detailed discussion of the ultrasound criteria differentiating between benign and malignant ascites is found in the section on "Wall Structures" below.

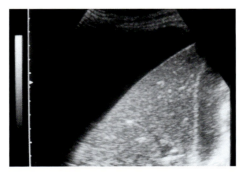

▲ *Fig. 8.17* Anechoic ascites enveloping the liver in peritoneal carcinomatosis of metastatic gastric cancer. Most often peritoneal carcinomatosis will display echoes within the fluid, but it may also be anechoic.

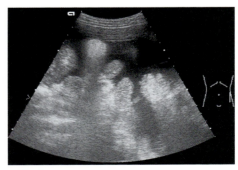

▲ *Fig. 8.18* Anechoic malignant ascites in advanced gastric cancer. The retracted mesentery pulls together the bowel loops quite clearly.

▶ Hemoperitoneum

During its early phase, acute bleeding into the peritoneal cavity after blunt abdominal trauma, iatrogenic injury, in ectopic pregnancy, or drug induced (e.g., anticoagulation therapy) will also demonstrate an anechoic fluid collection (**Fig. 8.19**). However, as time passes (hours) there will be echogenic internal echoes due to strands of fibrin that are formed while coagulation sets in. History, clinical signs, and the changing ultrasound image will firm up the diagnosis in 95–98% of cases.

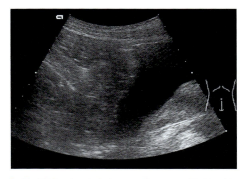

▲ **Fig. 8.19 a** Anechoic hemoperitoneum with blood in the lesser pelvis after blunt abdominal trauma. With the passage of time there will be echoes and strands of fibrin, indicating the beginning of organization.

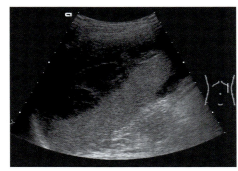

▲ **b** This massive hemoperitoneum was caused by a marked splenic lesion. The hematoma encompasses more than 50% of the organ, while at the inferior pole of the spleen there is free blood indicating open rupture.

Hypoechoic Structure

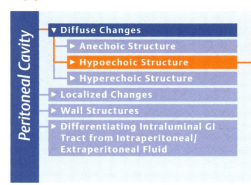

- ▶ Pancreatitis
- ▶ Cirrhosis of the Liver with SBP (Spontaneous Bacterial Peritonitis)
- ▶ Peritoneal Carcinomatosis
- ▶ Purulent Peritonitis
- ▶ Tuberculosis
- ▶ Choleperitoneum
- ▶ Hemoperitoneum
- ▶ GI Tract perforation
- ▶ Chyloperitoneum

Exudate. In most cases, the hypoechoic intra-abdominal liquid structure displaying fine internal echoes or septation will be an exudate. Strandlike structures adhering to the lateral abdominal wall or the visceral peritoneum are also rather characteristic. These strands of fibrin will demonstrate a classic swinging or undulating motion with the shifting intra-abdominal fluid. Examples of echogenic ascites are pancreatogenous ascites and the ascites in purulent peritonitis. Ascites permeated by fine floating echoes may be present in spontaneous bacterial peritonitis (SBP), a classic complication of decompensated cirrhosis of the liver. However, echogenic internal echoes within the fluid have been demonstrated in peritoneal carcinomatosis as well.

▶ Pancreatitis

In many cases of acute or recurrent pancreatitis exudation into the free peritoneal cavity will be seen. This is more true for necrotizing pancreatitis than for the hemorrhagic type. In severe cases, all compartments are involved, presenting the full-blown picture of pancreatogenous ascites. The latter may be anechoic, although internal echoes and septation as well as irregularities in the walls are much more common (**Figs. 8.20 and 8.21**). The ultrasound image is characterized by floating strands of fibrin. The inflammatory changes in the pancreas itself (necrosis and other signs of pancreatitis as well as vascular changes) are also important for the diagnosis. If the clinical signs and ultrasound study do not result in a firm diagnosis, ultrasound-guided fine-needle paracentesis, with high levels of amylase and lipase in the ascites will prove the pancreatic origin.

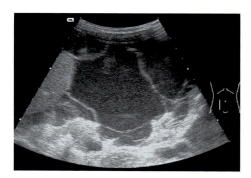

▲ **Fig. 8.20** Echogenic ascites with numerous strands of fibrin ("waving flag") resulting in septation; pancreatogenous ascites in acute necrotizing pancreatitis.

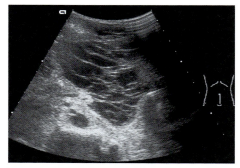

▲ **Fig. 8.21** Complete septation in the lower abdomen, classic honeycomb pattern in pancreatogenous ascites (necrotizing pancreatitis). Similar images will also be seen in tuberculous ascites.

▶ Cirrhosis of the Liver with SBP (Spontaneous Bacterial Peritonitis)

Decompensated cirrhosis of the liver is usually characterized by anechoic ascites, although fine echoes floating in the fluid can be demonstrated in up to 20% of patients (**Fig. 8.22**). In some marked cases there will be septation, mural strands of fibrin, and partially septated ascites. Ultrasound-guided fine-needle paracentesis and the subsequent laboratory workup (granulocyte count and bacterial culture) will firm up the diagnosis. Intractable echogenic ascites in cirrhosis of the liver does imply SBP and warrants further study.

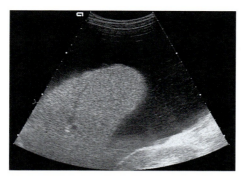

▲ **Fig. 8.22 a** Characteristic image of micronodular cirrhosis of the liver with marked ascites. The diffusely distributed fine echoes could be due to spontaneous bacterial peritonitis (SBP).

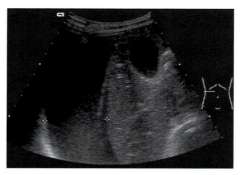

▲ **b** Echogenic ascites lateral to the right hepatic lobe with a single strand of fibrin in SBP.

▶ Peritoneal Carcinomatosis

Peritoneal carcinomatosis is characterized by echogenic ascites with fine echoes, irregular margin, septation, retraction of the mesentery, and solid structures on the peritoneum itself (**Fig. 8.23** and ▣ **8.3**). Differentiating between benign and malignant ascites resembles putting together a puzzle and will be explained further on (**see Tables 8.6 and 8.7,** ▣ **8.6**). The sensitivity of a single ultrasound-guided fine-needle puncture is unacceptably low (50–60%). If there is a definite case for suspected malignancy, repeat cytology is called for (at least three times). Peritoneal carcinomatosis can be like a chameleon; it is detailed further in ▣ **8.3**.

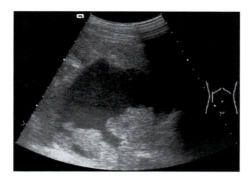

◀ **Fig. 8.23** Echogenic ascites and markedly thickened as well as irregularly delineated peritoneum in peritoneal carcinomatosis due to advanced cancer of the colon.

▣ 8.3 Echogenic Ascites in Peritoneal Carcinomatosis

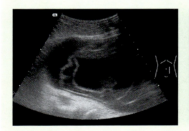

a Strandlike structures originating from the peritoneum in ovarian malignancy with peritoneal carcinomatosis.

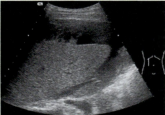

b "Turbid" echogenic ascites and fibrin apposition in peritoneal carcinomatosis of metastasizing gastric cancer. Normal hepatic texture; smooth margins.

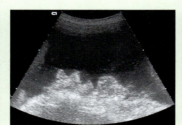

c Malignant ascites with fine internal echoes and a markedly retracted mesentery: peritoneal carcinomatosis in cancer of the colon.

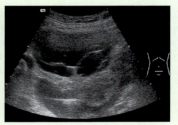

d Ascites with honeycomb septation in cystic ovarian malignancy. This aspect without acute symptoms is characteristic of a gynecological process.

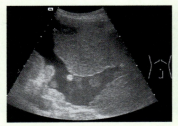

e Marked thickening of the abdominal wall with tumor masses adhering to the peritoneum: peritoneal carcinomatosis in colon cancer.

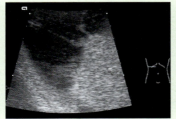

f Echogenic ascites and fine appositions on the parietal peritoneum in peritoneal carcinomatosis (gastric cancer).

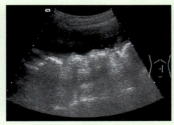

g Markedly pushed-back mesentery and air-filled bowel. Increased distance between omentum/bowel and abdominal wall, indicating peritoneal carcinomatosis.

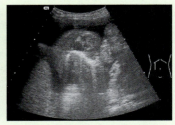

h Thickened visceral peritoneum in peritoneal carcinomatosis (gastric cancer) mimicking a pathological gut signature.

▶ Purulent Peritonitis

The ultrasound image of purulent peritonitis is characterized by inhomogeneous hypoechoic structures displaying a varied echo texture and lacking a definite interconnection (**Fig. 8.24**). During repositioning of the patient, the septation and adhesions will not permit free shifting of the putrid ascites. The clinical symptoms take puncture over any other modality. Ultrasound studies are of limited value in the primary diagnosis and are much more useful in identifying walled-off abscesses. Most often treatment is by surgery.

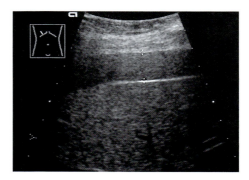

◀ *Fig. 8.24* Purulent peritonitis. Structured fluid (calipers) enveloping the liver. Clinically: perforated duodenal ulcer.

▶ Tuberculosis

The sonographic morphology of tuberculous ascites resembles that in necrotizing pancreatitis. As well as echoes within the fluid there is also septation and the wall is irregular in outline. If the paracentetic specimen is hemorrhagic, this is also indicative in terms of diagnosis.

▶ Choleperitoneum

Bile leakage may be due to a perforated hydropic or empyemic gallbladder as rare complication of cholecystolithiasis. Localized perforation is much more common than free bile leakage into the abdominal cavity (choleperitoneum). Other causes may be intraoperative lesions to the biliary tree or iatrogenic endoscopic injury. Another quite common complication after external PTCD (percutaneous transhepatic bile duct drainage) for palliation of a stenosing malignancy is dislocation of the drain with subsequent bile leakage.

Initially the leaking bile is anechoic, but after a few hours the characteristic streaks and septa will appear that induce layering and which are pathognomonic (**Fig. 8.25**). In those few cases with uncertain diagnosis, ultrasound-guided fine-needle puncture will confirm the free intra-abdominal bile (gross assessment and bilirubin panel).

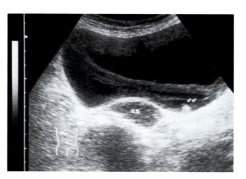

▲ *Fig. 8.25 a* Anechoic intra-abdominal formation with streaks of internal structures in choleperitoneum due to a perforated gallbladder (GB).

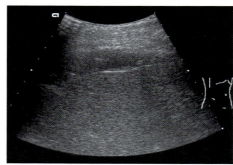

▲ *b* Thin hypoechoic film around the right hepatic lobe due to intra-abdominal collection of bile in biliary leakage after a dislocated PTCD.

▶ Hemoperitoneum

Within a few hours after hemorrhage, the organizing hemoperitoneum will become more and more echogenic, comprising internal echoes, strands of fibrin, and septation. The effusion will become more hyperechoic and inhomogeneous (**Figs. 8.26 and 8.27**). If there is no increase in volume, ultrasonography lends itself quite easily to the morphological follow-up. The advancing organization will be accompanied by absorption, and sometimes some regions will undergo re-liquefaction.

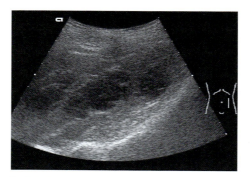

▲ *Fig. 8.26* Anechoic inhomogeneous structures in intra-abdominal and retroperitoneal hemorrhage under anticoagulant therapy.

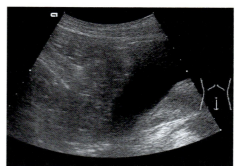

▲ *Fig. 8.27* Anechoic collection of fluid in the lesser pelvis after blunt abdominal trauma with ruptured spleen. The blood will collect at the most dependant part of the abdominal cavity; initially it is anechoic, becoming echogenic later.

GI Tract Perforation

The cardinal symptom of GI tract perforation is the demonstration of free gas within the peritoneal cavity. However, there may also be fluid leaking from the stomach or bowel. This fluid is permeated by echoes and displays gas inclusion (Fig. 8.28). Demonstration of the actual site leaking gas and fluid is a rare feat. The preferred localization of fluid collections in a perforated upper GI tract is around the stomach and duodenum as well as around both hepatic lobes. In perforation of the more downstream intestinal regions, the free gas tends to accumulate more in the lower abdomen.

It should be kept in mind that the combination of free gas and free fluid may be indicative for GI tract perforation.

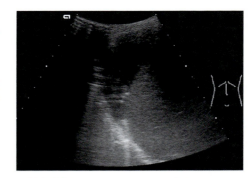

Fig. 8.28 Demonstration of echogenic fluid and some free gas after upper GI tract perforation (duodenal ulcer).

Chyloperitoneum

Chyle leaking into the abdominal cavity is a rare event, its cause possibly being traumatic or a postoperative complication. Chyloperitoneum has also been demonstrated in malignant lymphoma. Ultrasound will depict homogeneous ascites permeated by fine echoes, resulting in a "milky" image. After ultrasound-guided fine-needle puncture, chyloperitoneum permits diagnosis at a glance: milky white turbid lymph!

Hyperechoic Structure

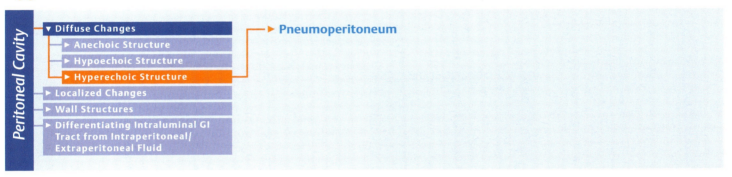

Pneumoperitoneum

A collection of free intra-abdominal gas (pneumoperitoneum) is visualized as a hyperechoic structure with characteristic reverberation echoes and appears, for example, in free perforations of the GI tract. However, in general a frank perforation is a rare event (frequency only 1–2%).

Cause. The most common causes are:
- Duodenal/gastric ulcer
- Inflammatory bowel disease (appendicitis, diverticulitis, etc.)
- Postoperative, anastomotic/suture line leakage
- Iatrogenic (endoscopy, excision biopsy and polypectomy, contrast enema)
- Trauma, foreign body
- Tumor (stomach, colon)

The most common cause of a free perforation is gastric or duodenal ulcer. In complicated diverticulitis of the colon, the leading symptom tends to be localized peritonitis of the left lower quadrant.

Sonographic morphology. In the hands of the expert the signs of a free collection of intra-abdominal gas are easy to recognize (sensitivity 80–90%), while the less experienced sonographer can reproduce these findings in postoperative patients after laparoscopic surgery and with vestiges of pneumoperitoneum. Follow-up studies of these patients provides excellent training. The most important signs of free intra-abdominal gas will be discussed below (8.4).[4]

- The characteristic localizations have already been mentioned above. If the echoes (gas) rise on patient repositioning, this is pathognomonic.
- The reverberation echoes at the preferred localizations already mentioned are characteristic of perforation.
- The additional leakage of fluid, quite often with internal echoes, is another sign of GI tract injury.
- Compared with intraluminal gas collections in the GI tract, marked breathing movement will not result in positional changes (constant respiratory position).
- Furthermore, in the left lateral position there is a discontinuity between the gas in the distal segments of the lungs and the free gas anterior to the liver.
- In the more superior recesses, however, e.g., below the diaphragm with the patient upright or below the abdominal wall with the patient supine, the echoes there will shift when repositioning the patient.

8.4 The Ultrasound Signs of Free Intra-abdominal Gas

- Multiple reverberation echoes
- Characteristic localizations (see above)
- Additional fluid with internal echoes
- No change in position with breathing movements
- Pleuroperitoneal discontinuity
- Hyperechoic echoes in the superior recesses

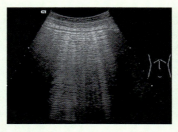

a Hyperechoic intra-abdominal collection of gas. No organs can be visualized behind the curtain of free gas, characteristic reverberation echoes.

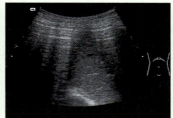

b Hyperechoic collection of gas anterior to the left and right hepatic lobe; parts of the liver are masked. Status post perforation of a duodenal ulcer.

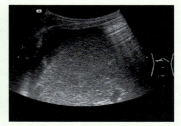

c Apart from the free perihepatic gas on the right of the liver, there is also echogenic free fluid. Free gas + fluid is indicative of a perforated GI tract (here, perforated duodenal ulcer).

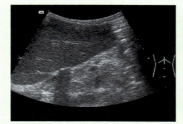

d At the lower margin of the left hepatic lobe: hyperechoic structure (free gas). Posterior to the left hepatic lobe: intense echo complex with posterior shadowing marking the site of the perforation (duodenal ulcer).

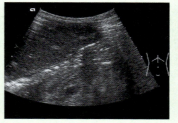

e Anterior to and at the lower margin of the left hepatic lobe: free gas (hyperechoic). Posterior to the left hepatic lobe: a string of small hyperechoic gas bubbles.

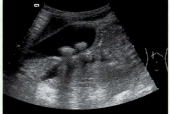

f In the longitudinal plane: some free gas anterior to and to the right of the calculous gallbladder.

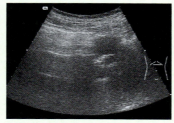

g In the transverse plane of the epigastric region: a small section of the left hepatic lobe. The rest of the organ is masked by the free gas. Status post perforation of the colon in cancer of the hepatic flexure.

Localized Changes

"Pseudoascites." Diagnosis of anechoic and hypoechoic intra-abdominal structures has to differentiate them from fluid structures without connection to the abdominal cavity. The latter are also called "pseudoascites." This term is something of a misnomer since the fluid is not actual ascites but rather structures outside the abdominal cavity that are not interconnected with it. This includes quite a number of fluid collections discussed elsewhere, the most important being (8.5):

- Abscess
- Hematoma
- Cysts (liver, kidney, pancreas pseudocysts, ovaries)
- Ovarian cystoma and other cystic masses (cystadenoma, cystadenocarcinoma)
- Mesothelioma, lymphangioma
- Preformed hollow viscera (urinary bladder, gallbladder hydrops)
- Aortic aneurysm
- Hydronephrosis
- Ileus and gastric outlet obstruction
- Hypoechoic masses
- Fluid processes within the abdominal wall.

8.5 Differentiating Fluid Masses from Ascites

- Liver
- Abdominal wall

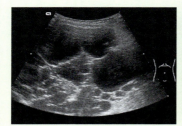 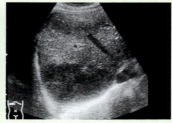 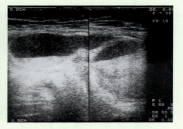

a Polycystic liver: to be differentiated from septated ascites in the upper quadrants.

b Large irregularly defined collection of fluid: large abscess in the right hepatic lobe as sequela of pyogenic cholangitis.

c Septated collection of fluid with some sedimentation of the contents: massive hematoma after heparin induced thrombocytopenia, totally within the abdominal wall and therefore extraperitoneal in location.

- Pancreas
- Spleen
- Kidney

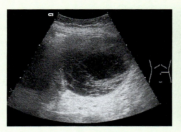 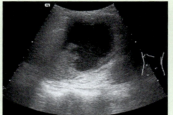 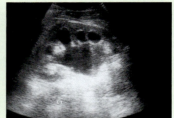

d Localized cystic mass in the left upper quadrant, permeated by septumlike structures; no walled-off pancreatogenous ascites but cystic malignancy of the pancreas (cystadenocarcinoma).

e Irregularly defined collection of fluid within the spleen: invasion of a pancreatic pseudocyst.

f Massively dilated renal calices and pelvis. No parenchymal margin to be visualized; hydronephrotic nephrectasia; no interconnection with the abdominal cavity.

Anechoic Structure

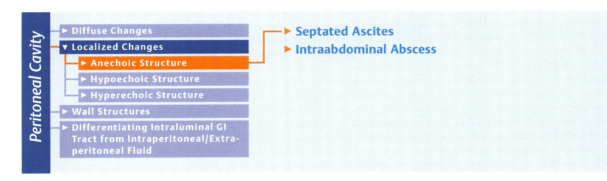

▶ Septated Ascites

If there is no unrestricted intercompartmental connection, e.g., as may be the case in the presence of adhesions, the collection of intraabdominal fluid will be localized. Classic examples are the septated ascites in peritoneal carcinomatosis with adhesions (**Fig. 8.29**) and in pancreatitis (**Fig. 8.30**). The example of septated ascites in the omental bursa has already been demonstrated (**8.2e**).

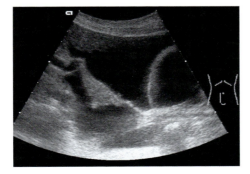 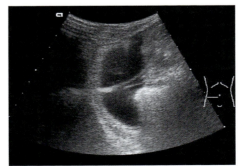

▲ **Fig. 8.29** Septated ascites in peritoneal carcinomatosis (ovarian malignancy). The septa may compartmentalize the fluid, which then will not shift freely on repositioning of the patient.

▲ **Fig. 8.30** In necrotizing pancreatitis, septation may also result in compartmentalization, thus "trapping" the ascites. Here, too, the fluid cannot shift freely on repositioning of the patient.

▶ *Intra-abdominal Abscess*

Inflammatory adhesions may also wall off intra-abdominal collections of fluid, for instance in abscesses. However, these structures are rarely anechoic but more commonly tend to be hypoechoic.

Hypoechoic Structure

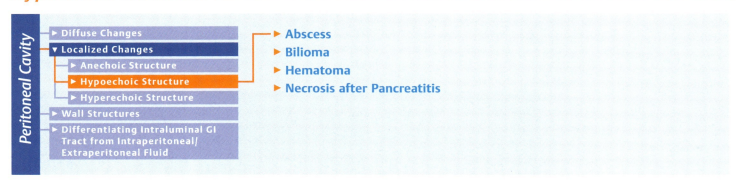

▶ Abscess

Intra-abdominal abscess, e.g., between the bowel loops, subphrenic, or subhepatic, is hypoechoic and displays an inhomogeneous structure. In most cases the margin is irregular (**Figs. 8.31 and 8.32**). Less frequently the abscess may be anechoic or hyperechoic; this is particularly true in gas abscess due to bacterial colonization. The diagnosis is facilitated by the presence of the appropriate clinical symptoms with markedly elevated blood markers, fever, and pain.

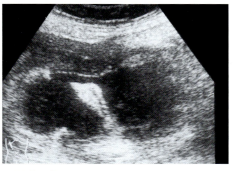

▲ **Fig. 8.31** Two large, irregularly defined hypoechoic abscesses below the liver after cholecystectomy. The narrow interconnection between the abscess permits the fluid to communicate; successful interventional treatment with two drains.

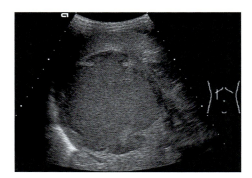

▲ **Fig. 8.32** Localized, irregularly defined echogenic process around the right liver after pancreatitis: abscess.

▶ Bilioma

Biliary leakage or perforation does not necessarily result in the full-blown picture of choleperitoneum. Much more common is the localized collection of bile, the so-called bilioma. The internal texture of the bilioma is echogenic, or it may be characterized by streaking (**Fig. 8.33**). Only "fresh" bile will be anechoic. Biliomas are found in the vicinity of the biliary tree.

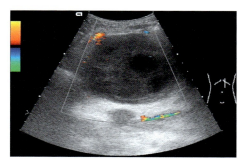

◀ **Fig. 8.33** Localized anechoic liquid structure below the liver after dislocated left-sided PTCD, corresponding with a bilioma. Color-flow Doppler imaging will help differentiate it from a solid mass.

▶ Hematoma

If there is no frank hemorrhage into the abdominal cavity, a hematoma may be formed within the smaller compartments. With aging, the intra-abdominal hematoma will become more and more hyperechoic and will display an internal texture. Over the course of the hematoma, it may demonstrate not only the more organized echogenic parts but also liquid regions undergoing liquefaction (**Fig. 8.34**).

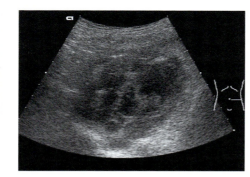

◀ **Fig. 8.34** Status post hemorrhage under anticoagulant therapy: hypoechoic inhomogeneous paracolic structure, corresponding with a localized hematoma becoming organized.

▶ Necrosis after Pancreatitis

Necrosis as sequela of necrotizing pancreatitis (see Chapter 4, "Pancreas") is frequently localized in the retroperitoneum, but it may also arise within the abdominal cavity apart from the pancreas, resulting in the image of a circumscribed hypoechoic mass (**Fig. 8.35**). The necrosis is irregularly defined and inhomogeneous. In addition, there are clear signs of pancreatitis at the organ itself. Ultrasound can demonstrate peripancreatic as well as paracolic necrosis and necrosis invading parenchymal organs, such as the liver or spleen.

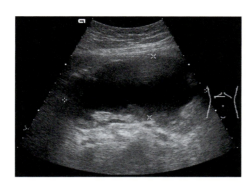

◀ **Fig. 8.35** Large anechoic mass with hyperechoic posterior sections: marked necrosis of the pancreas.

Hyperechoic Structure

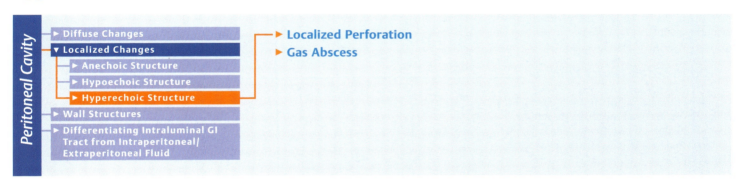

In the case of a localized hyperechoic structure, the sonographer should primarily think of accumulated gas—for instance, localized perforation or gas abscess between the bowel loops.

▶ Localized Perforation

If the gas leak is small and the perforation in the GI tract is well localized, there will not be any frank perforation. The hyperechoic collection of gas with its characteristic reverberation echoes is truly local and will not shift on patient repositioning. Most of the localized hyperechoic collections of gas will be seen in the immediate vicinity of the GI tract and will be difficult to differentiate from the intraluminal gas collections (**Fig. 8.36**). Apart from the intracavitary hyperechoic structures of the perforation, there may be fluid as well (mixed with hypoechoic regions), resulting in a mixed image.

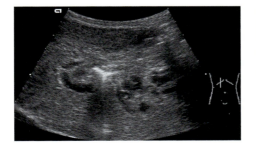

▲ **Fig. 8.36 a** Localized hyperechoic structure with reverberation echoes and posterior shadowing around the hepatic portal (subhepatic left) in a localized perforated duodenal ulcer.

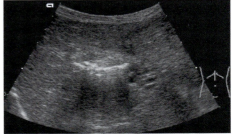

▲ **b** Hyperechoic structures in localized perforation.

▶ Gas Abscess

In a gas abscess the hypoechoic regions of the liquid components may be predominant. The gas produced by the bacteria is characterized by individual marked echo complexes increasing over the course of the abscess (**Fig. 8.37**). In most cases it displays an irregular margin. Differential diagnosis is based on the clinical picture supplemented by fine-needle puncture.

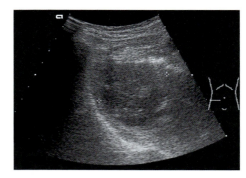

◀ **Fig. 8.37** Localized hypoechoic, rather smoothly defined structure with a hyperechoic region corresponding with gas; the "curtainlike" appearance and the posterior shadowing are indicative. Large paracolic gas abscess on the right complicating necrotizing pancreatitis.

Wall Structures

Smooth Margin

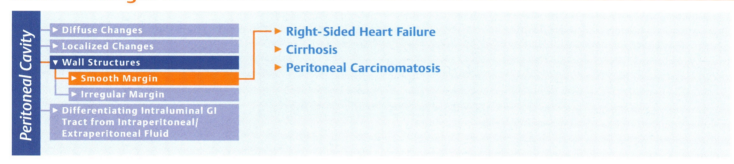

The peritoneum can only be visualized indirectly (see above). Usually the peritoneum is smoothly defined.

▶ Right-Sided Heart Failure

In right ventricular failure the intra-abdominal collection of fluid is a transudate. The outline of the peritoneum is always smooth and lacks any juxtaposition, while the ascites is anechoic (**Fig. 8.15**).

▶ Cirrhosis

Decompensated cirrhosis of the liver with ascites is characterized by a smoothly delineated peritoneum. The ascites is anechoic. The liver displays the changes in shape and texture, among others, characteristic of cirrhosis (**Fig. 8.38**).

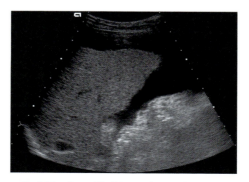

▲ **Fig. 8.38 a** Smoothly delineated visceral and parietal peritoneum in decompensated alcoholic cirrhosis of the liver.

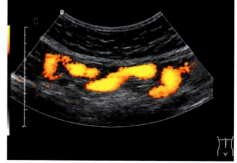

▲ **b** In Medusa's head, the tortuous course of the blood vessels on the inside of the abdominal wall is a sure sign of portal hypertension in cirrhosis.

▶ Peritoneal Carcinomatosis

In peritoneal carcinomatosis the peritoneum may still be smoothly delineated and appear absolutely normal (**Fig. 8.9**). However, much more common are irregularities, septation, and tumor masses on the peritoneum itself. The findings are considered as cardinal signs of malignancy.

Irregular Margin

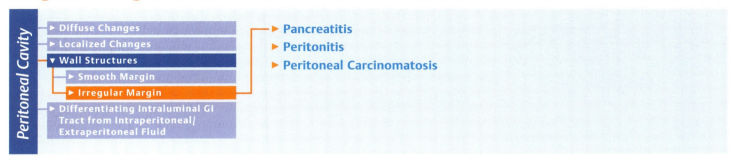

▶ Pancreatitis

The intra-abdominal collection of fluid in pancreatitis is characterized not only by its internal echoes but, as has already been stated above, quite often by septation and strands of fibrin. These originate from the peritoneum and will lead to an irregular outline. "Fluttering fibrin strands" originating from the peritoneum may be found in pancreatitis as well as peritonitis (**Figs. 8.39 and 8.40**).

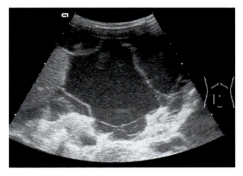

▲ **Fig. 8.39** "Flags" of fibrin coating the peritoneum and dominating the picture in necrotizing pancreatitis (exudate).

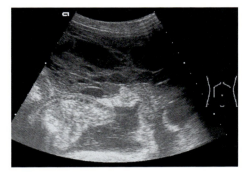

▲ **Fig. 8.40** The septation may become almost complete and can mask all of the peritoneum. Honeycomb texture due to strands of fibrin in necrotizing pancreatitis.

▶ Peritonitis

Bacterial peritonitis is not necessarily accompanied by ascites. In the classic case, the peritoneum is lined by inflammatory accretions and will display an irregular outline on ultrasonography. In addition, there may be strand-like extensions and irregular thickening.

▶ Peritoneal Carcinomatosis

In peritoneal carcinomatosis the peritoneum may be thickened and display an irregular outline. These irregularities in the contour, including tumor masses on the peritoneum, are indicative of advanced peritoneal carcinomatosis. The more ascites the better the irregularities will be visualized. Usually, these changes are easier to demonstrate on the visceral peritoneum (**Figs. 8.41, 8.42, Fig. 8.23, and 8.3**).

The peritoneum is a frequent site for metastases. Eighty percent of all malignancies can result in peritoneal carcinomatosis; the most common origin is gastrointestinal and gynecological tumors (**Table 8.5**). However, diagnostic ultrasound in peritoneal carcinomatosis is not

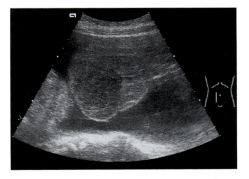

▲ **Fig. 8.41** Inhomogeneous solid tumor masses lining the parietal (anterior) peritoneum, which on the whole is displaying an irregular outline.

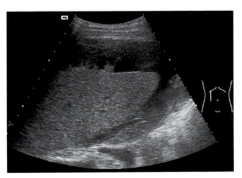

▲ **Fig. 8.42** Juxtapositions and strands of fibrin on the visceral peritoneum (liver and bowel) destroying an otherwise smooth contour: peritoneal carcinomatosis in advanced gastric cancer.

without pitfalls. Its sensitivity is only 50–60%, one of the prime reasons being the fact that only about 50% of all cases with peritoneal carcinomatosis will present with ascites! The optimum diagnostic modality is laparoscopy. But some criteria for ultrasound morphology can be quite useful for differentiating benign from malignant ascites (**Table 8.6 and 8.7, Fig. 8.43, ▣ 8.6**).

The importance of ultrasound-guided fine-needle puncture in the precise assessment of the fluid has already been discussed. In malignant ascites this is an exudate that quite often has high cholesterol levels. Malignant cells will be found in 50–70% of cases. Repeat paracentesis and cytological evaluation will increase the sensitivity to 70–80%.[3]

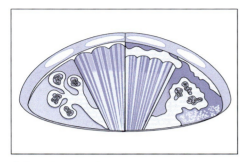

▲ **Fig. 8.43** Schematic representation of the characteristic signs in benign (left) and malignant (right) ascites (based on reference 6).

Table 8.5 Primary malignancies in peritoneal carcinomatosis

GI tract (stomach, pancreas, colon)	34%
Ovaries	27%
Breast	14%
Lymphoma	4%
Sarcoma, kidney, uterus, unknown primary	18%

Table 8.6 Signs of peritoneal carcinomatosis (based on reference 8)

Thickened omentum	97%
Peritoneal mass	19%
Interrupted peritoneum	16%
Mesenteric adhesions	16%
Hepatic metastases	24%
Ascites	49%

Table 8.7 Ultrasound in the differential diagnosis of benign and malignant ascites

Ultrasound morphology	**Benign**	**Malignant**
Echogenicity of the ascites ▸ Anechoic ▸ Internal echoes (echogenic) ▸ Septation	++ + +	+ ++ ++
Fluid shift on repositioning	Unrestricted	Limited
Septation	Unrestricted	Walled off, encapsulated
Peritoneal margin	Smooth	Irregular, mass
Greater omentum	Thin	Thickened, rigid
Mesentery	Unrestricted	Retracted
Small-bowel loops	"Sea anemone," "creepers"	Conglomerate
Abdominal wall	Thin, mobile	Thickened, rigid
Bowel—abdominal wall	Unrestricted	Adherence
Other signs of disease	Cirrhosis Pancreatitis Right ventricular failure	Metastases; malignancy of the bowel, pancreas, uterus, ovaries
Lymph node and hepatic metastases	None	++

▣ 8.6 Differential Diagnosis of Benign and Malignant Ascites

▸ **Benign ascites**

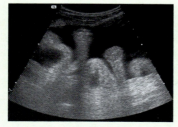
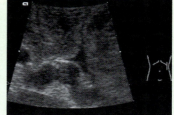
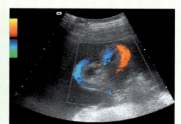

a Smooth peritoneum and freely floating loops of bowel ("sea anemone" phenomenon) in benign ascites: decompensated cirrhosis.

b 'Angle of ascites' and mesenteric collaterals (shunts) in portal hypertension point to benign ascites: portal hypertension.

c The 'heart' in the lower abdomen, resulting from the tortuous collaterals in portal hypertension with shunts, points to benign ascites.

8.6 Differential Diagnosis of Benign and Malignant Ascites

▶ **Malignant ascites**

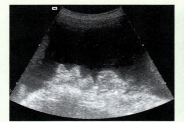 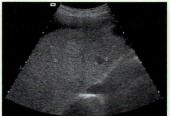 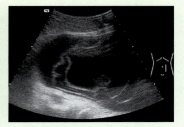

d Internal echoes and a clearly retracted mesentery signifying malignant ascites, compared with the "sea anemone phenomenon" in benign ascites.

e The presence of hepatic metastasis usually proves the malignant origin of the ascites: small hepatic metastasis in pancreatic cancer.

f Marked septation and strandlike structures originating from the peritoneum (here, ovarian malignancy) tend to be indicative of malignant rather than benign ascites.

▶ **Peritoneal tumor masses**

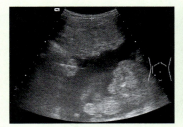 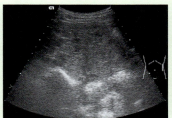 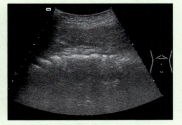

g Peritoneal tumor masses are a certain sign in the differential diagnosis: peritoneal carcinomatosis in advanced cancer of the colon.

h Peritoneal carcinomatosis without ascites (about 50%). Peritoneal tumor masses are the cardinal sign in sonography.

i Increased separation of colon and abdominal wall because of the peritoneum and greater omentum. This is a cardinal sign even if ascites is not present.

Differentiating Intra- and Extraluminal GI Tract Fluid

In the differential diagnosis of intra-abdominal and extra-abdominal fluid the pathological collection of fluid within the GI tract plays a special role and therefore will be discussed separately. This topic includes especially the impaired intragastric and intraintestinal transport, where there is no definite peristalsis facilitating the assessment "within the GI tract lumen" but where the fluid simply sits (**Table 8.8**).

Assessment is possible when considering the following signs:
- Demonstration of the GI tract wall
- Peristalsis
- Characteristic localization and shape
- Characteristic intraluminal structures, e.g., haustration and Kerckring's folds

Table 8.8 Possible causes of impaired GI tract transport

Stomach	Bowel
▶ Ulcer	▶ Peritoneal carcinomatosis
▶ Tumor	▶ Inflammatory stenosis (Crohn disease)
	▶ Tumor
	▶ Intussusception
	▶ Mechanical ileus (adhesions)
	▶ Volvulus

Intragastric Processes

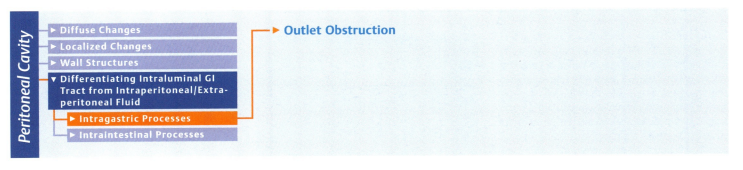

▶ Gastric Outlet Obstruction

The stomach is easily delineated because of its location (subhepatic, anterior to the pancreas). A massively fluid-filled stomach concomitant with a lack of fluid in the duodenum suggests gastric outlet obstruction. With the upper abdomen upright, the fluid that will not drain becomes clearly visible, while the impeding gas will rise cephalad (gastric bubble, fornix). This disorder is characterized by small rising gas bubbles producing the image of a "starry sky" with the paradoxical fact that there are not falling but rising stars **(Fig. 8.44)**. The most common origins of gastric outlet obstruction are ulcers and tumors. In this case ultrasound will be able to demonstrate the signs of a pathological gut signature (see Chapter 7, "Gatrointestinal Tract," pp. 229, Focal Wall Changes).

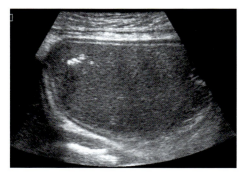

▲ **Fig. 8.44** Small gas bubbles rising in the massively fluid-filled stomach (fermentation), producing the image of the "star studded stomach": gastric outlet obstruction.

Intraintestinal Processes

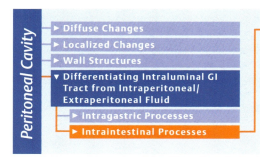

- ▶ Duodenal Stenosis
- ▶ Small Bowel Obstruction
- ▶ Large Bowel Obstruction

▶ Duodenal Stenosis

If impaired gastric emptying is accompanied by a rather distended and fluid-filled duodenum, while the other parts of the small and large intestine are without pathological findings, the stenosis or obstruction will be in the more distal duodenum **(Fig. 8.45)**. This condition will always be accompanied by collections of fluid in the duodenum as well as the stomach, and the most common causes are tumors and inflammation at the head of the pancreas.

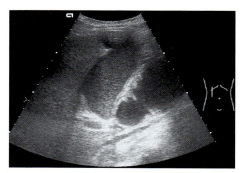

▲ **Fig. 8.45 a** Duodenal stenosis: massive collection of fluid and distension of the duodenum (posterior to a hydropic gallbladder) in distal duodenal obstruction due to cancer of the pancreas.

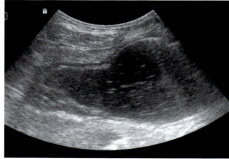

▲ **b** Distal duodenal obstruction is characterized by a fluid-filled stomach and distended duodenum, while the other sections of the small bowel do not exhibit any luminal filling.

▶ Small Bowel Obstruction

Classic small bowel obstruction is characterized by distended bowel loops with their typical Kerckring's folds, the so-called "piano key phenomenon" **(Figs. 8.46–8.48)**. Depending on the stage and origin of the ileus, massive resistance-induced peristalsis, pendulating peristalsis, or no peristalsis at all can be demonstrated. The most common causes are inflammatory changes of the intestinal wall (see Chapter 7, pp. 245) and peritoneal carcinomatosis.

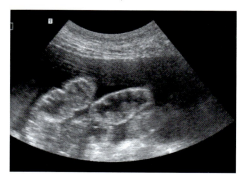

◀ **Fig. 8.46** Differential diagnosis is not always as easy as in this case with its peritoneal carcinomatosis and ileus.

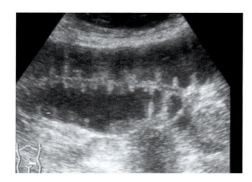
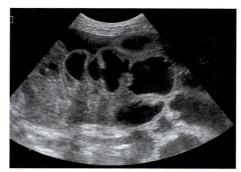

◄◄ **Fig. 8.47** Small-bowel obstruction. Distended intestine and the loops of the small bowel are identified by their Kerckring's folds projecting into the lumen, the so-called "piano key" or "Jacob's ladder" phenomenon.

◄ **Fig. 8.48** Small-bowel obstruction. Tentative "piano key phenomenon" in ileus due to peritoneal carcinomatosis in cancer of the pancreas. Also note the free ascites outside the bowel.

► Large Bowel Obstruction

In the presence of a distended and rather fluid-filled intestinal lumen, large bowel obstruction is characterized by the haustra coli and the typical course of the intestine (fixed colic position) (**Fig. 8.49**). The segments of bowel upstream will also be affected. The most common causes are tumors and inflammatory stenosis.

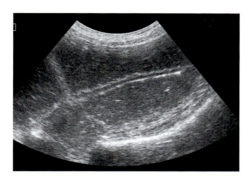
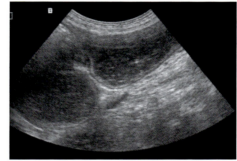

▲ **Fig. 8.49 a** Large-bowel obstruction: well distended lumen and marked intraluminal fluid filling.

▲ **b** Severe large-bowel obstruction with demonstration of the ileocecal valve in a stenotic sigmoid mass.

References

1. Beyer D, Mödder U. Diagnostik des akuten Abdomens mit bildgebenden Verfahren. Berlin: Springer 1985.
2. Bilger R. Klinische abdominelle Ultraschalldiagnostik. Stuttgart: Fischer 1989.
3. Gerbes A. Ascitic fluid analysis for the differentiation of malignancy-related and nonmalignant ascites. Cancer 1991;68:1808.
4. Kainberger P, Zukriegel M, Sattlegger P, Forstner R, Schmoller H.J. Ultrasound detection of pneumoperitoneum based on typical ultrasound morphology. Ultraschall Med 1994; 3: 122-5.
5. Kremer H, Dobrinski W. Sonographische Diagnostik. 4th ed. Munich: Urban & Schwarzenberg 1994.
6. Meckler U. Ultraschall des Abdomens. 3rd ed. Cologne: Deutscher Ärzteverlag 1998.
7. Rettenmaier G, Seitz KH. Sonographische Differentialdiagnose. Stuttgart: Thieme 2000.
8. Rioux M. Sonographic detection of peritoneal carcinomatosis. Abdom Imaging 1995;20:47–51.
9. Schölmerich J. Diagnostik und Therapie des Aszites. Internist 1987;28:448–58.
10. Thomas L. Diagnostik des Aszites In: Labor und Diagnose. 5th ed. Frankfurt/M.: TH-Books Verlagsgesellschaft 1998.

9 Kidneys

Kidneys 275

▼ Anomalies, Malformations — 276

▶ Aplasia, Hypoplasia — 276
- ▶ Renal Agenesis
- ▶ Hypoplasia

▶ Cystic Malformation — 277
- ▶ Polycystic Kidney Disease

▶ Anomalies of Number, Position, or Rotation — 278
- ▶ Duplex Kidney
- ▶ Ectopic Kidney
- ▶ Malrotation

▶ Fusion Anomaly — 280
- ▶ Horseshoe Kidney

▶ Collecting System Anomaly — 281
- ▶ Caliceal Diverticula
- ▶ Megacalicosis

▶ Vascular Anomaly — 281
- ▶ Aberrant Vessels
- ▶ Renovascular Malformations

▼ Diffuse Changes — 282

▶ Large Kidneys — 282
- ▶ Constitutional/Acromegaly
- ▶ Duplex Kidney, Single Kidney
- ▶ Diabetic Nephropathy
- ▶ Polycystic Kidney Disease
- ▶ Acute Renal Failure, Shock Kidney
- ▶ Septic-Toxic Kidneys
- ▶ Acute Urinary Retention, Acute Outflow Obstruction
- ▶ Renal Congestion due to Heart Failure
- ▶ Renal Vein Thrombosis
- ▶ Acute Glomerulonephritis
- ▶ Acute Pyelonephritis
- ▶ AIDS- and Heroin-induced Nephropathy
- ▶ Amyloidosis/Paraprotein Kidney
- ▶ Pyonephrosis
- ▶ Renal Tumor
- ▶ Renal Allograft, Allograft Rejection

▶ Small Kidneys — 287
- ▶ Hypoplasia
- ▶ Renal Artery Stenosis, Embolism
- ▶ Arteriosclerosis, Arteriolosclerosis
- ▶ Chronic Pyelonephritis
- ▶ Analgesic Nephropathy
- ▶ Chronic Glomerulonephritis
- ▶ Diabetic Nephropathy

▶ Hypoechoic Structure — 289
- ▶ Acute Renal Failure
- ▶ Acute Nephritis
- ▶ Right Heart Failure
- ▶ Renal Vein Thrombosis

▶ Hyperechoic Structure — 290
- ▶ Hypoxemic Renal Shock
- ▶ Diabetic Nephropathy
- ▶ Acute and Chronic Glomerulonephritis
- ▶ Chronic Pyelonephritis
- ▶ Analgesic Nephropathy
- ▶ Septic-Toxic Kidneys

Diffuse Changes (Continue)

Hyperechoic Structure — 290
- Severe Metabolic Disorders
- Light-Chain Deposition Disease, Waldenström Disease
- Amyloidosis
- Infiltration by Lymphoma
- Atrophic Kidneys

Irregular Structure — 295
- Analgesic Nephropathy
- Diffuse Tumor Infiltration
- Suppurative Pyelonephritis, Pyonephrosis

Circumscribed Changes — 296

Anechoic Structure — 296
- Renal Cysts, Polycystic Kidney
- Perirenal Cystic Masses
- Lymph Cysts
- Cystic Renal Cell Carcinoma, Intracystic Carcinoma
- Papillary Necrosis, Cystic Degeneration of the Medullary Pyramids
- Cavities
- Abscess
- Organized Hematoma
- Urinoma, Seroma
- Vascular Dilatations
- Hydrocalices, Pyelectasis, Hydronephrosis

Hypoechoic or Isoechoic Structure — 301
- Dromedary Hump, Fetal Lobulation
- Abscess
- Hemorrhagic Cyst
- Fresh Renal Infarct
- Hematoma
- Renal Cell Carcinoma
- Urothelial Carcinoma
- Malignant Lymphoma
- Metastasis
- Adenoma, Inflammatory Tumor

Complex Structure — 307
- Abscess, Pyonephrosis
- Xanthomatous Pyelonephritis
- Hematoma, Intracystic Hemorrhage
- Renal Cell Carcinoma, Cystic Renal Carcinoma, Malignant Lymphoma

Hyperechoic Structure — 309
- Renal Abscess, Carbuncles
- Hemorrhagic Cyst
- Renal Cell Carcinoma
- Angiomyolipoma
- Scars

Echogenic Structure — 311
- Papillary Calcification
- Interlobar and Arcuate Arteries
- Bacterial Gas Bubbles
- Parenchymal Calcification
- Nephrocalcinosis, Medullary Sponge Kidney
- Renal Tuberculosis, Putty Kidney
- Pyelocaliceal Stone, Staghorn Calculus

9 Kidneys

G. Schmidt

Anatomy

Anatomical structures
- Renal hilum
- Renal cortex and medulla
- Medullary pyramids and papillae
- Renal vessels

Size
- Length 10–11.5 cm
- Width 5–7 cm
- Thickness 3–4 cm

The convex anterior surface of the kidney and its smooth posterior surface unite at the rounded lateral border. On the medial border they form a central fissure, the renal hilum, where the renal vein, renal artery, and ureter enter and leave the organ. The anatomical subdivision into the renal cortex and medulla is clearly appreciated at ultrasound.

Cortex. The renal cortex is a 6 to 10 mm-wide strip located just beneath the fibrous renal capsule. Its boundary is formed by an imaginary line along the bases of the medullary pyramids. Extensions of the renal cortex, called the renal columns, extend between the seven to nine pyramids that make up the renal medulla. The renal cortex contains the renal (malpighian) corpuscles, composed of a glomerulus and Bowman capsule, and the renal tubules.

Medulla. The renal medulla consists of the renal pyramids with their collecting ducts and more central papillary ducts, which unite at the papilla. The papillae project into the renal calices. Due to the high fluid content of the collecting ducts, the medullary pyramids appear markedly less echogenic at ultrasound than the renal cortex (**Fig. 9.1**).

Vessels. The vessels of the kidney, the renal artery and vein, divide into an anterior and a posterior branch at the renal hilum while still outside the kidney. Further branching into four segmental arteries and veins occurs in the fatty renal sinus. From there the vessels run along the columns between the medullary pyramids to the renal cortex as the interlobar arteries and veins (**Figs. 9.2, 9.3**). There they divide into the arcuate arteries, which run horizontally parallel to the bases of the pyramids, and the interlobular arteries, which pass radially into the renal cortex. The individual vessels are displayed particularly well by color Doppler ultrasound. The veins run parallel to the named arteries. The entire vascular system is also clearly demonstrated by 3D imaging.

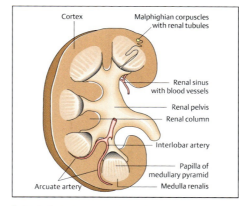

▲ **Fig. 9.1** Renal cortex and medulla.
a Diagram showing the medullary pyramids, vessels, and a malpighian corpuscle.

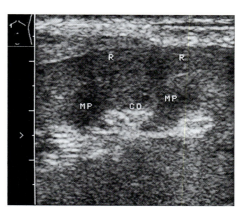

▲ **b** Close-up view of the right kidney, showing the relatively hypoechoic medullary pyramids (MP) and the cortex (R), bounded by an imaginary line connecting the bases of the pyramids. Between the medullary pyramids are the renal columns (CO).

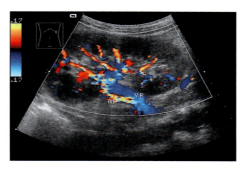

▲ **Fig. 9.2** Radial branching of the segmental arteries into the interlobar vessels. Left kidney (enlarged following a right nephrectomy). AR = renal artery; VR = renal vein.

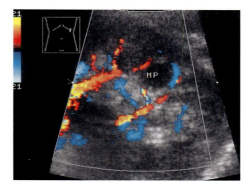

▲ **Fig. 9.3** Detail view of a medullary pyramid (MP) with the surrounding interlobar vessels, which turn horizontally at the bases of the pyramids to form the arcuate vessels.

Topography

Relations
- The kidneys are retroperitoneal, lying anterior to the lumbar muscles.
- Colic flexures overlie the lower renal poles; liver and stomach overlie the upper poles.
- The spleen and pancreatic tail are in contact with the upper pole of the left kidney.

Both kidneys are located in the retroperitoneal space, one on either side of the spinal column, and are anterior to the lumbar muscles (psoas major, quadratus lumborum, and transversus abdominis). They project past the 12th rib into the last intercostal space, so that part of the kidneys extends into the chest between the diaphragm and chest wall. The central portion of each kidney is anterior to the diaphragm at the level of the lateral part of the 12th rib, and the lower portion extends down past the 12th rib (**Fig. 9.4a**).

At the medial, concave border of the kidney is the hilum with the renal vessels. The vein is anterior, the artery is behind it, and the upper ureter is posterior. In the right kidney, this region borders on the descending part of the duodenum. The anterior surface of the kidney

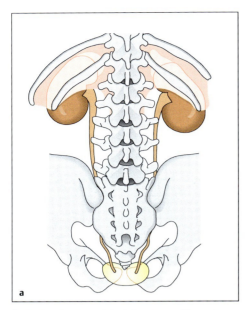
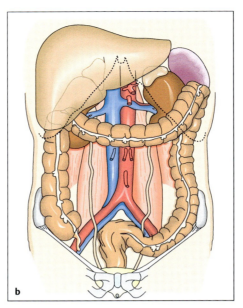
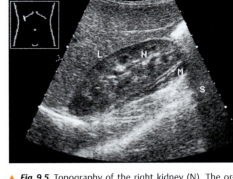

▲ **Fig. 9.5** Topography of the right kidney (N). The organ is retroperitoneal, lying anterior to the musculature (M). Its anterior surface is related to the liver (L), which bears the renal impression. The lower pole of the kidney extends anteriorly downward and is partially obscured by high-level echoes from the right colic flexure, which casts an acoustic shadow (S).

▲ **Fig. 9.4** Relations of the kidney to neighboring structures.
 a Ribs and spinal column (from a dorsal point of view).

▲ **b** Organs in the upper and lower abdomen.

forms the renal impression in the right lobe of the liver. The right and left colic flexures overlie the lower renal poles (**Figs. 9.4b, 9.5**). The upper portion of the left kidney borders on the spleen, while the tail of the pancreas and the posterosuperior gastric surface overlie it. Cystic areas arising from the spleen, kidney, or tail of the pancreas may be found in the renal-splenic angle; they are difficult to localize to a specific organ in ultrasonography (**see ▣ 9.2h**).

Anomalies, Malformations

Anomalies and malformations are based on a congenital disturbance of fetal renal development. Their severity depends on the timing of their occurrence, i.e., the period ranging from the metanephrogenic blastema and the ureteric bud (agenesis) to the fully formed kidney (postrenal urinary tract anomaly).

Not every presumed malformation is actually classified as such. A number of "malformations" are actually normal variants, such as a dromedary hump in the lateral border of the left kidney (**see Fig. 9.66b**).

Aplasia, Hypoplasia

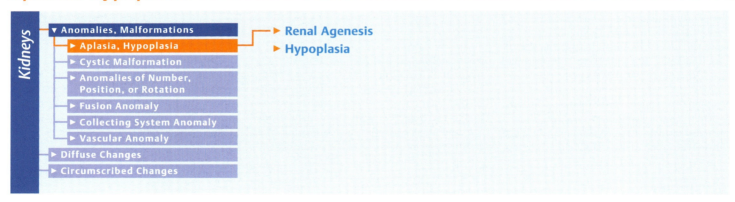

▶ Renal Agenesis

Inability to visualize the kidney with ultrasound is not unusual. Most of these cases involve an ectopic kidney, whereas actual renal agenesis is very rare. In both cases the kidneys are not found in the renal fossa. An ectopic kidney and renal agenesis are easily differentiated with ultrasound, because the contralateral kidney is enlarged in agenesis but is of normal size in ectopia (except in patients with ectopic hypoplastic kidneys, which also leads to compensatory enlargement of the opposite kidney if there is much functional impairment). The measurement of renal size, then, is as important as the search for an ectopic kidney (**Fig. 9.6**). The latter is most easily found by looking caudal to the "normal location" along the line of ascent (pelvic, lumbar, abdominal dysplasia). Renal agenesis in one-third of patients is associated with cystic seminal vesicles or unilateral seminal-vesicle agenesis.

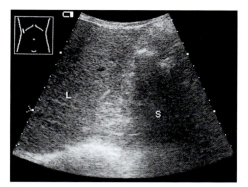
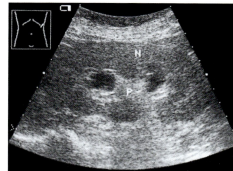

◄◄ **Fig. 9.6** Aplasia of the right kidney with compensatory enlargement of the left kidney (N).
a The right renal fossa is empty. L = liver, S = Shadowing from gas in the colon.

◄ **b** Left kidney with two parapelvic cysts. P = pyelon.

▶ Hypoplasia

Hypoplastic renal dysplasia appears sonographically as abnormal development of the renal tissue with associated disturbances of normal renal architecture. The kidney is small or very small, and some hypoplastic kidneys are too small to be defined with ultrasound. Differentiation from an atrophic kidney is not always possible, but most hypoplastic kidneys exhibit normal parenchyma and normal central hilar echoes. Calcifications or multicystic changes may be found (**Fig. 9.7, Fig. 9.14 b**).

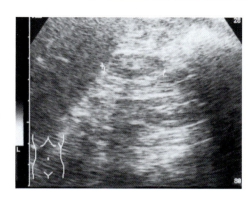

◄ **Fig. 9.7** Renal hypoplasia. The apparent "missing left kidney" is probably a tiny hypoplastic kidney (cursors).

Cystic Malformation

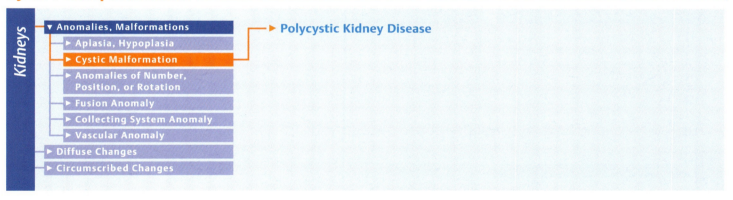

▶ Polycystic Kidney Disease

Polycystic kidney diseases fall in the category of ontogenic renal lesions. They are frequently associated with cystic changes in other organs and are caused by increased intratubular pressure due to distal tubular obstructions and by tubular epithelial dysplasia. The cystic lesions thus represent tubular retention cysts. Cysts located in the area of the renal sinus are generally lymphatic cysts. Secondary cysts may be found in the setting of chronic renal diseases (see below). The various types of renal cyst are reviewed in **Table 9.1**.

Sonographic features. Renal cysts appear sonographically as round, anechoic, smooth-bordered masses that are lined with epithelium, forming a cyst wall. For physical reasons, they cause posterior acoustic enhancement. Simple solitary or multiple cysts and adult-type polycystic kidneys (Potter type III) are of particular interest for routine scanning in internal medicine.

Polycystic kidneys contain multiple anechoic masses of varying size, usually causing considerable organ enlargement. The cysts produce an undulating renal outline with no discernible capsule, causing poor delineation of the kidney. Large bullous cysts obscure the residual intact parenchyma through a "blooming effect," so that the kidney appears to consist almost entirely of cystic areas. Microcystic kidneys still display numerous areas of renal parenchyma. This pattern requires differentiation from multiple renal cysts. In this case the parenchyma is still clearly visible and generally the kidneys are not enlarged (**Figs. 9.8 and 9.9**; see also Circumscribed Changes).

Table 9.1 Types of renal cysts (after reference 11)

Type of cystic kidney (Potter)	Age at symptom onset, location	Morphology	Complications, associated disorders
Infantile polycystic nephropathy (type I)	Newborn, infants Bilateral	Kidneys greatly enlarged, with collecting ducts 1–2 mm in size	Renal failure, hepatic fibrosis
Dysplastic cystic kidney (type II)	Infants, small children Unilateral or bilateral	Polycystic kidneys, cortical cysts	Obstructive ureteral or bladder anomalies, recurrent urinary tract infections
Adult polycystic nephropathy (type III)	20–40 years of age Bilateral	Kidneys greatly enlarged, with cysts in all nephrons	Frequent hepatic cysts, pyelonephritis, hypertension, uremia
Familial nephronophthisis	Adolescents, adults Bilateral	Small kidneys, sclerosing interstitial nephropathy with distal tubular cysts	Mental deficiency, hepatic fibrosis, ataxia, uremia
Medullary sponge kidney	Adults 80% bilateral	Collecting duct cysts in the papillae with calculi	Recurrent urinary tract infections, urolithiasis
Simple renal cysts	Any age Unilateral or bilateral	Solitary or multiple cysts up to 5 cm in size	Rarely, pyelonephritis

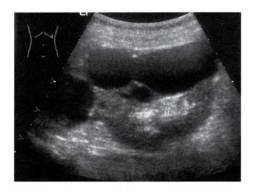 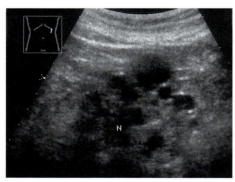 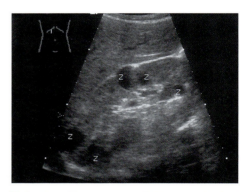

▲ **Fig. 9.8** Polycystic renal degeneration (Potter type III adult polycystic disease). Cystic renal degeneration (N). The parenchyma is difficult to identify due to the many anechoic spaces.
a Macrocystic-bullous form.

▲ **b** Predominantly microcystic form.

▲ **Fig. 9.9** Multiple renal cysts (Z). The kidney is still of normal size, and the parenchyma is clearly visible; dialysis.

Anomalies of Number, Position, or Rotation

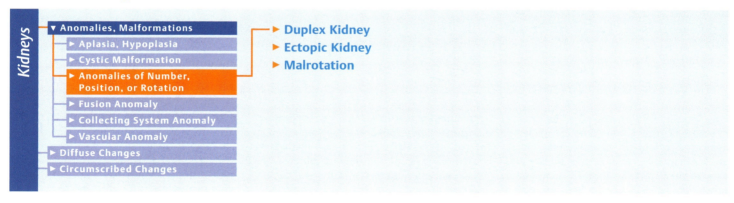

▶ Duplex Kidney

Duplex kidney is the most common renal anomaly, occurring in 1% of the general population. It is characterized by duplicated renal pelves and two ureters that unite somewhere between the kidney and bladder. The duplex kidney is also enlarged. When the ureters have different insertions, the ureter with the more distal insertion belongs to the upper moiety according to the Meyer–Weigert rule. The ureter belonging to the lower moiety consistently empties proximal to that site. In a duplex kidney with hydronephrosis, then, the upper ureter (e.g., megaureter, see Chapter 11) and associated pelvis will be obstructed owing to the ectopic insertion (caution: upper-pole cyst). But if the lower ureter is affected, the obstruction is not due to an ectopic insertion but to some other obstructive process.

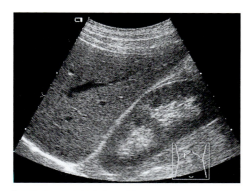

▲ **Fig. 9.10** Duplex kidney: 12 cm-long kidney with two pelves separated by a band of parenchyma.

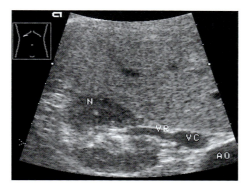

▲ **Fig. 9.11** Duplicated renal hilum. VC = vena cava; AO = aorta; N = kidney; VR = renal vein.
a Upper renal vein.

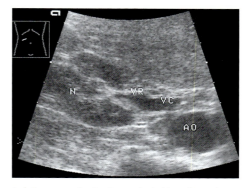

▲ **b** Lower renal vein, demonstrated by a lower transverse scan.

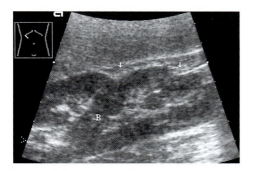

▲ **Fig. 9.12** Duplex kidney. The two moieties are separated by a parenchymal band (B), where a notch is visible in the renal outline (arrows; the lower arrow marks the hilum of the lower renal segment).

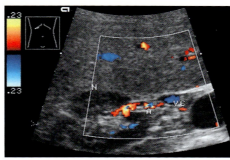

▲ **Fig. 9.13** Color duplex image showing two renal pelves. N = kidney; VC = vena cava.
a Upper renal artery (A).

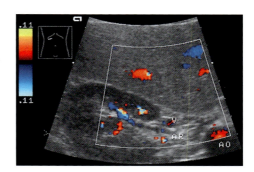

▲ **b** Lower renal artery (AR).

It is common to find an ectopic insertion of the lower moiety with an associated ureterocele, leading to vesicorenal reflux or ureteral obstruction that again affects the upper moiety (with a ureterocele, it cannot be determined with ultrasound whether the ureter runs within or outside the detrusor muscle).

The ultrasound features of a duplex kidney are as follows (**Figs. 9.10–9.13**):

▶ Longitudinal enlargement with a normal organ thickness

▶ A band of parenchyma separating the upper and lower collecting systems
▶ Usually, a notch at the level of the parenchymal band
▶ Duplication of the renal hilum

▶ Ectopic Kidney

Most ectopic kidneys are located low in the pelvis; high ectopic kidneys are very rare[3].

A lumbar kidney is the most common form of renal ectopia, with ultrasound revealing the ectopic kidney in the anterior iliac fossa. The key sonographic landmark is the iliac artery—the ectopic kidney will generally be found anterior to that vessel. The less common pelvic kidney lies anterior to the sacrum and below the aortic bifurcation. Abdominal ectopia is the easiest form to detect, as the affected kidney is markedly lower than its counterpart; but in contrast to the lumbar and pelvic forms, usually the kidney is not small or malrotated (**Fig. 9.14**).

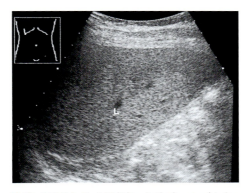

▲ **Fig. 9.14** Ectopic right kidney in the lesser pelvis (renal pelvic dysplasia).
a The right kidney is not found at its usual site posterior to the liver (L) (no renal impression!).

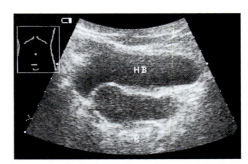

▲ **b** The dysplastic right kidney is located in the lesser pelvis between the bladder (HB) and rectum (R).

▶ Malrotation

Malrotation is an anomaly in which the renal hilum faces anteriorly (caution: this makes the vessels vulnerable to a percutaneous needle!). Otherwise difficult to detect, a malrotated kidney can be positively identified by the location of its hilum (**Fig. 9.15**).

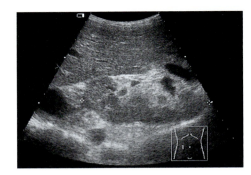

◀ *Fig. 9.15* Malrotated kidney in a slightly ectopic location (cursors). The renal hilum faces anteriorly.

Fusion Anomaly

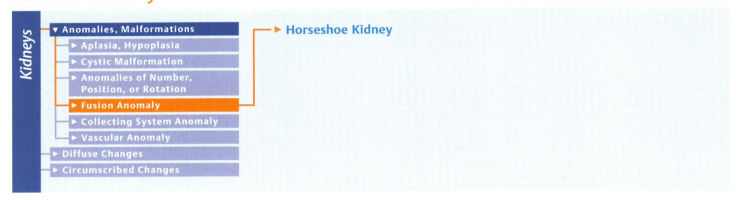

▶ Horseshoe Kidney

In the most common fusion anomaly, the symmetrical horseshoe kidney, the lower poles of the kidneys are fused together across the midline. Horseshoe kidney has an incidence of 1:425 in the general population. The descriptive term is best understood in the excretory urogram, where an AP view displays the typical horseshoe pattern (**Fig. 9.16**).

It is not unusual for horseshoe kidney to be missed at ultrasound, as the scan planes may not completely define the inferior outline of the lower pole. A lower pole that "keeps going" should always raise suspicion of the anomaly. Ultrasound may suggest a misdiagnosis of preaortic lymphoma unless horseshoe kidney is considered in the differential diagnosis. The apparent "tumor mass" in these cases is the isthmus joining the two lower poles, which may consist of renal parenchyma or a fibrous band (**Fig. 9.17**). Color Doppler usually establishes the diagnosis by demonstrating the typical vascular configuration.

Incomplete horseshoe kidney is diagnosed when ultrasound shows the typical medial extension of the lower pole, often crossing the aorta, but the contralateral kidney is absent. Morphologically, this results in an elongated L-shaped or sigmoid kidney. Fusion of the upper and lower poles results in a ring-shaped kidney. A cake kidney results when the fusion occurs over broader areas, producing an irregularly shaped organ.

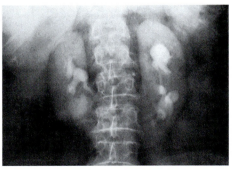

▲ *Fig. 9.16* Radiograph of a horseshoe kidney. The horseshoe shape of the kidney is appreciated in this AP view following intravenous contrast administration.

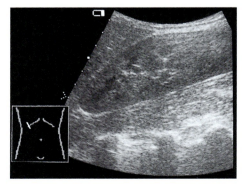
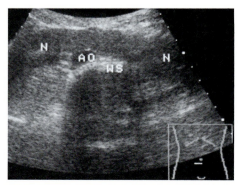
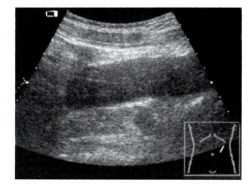

▲ *Fig. 9.17* Horseshoe kidney.
   a Right kidney with an unbounded lower pole.   ▲ **b and c** The renal parenchyma (N) continues to the left across the aorta (AO) and spinal column (WS).

Collecting System Anomaly

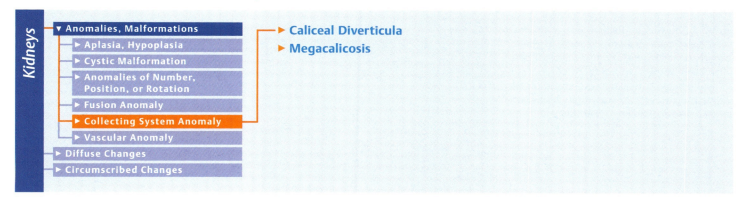

▶ Caliceal Diverticula

Caliceal diverticula are epithelialized protrusions of caliceal tissue that often contain crystalline precipitate and stones as a result of flow stasis (**Fig. 11.10, p. 335**). They require differentiation from caliectasis due to obstructing caliceal stones, which are more common in older patients.

▶ Megacalicosis

This is a congenital dilatation of the calices, which is usually asymptomatic.

Vascular Anomaly

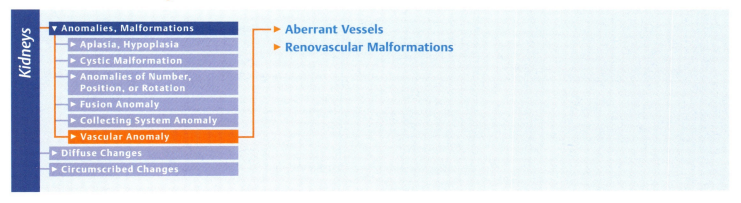

▶ Aberrant Vessels

A crossing interlobar artery will occasionally narrow the neck of the calix, causing prestenotic dilatation of the upper calix. Ultrasound then shows an abnormal expansion of the affected calix with no visible outflow obstruction (stone).

A more common aberrant configuration is a lower pole artery arising separately from the aorta and narrowing the upper ureter, causing pyelectasis. Ultrasound shows an anechoic mass in the pyelocaliceal system obstructing the proximal ureter but does not demonstrate a causative lesion (tumor, stone). This anomaly should always be suspected in cases of this kind (**Fig. 11.11, p. 335**). The differential diagnosis should also include pyelectasis due to an ampullary renal pelvis and a hypermobile kidney with proximal kinking of the ureter.

▶ Renovascular Malformations

These include intrarenal or extrarenal aneurysms, arteriovenous fistulas, and extrarenal vessels that take an atypical course. The latter are occasionally found at routine ultrasonography. Color duplex scanning should be performed whenever unexplained ectatic vessels, indeterminate cystic lesions, or atypical vascular courses are discovered (**Fig. 9.18**).

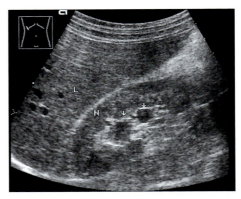
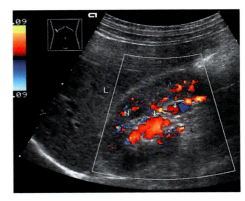

▲ **Fig. 9.18** Intrarenal vascular ectasia. Arteriovenous malformation appears as an echo-free mass within the kidney. L = liver; N = kidney.
a B-mode image demonstrates cystic masses in the renal sinus echo (arrows).

▲ **b** Color duplex scan identifies the cystic masses as ectatic intrarenal arterial vessels, probably arteriovenous malformations of the renal artery. (Doppler spectral analysis with resistance index [after Pourcelot: $V_{max} - V_{min} = V_{max}$] determination yields additional information on the nature of the vascular ectasia.)

Diffuse Changes

Large Kidneys

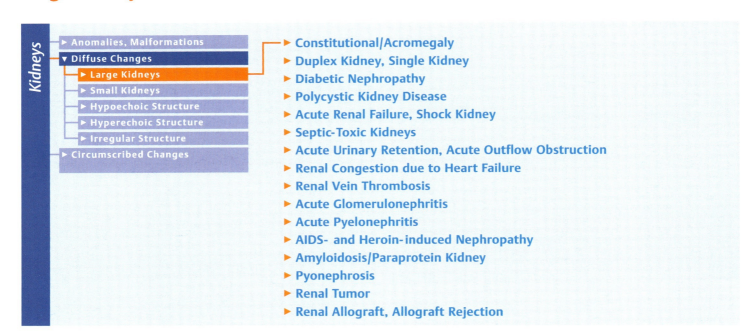

Sonographic Determination of Renal Size

The sonographic estimation of renal size is unreliable. Whether a kidney appears large or small at ultrasonography depends very much on the selected field of view, i.e., an undersize kidney may appear large because it is displayed in a large scale, and vice-versa (**Fig. 9.19**). For some investigations, then, it is necessary to measure at least the longitudinal renal diameter and parenchymal thickness.

Anatomically, the adult kidney measures 1 cm over the sonographic diameter, 10–11.5 cm in length, 5–7 cm in width, and 3–4 cm in thickness, while for physical reasons, radiographic measurements of the kidney add approximately 1.5 cm to its length and 1 cm to its width. Sonographic measurements are slightly smaller than the true dimensions because the kidneys occupy planes that are angled laterally and anteromedially and do not coincide precisely with the planes used for routine scanning.

The size ratio of the renal parenchyma to the central sinus echo provides an index for evaluating parenchymal thickness. **Table 9.2** shows how the normal ratio of the anterior and posterior parenchyma to the central sinus echo (the parenchymal–pelvic ratio) changes with aging.

Table 9.2 Dependence of the parenchymal–pelvic ratio on age (after reference 6)

Age (years)	Ratio
< 40	1.8 : 1–2.0 : 1
40–60	1.7 : 1
> 60	1.1 : 1

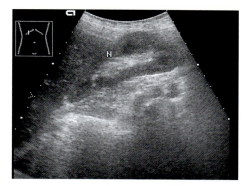
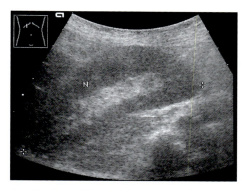

▲ **Fig. 9.19** Subjective assessment of renal size.
a In a large field of view, the kidney (N) appears small in relation to the overall image.

▲ **b** The kidney (N) appears larger in an enlarged view. According to measurements, this kidney is small but still within normal limits for the patient's body size.

▶ Constitutional/Acromegaly

Renal size is dependent on the patient's constitution or body size. As a result, the renal dimensions may be above or below normal, but the shape and parenchymal–pelvic ratio will still be within normal limits (**Table 9.2**). Lengths from 9.6 to 13 cm may still be considered normal, depending on body size (**Fig. 9.20**). Nomograms plotted for children (by Weitzel and Tröger) show a direct correlation with body size.

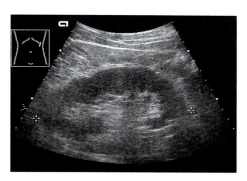
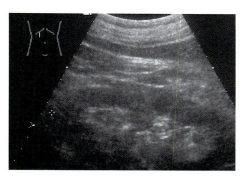

▲ **Fig. 9.20 a** Constitutionally large kidney (13.5 cm, contralateral 13.0 cm) in a 47-year-old man with a height of 196 cm and body weight of 111 kg.

▲ **b** Enlarged kidneys in acromegaly (13.7 cm).

▶ Duplex Kidney, Single Kidney

Duplex kidney. One of the most common types of renal enlargement involves duplex kidneys, whose sonographic features are described above. Their shape at ultrasound resembles that of a pretzel. The longitudinal diameter may be normal or increased up to 15 cm, with a normal width. The overall thickness may be increased if the duplicated kidneys are arranged side by side (**Fig. 9.21**), creating a tumorlike appearance. The moieties can be distinguished from a tumor by color Doppler sonography, which shows a normal duplex vascular pattern.

Single kidney. A single kidney undergoes compensatory physiological enlargement in response to contralateral hypoplasia or aplasia, contralateral nephrectomy, a nonfunctioning opposite kidney, or a renal allograft (**Fig. 9.22**).

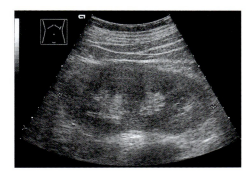
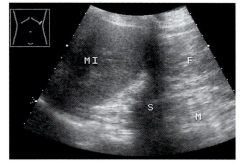
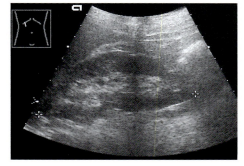

▲ **Fig. 9.21** Large duplex kidney with multiple parenchymal bands.

▲ **Fig. 9.22** Renal aplasia.
a Absent left kidney, empty renal fossa below the spleen (Ml) on the left side. F = fatty tissue; M = musculature; S = shadow.

▲ **b** Compensatory enlargement of the right kidney (12.3 cm, cursors).

▶ Diabetic Nephropathy

Another common but less familiar form of renal enlargement occurs in diabetic nephropathy. In its later stages, it is the most frequent indication for hemodialysis. In the early stage, which marks the onset of a progressive function impairment leading to frank renal failure, the kidneys are enlarged as a result of hyperperfusion. According to studies of diabetic nephropathy in type I diabetics, the enlargement is based on a volume increase[1] affecting both the longitudinal diameter and thickness of the organ.

In cases where diabetes and blood pressure are effectively controlled, the early changes (Mogensen stages I–III [8]) are reversible, which is why early detection at the hyperperfusion stage critically influences the prognosis. Other criteria of diabetic nephropathy are not present in stages I and II, and the only sign of hyperperfusion is an elevated creatinine clearance rate in excess of 120 ml/min.

Sonographic features. At ultrasound, the renal parenchyma is thickened and often shows increased sonodensity. The medullary pyramids appear bulky and less echogenic than the adjacent parenchyma, which often but not always shows increased echogenicity. The kidney should therefore be measured in patients evaluated for diabetic nephropathy. It is not until an advanced stage, when the patient requires hemodialysis, that the kidney shrinks in size and shows obvious structural changes. Other signs of diabetic nephropathy are swollen, hypoechoic medullary pyramids. In advanced stages (Mogensen stages IV–V, here with frank renal failure), the parenchyma shows increased echogenicity (**Figs. 9.23 and 9.24**).

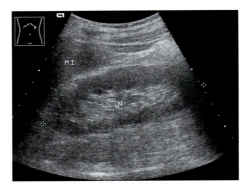

▲ *Fig. 9.23* Stage IV diabetic nephropathy with a large kidney (N) (12.1 cm) and proteinuria. Long history of type II diabetes mellitus. Six months later, persistent diarrhea and reversible decompensation with creatinine of 8 mg/dl. MI = spleen.

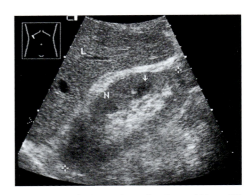

▲ *Fig. 9.24* Diabetic nephropathy. Large kidney (N) (12.5 cm) with prominent hypoechoic medullary pyramids (arrow). L = liver.

▶ Polycystic Kidney Disease

Besides multiple anechoic lesions and ill-defined borders, polycystic kidneys are conspicuous by their impressive enlargement due to the mass effect of the cysts (**Fig. 9.8**).

▶ Acute Renal Failure, Shock Kidney

In the setting of acute renal failure and renal shock or severe hypovolemia, ultrasound usually shows an increased parenchymal volume and a decrease (or increase) in echogenicity with enlargement of the kidneys and consequent narrowing of the sinus echo complex (**Fig. 9.25**).

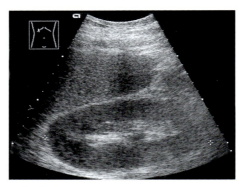

▲ *Fig. 9.25 a* Acute prerenal renal failure. Creatinine 8.2 mg/dl (alcohol-related disease, persistent vomiting and diarrhea). The kidney is greatly enlarged (16.1 cm) with a hypoechoic, ill-defined structure.

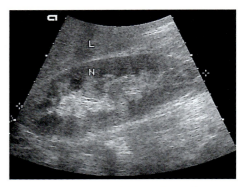

▲ *b* Sepsis, alcohol-related disease, kidney (N) enlarged to 13.0 cm. Renal echogenicity is slightly decreased. The medullary pyramids are swollen and very hypoechoic. L = liver.

▶ Septic-Toxic Kidneys

Renal enlargement also occurs occasionally in sepsis. The kidneys tend to show increased echogenicity, probably due a suppurative, leukocytic reaction to septicopyemic foci in the organs. The reaction may also be a result of dehydration (**Fig. 9.26**).

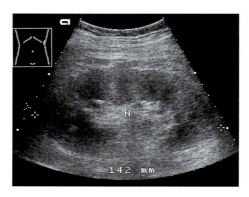

◀ *Fig. 9.26* Septic-toxic kidneys with renal failure: greatly enlarged kidney (N) with parenchymal swelling. The medullary pyramids are markedly enlarged and hypoechoic.

Acute Urinary Retention, Acute Outflow Obstruction

In this situation as well, the kidneys often react with enlargement and decreased echogenicity due to interstitial edema. The medullary pyramids may show signs of conspicuous swelling. Often the bladder is greatly distended. The sonographic renal changes are the same as those seen in renal congestion resulting from heart failure.

Renal Congestion due to Heart Failure

The fluid build-up that occurs in severe congestive heart failure leads to swelling and increased echogenicity of the renal parenchyma secondary to edema and hemorrhage. This swelling is another cause of renal enlargement (**Fig. 9.27**).

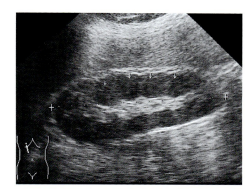

◂ *Fig. 9.27* Acute prerenal renal failure: enlarged kidneys (13.0 cm), hypoechoic parenchyma, and swollen, hypoechoic medullary pyramids (arrows).

Renal Vein Thrombosis

Acute renal vein thrombosis also leads to enlargement and unilateral hypoechoic swelling of the parenchyma (**Fig. 9.28**). The diagnosis is supported by:

▸ A broadened renal vein that contains intraluminal echoes and is devoid of color flow
▸ A high resistance index (after Pourcelot: $V_{max} - V_{min} = V_{max}$) in the intrarenal renal arteries
▸ Reverse flow (hard, negative systolic signal in the renal artery)

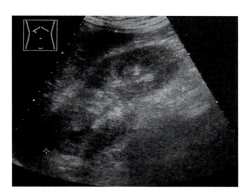

▴ *Fig. 9.28 a* Renal vein thrombosis secondary to suppurative pyelitis. The kidney is greatly enlarged to 142 mm (cursors) with a hazy, irregular hypoechoic structure.

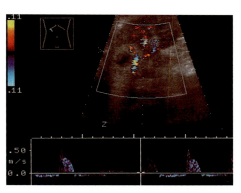

▴ *b* Spectral analysis in renal vein thrombosis indicates an extremely high resistance index of 0.96.

Acute Glomerulonephritis

In acute glomerulonephritis there may be significant broadening of the renal cortex with greatly increased echogenicity due to hyaline casts, leukocyte infiltration, glomerular obliteration, and tubular atrophy[5]. The increased cortical echogenicity is in stark contrast with the low echogenicity of the medullary pyramids (**Fig. 9.29, Fig. 9.41**).

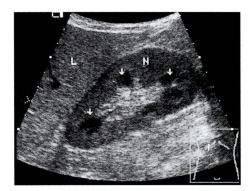

◂ *Fig. 9.29* Acute IGA (immune globulin A) nephritis: slightly enlarged, swollen kidney (N) with prominent medullary pyramids (arrows).

Acute Pyelonephritis

A different picture is seen with severe acute septic pyelonephritis, in which one or both kidneys are enlarged and generally show a decrease in parenchymal echogenicity. Often there are accompanying abscesses, pyonephrosis, or merely circumscribed anechoic to hyperechoic lesions in the parenchyma, renal pelvis, or renal sinus representing abscesses or infected, purulent urine. Swelling of the renal pelvic walls is also occasionally seen (**Fig. 9.30**). Other characteristic findings are urothelial thickening to more than 2 mm and hypoechoic foci in the parenchyma.

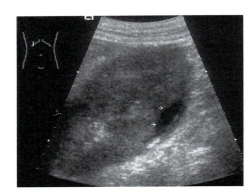 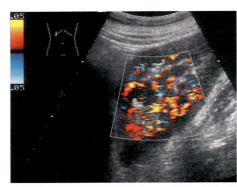

Fig. 9.30 a Acute septic pyelonephritis: slightly enlarged kidney with swollen, hypoechoic parenchyma. The sinus echo has largely disappeared. Focal abscess (arrows).

b Color duplex shows inflammatory hypervascularity.

▶ AIDS- and Heroin-induced Nephropathy

As in other forms of renal enlargement, these cases show increased cortical echogenicity that heightens the contrast with the unchanged, hypoechoic medullary pyramids.

▶ Amyloidosis/Paraprotein Kidney

The sonographic changes in amyloidosis are like those seen in AIDS-related and heroin-related nephropathy and acute glomerulonephritis. These conditions are indistinguishable by their sonographic features (**Fig. 9.31, Fig. 9.50**).

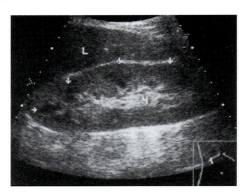

Fig. 9.31 Paraprotein kidney (lymphoplasmacytic immunocytoma with Bence Jones proteinuria). Enlarged kidney (N) shows slightly increased echogenicity relative to the liver (L). The medullary pyramids (arrows) are markedly swollen and show patchy low echogenicity due to protein-filled tubules, with the formation of hyaline casts in the distal tubules (creatinine 3.0 mg/dl).

▶ Pyonephrosis

If the purulent collection in the renal pelvis takes up the entire central echo complex, the pyonephrotic mass leads to overall renal enlargement. The affected kidney has a tumorlike appearance and is hardly distinguishable from a large tumor by its ultrasound features (**Fig. 9.76;** ▣ **11.3g–i**).

▶ Renal Tumor

The characteristic appearance of a malignant renal tumor is that of a circumscribed, hypoechoic mass. Renal cell carcinoma appears as a sharply circumscribed bulge in the renal outline, while urothelial carcinoma forms a hypoechoic mass in the central sinus echo. With extensive tumor infiltration, the kidney appears substantially enlarged and broadened. Its structure is markedly nonhomogeneous owing to intrarenal pyelectasis and the presence of calcifications (**Fig. 9.32**).

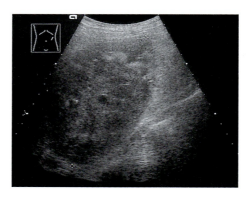

Fig. 9.32 Greatly enlarged kidney completely permeated by tumor. The kidney shows a heterogeneous, predominantly hypoechoic structure. Histological diagnosis: high-grade non-Hodgkin lymphoma.

▶ Renal Allograft, Allograft Rejection

As a solitary functioning kidney, the renal allograft is enlarged owing to adaptive hypertrophy. Additional enlargement occurs in association with allograft rejection. Enlargement is not a dependable sign of rejection, however. A more definitive sign is occlusive vasculopathy, which can be demonstrated with Doppler ultrasound.

Complications consist of renal artery stenosis, renal vein thrombosis, and arteriovenous fistulas. The resistance index (RI) in these cases is greater than 0.9 and the pulsatility index (PI) is greater than 1.6. Published reports on sensitivity and specificity range from 14% to 98%! (**Fig. 9.33**).

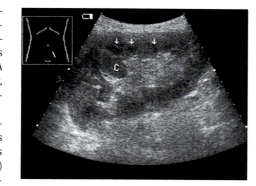

◀ *Fig. 9.33* Renal transplant. The allograft is enlarged to 13.0 cm, with accentuated renal columns (C) and prominent hypoechoic medullary pyramids (arrows).

Small Kidneys

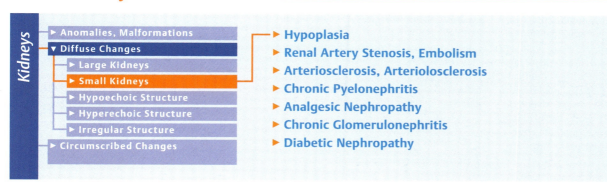

▶ Hypoplasia

Renal hypoplasia is characterized by a small kidney with essentially normal parenchyma accompanied by compensatory contralateral enlargement and often showing ectopia or malrotation. These features serve to distinguish a hypoplastic kidney from other, secondary forms of small kidney with associated structural and contour changes (**see Fig. 9.7**).

▶ Renal Artery Stenosis, Embolism

When a small kidney is due to renal artery stenosis, generally the stenosis is severe and of long duration and is associated with chronic hypertension.

Renal artery stenosis may be classified as atherosclerotic (85% of cases) or fibromuscular (15%). Accessory renal arteries occur in up to 28% of cases, so that when renovascular hypertension is diagnosed, these vessels should be included in diagnostic considerations.

Sonographic features. The parenchyma may appear normal or thinned at ultrasound. The structure is largely normal. The maximum flow velocity rises to values above 180 cm/s at the stenosis, and there is concomitant spectral broadening and aliasing. The resistance index associated with stenosis or occlusion of the segmental arteries is less than 0.5 with a sensitivity of 95% and a specificity of 97%[2].

The following signs indicate an occlusion:
▶ No intraluminal color or flow signals in the color Doppler image
▶ Markedly decreased flow velocity and RI in intrarenal branches relative to the opposite side
▶ Renal length decreased to less than 9 cm

With a renal arterial trunk embolism, a large portion of the kidney may become anemic and diminished in size, accompanied by an increase in echogenicity (**Fig. 9.34**).

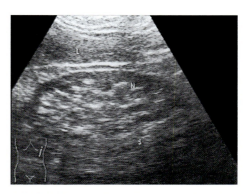

▲ *Fig. 9.34* Small, nonfunctioning kidney with a filiform renal artery stenosis.

▸ Arteriosclerosis, Arteriolosclerosis

While arteriolosclerosis leads to a decrease in renal size with thinning of the cortex, arteriosclerosis causes an irregular surface with areas of parenchyma thinning but a normal overall renal size. Similar changes are seen as a result of multiple infarcts in panarteritis nodosa (**Fig. 9.35**).

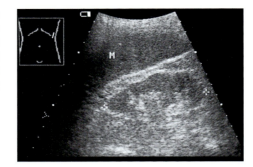

◂ **Fig. 9.35** Left kidney is atrophic probably due to arteriolosclerosis. Note the wavy surface contour. M = spleen.

▸ Chronic Pyelonephritis

Chronic pyelonephritis is a chronic interstitial (bacterial), episodic inflammatory process characterized by the scarring and destruction of renal parenchyma. In bilateral cases that have progressed to a stage requiring dialysis, the kidneys are significantly smaller than normal, especially in their longitudinal dimension[9]. Additional features are focal changes such as stones (33%) and cysts (31%) and changes in cortical structure with a significant increase in echogenicity (◨ **9.2g**). In interstitial renal diseases, a correlation exists between the echogenicity of the renal cortex and histological changes such as sclerosis, tubular atrophy, hyaline casts, and focal leukocyte infiltration[5].

A small or atrophic kidney in pyelonephritis is more often unilateral than bilateral, and it can be difficult in these cases to establish a cause. In the advanced stage of renal atrophy when the longitudinal size of the kidney has dwindled to approximately 6–7 cm, ultrasound generally is no longer helpful in diagnosing the cause. In addition to these changes, abscesses may form in the renal pelvis, appearing as hypoechoic masses. This is especially common in diabetics with an acute infection (**Figs. 9.36 and 9.61**, ◨ **9.5d**).

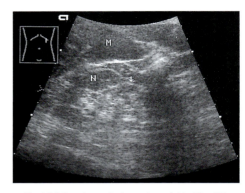

▴ **Fig. 9.36** Renal atrophy in pyelonephritis. The kidney is difficult to detect, consisting only of residual parenchyma (N) and scars (arrows). The patient had a history of recurrent pyelonephritis and analgesic use. M = spleen.

▸ Analgesic Nephropathy

The term analgesic nephropathy refers to a chronic, abacterial, interstitial, bilateral nephritis that is incited by the use of analgesic medication. The histological features are a lumen-occluding capillary sclerosis, tubular and papillary necrosis, and papillary necrosis with calcification of the papillary tips.

The sonographic features reflect the histological changes in the form of decreased renal size, increased echogenicity, wavy contours, and fine calcifications at the tips of the medullary pyramids. Some cases present with secondary microcysts, usually resulting from the cystic degeneration of medullary pyramids, or with tubular retention cysts (detectable in 50% of cases)[9] (**Fig. 9.37**).

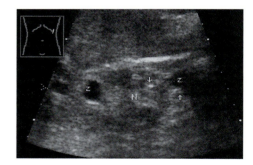

▴ **Fig. 9.37** Analgesic nephropathy (N). Marked parenchymal rarefaction with a hazy structure and fine calcifications projected over the papillary tips (arrows). Secondary cyst (Z). Patient had a 30-year history of daily analgesic use and known pyelonephritis. Creatinine 4.8 mmol/l. Harmonic imaging.

▸ Chronic Glomerulonephritis

Chronic glomerulonephritis and diabetic nephropathy (glomerulosclerosis) are both characterized by a decrease in renal size that does not occur until an advanced stage. In both diseases, the longitudinal diameter of the kidney is within normal limits in patients who have reached the dialysis stage[9]. The authors found cystic lesions in 14% of cases.

Sonographically, the kidney shows markedly increased echogenicity due to glomerular hyalinization and tubular atrophy. The medullary pyramids may still be appreciated as hypoechoic areas, but in most cases they disappear owing to histologically demonstrable tubular atrophy. In advanced stages the renal structural change may no longer be helpful in identifying the cause of the disease (**Figs. 9.38, 9.41, and 9.42**).

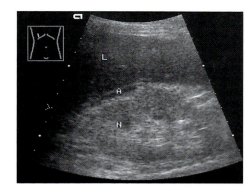

▲ *Fig. 9.38* Small, hyperechoic right kidney (N) due to an unknown cause. Left-sided hydronephrosis (following ureteral ligation). Renal failure with creatinine of 5.6 mg/dl. L = liver; A = ascites.

▶ Diabetic Nephropathy

In our own observations of diabetics with nephropathy, we found that the renal sizes in stage I to stage IV cases of diabetic nephropathy[8] were consistently above normal, with lengths up to 13.5 cm. In stage V disease, the kidneys are either normal or slightly decreased in size, and small kidneys are not seen until the later dialysis stage.

Ultrasound at that stage demonstrates rarefied areas in the cortex and increased echogenicity. Microcysts are also found, consisting mainly of medullary pyramids that have undergone cystic degeneration. The end stage is marked by atrophic kidneys with complete parenchymal destruction, and the nature of the disease can no longer be determined from sonographic findings (**Fig. 9.39**).

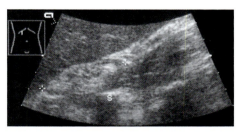

▲ *Fig. 9.39* Atrophic kidney (cursors) in diabetic nephropathy requiring dialysis. The kidney, which is very difficult to identify, has an irregular structure and contains calcifications with acoustic shadows (S).

Hypoechoic Structure

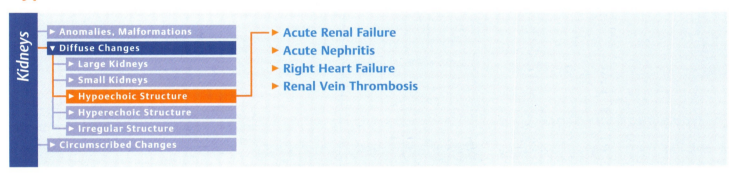

Many renal diseases marked by structural changes are also associated with a change in renal size. Thus, some of the following disorders have already been described above and will be merely outlined here. It should also be noted that while the features listed are suggestive of the various diseases, they do not necessarily mean that ultrasound can sensitively detect the disease in question.

▶ Acute Renal Failure

If there are any characteristic changes in acute renal failure, they are renal enlargement and decreased echogenicity. In many cases, however, no significant abnormalities are seen (**Fig. 9.25**).

▶ Acute Nephritis

Besides renal enlargement, decreased parenchymal echogenicity is frequently seen as a result of inflammatory edema (**Fig. 9.29**).

► Right Heart Failure

Characteristic features are enlargement and decreased echogenicity, accompanied by congestion of the vena cava and renal veins (**Fig. 9.27**).

► Renal Vein Thrombosis

Renal vein thrombosis may be unilateral or bilateral. Besides the enlargement noted above, the renal parenchyma generally appears hypoechoic (**Fig. 9.28**). Color duplex evaluation of the renal veins is diagnostic.

Hyperechoic Structure

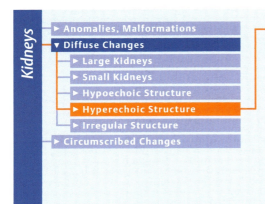

- Hypoxemic Renal Shock
- Diabetic Nephropathy
- Acute and Chronic Glomerulonephritis
- Chronic Pyelonephritis
- Analgesic Nephropathy
- Septic-Toxic Kidneys
- Severe Metabolic Disorders
- Light-Chain Deposition Disease, Waldenström Disease
- Amyloidosis
- Infiltration by Lymphoma
- Atrophic Kidneys

► Hypoxemic Renal Shock

A septic-toxic illness or hypoxemia can cause severe kidney damage with renal failure, leading to subtle but definite changes consisting of a diffuse increase in cortical echogenicity and very echopenic medullary pyramids. These changes are caused by diffuse tubular damage and necrosis, and also by decreased vascularization in cases with severe hypoxemia, so that hypovascular or avascular areas are found at color duplex scanning (**Fig. 9.40**).

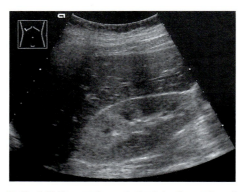

▲ **Fig. 9.40** Hypoxemic renal shock in the setting of acute cardiac and renal failure. The patient was resuscitated for ventricular fibrillation (after sniffing butane gas, with a fatal outcome).
a The parenchyma is broadened and hyperechoic, resulting in a narrow sinus echo complex. Prominent hypoechoic medullary pyramids.

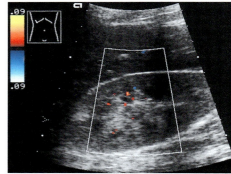

▲ **b** Color Doppler shows scant color signals, reflecting the marked decrease in vascularity.

► Diabetic Nephropathy

Diabetic nephropathy has become the most frequent indication for hemodialysis. Renal ultrasound examination in glomerular diseases, including diabetic glomerulosclerosis (known also as Kimmelstiel–Wilson syndrome), shows increased cortical echogenicity due to histopathological changes in basement membrane collagenization, glomerular enlargement, mesangial cell proliferation, and subsequent glomerulosclerosis. The lucency of the medullary pyramids stands in sharp contrast to the very echogenic cortex (◼ **9.1**) (**Table 9.3, 9.4**).

9.1 Diabetic Nephropathy (after reference 8)

▶ **Stages I and II** — Hyperperfusion with a volume increase

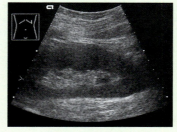

a Large kidneys, normal structure.

▶ **Stage III** — Incipient nephropathy with microalbuminuria (hyperperfusion with a volume increase)

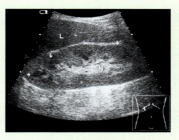

b Enlarged kidneys (N), normal width, incipient hyperechoic cortex, prominent hypoechoic medullary pyramids (arrows). L = liver.

▶ **Stage IV** — Overt nephropathy (proteinuria)

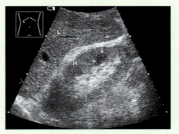

c Normal-size kidneys (N), parenchymal thickness still normal, increased cortical echogenicity; broadened, hypoechoic medullary pyramids.

▶ **Stage V** — Renal failure (nephrotic syndrome)

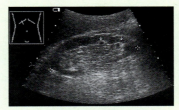

d Renal size still normal, rarefied cortex, markedly hypoechoic "cystic" pyramids with echogenic demarcation.

▶ **Stage V with dialysis**

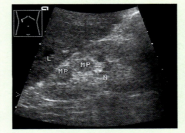

e Small kidneys (N) (8.7 cm), rarefied cortex, degeneration or disappearance of the medullary pyramids (MP), parenchymal destruction (possible secondary cysts, calcifications). Spotty, deformed vascular segments. L = liver.

Table 9.3 Sonographic changes seen in different stages of diabetic nephropathy

Early stage	Advanced stage	End stage
▶ Renal enlargement (volume increase) ▶ Increased cortical echogenicity ▶ Markedly hypoechoic medullary pyramids	▶ Normal renal size with rarefied parenchyma ▶ Increased cortical echogenicity ▶ Cystic transformation or disappearance of medullary pyramids ▶ Wavy contours	▶ Small kidneys ▶ Intensely hyperechoic parenchyma ▶ Disappearance of medullary pyramids ▶ Secondary cysts, calcifications

Table 9.4 Histopathology of chronic diabetic, glomerular and interstitial nephropathy (after reference 11)

Diabetic nephropathy	**Early stage** ▶ Glomerular enlargement, mesangial cell proliferation ▶ Basement membrane collagenization **Late stage** ▶ Glomerulosclerosis ▶ Broadened mesangium with deposits ▶ Arteriosclerosis ▶ Glycogen storage in tubules ▶ Papillary tip necrosis
Chronic glomerulonephritis	▶ Mesangial cell proliferation ▶ Glomerular enlargement ▶ Basement membrane thickening ▶ Mesangial, capillary, tubular deposits ▶ Cellular infiltrates
Chronic pyelonephritis	▶ Interstitial scarring ▶ Lymphoplasmocytic infiltrates ▶ Tubular atrophy ▶ Tubular protein deposits ▶ Scarring of the pyelocaliceal system
Analgesic nephropathy	▶ Papillary necrosis ▶ Broadening of the capillary basement membrane in the renal medulla (capillary sclerosis) ▶ Lipofuscin deposits in tubules ▶ Lymphoplasmohistiocytic infiltrate with fibrosis, sclerosis

▶ Acute and Chronic Glomerulonephritis

Both acute and chronic (bilateral) glomerulonephritis are associated with increased cortical echogenicity, which is more distinct than in diabetic nephropathy[9]. Again, the medullary pyramids appear markedly hypoechoic relative to the cortex. The kidney is enlarged in acute glomerulonephritis and is of normal size in chronic glomerulonephritis (**Figs. 9.41 and 9.42**).

The usually pronounced increase in echogenicity is caused by histological changes. It has been shown that cortical echogenicity correlates with histological criteria such as sclerosis, tubular atrophy, hyaline casts, and focal leukocytic infiltration[5] (**Table 9.4**).

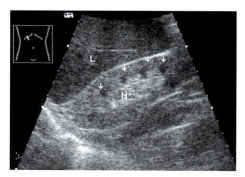

▲ *Fig. 9.41* Acute glomerulonephritis: enlarged kidneys (N) with markedly increased cortical echogenicity and very prominent, hypoechoic medullary pyramids (arrows).

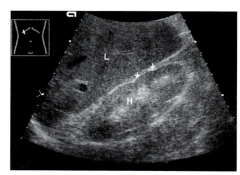

▲ *Fig. 9.42* Chronic glomerulonephritis (prior history of rheumatic fever) and chronic renal failure: small kidney (N), hyperechoic cortex, disappearance of the medullary pyramids, shallow notches due to scarring (arrows). L = liver.

▶ Chronic Pyelonephritis

Chronic pyelonephritis is also associated with increased echogenicity. The kidney is generally small, however, compared with the inflammatory conditions listed above, and scarring leads to areas of parenchymal thinning (**Fig. 9.43, Table 9.4**).

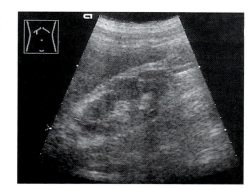

◀ **Fig. 9.43** Old chronic pyelonephritis: small kidney with multiple echogenic sites of parenchymal retraction due to scarring.

▶ Analgesic Nephropathy

Of all the chronic renal diseases, analgesic nephropathy shows the greatest increase in echogenicity. As in the other diseases above, this results from underlying histological changes, chiefly fibrosis, sclerosis, and calcifications. Sonographically, the changes cause scarring with contour irregularities, lack of demarcation, a decrease in renal size, anechoic areas (secondary cysts), and very hyperechoic areas with associated acoustic shadows, especially from calcifications at the tips of the papillae (**Fig. 9.37, Fig. 9.44, Table 9.4**).

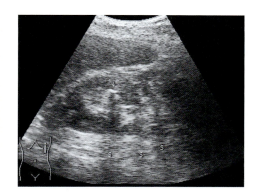

◀ **Fig. 9.44** Analgesic nephropathy: nonhomogeneous, hyperechoic parenchyma with ill-defined contours. Note the hyperechoic areas at the tips of the medullary pyramids (calcifying papillary necrosis, acoustic shadows S).

▶ Septic-Toxic Kidneys

Severe septic-toxic disease states are characterized by a markedly hyperechoic, swollen renal cortex. The changes are usually associated with renal enlargement. Direct septic-toxic tissue effects such as necrosis, lympholeukocytic infiltration, or ischemic vascular changes can occur. Similar changes are found in acute tubular obstruction by urates in the chemotherapy of malignant lymphoma, also in acute renal failure, lupus erythematosus, hemolytic-uremic syndrome, and acute glomerular renal diseases. After the systemic manifestations have subsided, the diffuse structural changes also regress (**Figs. 9.45 and 9.46**).

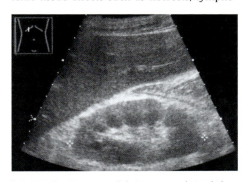

▲ **Fig. 9.45** Septic-toxic abdomen: normal-size kidney with increased cortical echogenicity and prominent hypoechoic medullary pyramids.

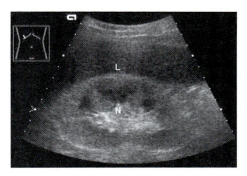

▲ **Fig. 9.46** Septic-toxic renal failure.
a The kidney (N) shows greatly increased echogenicity relative to the liver (L). Note the prominent, hypoechoic medullary pyramids.

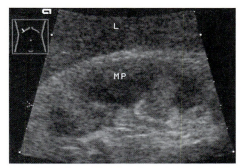

▲ *b* Enlarged view shows massive swelling and decreased echogenicity of the medullary pyramids (MP).

▶ Severe Metabolic Disorders

Severe metabolic disorders such as untreated diabetes mellitus, with or without diabetic coma, are occasionally associated with pronounced renal structural changes. Possible causes are severe dehydration, tubular glycogen storage or other storage disorders, as well as glomerular/tubular changes that do not always have a discernible cause, especially if the case cannot be evaluated histologically (**Figs. 9.47 and 9.48**).

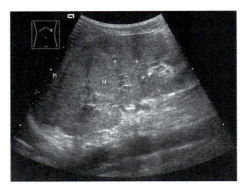

▲ **Fig. 9.47** Neglected case of type I diabetes mellitus: massive parenchymal swelling, increased echogenicity (relative to the spleen M), prominent hypoechoic pyramids (arrows). Lateral flank scan displays the aortic band at the bottom of the image. N = kidney.

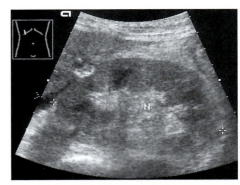

▲ **Fig. 9.48** Toxic renal failure secondary to extensive thrombosis of the portal venous system: large, echogenic kidney (N), prominent hypoechoic pyramids, perirenal ascites.

▶ Light-Chain Deposition Disease, Waldenström Disease

Light-chain deposition disease is a nonspecific condition that leads to renal failure based on the precipitation of light-chain paraproteins in the distal tubules, a hypercalcemic tubulopathy in hypercalcemia syndrome, and/or an accompanying deposition of amyloid. Similar changes are encountered in Waldenström disease and amyloid kidney.

Ultrasound may demonstrate renal enlargement and increased cortical echogenicity. Often there is only mild enlargement with an indistinct parenchymal texture (**Fig. 9.49**).

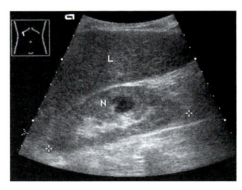

▲ **Fig. 9.49** Light-chain deposition disease, hypercalcemic crisis, renal failure.
a Right kidney (N): parenchyma has a somewhat indistinct structure and appears slightly hyperechoic to the liver (L). Prominent medullary pyramids.

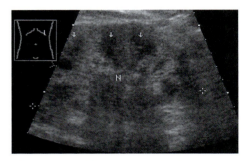

▲ ***b*** Acute renal failure requiring dialysis in a patient with paraproteinemia (and initial hypercalcemia) and a plasmacytoma. The kidneys are still of normal size (N, cursors). The parenchyma shows markedly increased echogenicity with enlarged, hypoechoic to anechoic medullary pyramids (arrows).

▶ Amyloidosis

Amyloidosis is also associated with an increase in cortical echogenicity and prominent hypoechoic pyramids. We see, then, that these diffuse structural changes occur in a variety of diseases and cannot be considered specific sonographic features; indeed, they are very nonspecific. Only if the underlying disease is known can the echogenicity changes be referred to a specific renal complication (**Fig. 9.50**).

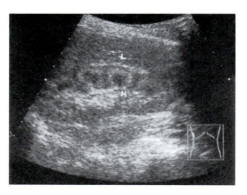

◀ **Fig. 9.50** Presumed renal amyloidosis: echogenic renal cortex with increased parenchymal volume causing slight narrowing of the sinus echo complex. Hypoechoic, ill-defined medullary pyramids (rheumatoid arthritis, renal failure with nephrotic syndrome). L = liver; N = kidney.

▶ Infiltration by Lymphoma

The infiltrating lymphomatous tissue leads to renal enlargement (see above). Increased echogenicity may be seen, but the bulges in the renal outline, frequent nonhomogeneous structure, and irregular tumor vascularity serve to distinguish this disease from those listed above (**Fig. 9.32 and Fig. 9.79**).

▶ Atrophic Kidneys

Generally the detection of renal atrophy does not point to a specific cause (**Fig. 9.51**), although bilateral atrophic kidneys are more likely to have a diabetic etiology (only in the late dialysis stage) or a glomerular cause or may result from analgesic nephropathy.

Unilateral renal atrophy, or bilateral atrophy that differs in severity between the sides, usually has a different cause such as pyelonephritis or vasopathy (**Fig. 9.52**).

As the name implies, the kidneys appear small at ultrasound. The parenchyma is thinned, and the renal outlines are smooth (glomerular, diabetic) or wavy (pyelonephritis or analgesic nephropathy). The structure is usually echogenic (except with renal artery stenosis). In the end stage of tuberculous kidneys ("putty kidney"), very hyperechoic areas are also seen. Calcifications and secondary stones are additionally found in some atrophic kidneys (**Figs. 9.53, 9.37, 9.39, and 9.94**).

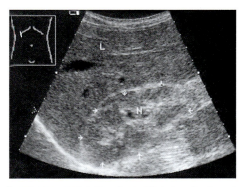
▲ **Fig. 9.51** Small, hyperechoic right kidney (N, arrows) due to an unknown cause. Slight structural irregularity. L = liver.

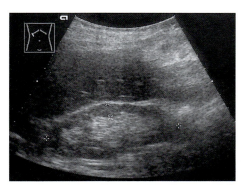
▲ **Fig. 9.52** Renal atrophy (85 mm) due to arteriosclerosis and arteriolosclerosis: irregular, rarefied, slightly hyperechoic parenchyma (cursors) with a correspondingly broadened sinus echo.

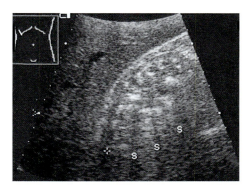
▲ **Fig. 9.53** Severely atrophic kidney with calcifications and acoustic shadows (S). Diabetic nephropathy, transplantation.

Irregular Structure

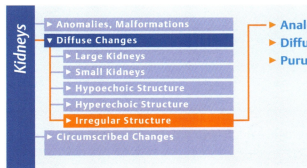

▶ Analgesic Nephropathy

The kidney in analgesic nephropathy also acquires an irregular echo structure as a result of fibrosis, papillary calcifications, and secondary cystic and calcifying changes (**Figs. 9.37, 9.44**).

▶ Diffuse Tumor Infiltration

Secondary changes such as liquefaction, calcification, and fresh tumor growth lead to irregular structural changes in the kidney. Renal enlargement and contour irregularities are also present (**Fig. 9.32**).

▶ Suppurative Pyelonephritis, Pyonephrosis

In cases with extensive pyelonephritis involving much of the renal pelvis and parenchyma, the hypoechoic inflammatory changes will be accompanied by a generally irregular structure like that associated with other types of abscess formation (**Fig. 9.54; see also** ◉ **11.3, p. 344**). The central sinus echo complex is poorly defined. In pyonephrosis caused by an ascending infection, the pyelocaliceal system is completely filled with pus.

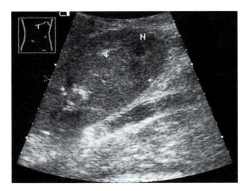

◀ *Fig. 9.54* Suppurative pyelonephritis (arrows): heterogeneous mass in the renal sinus echo complex with hyperechoic areas (bacterial gas bubbles? residual sinus echoes?). N = kidney.

Circumscribed Changes

Anechoic Structure

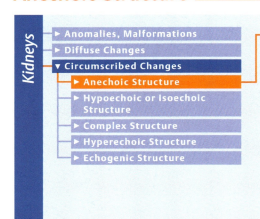

- ▶ Renal Cysts, Polycystic Kidney
- ▶ Perirenal Cystic Masses
- ▶ Lymph Cysts
- ▶ Cystic Renal Cell Carcinoma, Intracystic Carcinoma
- ▶ Papillary Necrosis, Cystic Degeneration of the Medullary Pyramids
- ▶ Cavities
- ▶ Abscess
- ▶ Organized Hematoma
- ▶ Urinoma, Seroma
- ▶ Vascular Dilatations
- ▶ Hydrocalices, Pyelectasis, Hydronephrosis

▶ Renal Cysts, Polycystic Kidney

Simple cysts (dysontogenic). Round, sharply circumscribed, anechoic masses located in or on the kidney and showing posterior acoustic enhancement can be confidently identified as primary (dysontogenic) cysts if, in addition to the usual cystic criteria, they show an absence of vascularity on color duplex scanning and there are no additional structural abnormalities in the affected kidney. Whether single or multiple, they represent tubular retention cysts that have resulted from dilatation of the Bowman capsule or proximal tubules. Consequently, they have a cyst wall that produces typical entrance and exit echoes at ultrasound but cannot always be directly visualized. Primary dysontogenic cysts display a typical location (**Table 9.5**) (◉ **9.2a–d**).

Multiple cysts (dysontogenic). Kidneys that contain multiple cysts are usually of normal size. In contrast to a polycystic kidney, the renal cortex, medullary pyramids, and renal sinus are clearly defined (◉ **9.2e, Fig. 9.9**).

Polycystic kidney (dysontogenic). This disease involves a polycystic malformation of the distal renal tubules, tubular epithelium, or tubular walls leading to a predominantly bilateral polycystic transformation of the kidneys. At ultrasound the kidneys are considerably enlarged and contain numerous cysts that completely alter the contours of the renal capsule and cause poor delineation of the renal borders. There is variable rarefaction of the parenchyma due to a combination of cyst compression, blooming effects, and interstitial fibrosis. Polycystic kidneys are commonly associated with cysts in the liver and other organs, and the initial ultrasound findings are unmistakable (**Fig. 9.8**).

Atypical or secondary cysts. Atypical or secondary cysts differ from simple, uncomplicated cysts in their shape, location, or contents. They may be elliptical, polygonal, or oblong; they may show a parapelvic or extrarenal location; and they may contain internal echoes (thickened walls, septa, sedimentation, flakes, or clots) and blood vessels in malignant tumors (◉ **9.2g, Fig. 9.55**).

Septated cysts. Renal cysts occasionally show fine septations that subdivide the cysts into separate compartments. Septated cysts require

Table 9.5 Classification of renal cysts by their location and strucure (after Bosniak)

Classification	Type of cyst
Bosniak I	Simple cyst
Bosniak II	Minimally complicated cyst (minimal septae)
Bosniak III	More complicated cyst (multiple septae)
Bosniak IV	Lesion probably malignant

careful scrutiny at ultrasound to differentiate them from cystic renal cell carcinoma (◉ **9.2a, Fig. 9.56**). Lesions having this appearance require surveillance and possible surgery. The differential diagnosis should also include a hydatid cyst and, in young boys, multilocular cystic nephroma (benign cystic nephroma), wich demonstrate in ultrasonography a complex renal mass with numerous anechoic cysts separated by echogenic septae ◉ **9.3g, h**.

9.2 Renal Cysts and Perirenal Cystic Masses

▶ **Perirenal cysts**

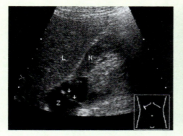 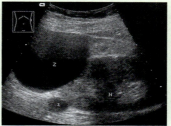 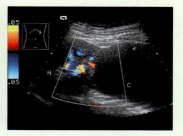

a Septated right upper pole cyst: slightly irregular cystic mass (Z) subdivided by an echogenic septum (arrows); Differential diagnosis: cystic renal cell carcinoma. L = liver; N = kidney.

b Two subcapsular cysts (Z, z) appear as anechoic masses "piggybacked" on the left kidney (N).

c Perirenal cyst, no vascularization. Left lower pole cyst (C).

▶ **Cortical and parapelvic cysts**

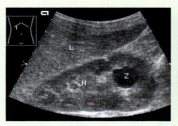 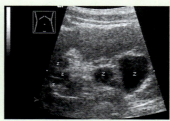 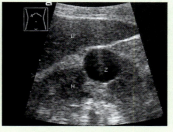

d Peripelvic cyst (Z): round, anechoic mass located in the renal sinus; apparently a cortical cyst protruding into the renal sinus. L = liver; N = kidney.

e Multiple renal cysts: some of the cysts (Z, z) are round; others are triangular or bandlike.

f Renal cortical cyst displaying all criteria: anechoic mass with smooth margins, a capsule (bright entry echo at the cyst apex), and distal acoustic enhancement; dysontogenic tubular retention cyst. L = liver; N = kidney.

▶ **Differential diagnosis of cystic masses**

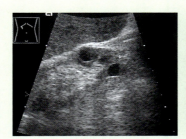 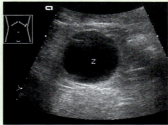 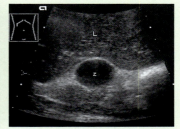

g Secondary cysts (arrows) in an atrophic kidney with a hyperechoic rim of residual parenchyma. The patient presented clinically with a plasmacytoma.

h und i Differential diagnosis of a perirenal cystic mass.
h Large echo-free mass (cyst, Z) in the triangle between the kidney, spleen, and pancreatic tail. Differential diagnosis: cyst of the kidney, spleen, or pancreatic tail.

i "Cystlike" metastasis (Z) from a high-grade adrenal non-Hodgkin lymphoma (see also **Fig. 9.79**). The indentation of the posterior hepatic surface suggests a solid mass. L = liver.

Retention cysts due to scarring. Secondary retention cysts develop in one-third to one-half of all patients with chronic interstitial nephritis requiring dialysis. These cysts result from scarring of the renal tubules. Many of the cysts are misshapen and rather small, and most are related to the cortex (**9.2g, Fig. 9.37**).

Hydatid cyst. Both the dog tapeworm (*Echinococcus granulosus*), which forms a primary cyst containing internal daughter cysts, and the fox tapeworm (*Echinococcus multilocularis*), in which the daughter cysts invade and destroy the host tissues from the primary cyst, can cause hydatid disease in humans. The most frequently infected organ is the liver but other sites may be affected, including the kidneys. Sonographically, the cysts are outlined by an echogenic wall. Daughter cysts produce a rosette-like pattern. *Echinococcus multilocularis* may also appear as a solid tumor mass. Hydatid cysts require differentiation from cysts with internal septations (**see Fig. 2.53 and Fig. 5.26**).

▶ ***Perirenal Cystic Masses***

Cystic renal lesions also require differentiation from other anechoic masses in neighboring organs and from adjacent cystic processes. Perirenal cystic masses may represent adherent bowel loops, the gallbladder, loculated ascites, cystic/liquid adrenal processes, and splenic or pancreatic-tail cysts or abscesses. In the case of adherent fluid-filled bowel loops, the correct diagnosis is supplied by using real-time ultrasound to observe the moving bowel contents.

Equivocal findings require further investigation, such as ultrasound-guided fine-needle aspiration biopsy (FNAB) (**9.2h and i**).

▶ Lymph Cysts

Parapelvic (peripelvic) lymph cysts. Parapelvic cysts generally represent lymph cysts, which have an epithelial lining. Projecting into the renal sinus, they present as flattened, usually elliptical cystic lesions. Generally these cysts are multiple.

When they are bilateral and show a finger-like arrangement extending toward the renal hilum, they are classified as multiple parapelvic cysts or benign cystic lymphangioma. Between the elliptical, anechoic lesions tapering toward the hilum are hyperechoic, septumlike partitions formed by the compressed sinus tissue and pyelocaliceal system (**9.3a–e**). Differentiation is required from renal pelvic dilatation due to a low urinary tract obstruction, but the absence of ureteropelvic junction dilatation serves to exclude that condition. Occasionally there is no alternative to excretory urography for establishing a diagnosis. In the case of lymph cysts, the urogram will show sharply circumscribed impressions on the pyelocaliceal system.

Intrarenal or perirenal lymphoceles. Intrarenal or perirenal cystic lesions may also be lymphoceles, depending on the cause of the disease. They occur after surgery, in rejection episodes after renal transplantation, and also in chronic progressive renal diseases such as renal failure requiring dialysis. When they present as a perirenal mass, lymphoceles have an anechoic, cystic appearance. They may also contain septations (**9.3f**).

▶ Cystic Renal Cell Carcinoma, Intracystic Carcinoma

Renal cell carcinoma. Cystic renal cell carcinoma (RCC) is a rare form of renal carcinoma (see **Table 9.6**). It shows a predominantly anechoic, cystic structure with more or less pronounced solid components. Foci of necrobiotic tumor liquefaction are common, especially in tumors of long duration (**Fig. 9.55**).

Intracystic carcinoma. Another type of cystic renal tumor is renal carcinoma that arises inside a cyst. Because intracystic carcinoma is extremely rare, it does not justify regular sonographic or CT follow-ups in patients with known cysts (**Figs. 9.56–9.58 and Fig. 9.78**).

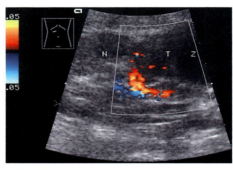

▲ **Fig. 9.55** Cystic renal cell carcinoma. No histology because of earlier nephrectomy on the left side.
a Transverse scan through the right upper abdomen: solid and cystic tumor components with pathological intratumoral vessels (compare with **Fig. 11.7, p. 334**). N = kidney.

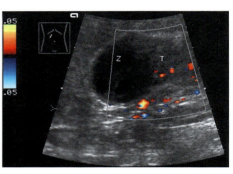

▲ **b** Oblique scan through the right upper abdomen: the solid tumor component (T) again shows internal vascularity, which is absent in the cystic component (Z) with an atypical internal structure.

9.3 Lymph Cysts

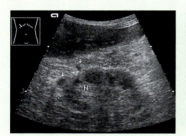 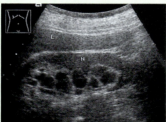 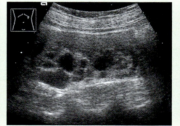 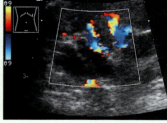

a Perirenal lymph cysts (arrows): small cysts, some showing a string-of-beads arrangement (varied at follow-ups). The patient presented clinically with severe right heart failure and erythrocytosis. N = kidney.

b and c Multiple parapelvic cysts on both sides: "benign cystic lymphangioma."
b Right kidney (N): elliptical cysts radiating toward the hilum in a fan-shaped pattern. L = liver.

c Left kidney: a less obvious alignment toward the hilum.

d Benign cystic lymphangioma: fragmented color pixels among the cysts, representing vessels in the renal sinus; no typical tumor vessels (clinical presentation: advanced colon carcinoma!).

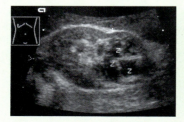 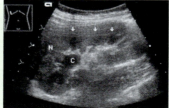 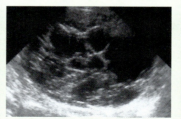 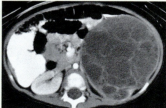

e Cystic renal cell carcinoma? Atypical cysts (Z), septumlike internal structures, contour distortion (arrow). Requires cytohistological workup! (Given the bilateral occurrence of parapelvic cysts, an atypical benign cystic lymphangioma is likely.)

f Postoperative lymphocele (C) following stone surgery with postoperative bleeding; very conspicuous medullary pyramids (arrows). Left nephrectomy. N = kidney.

g, h Differential diagnosis. Multilocular cystic nephroma.
g Longitudinal scan of the left kidney shows numerous anechoic locules separated by echogenic septae.

h Contrast-enhanced CT confirms a multilocular mass with enhancing septations replacing the renal parenchyma.

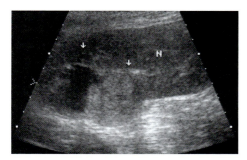

▲ *Fig. 9.56* Cyst-associated renal cell carcinoma (RCC) (arrows). Histology: chromophobe clear-cell RCC. N = kidney.

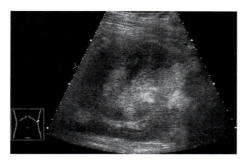

▲ *Fig. 9.57* Extensive tumor necrosis and cystic intratumoral hemorrhage (90%) in a chromophil renal cell carcinoma (histology). Woman 47 years of age presented with a cystic-solid mass. Ultrasound findings suggested xanthogranulomatous pyelonephritis. CT revealed intracystic hemorrhage. Intracystic carcinoma?

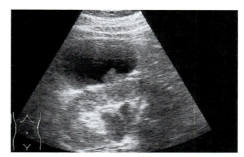

▲ *Fig. 9.58* Large perirenal cyst with papillomatous tumor infiltration of the cyst floor (no histology). Associated finding: parapelvic cysts.

▶ Papillary Necrosis, Cystic Degeneration of the Medullary Pyramids

Papillary necrosis and caliceal cysts most commonly develop in a setting of purulent or nonpurulent interstitial chronic nephritis. They present as small cystic lesions projecting toward the calices.

In advanced diabetic nephropathy, it is not uncommon to find cystic degeneration of the medullary pyramids, which exhibit classic cystic features. Often they are located next to very hypoechoic medullary pyramids that may eventually undergo complete cystic transformation. The medullary pyramids disappear in the dialysis stage, often to be replaced by multiple small, secondary cysts that were once pyramids (**Fig. 9.59**, ▣ **9.1 d**).

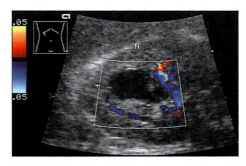

▲ *Fig. 9.59* Irregular cystic mass in the area of a medullary pyramid. Color Doppler shows no vascularity. Diabetes mellitus. Probably the cystic transformation of a medullary pyramid. N = kidney.

▶ Cavities

Hematogenous spread of renal tuberculosis gives rise to cortical tubercles that descend into the tubules, papillae, and associated calices where they form ulcer cavities.

These cavities have a cystic appearance at ultrasound. While a purely cavernous-cystic process cannot be recognized sonographically as a tuberculous cavity, the late stage is additionally marked by the formation of scars and calcifications. This combination allows for a presumptive sonographic diagnosis (**Figs. 9.60, 9.92, and 9.93**).

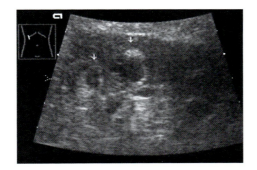

◀ *Fig. 9.60* Old cavernous (?) medullary pyramids that have undergone secondary cystic transformation (arrows). Ultrasound shows irregular, echo-free masses with a hyperechoic rim projected at the site of the medullary pyramids (see also **Fig. 9.92**). Patient had a known history of spinal tuberculosis.

▶ Abscess

Renal abscess generally appears as a predominantly hypoechoic mass with internal echoes that distinguish it from a cystic lesion. Some abscesses, however, may be so hypoechoic that they mimic cystic lesions. A color void is seen on color Doppler scanning (**Fig. 9.61**, ▣ **9.5 d**, and ▣ **11.3 d–f, p. 344**).

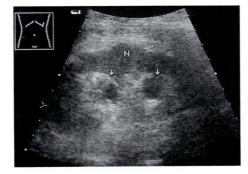

▲ *Fig. 9.61* Bilateral abscesses in a patient with septic urinary tract infection and diabetes mellitus. N = kidney.
a Left kidney: predominantly echo-free cystic abscesses with irregular margins (arrows).

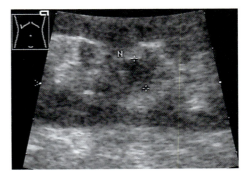

▲ *b* Right kidney in magnified view: cystic mass with irregular margins (cursors) in the renal sinus echo complex.

▶ Organized Hematoma

Whereas fresh hematomas appear as echogenic, heterogeneous masses at ultrasound (see below), older hematomas appear increasingly hypoechoic to anechoic. Besides circumscribed parenchymal destruction, hematomas usually produce a subcapsular mass caused by the subcapsular extravasation of blood. This mass presents sonographically as perirenal fluid (**Fig. 9.62**). Color Doppler shows decreased perfusion in areas of renal contusion, while it shows an absence of perfusion in a hematoma.

The history and clinical presentation give additional information on the cause of these cystic lesions. Equivocal cases should be evaluated by CT, which is superior to ultrasound for this type of investigation.

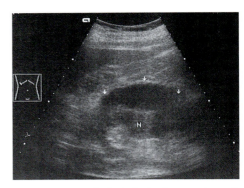

▲ *Fig. 9.62* Perirenal, elliptical echo-free mass (arrows): urinoma, hematoma following renal trauma. N = kidney.

▶ Urinoma, Seroma

Urinoma. The presence of a urinoma signifies leakage from the renal pelvis or ureter in a setting of renal colic or trauma. Accordingly, it appears sonographically as an anechoic, triangular or crescent-shaped perirenal mass. It is typically associated with flank pain, and pyelocaliceal obstruction is always detectable with ultrasound (**Fig. 11.27, p. 339**).

Seroma. A seroma is a collection of blood, serum, or lymph in a postsurgical cavity. For this reason, the nature of the mass can generally be inferred from the patient's history. It is usually anechoic with somewhat irregular margins, but some seromas contain internal echoes.

▶ Vascular Dilatations

Aneurysm or intrarenal arteriovenous malformation. Aneurysms or arteriovenous malformations of the renal artery can mimic a cyst when located within the kidney. The nature of the lesion can be established by color Doppler scanning and spectral analysis. Arterial signals are typically recorded from aneurysms, while arteriovenous malformations exhibit high flow velocities up to 180 cm/s and low resistance indices (RI 0.32–0.25)[12] (**Fig. 9.18**). Renal artery aneurysms located outside the kidney are relatively easy to identify.

Renal vein ectasia or congestion. An ectatic or congested renal vein has the same sonographic appearance as an aneurysm or arterial-veinous malformation (AVM), and the color Doppler examination is diagnostic. The vein can be confidently distinguished from an arterial aneurysm by spectral analysis (**Fig. 9.63**).

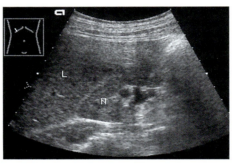

▲ *Fig. 9.63* Ectatic branches of the renal vein. L = liver; N = kidney.
a B-mode image: irregular cystlike areas in the sinus echo complex.

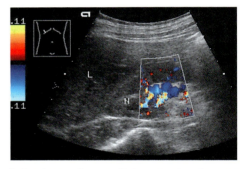

▲ *b* Color Doppler: vascularity consistent with ectatic renal veins.

▶ Hydrocalices, Pyelectasis, Hydronephrosis

Certain planes of section through distended calices in obstructive pyelocaliceal dilatation can create the impression of multiple renal cysts. In this case an oblique longitudinal scan, preferably from the posterior side (ureter!), will demonstrate the cystic enlargement of the calices.

Hydrocalices and hydronephrosis are seen in association with ureteral obstructions. Hydrocalices may also be congenital or secondary to caliceal stones or nephrocalcinosis (**Figs. 9.64 and 9.65, and Fig. 11.10, p. 335**).

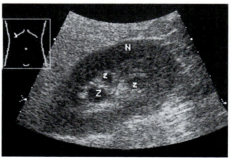

▲ *Fig. 9.64* Obstructive caliectasis. N = kidney.
a Scan through the calices, which resemble cysts (Z) in this plane.

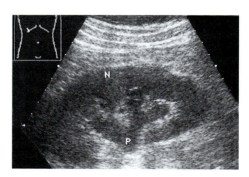

▲ *b* Oblique scan demonstrates the dilated pyelocaliceal system (P).

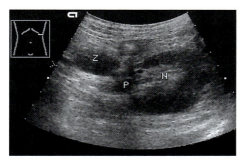

▲ **Fig. 9.65** Cyst combined with obstructive caliceal and pelvic ectasia. N = kidney.
a Transverse ultrasound scan through the left kidney: cyst (Z), pyelectasis (P).

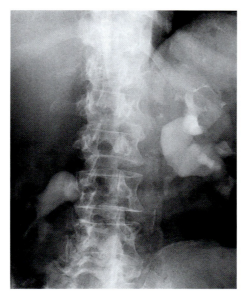

◀ ***b*** Excretory urogram: curved medial and lateral indentations in the upper portions of the calices. Renal pelvic indentation and congestion due to subpelvic obstruction (by a tumor?).

Hypoechoic or Isoechoic Structure

Kidneys
- Anomalies, Malformations
- Diffuse Changes
- ▼ Circumscribed Changes
  - Anechoic Structure
  - **Hypoechoic or Isoechoic Structure**
  - Complex Structure
  - Hyperechoic Structure
  - Echogenic Structure

- Dromedary Hump, Fetal Lobulation
- Abscess
- Hemorrhagic Cyst
- Fresh Renal Infarct
- Hematoma
- Renal Cell Carcinoma
- Urothelial Carcinoma
- Malignant Lymphoma
- Metastasis
- Adenoma, Inflammatory Tumor

▶ Dromedary Hump, Fetal Lobulation

Dromedary hump. The physiological dromedary hump in the left kidney appears as a hypoechoic "mass" that is occasionally difficult or impossible to distinguish from a tumor. It is helpful to inspect the structure closely in a zoomed view and note the normal renal architecture, and to obtain a color Doppler view showing an absence of irregular tumor vessels and an abnormal vascular rim.

Fetal lobation. Fetal lobation is a developmental anomaly based on incomplete fusion of the fetal nephrons. It is characterized by a normal but undulating parenchyma that bulges outward and also toward the renal sinus. The constricted areas between the bulges represent sites of normal parenchymal thickness and are not rarefied areas like those caused by scarring (**Fig. 9.66**).

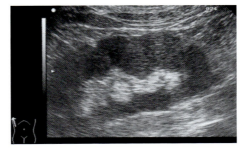

▲ **Fig. 9.66** Renal contour distortion.
a In fetal lobation.

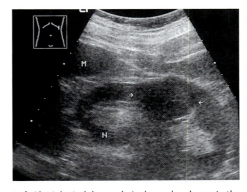

▲ ***b*** Physiological, hypoechoic dromedary hump in the left renal border, indistinguishable from a tumor (see 9.4). M = spleen; N = kidney.

▶ *Abscess*

Abscesses in and about the kidney can result from local abscessation (pyelonephritis, usually *E. coli*) or from the hematogenous spread of infection (usually staphylococcal). They can spread beyond the renal capsule to form a perinephritic abscess, or they may spread into the perirenal fat, forming a paranephritic abscess.

Their sonographic features are diverse. A simple abscess produces a mass effect creating a bulge in the renal outline. It shows a hypoechoic to heterogeneous echo structure and usually has ill-defined margins. The sonographer should look for gas bubbles, which are a common phenomenon and appear as focal echogenic inclusions with or without reverberations (**Figs. 9.67 and 9.30**).

Perirenal abscesses appear as ill-defined masses that may spread in an inferior or lumbar direction. Emphysematous and xanthogranulomatous pyelonephritis are special forms.

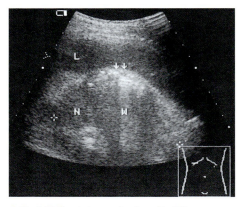

▲ *Fig. 9.67* Renal abscess. L = liver; N = kidney.
a Echogenic bacterial gas bubbles with reverberations (arrows, W) before medical treatment.

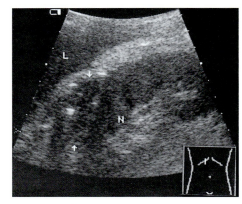

▲ *b* After antibiotic treatment: hypoechoic mass (arrows), contour distortion, ill-defined margins, and scattered echogenic gas bubbles.

▶ *Hemorrhagic Cyst*

While some cyst criteria such as smooth margins and a round shape are maintained in a hemorrhagic cyst, the bleeding causes the initial anechoic mass to become more reflective. This makes the cyst difficult to distinguish from a tumor. The diagnosis can be established by fine-needle aspiration biopsy or CT (**Figs. 9.68 and 9.77**).

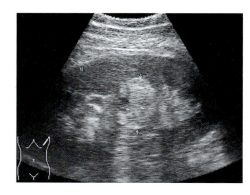

◀ *Fig. 9.68* Hemorrhagic cyst (ultrasound-guided aspiration): elliptical, isoechoic to hyperechoic mass in the renal sinus. The patient presented clinically with metastatic colon cancer. N = kidney.

▶ *Fresh Renal Infarct*

A fresh renal infarct is seldom diagnosed clinically and is usually detected incidentally at imaging. In the acute stage, it displays a typical wedge shape with the base directed toward the renal capsule. The late stage is marked by surface retractions and focal rarefied areas in the parenchyma due to scarring and fibrous contracture (**Fig. 9.69**).

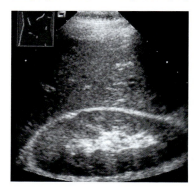

▲ *Fig. 9.69* Fresh renal infarct.
a Survey scan shows increased echogenicity in the upper pole of the right kidney.

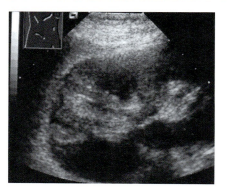

▲ *b* Close-up view shows a sharply defined, wedge-shaped hypoechoic region.

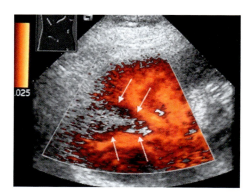

▲ *c* Color Doppler: the wedge-shaped avascular region (arrows) confirms the infarct. The patient presented clinically with flank pain.

▶ Hematoma

Like renal infarcts and hematomas at other locations, a renal hematoma or contusion undergoes structural changes over time. It appears initially as a hyperechoic or isoechoic mass that causes a bulge in the renal outline. The echo structure of the mass is somewhat irregular compared with the normal renal parenchyma. Later the hematoma becomes less echogenic and may culminate in a residual secondary cyst or pseudocyst (**Fig. 9.77 c**).

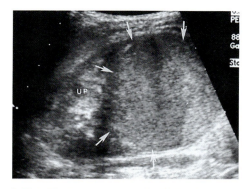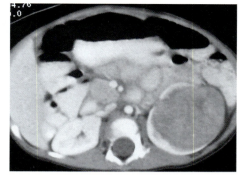

▲ *Fig. 9.77 c* Common sonographic findings include an echogenic intrarenal mass with a homogeneous or heterogeneous appearance reflecting varying degrees of hemorrhage and necrosis; increased vascularity is noted on color doppler sonography.[13]

▶ Renal Cell Carcinoma

Forms. Renal cell carcinoma (RCC) occurs in three different forms:
- ▶ Ordinary solid renal cell carcinoma (most common form)
- ▶ Tubulopapillary form
- ▶ Cystic renal cell carcinoma (rare)

Based on the international WHO classification of 1998, renal cell carcinomas are classified histologically as epithelial or nonepithelial types as shown in **Table 9.6**. Since RCC arises from the renal parenchyma, it displays the immunohistochemical features of uropoietic tubular epithelium[11].

Sonographic features. The ultrasound appearance of RCC varies greatly with its stage and histological classification.

The most common and characteristic appearance of RCC is that of a round, isoechoic mass in the renal parenchyma that creates a bulge in the renal outline. Hypoechoic tumors are also seen. Atypical hyperechoic tumors are found in 30% of cases; most of these are early-stage tumors (**see Figs. 9.81 and 9.82**). Cystic RCC displays cystic features along with solid elements or septations (**Fig. 9.55, Fig. 9.78**).

The echo texture of RCC is homogeneous to irregular. Advanced tumors show regressive changes in the form of liquefaction, hyperechoic areas, and calcifications (◨ **9.4c**). With its wide spectrum of features, RCC can be characterized as a chameleon in its sonographic appearance (◨ **9.4**).

A narrow, anechoic rim (displaced vessels) is consistently present around the tumor. If this is accompanied by irregular internal tumor vessels within the mass (color Doppler), the ultrasound diagnosis may be considered established and the patient can be referred at once for surgical treatment without further tests. Contrast-enhanced color duplex scanning demonstrates increased vascularity with arteriovenous shunts. Spectral analysis shows a high Doppler shift > 1 m/s with high diastolic flow.

Diagnostic procedure. At present, renal cell carcinoma is detected incidentally at routine ultrasound in 70–80% of cases. It is rarely diagnosed by a targeted search in patients who already have metastatic symptoms. Metastasis may occur by the hematogenous route or by contiguous spread into the renal vein (20%) and inferior vena cava (5%)[4]. Tumor thrombi may occur in the right heart. It is essential, therefore, to closely inspect the renal veins, vena cava, and locoregional lymphatics during ultrasound examination. On the left side, a dromedary hump should be included in the differential diagnosis.

Wilms tumor. A special type of renal tumor in children is nephroblastoma (Wilms tumor; see **Table 9.6**), which usually presents as a rapidly enlarging mass that becomes symptomatic (**Fig. 9.70**).

Table 9.6 International classification of renal parenchymal tumors (after reference 10)

Benign forms	Malignant forms
Epithelial tumors	**Epithelial tumors**
▶ Papillary and tubulopapillary adenoma	▶ Renal cell carcinoma
▶ Oncocytic adenoma	▶ Clear cell carcinoma
▶ Metanephric adenoma	▶ Granular cell carcinoma
	▶ Chromophobe cell carcinoma
	▶ Spindle cell carcinoma
	▶ Cyst-associated renal cell carcinoma
	– Renal cell carcinoma originating in a cyst
	– Cystic renal cell carcinoma
	▶ Papillary renal cell carcinoma
	▶ Collecting-duct carcinoma
Nonepithelial tumors	**Nonepithelial tumors**
▶ Angiomyolipoma	▶ Malignant soft-tissue tumors
▶ Leiomyoma	
▶ Lipoma	
▶ Renomedullary interstitial cell tumor	
▶ Hemangioma	
▶ Lymphangioma	
▶ Juxtaglomerular cell tumor	
Nephroblastic lesions (pediatric tumors)	
▶ Nephroblastoma (Wilms tumor)	
▶ Benign or malignant cystic nephroma	
▶ Cystic, partially differentiated nephroblastoma	
▶ Other pediatric tumors	

9.4 Renal Cell Carcinoma (RCC)

▶ **Varying echogenicity**

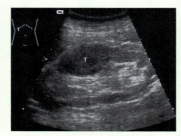 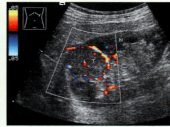 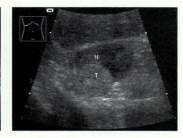

a Hypoechoic tumor (T) with ill-defined margins. Bulging renal outline.

b Isoechoic mass (T) at the upper pole of the kidney, pathognomonic: vascular rim and intratumoral vessels (arrows).

c Hyperechoic tumor (T). N = renal parenchyma.

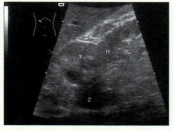 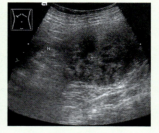 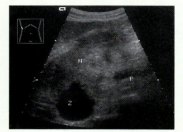

d Partially cystic (Z) transformed tumor. N = kidney.

e Areas of necrobiotic liquefaction. N = kidney; T = tumor.

f Complex structured tumor mass with hyper- and anechoic (Z) portions of the right kidney (N). P = pyelon.

▶ **Route for tumor metastasis**

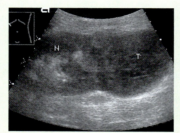 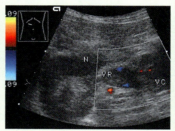 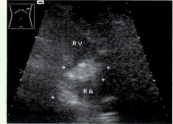

g and *h* **Advanced RCC.**
g Large, hypoechoic tumor (T). Partial hypoechoic transformation of sinus echo due to tumor vein thrombosis. N = kidney.

h Extension of tumor into the central echo complex. The tumor has invaded and thrombosed the renal vein (VR). Color Doppler shows patchy tumor vascularity. A tumor thrombus is also present in the vena cava (VC).

i Another echogenic tumor thrombus is in the right atrium (RA), making the RCC inoperable. RV = right ventricle.

▶ **Urothelial Carcinoma**

Carcinomas of the renal pelvis, ureter, and bladder differ fundamentally from renal tumors. They arise from the urothelium, or transitional epithelium, and occur as papillary and solid tumors. Renal pelvic carcinoma is three times more common than ureteral carcinoma. The tumor presents clinically with hematuria.

Urothelial carcinoma forms a hypoechoic, polypoid mass that fills the lumen of the renal pelvis to produce a hypoechoic, butterfly-like figure. The tumor usually has a homogeneous echo texture, but the added presence of liquefied foci and calcifications give the tumor a nonhomogeneous appearance (**Fig. 9.71**). Unlike an infected obstruction and other masses in the central sinus echo complex, the tumor exhibits vascularity on color duplex examination. It is difficult to distinguish from renal cell carcinoma that has invaded or displaced the renal sinus or renal pelvis (◨ **9.5f, g, Figs. 11.34 and 11.35** in Chapter 11).

Given the major importance of hypoechoic masses in the renal sinus echo complex, the differential diagnostic features of these masses are reviewed in ◨ **9.5**.

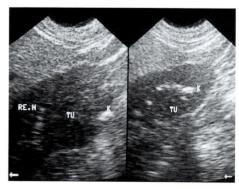

▲ *Fig. 9.71* Urothelial carcinoma: hypoechoic mass (TU) in the renal sinus echo complex with calcification (K). RE.N = right kidney.

9.5 Differential Diagnosis of Hypoechoic Masses in the Renal Sinus Echo Complex

▶ **Renal column**
- ▶ Conical extension between the medullary pyramids
- ▶ Isoechoic to the renal cortex
- ▶ No vascularity

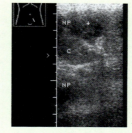

a Hypertrophic renal column (C) next to large, hypoechoic medullary pyramids; renal transplant. NP = parenchyma.

▶ **Duplex kidney**
- ▶ Notch in the renal outline
- ▶ Enlarged, elongated kidney
- ▶ Normal echo structure (or hypoechoic with overlying parenchyma)
- ▶ Normal vascularity
- ▶ Duplicated renal pelvis
- ▶ Duplicated ureters (visible only with obstruction)

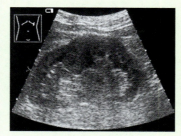

b Tumorlike nub of parenchyma extending into the central echo complex.

▶ **Sinus lipomatosis**
- ▶ Hypoechoic, nodular mass with ill-defined margins
- ▶ Confined to the sinus echo complex
- ▶ Parenchymal–pelvic ratio shifted in favor of renal sinus
- ▶ No vascularity
- ▶ Bilateral

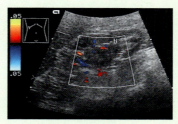

c Hypoechoic tumorlike transformation of the sinus echo complex; no vascularity in the mass. N = kidney.

▶ **Infected obstruction, abscess**
- ▶ Infected obstruction
- ▶ Hypoechoic to anechoic area conforming to the pyelocaliceal system and extending into the ureter
- ▶ No vascularity

Abscess, pyonephrosis
- ▶ Round or polygonal, nonhomogeneous mass, usually with ill-defined margins
- ▶ No vascularity

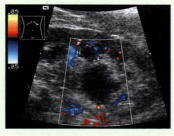

d Renal pelvic abscess: hypoechoic mass with ill-defined borders. Clinically, the patient had poorly controlled diabetes. N = kidney.

▶ **Parapelvic cysts, atypical cysts**
- ▶ Multiple round to oval masses with ill-defined margins
- ▶ Anechoic to hypoechoic (in small cysts with flat bases)
- ▶ Echogenic walls
- ▶ Distal acoustic enhancement
- ▶ Frequently bilateral (always bilateral with benign cystic lymphoma)

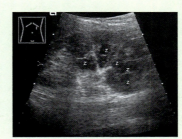

e Atypical parapelvic cysts (z) with septations (cystic carcinoma?); here, benign cystic lymphoma.

9.5 Differential Diagnosis of Hypoechoic Masses in the Renal Sinus Echo Complex

▶ Renal pelvic carcinoma
- ▶ Hypoechoic mass in the central echo complex
- ▶ Polygonal margins
- ▶ Detectable tumor vessels

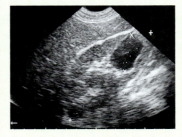

f Liquefied area in a renal pelvic carcinoma (cursors). Histology: urothelial carcinoma.

▶ Renal cell carcinoma
- ▶ Well-demarcated mass that may be hypoechoic, isoechoic, or hyperechoic to the renal parenchyma
- ▶ Connection with cortical substance
- ▶ Detectable tumor vessels

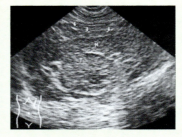

g Renal cell carcinoma (T) that has invaded the renal sinus and renal pelvis. Perirenal abscess with gas bubbles (arrows) in emphysematous pyelonephritis. N = kidney.

▶ Malignant Lymphoma

Another hypoechoic renal tumor is malignant lymphoma. It may occur as a diffuse hypoechoic or heterogeneous mass (high-grade lymphoma) or as a smaller, circumscribed, round or oval tumor (renal involvement by low-grade lymphoma) (**Figs. 9.72, 9.32, and 9.79**).

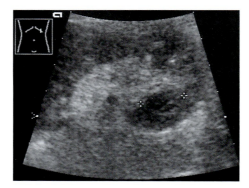

◀ **Fig. 9.72** Renal involvement by low-grade non-Hodgkin lymphoma (cursors): elliptical hypoechoic tumor as the junction of the renal sinus and parenchyma.

▶ Metastasis

It is not uncommon for tumors to metastasize to the kidney by the hematogenous route. Metastases most often originate from the breast, bronchi, or gastrointestinal tract, or from the lymphogenous or hematogenous spread of ipsilateral or contralateral renal cancers.

Renal metastases appear sonographically as round, nodular, relatively homogeneous, hypoechoic masses located in the renal parenchyma or the sinus echo complex (**Fig. 9.73**).

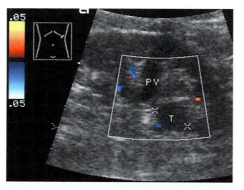 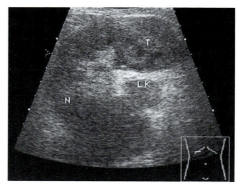

▲ **Fig. 9.73** Renal metastases.
a Metastasis (T) from small-bowel carcinoma, with focal pyelectasis (PV).

▲ *b* Ipsilateral metastasis (LK) of renal cell carcinoma (T). Round, isoechoic, homogeneous mass in the renal sinus. N = kidney.

▶ Adenoma, Inflammatory Tumor

Adenoma. Adenoma (classification in **Table 9.6**) is a benign, slow-growing renal tumor that can reach considerable size. Regressive changes are common, and progression to carcinoma can occur.

Sonographically, adenoma appears hypoechoic and nonhomogeneous but occasionally may be hyperechoic. It has smooth margins. No reliable sonographic criteria are available (**Fig. 9.74**).

Inflammatory tumor. By contrast, inflammatory tumors are rare lesions that tend have ill-defined margins and a nonhomogeneous, hypoechoic structure (**Fig. 9.75**). Inflammatory tumors in the sinus echo complex are virtually indistinguishable from masses due to bacterial inflammation, although the former show intense vascularity on color duplex examination.

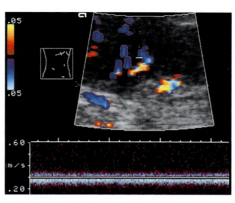
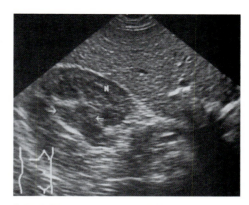

▲ **Fig. 9.74** Renal adenoma (CT, operation).
a Sharply circumscribed, very hypoechoic mass. Based on ultrasound morphology, the fine echogenic wall (arrows) is suggestive of a hemorrhagic cyst. N = kidney.

▲ **b** Color Doppler shows subtle but constant vascularity, ruling out a cyst or abscess in favor of a solid mass.

▲ **Fig. 9.75** Inflammatory tumor in the renal sinus complex: elliptical mass with an irregular echo structure. Histology identified the mass as tumor-simulating vasculitis. Clinical presentation: dysplastic syndrome; inflammatory lung tumor was detected incidentally; operation. N = kidney.

Complex Structure

Kidneys
- ▶ Anomalies, Malformations
- ▶ Diffuse Changes
- ▼ Circumscribed Changes
  - ▶ Anechoic Structure
  - ▶ Hypoechoic or Isoechoic Structure
  - ▶ **Complex Structure**
  - ▶ Hyperechoic Structure
  - ▶ Echogenic Structure

- ▶ **Abscess, Pyonephrosis**
- ▶ **Xanthomatous Pyelonephritis**
- ▶ **Hematoma, Intracystic Hemorrhage**
- ▶ **Renal Cell Carcinoma, Cystic Renal Carcinoma, Malignant Lymphoma**

▶ Abscess, Pyonephrosis

Large abscesses and pyonephrosis present sonographically as an irregular mass that destroys the normal renal architecture while forming hyperechoic and hypoechoic areas. They may contain bizarre, anechoic components. The diagnosis is based on the clinical presentation, fine-needle aspiration, CT, or the histological analysis of surgical specimens (**Fig. 9.61, 9.76**, and 11.3g–i in Chapter 11).

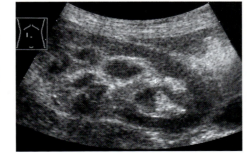

◀ **Fig. 9.76** Pyonephrosis: hypoechoic mass with ill-defined margins, partially filled with echogenic material (debris, inspissation).

▶ Xanthomatous Pyelonephritis

This is a subacute or chronic pyelonephritis in which the usual pyelonephritic structural changes are accompanied by the presence of lipid-laden foam cells, granulomas, and giant cells. At ultrasound, these elements (sometimes combined with focal urinary tract obstruction and phosphate stones) can produce a heterogeneous mass that resembles a tumor.

▶ Hematoma, Intracystic Hemorrhage

Depending on its stage, a hematoma may contain anechoic to hyperechoic components that create an irregular echo pattern. Intracystic hemorrhage leads to a hypoechoic (rare), heterogeneous, or hyperechoic structure, raising serious problems of sonographic differential diagnosis, especially since renal carcinomas also tend to bleed and may be masked by intracystic hemorrhage (**Figs. 9.77, 9.68, and 9.70**).

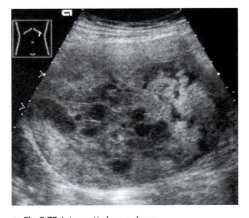
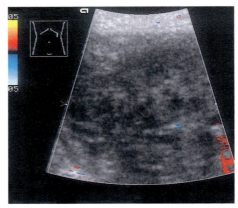
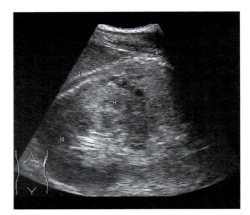

▲ **Fig. 9.77** Intracystic hemorrhage.
 a Large, sharply circumscribed, irregular structure with cystic and solid components.

▲ **b** Color duplex shows no vascularity even at a low pulse repetition frequency. This means that a tumor is unlikely.

▲ **c** Traumatic renal hematoma (H): isoechoic (to slightly hyperechoic) mass causing circumscribed parenchymal destruction and a bulge in the renal outline (arrows). N = kidney.

▶ Renal Cell Carcinoma, Cystic Renal Carcinoma, Malignant Lymphoma

Diffuse RCC, cystic renal cell carcinoma, and high-grade lymphoma are additional lesions that can acquire a heterogeneous echo texture as they enlarge.

Predominantly regressive tumor changes in the form of calcifications and cystic tumor liquefaction determine the ultrasound appearance of the affected kidneys. Anechoic elements may also represent displaced blood vessels or focal obstructions of the pyelocaliceal system (**Figs. 9.78, 9.79, 9.55, and ◩ 9.4**).

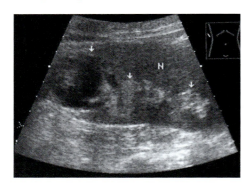
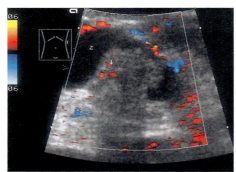

◀◀ **Fig. 9.78** Cyst-associated renal cell carcinoma (arrows). Histology: chromophobe clear-cell renal cell carcinoma (pseudocystic transformation to cystic RCC occurs only in clear-cell and papillary carcinomas).
 a Nonhomogeneous, hyperechoic tumor areas accompanied by partially infiltrated, tumor-compressed cysts with irregular margins. N = kidney.

◀ **b** Cyst-associated renal cell carcinoma: cystically transformed (necrosis, hemorrhage, Z) clear cell carcinoma. Color duplex shows scant vascular signals.

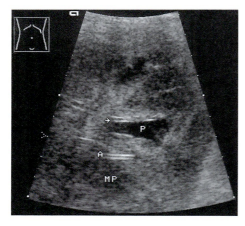
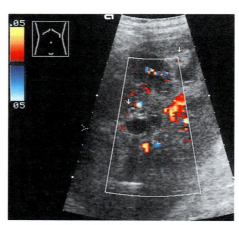

◀◀ **Fig. 9.79** High-grade renal lymphoma (enlarged view).
 a Irregular mass with echo-free components (obstructive pyelectasis, P) and vascular structures (arrow, A) along with intact, hypoechoic medullary pyramids (MP).

◀ **b** Color Doppler: echo-free to hyperechoic areas (arrows), irregular tumor vessels.

Hyperechoic Structure

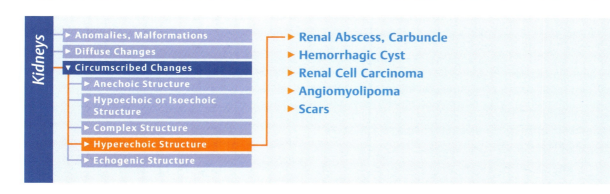

▶ Renal Abscess, Carbuncles

Renal abscesses, like hepatic abscesses, often acquire a structure that is hyperechoic to the normal parenchyma. Renal carbuncles are staphylococcal abscesses that arise in the kidney owing to hematogenous spread (**Fig. 9.80**).

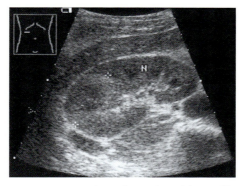

▲ *Fig. 9.80* Mass in the renal parenchyma (N) caused by abscessation.
a Circumscribed mass with an echogenic border (cursors).

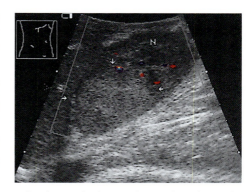

▲ *b* Color Doppler shows an absence of vascularity in the abscess structure (arrows), which is surrounded by displaced normal parenchyma (N). The kidney is generally enlarged with a washed-out appearance. Patient presented clinically with headache and septic fever.

▶ Hemorrhagic Cyst

A hemorrhagic cyst can also show increased echogenicity relative to the surrounding parenchyma. Hemorrhagic cysts, angiomyolipomas, and renal cell carcinomas appear as almost identical masses and are very difficult to distinguish from one another. A cyst always has smooth margins. The sonographic features of angiomyolipoma are listed in **Table 9.7** (**Fig. 9.68**).

▶ Renal Cell Carcinoma

RCCs with a dense echo pattern are less common than the isoechoic tumors cited above. Echogenic RCCs always raise formidable problems of differential diagnosis. The lesion can be correctly identified by the appearance of its peripheral rim and fine internal vascularity or, if necessary, by ultrasound-guided fine-needle aspiration biopsy with cytological or histological analysis and/or CT scanning (**Figs. 9.81 and 9.82**).

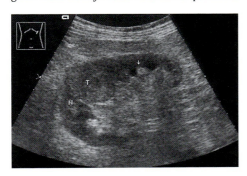

▲ *Fig. 9.81* Two renal tumors: the large tumor (T) is a renal cell carcinoma (RCC), appearing as an oval mass isoechoic or slightly hyperechoic to the renal parenchyma (N). It has a faint peripheral rim and creates an outward bulge in the renal sinus. These features are typical of RCC (and could justify surgery without further testing). The second mass is a small, echogenic tumor (arrow), most likely a benign nonepithelial tumor.

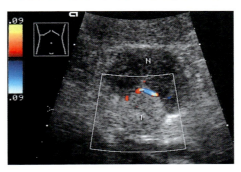

▲ *Fig. 9.82* Echogenic renal cell carcinoma (T). The differential diagnosis includes angiomyolipoma, and therefore CT should be performed.
a Transverse scan through the right upper quadrant shows a sharply circumscribed, homogeneously echogenic mass with a vascularized rim. N = kidney.

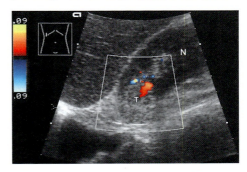

▲ *b* Flank scan reveals intratumoral vessels. The vascular rim and intratumoral vessels are consistent with renal cell carcinoma, not angiomyolipoma. N = kidney.

▶ Angiomyolipoma

Angiomyolipomas are a common type of benign nonepithelial tumor. They contain thick-walled vessels, smooth muscle, and fatty tissue in varying proportions.

The tumor can confidently be diagnosed by the fat attenuation observed on CT, but this study is unnecessary when typical ultrasound findings are present. The accuracy of CT is compromised by an absence of fat in some tumors (< 10%). When characteristic ultrasound features are noted (**Table 9.7**), the identity of the lesion can be appreciated at once (**Figs. 9.83 and 9.84**).

Multiple, bilateral angiomyolipomas occur in the setting of tuberous sclerosis (van Hippel–Lindau syndrome). This disease is frequently associated with clear-cell renal carcinomas, however, and so additional tests should be performed (**Fig. 9.85, Table 9.7**).

Table 9.7 Sonographic features of angiomyolipoma (after Helweg and Frauscher[13])

- ▶ Hyperechoic mass
- ▶ Size 1–3 cm (occasionally > 5 cm)
- ▶ Globular shape
- ▶ No distal acoustic shadow
- ▶ Solitary occurrence (except in tuberous sclerosis)
- ▶ Rarely causes a bulge in the renal outline
- ▶ Detectable vascularity
- ▶ Multiple in 80% of patients with tuberous sclerosis; only angiomyolipomas associated with this condition may undergo malignant transformation!

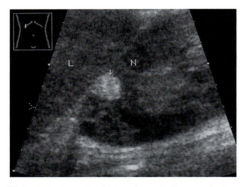

▲ **Fig. 9.83** Angiomyolipoma (arrow) showing distinctive sonographic features: echogenic intraparenchymal tumor with a fine, reticular internal structure and finely serrated contours. N = kidney; L = liver.

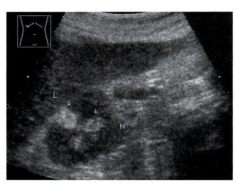

▲ **Fig. 9.84** Angiomyolipoma. Changing the scan angle demonstrates two additional echogenic tumors (arrows). Multiple angiomyolipomas, often in both kidneys, occur in Bourneville–Pringle disease.

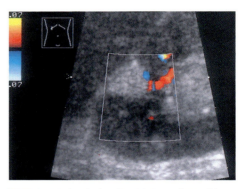

▲ **Fig. 9.85** Color duplex shows here no detectable internal vascularity.

▶ Scars

"Scar" refers to any circumscribed, fibrous area of postinflammatory or postinfarction contraction. The areas may be solitary or multiple and tend to undergo focal calcification, producing high-level entry echoes with acoustic shadowing. Scars may appear as linear or patchy lesions (▣ **9.6**).

Cause. It can be difficult to establish a cause in any given case (pyelonephritic abscessation, stone-related, tuberculous, or secondary to anemia or infarction), although funnel-shaped scars most likely result from an old renal infarction (▣ **9.6a**) while pyelonephritic scars tend to have an irregular shape (▣ **9.6d**).

Multiple wavy parenchymal notches and rarefactions are characteristic features of peripheral renal arteriosclerosis in a setting of long-standing hypertension (▣ **9.6b, c**). These cases show undulant thinning of the parenchyma with no overall decrease in renal size.

Rarely, sites of irregular scarring are also seen in panarteritis nodosa.

Scars in the setting of chronic, nondestructive interstitial nephritis are diffuse and therefore produce an irregular renal surface with indistinct outlines. Calcifications may occur.

True scars require differentiation from a parenchymal notch in duplex kidneys, a medially tilted scan plane through the renal hilum, and fetal lobulations (▣ **9.6e and f, Fig. 9.66a**).

▣ 9.6 Scars and Parenchymal Notching

▶ **Vascular scars**

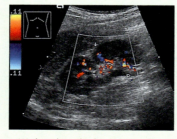 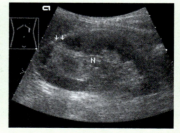 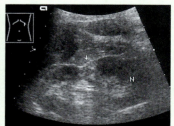

a Wedge-shaped infarction scar (arrows) in a patient with absolute arrhythmia in atrial fibrillation. P = pyelon.

b Vascular scar (arrows) with focal thinning of the parenchyma. The patient presented clinically with advanced atherosclerosis. N = kidney.

c Broad, echogenic atherosclerotic scar extending focally through the entire parenchyma (arrow) in a patient with chronic hypertension and generalized atherosclerosis. N = kidney.

9.6 Scars and Parenchymal Notching

▶ **Postinflammatory scars and differential diagnosis**

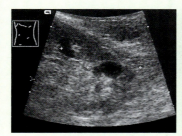 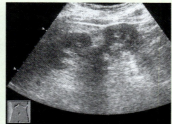 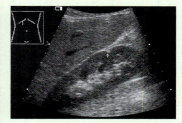

d Pyelonephritic scar (arrow). Cystic transformation of two medullary pyramids and a calix (arrows), appearing as "caliceal cysts" in the urogram.

e Broad, echogenic scar in the anterior parenchyma following renal tuberculosis.

f Anteroinferior notching of the parenchyma (arrow): scan plane cuts the renal hilum.

Echogenic Structure

Kidneys
- Anomalies, Malformations
- Diffuse Changes
- ▼ Circumscribed Changes
  - Anechoic Structure
  - Hypoechoic or Isoechoic Structure
  - Complex Structure
  - Hyperechoic Structure
  - ► **Echogenic Structure**

- ▶ Papillary Calcification
- ▶ Interlobar and Arcuate Arteries
- ▶ Bacterial Gas Bubbles
- ▶ Parenchymal Calcification
- ▶ Nephrocalcinosis, Medullary Sponge Kidney
- ▶ Renal Tuberculosis, Putty Kidney
- ▶ Pyelocaliceal Stone, Staghorn Calculus

▶ Papillary Calcification

Calcifications at the tips of the renal papillae are characteristic findings in analgesic nephropathy and diabetes mellitus. They appear only as echogenic flecks on ultrasound survey scans, where they often go undetected. They are easily detected and identified in strongly magnified views (**Fig. 9.86**).

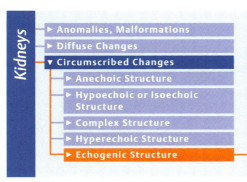

◀ **Fig. 9.86** Medullary (papillary) (MP) calcification (arrows) with an acoustic shadow. Clinical presentation: neglected type I diabetes.

▶ Interlobar and Arcuate Arteries

The renal artery itself, its branches in the renal sinus, and the interlobar and arcuate arteries tend to undergo atherosclerosis and calcification in patients with longstanding hypertension (arteriolosclerosis would affect the straight and interlobular arterioles arising from the arcuate artery along with the more distal afferent vessels and the postglomerular efferent vessels).

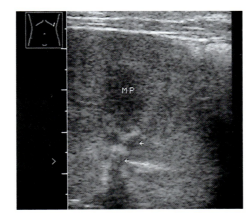

◀ **Fig. 9.87** Bright double echoes with a central, narrow echo-free band (arrow). Atherosclerosis of the arcuate artery at the base of the medullary pyramid (MP). N = kidney.

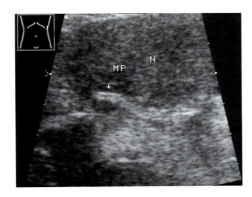

Ultrasound will occasionally demonstrate these thickened, echogenic vessels, some of which have shadowing wall calcifications (**Figs. 9.87 and 9.88**).

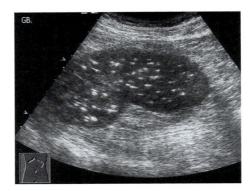

◂ **Fig. 9.88** Extensive atherosclerosis of the small renal arteries, close-up tangential parenchymal view in pseudoxanthoma elasticum.

▶ Bacterial Gas Bubbles

Small, vesicular, hoodlike echogenic masses may be observed in the setting of emphysematous (bacterial gas-forming) pyelonephritis; the shadowed region usually obscures the abscess itself. These findings indicate an urgent need for treatment (immediate broad-spectrum antibiotics or nephrectomy) due to existing or impending bacterial sepsis (**Fig. 9.89 and Fig. 9.67**).

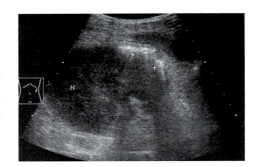

◂ **Fig. 9.89** Hoodlike bacterial gas collection (arrows) with associated reverberations. An actual abscess cannot be identified. Sepsis, emergency surgery, nephrectomy. N = kidney.

▶ Parenchymal Calcification

Parenchymal calcifications can have a variety of causes. They may reflect an old focal pyelonephritis, possibly in a setting of renal lithiasis, as well as calcifications in diabetic nephropathy or analgesic nephropathy. Some calcifications suggest a cystic etiology because of their shape. Calcifications also occur in the setting of tuberculosis (see below). Other calcifications develop as a sequel to old renal trauma, and others remain unexplained (**Fig. 9.90**).

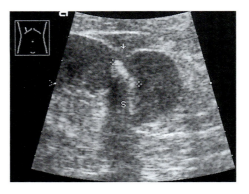

◂ **Fig. 9.90** Broad scar with calcification (arrows) of undetermined cause. Acoustic shadow (S).

▶ Nephrocalcinosis, Medullary Sponge Kidney

Nephrocalcinosis and medullary sponge kidney are different renal diseases that are associated with calcifications and have similar or identical ultrasound appearances.

Medullary nephrocalcinosis (medullary sponge kidney) is based on a dysontogenic disorder that can be broadly classified among the cystic diseases. It is characterized by a cystic dilatation of the collecting tubules in the renal papillae, leading to stone formation (a cauliflower or rosette pattern is seen in the i.v. pyelogram). Ultrasonography shows echogenic, rosettelike calcifications with acoustic shadows in the medullary pyramids.

Cortical nephrocalcinosis is marked by calcifications of the parenchyma and medullary pyramids and the formation of kidney stones. Calcifications of the medullary pyramids are the dominant feature. Nephrocalcinosis develops in a setting of hypercalcemia or tubular acidosis. A calcium excess is common to both disorders (increased supply or decreased tubular reabsorption).

If caliceal stones and renal pelvic/ureteral stones are also present, scans will show more or less intense, anechoic areas of caliceal and pelvic ectasia (**Fig. 9.91**).

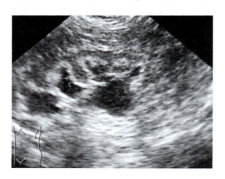
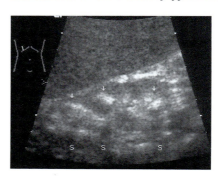

◂◂ **Fig. 9.91 a** Medullary nephrocalcinosis (renal tubular acidosis): echogenic medullary pyramids (arrows) and obstructive pyelocaliectasis (C) with multiple renal pelvic and ureteral stones. N = kidney.

◂ **b** Medullary nephrocalcinosis: annular calcifications in medullary pyramid projection (arrows). S = acoustic shadow.

▶ Renal Tuberculosis, Putty Kidney

Advanced stage III ulcerocavernous urogenital and renal tuberculosis leads to ulcerative, cavernous destruction of renal caliceal groups with stasis, calcifications, and the spread of caseous tuberculosis through the kidney.

The renal changes are impressive, and normal renal architecture is not observed. The ultrasound findings are diverse, with shadowing lesions of varying echogenicity that correlate with inspissated, calcified necrotic material and scar tissue (**Figs. 9.92–9.94**).

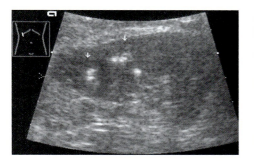

▲ **Fig. 9.92** Renal tuberculosis: focal parenchymal calcifications (arrows) around a presumably destroyed medullary pyramid (see also **Fig. 9.60**).

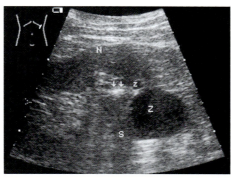

▲ **Fig. 9.93** Renal tuberculosis: calcifications (arrows, acoustic shadow S), cavernous cysts (Z). N = kidney.

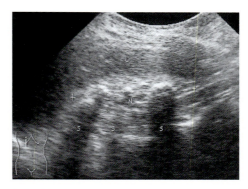

▲ **Fig. 9.94** Putty kidney (following tuberculosis): diffuse calcifications, acoustic shadow (S). An actual renal structure is not defined (N, cursors). L = liver.

▶ Pyelocaliceal Stone, Staghorn Calculus

Pyelocaliceal stones or staghorn calculi are easily diagnosed with ultrasound, which demonstrates the bright stone-surface echoes and associated shadows that are typical of stones and calcifications. Occasionally the stones are so small that their presence is revealed only by an acoustic shadow. This introduces a degree of uncertainty, as the shadowing focus may represent a vascular calcification.

Staghorn calculi in the renal pelvis may exhibit various shapes, depending on the orientation of the scan plane. If the scan is directed through the greatest width of the renal pelvis, it will display a broad, hard linear echo with an equally broad acoustic shadow. But if the plane cuts portions of the stone in the calices, multiple echoes and acoustic shadows will be seen (**Figs. 9.95 and 9.96**; see also Chapter 11).

Some small stones may be missed within the bright reflections of the sinus echo complex. A helpful guide in these cases is the "twinkling artifact" seen in color duplex scanning. It consists of red and blue color artifacts appearing within the shadow cast by calcified renal stones (or calcium stones in general; **Figs. 4.46 and 4.47** in Chapter 4). Reportedly, this phenomenon is seen even with very small stones[7].

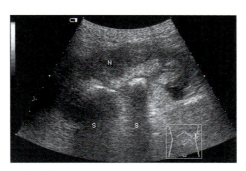

▲ **Fig. 9.95** Staghorn calculi in the renal pelvis with circumscribed pyelocaliectasis: multiple high-amplitude stone echoes (arrow) and acoustic shadows (S). N = kidney.

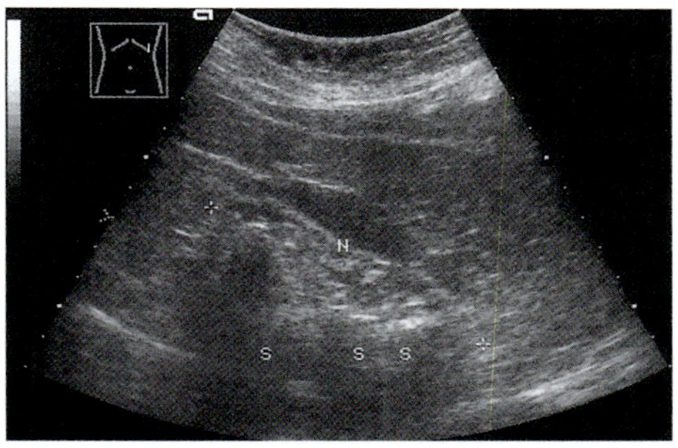

▲ **Fig. 9.96** Small atrophic kidney (N, cursors) due to renal pelvic stones or (unlikely here) multiple calcifications. Acoustic shadows (S). Excretory urogram showed a silent kidney with no focal opacities (urate stones?).

References

1. Banholzer P, Haslbeck M, Mehnert H. Sonographische Größenveränderungen der Nieren bei Typ-I-Diabetes als Früherkennungsmethode der diabetischen Nephropathie. Ultraschall 1988;9:255–9.
2. Bönhof JA, Meairs SP, Wetzler H. Duplex- und Farbdoppler-sonographische Kritrien von Nierenarterien-Stenosen. Ultraschall Klin. Prax. 1990; 5: 187.
3. Brühl P, Schäfer M. Fehlbildungen und spezielle Erkrankungen. In: Jocham D, Miller K (eds.). Praxis der Urologie. Stuttgart: Thieme 1994.
4. Hofmann R, Schütz R, Leyh H, Braun J. Sonographischer Nachweis von Nierenvenen- und Vena-cava-Thrombosen beim Adenokarzinom der Niere. Ultraschall 1985;6:312–5.
5. Hricak H, Cruz C, Romanski R et al. Renal parenchymal disease: sonographic-histologic correlation. Radiology 1982;144:141–7.
6. Hust W, Preim D, Bundschuh H. Parenchym-Pyelon-Index. Eine wertvolle Hilfe in der Beurteilung renaler Erkrankungen. In: Rettenmaier G (eds.). Ultraschalldiagnostik in der Medizin. Stuttgart: Thieme 1981.
7. Klauser A, Pallwein L, Frauscher F, Helweg G, Peschel R, Debus J. Die Wertigkeit des farbdopplersonographischen „Twinkling-Artefakts" in der Diagnostik der Nephrolithiasis. 24th Dreiländertreffen der ÖGUM, DEGUM, SGUM. Vienna 2000.
8. Mogensen CE. Diabetes mellitus and the kidney. Kidney Int 1982;21:673–5.
9. Mostbeck G, Derfler K, Walter R, Herold Ch, Mallek R, Tscholakoff D. Sonographie bei terminaler Niereninsuffizienz – ätiologische Rückschlüsse? Ultraschall 1988;9.
10. Mostofi FK, Davis CJ. Histological Typing of Kidney Tumours. 2nd ed. Berlin: Springer 1998.
11. Riede UN, Werner H. Nieren. In: Riede UN, Schaefer HE (eds.). Allgemeine und spezielle Pathologie. Stuttgart: Thieme 1995.
12. Takebayashi S, Aida N, Matsui K. Arteriovenous malformations of the kidney: diagnosis and follow-up with color Doppler sonography in six patients. Am J Roentgenol 1991;157:991–5.
13. Ultraschall 2000; 24. Dreiländertreffen SGUM/DEGUM/ÖGUM Wien 2000.
14. Van Campenhout J. Patriquin H. Malignant microvasculature in abdominal tumors in children: Detection with Doppler US. Radiology 1992;183: 445-448.

10 Adrenal Glands

Adrenal Glands 317

- **Enlargement** — 318
  - **Anechoic Structure** — 318
    - Adrenal Cyst
    - Intra-adrenal Hemorrhage
    - Adrenal Abscess
    - Cystic Tumor
  - **Hypoechoic Structure** — 320
    - Hyperplasia
    - Adenoma
    - Metastasis
    - Lymphoma
    - Adrenal Carcinoma
    - Incidentaloma
  - **Complex Echo Structure** — 324
    - Metastasis
    - Pheochromocytoma
    - Carcinoma
  - **Hyperechoic Structure** — 325
    - Lipoma, Myelolipoma
    - Calcification
    - Metastasis
    - Pheochromocytoma
    - Neuroblastoma

10 Adrenal Glands

D. Nuernberg

Anatomy

The adrenal glands are small, caplike glandular organs situated in close proximity to the kidneys. Often these "suprarenal" glands are incorrectly looked for above the kidneys, but the term "adrenal" correctly implies that each gland is predominantly medial to the upper pole of the associated kidney. The right adrenal gland has a linear or V shape, while the left adrenal gland is more V- or Y-shaped. The wings of each gland are 2–3 cm long and 6–8 mm thick. Their function is hormone production. The adrenal cortex secretes cortisol, aldosterone, and sex hormones, while the adrenal medulla secretes epinephrine and norepinephrine.

Shape
- Right: linear or V-shaped
- Left: V- or Y-shaped

Size
- Wings are 2–3 cm long and 6–8 mm thick.

Ultrasound Topography

Landmarks
- Right side: kidney and inferior vena cava
- Left side: aorta, lower pole of spleen, upper pole of kidney

Visualization
- Right side: subcostal flank scan or oblique scan
- Left side: intercostal flank scan through the spleen

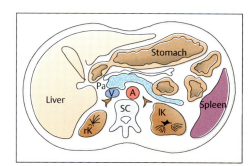

▲ **Fig. 10.1** Cross-sectional diagram at the level of the adrenal glands. The adrenal glands are the Y-shaped structures lying anteromedial to the kidneys. Pa = pancreas; rK = right kidney; lK = left kidney; A = aorta; V = inferior vena cava; SC = spinal column.

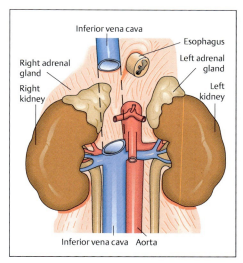

▲ **Fig. 10.2** Diagram of the adrenal glands showing their relations to neighboring organs.

The adrenal glands are located within the retroperitoneum. The right adrenal gland lies superomedial to the right kidney and posterolateral to the inferior vena cava. These are the principal landmarks on the right side. Typically the right adrenal gland is visualized behind the right lobe of the liver and anterior to the inferior (lumbar) crus of the diaphragm. The most favorable planes for ultrasound scanning are a right subcostal flank scan or oblique subcostal scan.

The left adrenal gland is inherently more difficult to scan than the right because it lacks the acoustic window of the liver and is obscured by air in the stomach. It is imaged with an intercostal flank scan directed through the spleen. The key landmarks are the aorta medially and the lower pole of the spleen or upper renal pole laterally.

Not infrequently, the adrenal glands extend down to the level of the renal hilum. Besides the kidneys, they are bordered by the liver and inferior vena cava on the right side and by the aorta and tail of the pancreas on the left side (**Figs. 10.1 and 10.2**). The adrenal region on each side appears as a triangular echogenic area bordered by the landmarks noted above (**Figs. 10.3 and 10.4**).

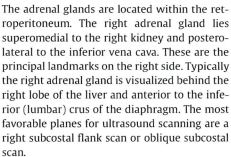

▲ **Fig. 10.3** The adrenal region is the space located posterior to the right lobe of the liver, lateral to the vena cava, and medial to the right kidney.

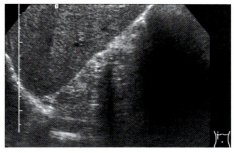

▲ **Fig. 10.4** In transverse section the adrenal region is posterior to the right lobe of the liver and medial to the right kidney. It is an echogenic area in which the gland itself is often not visualized.

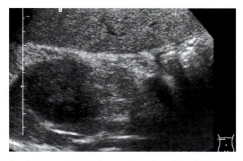

Ultrasound Morphology

The normal adrenal glands are difficult to visualize with ultrasound. This requires good scanning conditions, a high-resolution transducer, and a meticulous examination by a knowledgeable sonographer. It is more accurate, then, to speak of evaluating the "adrenal region" rather than the glands themselves. CT can consistently define the normal-size adrenal glands, giving this study a priority role in the primary imaging of these structures.

When the normal adrenal glands can be defined with ultrasound, they present a narrow, oblong shape with a hypoechoic cortex and medulla. The adrenal glands can almost always be visualized in newborns. The physiological hypertrophy at this stage of life results in relatively large glands that are easily identified at ultrasound and show clear corticomedullary differentiation (**Fig. 10.5a**).

In adults, however, the adrenal glands are usually visualized only when they are enlarged.

Some types of enlargement have pathological significance. Diseases of the adrenal glands may or may not be associated with endocrine symptoms (**Table 10.1**). Examination of the adrenal region is indicated for the staging of oncological disease and in endocrinological investigations. Adrenal abnormalities are often detected incidentally, however. In the absence of an underlying disease, an incidentally detected solid adrenal mass is called an incidentaloma (**Fig. 10.5b**).

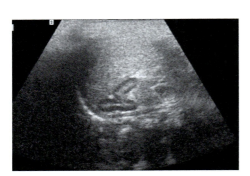

▲ *Fig. 10.5 a* Normal adrenal gland of an infant, consisting of a hyperechoic medulla and hypoechoic cortex.

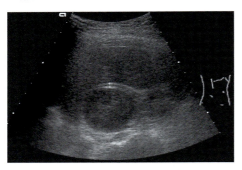

▲ *b* Medial to the upper pole of the right kidney is a sharply circumscribed, hypoechoic mass: typical adrenal incidentaloma.

Table 10.1 Sonographic features of adrenal diseases with or without endocrine symptoms (after reference 8)

	Sonographic appearance
Diseases with endocrine symptoms	
Addison disease	Adrenal atrophy not detectable with ultrasound; possible calcifications as evidence of prior tuberculosis
Conn disease	Unilateral adenomas, usually < 2 cm, not detectable with ultrasound
Cushing syndrome	In 80% of cases, bilateral hyperplasia due to pituitary (75%) or paraneoplastic (5%) ACTH overproduction; hyperplasia is usually not detectable with ultrasound
Pheochromocytoma	Can be localized with ultrasound in 80–90% of cases; extra-adrenal location is difficult, usually prevents identification
Diseases without endocrine symptoms	
Adrenal adenoma	Most common solid mass
Adrenal carcinoma	Often quite large (several centimeters) despite absence of symptoms; sometimes detected incidentally at ultrasound
Adrenal metastases	Common with bronchial carcinoma, malignant lymphoma, breast cancer, renal cancer, pancreatic cancer, and melanoma
Adrenal tumors and cysts	Detectable at 1–1.5 cm on the right side, at 1.5–2 cm on the left side

Enlargement

As mentioned, only enlarged adrenal glands can be clearly visualized with ultrasound.

Anechoic Structure

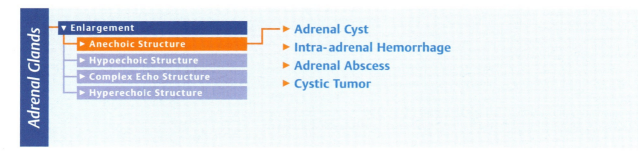

Masses adjacent to the adrenal glands. Anechoic adrenal masses require differentiation from anechoic structures that are located near the gland but are not related to it. These include the following:
- Renal cysts
- Pancreatic pseudocysts
- Splenic vessels

Renal cysts. Parietal cysts located in the upper pole of the kidney are particularly apt to be mistaken for adrenal cysts. They are distinguished by defining the relation of the cyst to the renal parenchyma.

Pancreatic pseudocysts and tumors. Pancreatic pseudocysts often form in the retroperitoneum following acute pancreatitis. The contents of the cysts may be completely anechoic, and the wall is usually irregular (**Fig. 10.6**). Fine-needle aspiration and laboratory analysis demonstrate high levels of pancreatic enzymes. Cystadenocarcinoma of the pancreas can also be a source of confusion (**Fig. 10.7**).

Splenic vessels. Tortuous and ectatic splenic vessels can mimic a cystic mass in the adrenal region. Shunt vessels in portal hypertension (e.g., secondary to splenic vein thrombosis) can also assume bizarre shapes.

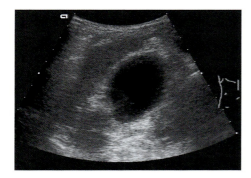

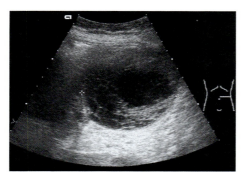

◂◂ **Fig. 10.6** Pancreatic tail pseudocysts are clearly visualized with transsplenic ultrasound and require differentiation from upper renal cysts and adrenal cysts. Diagnosis is aided by the history and ultrasound-guided fine-needle aspiration.

◂ **Fig. 10.7** A cystic, septated mass medial to the left kidney is localized to the pancreatic tail, not the left adrenal gland. Imaging and ultrasound-guided fine-needle aspiration identify the lesion as a cystadenocarcinoma of the pancreas.

▶ Adrenal Cyst

A cyst of the adrenal region is anechoic, has smooth margins, and shows distal acoustic enhancement. Its extent is variable. True cysts have regular walls and are filled with serous material (**Fig. 10.8**).

Most cystic masses in the adrenal region are secondary cysts that develop following pancreatitis, hemorrhage, or inflammation.

The greater mobility of adrenal cysts serves to differentiate them from hepatic cysts in the right adrenal region. Lack of contact with the renal parenchyma distinguishes them from a cyst of the upper renal pole.

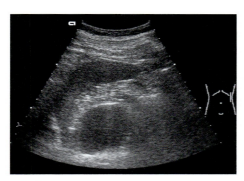

▴ **Fig. 10.8 a** Round, sharply circumscribed, echo-free mass located medial to the spleen and cranial to the left kidney: adrenal cyst. Ultrasound-guided fine-needle aspiration excluded pancreatic cyst, hemorrhage, etc.

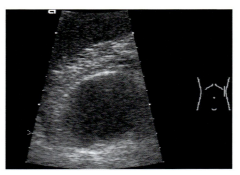

▴ **b** Typical cystic criteria: echogenic wall, echo-free contents, and distal acoustic enhancement characterize the adrenal cyst.

▶ Intra-adrenal Hemorrhage

Bleeding into an adrenal gland is anechoic in its early stage. It can occur in newborns due to obstetric trauma, hypoxia, or coagulation disorders. Intra-adrenal hemorrhage may correlate clinically with adrenal insufficiency. A large central hemorrhage (adrenal apoplexy) consistently leads to marked enlargement of the gland (**Fig. 10.9**). An older hemorrhage becomes increasingly echogenic over time and may eventually be completely absorbed. Differentiation is required from partially cystic neuroblastomas in small children.

Up to 25% of patients who sustain blunt abdominal trauma are discovered to have hematomas in the adrenal region. They also occur in patients on anticoagulant medication and can lead to hypocortisolism (Addison disease).

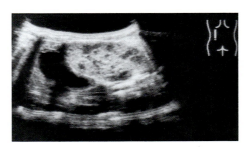

▴ **Fig. 10.9** Echo-free intra-adrenal hemorrhage in a newborn.

▶ Adrenal Abscess

An abscess of the adrenal glands is rarely anechoic. It is usually hypoechoic or has a complex echo structure. When the contents are anechoic, the clinical and laboratory findings can differentiate the lesion from an ordinary cyst. The wall is irregular, and distal acoustic enhancement may be present (**Fig. 10.10**).

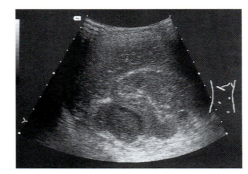

◀ *Fig. 10.10* Adrenal abscess. Circumscribed hypoechoic structure in the right adrenal region. Typical inflammatory laboratory findings. Ultrasound-guided fine-needle aspiration yielded pus.

▶ Cystic Tumor

A cystic tumor may be anechoic in rare cases, but usually it is hypoechoic. The walls are irregular in thickness and outline (some solid elements) (**Fig. 10.11**).

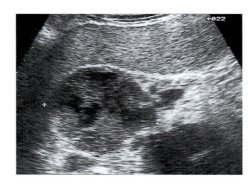

◀ *Fig. 10.11* Hypoechoic, partly cystic, predominantly solid tumor in the right adrenal gland: adrenal metastasis from bronchial carcinoma.

Hypoechoic Structure

Adrenal Glands
- ▼ Enlargement
  - ▶ Anechoic Structure
  - ▶ **Hypoechoic Structure**
  - ▶ Complex Echo Structure
  - ▶ Hyperechoic Structure

▶ **Hyperplasia**
▶ **Adenoma**
▶ **Metastasis**
▶ **Lymphoma**
▶ **Adrenal Carcinoma**
▶ **Incidentaloma**

▶ Hyperplasia

Hyperplastic adrenal glands are usually hypoechoic, especially in the cortical zone. They appear plump and elongated, may show low-level nodular echoes, and usually are only moderately enlarged (**Fig. 10.12**). Adrenal hyperplasia can occur, for example, as an adaptive response in ACTH-dependent Cushing syndrome. It may have a paraneoplastic cause, or it may occur in hyperaldosteronism. The hyperplasia is bilateral in most cases. The adrenal glands are poorly demarcated from their surroundings. Again, CT provides a better view of the hyperplastic adrenal glands, which usually cannot be detected with ultrasound.

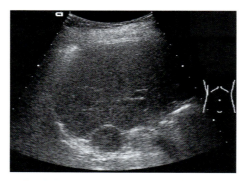

▲ *Fig. 10.12 a* Hypoechoic enlargement of the adrenal glands, identified as bilateral adrenal hyperplasia.

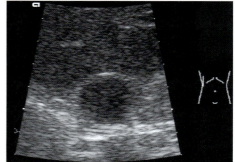

▲ *b* The hyperplastic adrenal gland is enlarged to approximately 2.5 cm. Affected glands may retain their normal triangular shape or may be rounded.

▶ Adenoma

Adenomas are uniformly hypoechoic with smooth margins and a round to oval shape, although some lesions have scalloped borders (**Fig. 10.13**). Adenomas occasionally have a nonhomogeneous appearance. Autopsy statistics indicate that they are quite common (10–20%), but most adenomas (90%) produce no endocrine symptoms and are too small to be seen with ultrasound. The average size of 23 operated adenomas in one study was 1.5 cm³, although they may exceed 5 cm in diameter. Adenomas are bilateral in a small percentage of patients. Functioning and nonfunctioning adenomas are indistinguishable by their sonographic features.

▲ **Fig. 10.13 a** Large, very hypoechoic, sharply circumscribed mass above the right kidney. Typical adrenal adenoma. If the gland measures more than 5 cm in diameter, laparoscopic adrenalectomy should be performed.

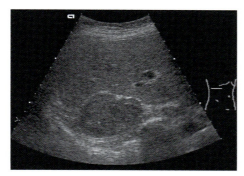

▲ **b** Hypoechoic, sharply circumscribed adenoma of the right adrenal gland discovered at routine ultrasound (confirmed by ultrasound-guided fine-needle aspiration).

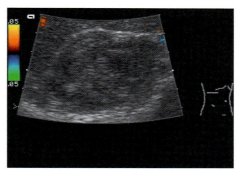

▲ **c** Scant vascularity on color Doppler.

▶ Metastasis

With their rich blood supply, the adrenal glands are the fourth most frequent site for hematogenous metastasis. Metastases to the adrenal glands account for the majority of solid adrenal tumors. These lesions are less homogeneous than adenomas and often have irregular margins (**10.1**). The most common primaries are bronchial carcinoma (15–25%) and breast carcinoma. Other possible sources are renal carcinoma, gastric carcinoma, pancreatic carcinoma, and malignant melanoma. Adrenal metastases are bilateral in up to 30% of cases, and this can produce the clinical manifestations of Addison disease. Bronchial carcinoma is virtually the only tumor that is associated with isolated adrenal metastases.

▣ 10.1 Adrenal Metastases

▶ **Primary tumors that can metastasize to the adrenal glands**
- ▶ Bronchial carcinoma
- ▶ Breast carcinoma
- ▶ Renal carcinoma
- ▶ Pancreatic carcinoma
- ▶ Malignant lymphoma

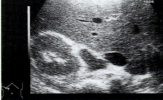
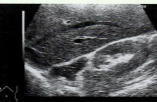
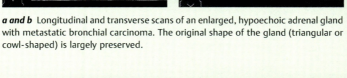

a and b Longitudinal and transverse scans of an enlarged, hypoechoic adrenal gland with metastatic bronchial carcinoma. The original shape of the gland (triangular or cowl-shaped) is largely preserved.

c Large hypoechoic, partially irregular metastasis from bronchial carcinoma on the left side, imaged by scanning through the spleen.

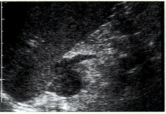
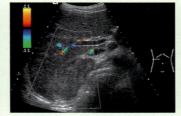
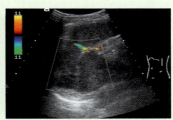

d Irregularly marginated tumor of the right adrenal gland located posterior to the right lobe of the liver: metastatic colon carcinoma.

e Metastases are generally hypovascular in the color Doppler image, whereas adrenal adenomas may be hypervascular. Metastatic tumor of the right adrenal gland.

f Left and right adrenal metastases from bronchial carcinoma. Negative on color Doppler.

Lymphoma

The adrenal region is a rare extranodal site of occurrence for lymphoma. Foci of lymphomatous infiltration have smooth borders and are hypoechoic (**Fig. 10.14**). Differentiation is required from lymphomas in the renal hilum (**9.2i, p. 297**). If invasion by lymphoma is suspected, other nodal stations should be scanned and commonly infiltrated organs should be closely scrutinized.

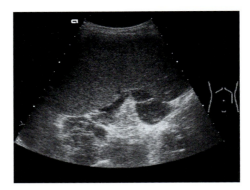

Fig. 10.14 Perisplenic lymphoma in the left adrenal region of a patient with B-cell lymphoma.

Adrenal Carcinoma

Adrenal carcinoma is usually hypoechoic with irregular margins. It frequently infiltrates its surroundings, and metastases can be demonstrated in the adrenal region and in other organs (e.g., the liver) (**Fig. 10.15**).

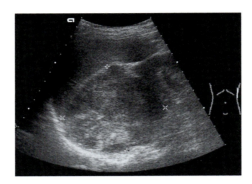

Fig. 10.15 Adrenal carcinoma may be hypoechoic or may have a complex echo structure. Usually it is relatively large when diagnosed (in this case 8 cm × 9 cm) and has irregular margins.

Incidentaloma

An incidentaloma is an adrenal tumor that is detected incidentally in an asymptomatic patient. Incidentalomas are found in 1% of CT examinations. They are much less common in ultrasound examinations, if only because of the difficulty in defining small lesions (**Fig. 10.16**). The predominantly hypoechoic tumors listed in **Table 10.2** account for the great majority of incidentalomas. **Figure 10.17** shows the algorithm used in the investigation of incidentalomas. The recommended endocrine work-up is detailed in **Table 10.3**. In some cases, ultrasound-guided fine-needle aspiration can also aid in the evaluation of incidentalomas (**Fig. 10.18**).

Hypoechoic tumors of the adrenal region require differentiation from other masses in that region such as a renal tumor (**Fig. 10.19**), accessory spleen (**Fig. 10.20**), lymphoma (**Fig. 10.21**), and gastric folds.

Table 10.2 Pathological classification of incidentalomas (n = 172) (after reference 8)

Diagnosis	n	%
Nonfunctioning adrenal adenoma	134	77.9
Cortisol-producing adenoma	14	8.1
Aldosteronoma	1	
Adrenal carcinoma (aldosterone-forming)	1	
Pheochromocytoma	5	2.9
Adrenal cyst	5	2.9
Myelolipoma	6	3.5
Ganglioneuroma	2	
Neurilemoma	1	
Hypernephroma	1	
Metastasis (thyroid carcinoma)	1	

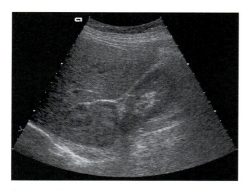

▲ **Fig. 10.16 a** Approximately 5 cm hypoechoic mass above the right kidney: typical incidentaloma without associated symptoms, detected at routine upper abdominal ultrasound. Histology identified the lesion as an adrenal adenoma (most common incidentaloma).

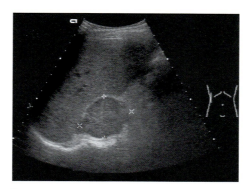

▲ **b** Hypoechoic tumor detected incidentally in the right adrenal region. Because of its irregular margins, biopsy was performed. Result: metastasis from a previously undiagnosed bronchial carcinoma.

Ultrasound-guided Fine-needle Aspiration of an Adrenal Lesion

Given the frequency of incidentally detected adrenal tumors, every case should undergo an initial endocrine work-up. If the tumor cannot be positively identified by laboratory tests and imaging (ultrasound, CT), ultrasound-guided fine-needle aspiration (UFNA) can supply a diagnosis in cases requiring treatment. The sensitivity of adrenal UFNA is between 90% and 95%. UFNA can furnish material for cytological or preferably histological analysis with a relatively low risk of complications. The procedure is performed in a lateral position. Access is more favorable for a right-sided lesion than a left-sided lesion, and the complication rate is also somewhat higher on the left side. UFNA is particularly indicated for the oncological investigation of tumors larger than 3 cm (**Fig. 10.18**).

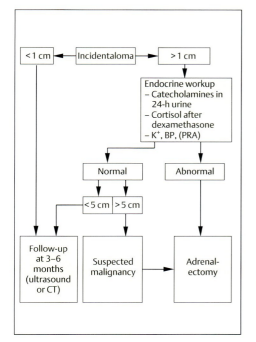

▲ **Fig. 10.17** Algorithm for investigating an adrenal incidentaloma (after reference 8).

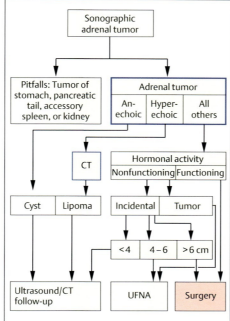

▲ **Fig. 10.18** Algorithm for "sonographic" adrenal tumors and the use of ultrasound-guided fine-needle aspiration (UFNA) (after reference 4).

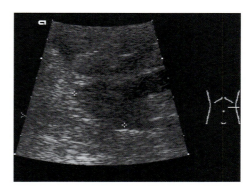

▲ **Fig. 10.19** Differential diagnosis: small, solid tumor on the upper pole of the left kidney. This lesion is definitely related to the kidney. Renal carcinoma.

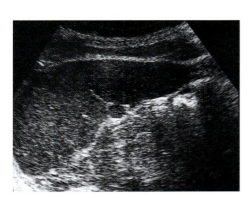

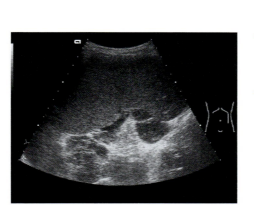

◂◂ **Fig. 10.20** A rounded mass having the same echogenicity as the spleen is sometimes found in the splenic hilum or at the inferior border of the spleen. It is not a left adrenal mass but an accessory spleen.

◂ **Fig. 10.21** Transsplenic scan of a large, hypovascular tumor.

Table 10.3 Endocrine laboratory work-up of adrenal incidentaloma (after reference 8)

Initial work-up

Mandatory	▸ Free catecholamines in 24 h urine ▸ Serum cortisol in dexamethasone suppression test (1 mg)
Optional	▸ Plasma renin activity after 30 min rest period ▸ Potassium excretion in 24 h urine

Extended work-up if initial findings are abnormal

Preclinical Cushing syndrome	▸ High-dose dexamethasone suppression test (8 mg) ▸ CRH stimulation test
Conn syndrome	▸ Aldosterone-18-glucuronide in 24 h urine ▸ Plasma renin activity and aldosterone at rest and orthostasis ▸ Selective renal vein catheterization with bilateral blood sampling for aldosterone and cortisol in adrenal venous blood

Complex Echo Structure

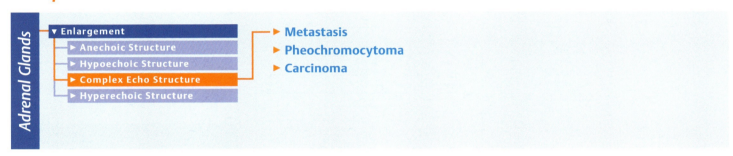

▸ Metastasis

Metastases are the adrenal tumors that are most frequently detected by ultrasound. Their appearance can be very diverse. Some metastases have a complex, nonhomogeneous echo structure and irregular margins (**Figs. 10.22–10.24**). The most common primary tumor is bronchial carcinoma. Other primary tumors have been mentioned above.

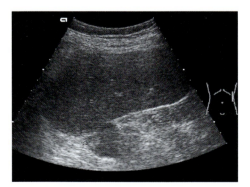

◂ **Fig. 10.22** Metastasis from advanced renal cell carcinoma in a left transsplenic scan. Complex internal structure.

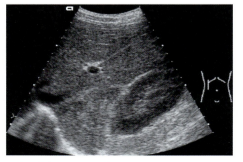
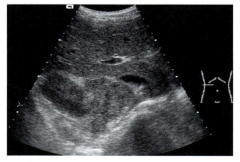
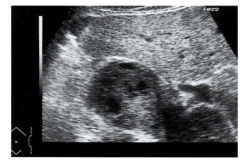

▴ **Fig. 10.23** Metastasis from bronchial carcinoma.
a Large, triangular mass with a complex echo structure located above the right kidney.

▴ **b** Transverse scan shows a metastasis with a complex echo structure "wedged" between the kidney, inferior vena cava, right lobe of the liver, and spinal column.

▴ **Fig. 10.24** Large metastasis from bronchial carcinoma on the right side, with a very nonhomogeneous internal structure. Solid components are seen along with liquid areas.

▶ Pheochromocytoma

Pheochromocytoma is a tumor of the adrenal medulla that is generally detected sonographically (80–90% of cases) following the appearance of clinical symptoms (hypertension and tachycardia caused by increased catecholamine secretion). Most pheochromocytomas are already several centimeters in diameter when diagnosed. They have smooth margins, a round shape, and a nonhomogeneous or complex echo structure. Hypoechoic liquid components are also observed. A spectrum of appearances may be seen (**Figs. 10.25 and 10.26**). Pheochromocytomas are bilateral in approximately 10% of cases and extra-adrenal in 10–20%. The "Zuckerkandl organ" should be looked for at the level of the origin of the inferior mesenteric artery, anterior to the aorta. Other extra-adrenal sites are the renal hilum, bladder wall, and thorax. Pheochromocytoma is occasionally seen posterior to the renal vein in transverse scans.

Rarely, pheochromocytoma is diagnosed in the setting of multiple endocrine neoplasia (MEN). From 2% to 5% of pheochromocytomas are malignant.

Owing to the risk of inciting a hypertensive crisis, fine-needle aspiration biopsy should definitely be avoided when a pheochromocytoma is suspected.

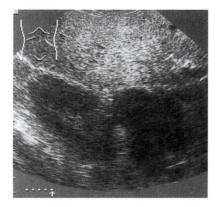

▲ **Fig. 10.25** Pheochromocytoma.
a Nonhomogeneous tumor with a hyperechoic center (positive endocrine test, increased catecholamine secretion).

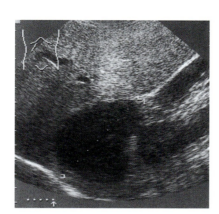

▲ **b** Large, functionally active pheochromocytoma (7.3 cm in diameter). The lateral scan bypasses the relatively hyperechoic tumor core.

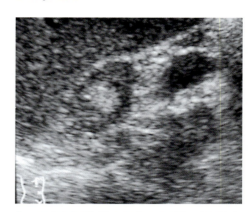

▲ **Fig. 10.26** Small, functionally active pheochromocytoma only 3 cm in diameter. Typical hyperechoic internal structure.

▶ Carcinoma

Adrenal carcinoma is a very rare (1:17 million), highly malignant tumor with a poor prognosis. Carcinomas have a hypoechoic to complex echo structure that is usually nonhomogeneous. The tumors have irregular margins and may infiltrate their surroundings. Adrenal carcinoma is indistinguishable sonographically from a metastasis, although the visualization of additional tumors can advance the differential diagnosis. Most adrenal carcinomas are hormone-producing. The tumor is usually detected only after it has reached considerable size (often > 8 cm). Intratumoral hemorrhage, necrotic foci, and calcifications may occur, adding to the variegated appearance (**Fig. 10.15**).

Hyperechoic Structure

Adrenal Glands
- ▼ Enlargement
  - ▶ Anechoic Structure
  - ▶ Hypoechoic Structure
  - ▶ Complex Echo Structure
  - ▶ Hyperechoic Structure
    - ▶ Lipoma, Myelolipoma
    - ▶ Calcification
    - ▶ Metastasis
    - ▶ Pheochromocytoma
    - ▶ Neuroblastoma

▶ Lipoma, Myelolipoma

Lipoma. A pure lipoma of the adrenal glands has smooth margins and high, homogeneous echogenicity. In contrast to the mixed tissues of myolipoma, posterior acoustic shadowing does not occur. Lipoma is rare and shows no proliferative tendency.

Myelolipoma. Adrenal myelolipoma has smooth margins and a homogeneous hyperechoic structure (but it may also be heterogeneous or hypoechoic depending on the medullary component) and it is well delineated; large fatty areas are defined by CT[7] (**Figs. 10.27 and 10.28**). It resembles a renal angiomyolipoma in its sonographic features. Posterior acoustic shadowing is often present. Malignant transformation is not known to occur. The tumor consists histologically of fat and bone marrow tissue (hematopoietic cells and reticular cells). Intratumoral hemorrhage and calcifications may be seen.

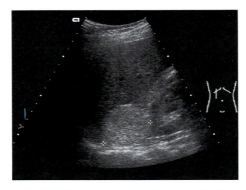

▲ **Fig. 10.27** Homogeneous, sharply circumscribed, hyperechoic tumor adjacent to the right kidney. Classic adrenal lipoma.

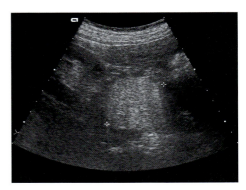

▲ **Fig. 10.28** Hyperechoic, homogeneous tumor above the right kidney represents a myelolipoma of the adrenal gland. Differentiation is mainly required from a renal angiomyolipoma.

▶ Calcification

Complete or partial calcification of the adrenal glands is characterized by a typical echo complex with a posterior acoustic shadow. Calcifications can result from a retained intra-adrenal hemorrhage or prior inflammatory process (e.g., tuberculosis). Patients occasionally show the clinical manifestations of Addison disease. Calcifications can also develop in tumors, however (carcinoma, metastases, pheochromocytoma, adenoma).

▶ Metastasis

Metastases can have a variety of ultrasound appearances, including high echogenicity. They tend to have irregular margins and a nonhomogeneous internal structure (**Figs. 10.29–10.32**). The most common primary tumor is bronchial carcinoma, which is associated with adrenal metastases in up to 25% of cases.

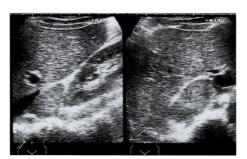

◀ **Fig. 10.29** Hyperechoic, relatively homogeneous metastasis from breast carcinoma.

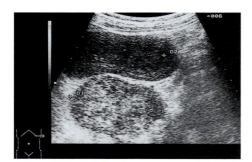

▲ **Fig. 10.30** Large, hyperechoic, nonhomogeneous tumor of the left adrenal gland: adrenal metastasis from bronchial carcinoma (cursor 1). The less echogenic mass in the spleen is a splenic metastasis (cursor 2).

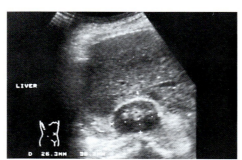

▲ **Fig. 10.31** Longitudinal scan shows a nonhomogeneous, hyperechoic tumor above the right kidney: metastasis from bronchial carcinoma.

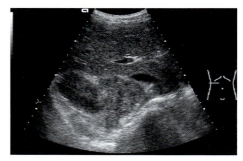

▲ **Fig. 10.32** An adrenal metastasis (e.g., bronchial carcinoma) can also appear hyperechoic, but it usually has a nonhomogeneous internal structure with irregular margins.

▶ Pheochromocytoma

Pheochromocytomas typically have a complex echo structure with hypoechoic elements, but some appear hyperechoic. The descriptions presented earlier under "Complex Echo Structure" also apply to the hyperechoic variant.

▶ Neuroblastoma

Neuroblastoma, like pheochromocytoma, arises from cells of the adrenal medulla. Next to Wilms tumor, it is the most common malignant abdominal tumor in children. Approximately 70% of neuroblastomas are located in the adrenal glands, the rest occurring at other sites in the sympathetic chain. Most neuroblastomas are very large and predominantly hyperechoic. Some may have cystic elements (due to hemorrhage) and calcifications. Laboratory tests usually show an increase in catecholamine secretion.

Considerably less common are benign neural tumors such as ganglioneuromas. They have been described only sporadically in the adrenal glands, occurring more commonly in the posterior mediastinum and at paravertebral sites.

References
1. Allolio B, Schulte HM. Praktische Endokrinologie. Munich: Urban & Schwarzenberg 1996.
2. Braun B. Nebennieren. In: Braun B, Günther R, Schwerk WB. Ultraschalldiagnostik. Lehrbuch und Atlas. Landshut: Ecomed 1983.
3. Burton S, Ros PR. Adrenal Glands. In: Stark D, Bradley WG (eds.). Magnetic Resonance Imaging. Mosby 1999.
4. Fröhlich E, Rufle W, Strunk H, Struckmann G, Seeliger H. Stellenwert der Feinnadelpunktion bei Nebennierentumoren. Ultraschall in Med 1995;16:90–3.
5. Görg C, Schwerk WB, Bittinger A, Euer B, Görg K. Sonographisch gesteuerte Feinnadelpunktion von Nebennierentumoren. DMW 1992;117:448–54.
6. Günther R. Sonographie der Nebennierenerkrankungen. Radiologe 1986;26:174.
7. Rao P., Kenney P, Wagner B, Davidson A. Imaging and pathological features of myelolipoma. Radiographics 1997;17;1373–85.
8. Reincke M, Allolio B. Das Nebennierenninzidentalom. Dtsch. Ärztebl. 1995;92:A764–A770.
9. Schmidt G. Ultraschall-Kursbuch. Stuttgart: Thieme 2004.

11 Urinary Tract

Urinary Tract 331

Malformations 333
Duplication Anomalies 333
- Duplex Kidney
- Duplex Ureter
- Bifid Ureter

Dilatations and Stenoses 334
- Caliceal and Ureteral Diverticula
- Megacalicosis
- Aberrant Arteries
- Megaureter
- Ureteropelvic Junction Obstruction

Dilated Renal Pelvis and Ureter 336
Anechoic 336
- Pyelectasis
- Subpelvic Ureteral Stenosis
- Urinary Stone Colic
- Chronic Urinary Stasis
- Retroperitoneal Fibrosis (Ormond Disease)
- Reflux

Hypoechoic 342
- Hemorrhage (Traumatic, Clot)
- Infected Obstruction
- Suppurative Pyelitis
- Pyonephrosis

Renal Pelvic Mass, Ureteral Mass 344
Hypoechoic 344
- Urothelial Carcinoma
- Ureteral Clots

Hyperechoic 345
- Caliceal Stones
- Renal Pelvic Stone
- Staghorn Calculus
- Ureteral Stone

Changes in Bladder Size or Shape 348
Large Bladder 348
- Urinary Retention
- Overflow Bladder, Neurogenic Bladder

Small Bladder 349
- Empty Bladder
- Residual Urine
- Shrunken Bladder

Altered Bladder Shape 351
- Partially Contracted Bladder
- Diverticulum, Pseudodiverticulum
- Indented Bladder, Operated Bladder

Intracavitary Mass 352
Hypoechoic 352
- Blood Clots
- Bladder Sludge
- Bladder Papilloma
- Polypoid Bladder Carcinoma
- Mesenchymal Tumors

Hyperechoic 355
- Urinary Catheter
- Blood Clots
- Polypoid Bladder Tumor
- Benign Prostatic Hyperplasia
- Lipoma, Fibroma, Myoma, Hemangioma
- Ureterocele
- Artifacts

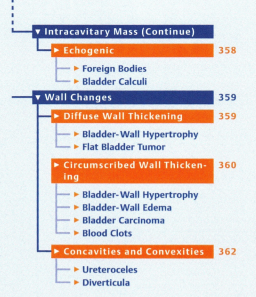

11 Urinary Tract

G. Schmidt

The excretory portion of the urinary tract begins with the collecting ducts of the renal parenchyma, where the secondary urine is formed through reabsorption. These ducts unite to form 10–30 papillary ducts, which open into the minor calices at the tips of the papillae. The papillae are lined with a single layer of epithelium that becomes stratified in its further course and lines a total of 8–10 minor calices, which collect the urine like funnels. They unite to form major calices, from which urine drains into the renal pelvis and thence to the ureter, bladder, and urethra.

Anatomy

> **Shapes and sizes**
> ▶ Shape of the renal pelvis
> ▶ Ureteral length and diameter
> ▶ Shape, volume, and size of the urinary bladder

Shape of the renal pelvis. The renal pelvis presents a spectrum of shapes ranging from the tubular (dendritic) form to the saclike "ampullary" form. The latter type is usually appreciated as a fluid-filled space at ultrasound, whereas the normal, non–fluid-filled pyelocaliceal system is not visible sonographically.

The renal pelvis is lined by a thin mucosa composed of special stratified, transitional epithelium ("urothelium," which also lines the ureter and bladder) and a muscular layer composed of smooth-muscle fibers. The mucosa can be distinguished from the renal sinus echo complex only when it is inflamed and swollen or when the pyelocaliceal system is filled with fluid (**Fig. 11.1**).

Ureteral length and diameter. The ureter similarly consists of an inner layer of mucosa, an intermediate layer of smooth-muscle fibers, and an outer adventitial layer. Normally it is not visualized with ultrasound owing to lack of contrast with the surrounding retroperitoneal tissue. The ureter is 30 cm long and 4–7 mm in diameter.

Shape, volume, and size of the bladder. The bladder wall consists of a thick muscular coat along with a mucous and submucous layer and a serosal layer. The three-layered structure of the bladder wall can be appreciated at ultrasound, especially in relation to the fluid-filled lumen.

The body or corpus of the bladder forms the anterosuperior roof, and the base or fundus of the bladder forms the posteroinferior floor. From the fundus, the bladder tapers in a funnel shape across the bladder neck to the urethra, which opens at the apex of the bladder trigone. The ureters pierce the muscular bladder wall and enter the bladder lumen at the ureteral orifices, located at the lateral angles of the trigone on the posterior wall of the fundus (**Figs. 11.2 and 11.3**). Sonographically, the submucous segments of the ureters appear as prominent ureteral ridges that protrude into the bladder lumen (**Fig. 11.3**).

The size of the bladder depends on its degree of distension. This also determines the shape of the bladder, which may appear round, squared with rounded corners, or elliptical (**Fig. 11.2**). The wall thickness of the full bladder is 1–3 mm. An urge to urinate is felt when the bladder is filled to approximately 350 ml, but the bladder can easily accommodate twice that volume.

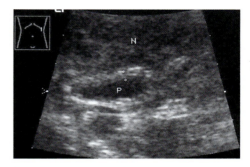

▲ **Fig. 11.1** Acute suppurative pyelitis with pelvic dilatation and hypoechoic wall thickening (cursors).

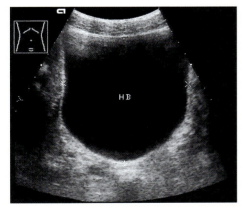

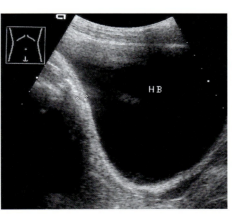

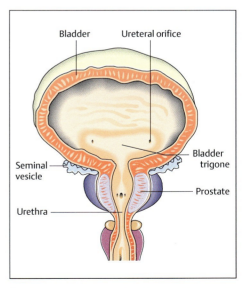

▲ **Fig. 11.2** Urinary bladder.
a Normal full bladder (HB) in a transverse scan through the lower abdomen: squared-off shape with rounded corners.

▲ **b** Full bladder in a longitudinal scan through the lower abdomen: oval shape with a tapered anterosuperior roof and posteroinferior floor. Normal wall thickness (cursors).

▲ **c** Diagram showing the anatomy and relations of the bladder, seminal vesicles, urethra, and prostate.

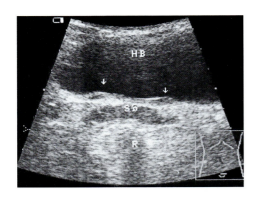
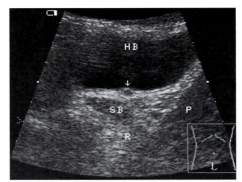

Fig. 11.3 Ureteral orifices at the lateral angles of the trigone (arrows) with a prominent "ureteral bud." SB = seminal vesicle; R = rectum; HB = urinary bladder; P = pelvis.
a Transverse scan.

b Longitudinal scan.

Topography

Locations
- Ureteropelvic junction
- Ureter anterior to the iliac vessels
- Prevesical ureter
- Bladder in the lesser pelvis

Ureteropelvic junction and course of the ureter. The ureter leaves the renal hilum posterior to the renal vein and artery. Hence it is best to scan the ureter from behind with the ultrasound beam directed anteriorly (**Figs. 11.4 and 11.5**). The ureter descends anteriorly to the iliopsoas muscle, following the lordotic curvature of the lumbar spine. Initially it takes a steep anterior and inferomedial course, then turns distally toward the lateral border of the bladder. As it descends, it crosses over the iliac vessels at the level of the origin of the deep iliac artery, follows the wall of the lesser pelvis, and finally opens into the bladder at the laterobasal ureteral ridges (**Fig. 11.5**).

Bladder. Figures 11.3 and 11.6 illustrate the relations of the bladder to the organs of the lesser pelvis and to the male reproductive tract.

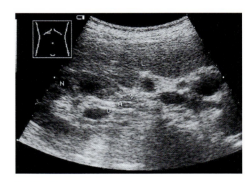

Fig. 11.4 Transverse scan of the right kidney (N). From anterior to posterior: the renal vein (V) followed by the renal artery (A) and upper ureter (U). L = liver.

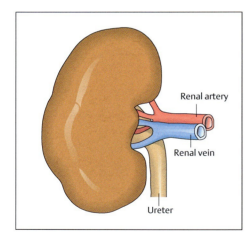
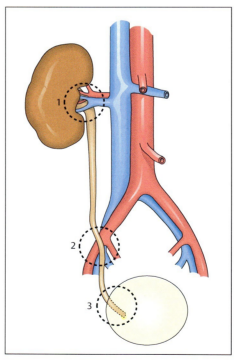

Fig. 11.5 Course and relations of the ureter.
a Proximal ureter.

b Course from the renal pelvis to the bladder trigone. 1 = ureteropelvic junction area; 2 = ureter crossing over the iliac vessels; 3 = supravesical segment.

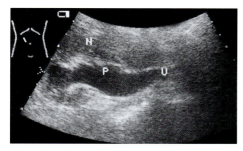 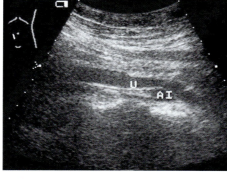 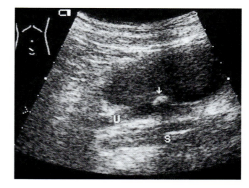

▲ **c–e** Course of the ureter (U) is visualized by ultrasound due to obstruction by a prevesical ureteral stone (arrow, acoustic shadow S).
c Junction of the ureter (U) with the dilated renal pelvis (P). N = kidney.

▲ **d** Ureteral segment anterior to the iliac artery (AI).

▲ **e** Prevesical ureter.

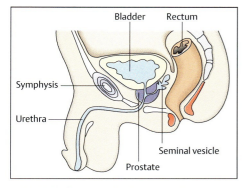 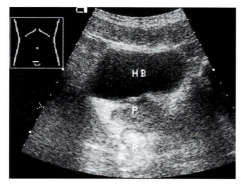 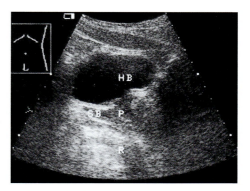

▲ **Fig. 11.6a** Diagram showing a sagittal section through the bladder and male reproductive tract.

▲ **b, c** Sonographic relationship of the bladder (HB), prostate (PR), seminal vesicle (SB; see **Fig. 11.3**), and rectum (R).
b Lower abdominal transverse scan.

▲ **c** Lower abdominal longitudinal scan.

Malformations

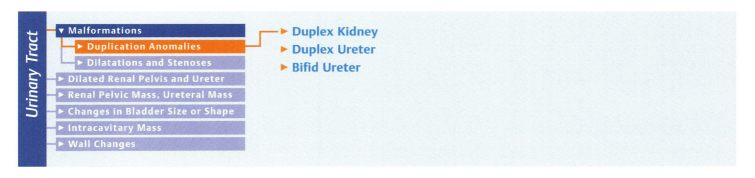

Duplication Anomalies

The renal collecting ducts, renal pelvis, and ureter are formed by the differentiation of the cranial end of the ureteral bud in the fourth to fifth week of gestation. The ureteral bud itself forms posteriorly and medially from the primary ureter, the Wolffian duct, before it opens into the urogenital sinus. The presence of a second, separate ureteral bud gives rise to a complete ureteral duplication, while division of the ureteral bud at the later stage results in a partial duplication. When two ureters are present, the Weigert–Meyer rule states that the upper-pole ureter inserts closer to the bladder neck, frequently at an ectopic site, owing to the medial and caudal rotation of the Wolffian duct that occurs during embryonic development. Meanwhile the lower-pole ureter inserts closer to the bladder roof. This accounts for the tendency for reflux to occur in the lower-pole system while the upper system is more susceptible to obstruction.

A ureterocele is another relatively common anomaly resulting from abnormal development of the initially higher ureteral bud, which drains the upper-pole system but opens in the bladder floor due to caudal rotation. This leads to frequent dysplasia with megaureter formation and hydronephrosis of the upper system.

▶ Duplex Kidney

Duplex kidney is an anomaly characterized by the presence of two renal pelves that are joined at the level of the ureteropelvic junction. Sonographically, the kidney appears elongated and the moieties are separated by a band of parenchyma, creating a visible notch in the renal outline (**Figs. 11.7 and 11.8**).

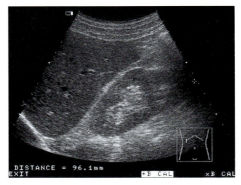

▲ **Fig. 11.7** Duplex kidney: normal renal size (33 cm), complete parenchymal band with a notch in the renal outline (cystic RCC was diagnosed five years later; **Fig. 9.55, p. 298**; contralateral kidney **Fig. 11.23**).

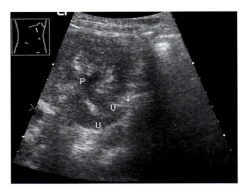

▲ **Fig. 11.8** Bifid ureter: the duplicated upper ureters (U) are joined at the level of the ureteropelvic junction (arrow), with a dilated renal pelvis (P). Urinary obstruction.

▶ Duplex Ureter

Duplex ureter refers to a complete ureteral duplication with two separate renal pelves. The ultrasound appearance is like that of a duplex kidney, because normally both ureters cannot be visualized. Ultrasound can confirm a duplex ureter only when urinary tract obstruction is present, but excretory urography can consistently demonstrate the anomaly.

▶ Bifid Ureter

Bifid ureter is a partial ureteral duplication in which the ureters arise from separate renal pelves and unite between the pelvis and bladder to form a single ureter (**Figs. 11.8 and 11.9**).

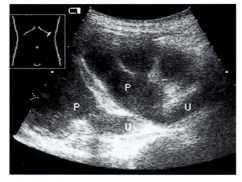

▲ **Fig. 11.9** Bifid ureter: both ureters (U) are obstructed.
a Oblique upper abdominal scan through the left kidney (P = renal pelvis).

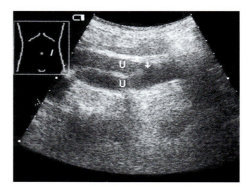

▲ *b* Oblique midabdominal scan on the left side, showing the site where the ureters join together.

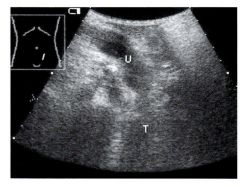

▲ *c* Oblique lower abdominal scan on the left side. Cause of the ureteral obstruction: metastatic tumor (T) of the left ovary.

Dilatations and Stenoses

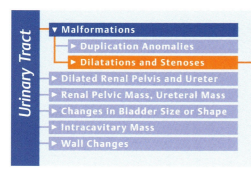

- ▶ Caliceal and Ureteral Diverticula
- ▶ Megacalicosis
- ▶ Aberrant Arteries
- ▶ Megaureter
- ▶ Ureteropelvic Junction Obstruction

▶ Caliceal and Ureteral Diverticula

Caliceal and ureteral diverticula are very rare, congenital lesions. Stone precipitation occurs in caliceal diverticula and can lead to clinical symptoms. Diverticula appear sonographically as anechoic masses in calices or along the course of a ureter (**Fig. 11.10**).

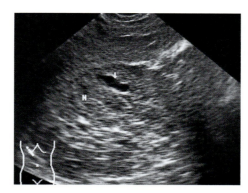

▲ *Fig. 11.10* Caliceal diverticulum (12-year-old boy).
a Oval, echo-free area of caliectasis. N = kidney.

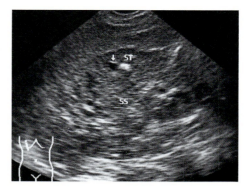

▲ **b** A stone (ST; arrow = acoustic shadow) is visible in the distended calix of a child with colicky episodes. It is likely that the caliectasis is primary and that the stone formed secondarily. SS = shadowing.

▶ Megacalicosis

Megacalicosis is an anomaly in which the calices in one kidney are dilated and increased in number. Most of these cases are clinically asymptomatic. Ultrasound examination reveals enlarged, dilated, fluid-filled calices.

▶ Aberrant Arteries

Aberrant arteries can occur in the necks of the calices and at the ureteropelvic junction. Ultrasound may show caliceal enlargement in cases where an interlobar artery leads to caliectasis, or it may show enlarged groups of calices when pyelectasis has developed due to tethering of the upper ureter by an aberrant renal artery. Color duplex examination can demonstrate an aberrant vessel in 91% of cases (**Fig. 11.11**).

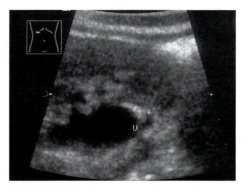

▲ *Fig. 11.11* Subpelvic ureteral stenosis. Ultrasound shows marked separation of the sinus echo complex by a bandlike, echo-free mass representing the fluid-filled renal pelvis (P). Vascular tethering?
a B-mode image: small, anechoic round feature by the ureteropelvic junction (U, arrow).

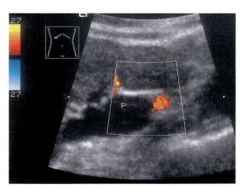

▲ **b** Color duplex: aberrant lower pole vessel. P = pelvis.

▶ Megaureter

Megaureters and megacalices are congenital anomalies involving the dilatation of urinary passages. The classification of Hohenfellner and Walz[3], as modified by Kröpfl[6], is shown below. Nowadays a congenital megaureter is generally diagnosed with antenatal ultrasound, but this modality is of limited value for classifying the lesion.

Primary idiopathic megaureter is caused by a perivesical fibrotic stenosis. Concomitant reflux is present. Primary refluxive megaureter is based on an anomalous insertion of the ureteral bud. Secondary refluxive and obstructive megaureters are usually caused by bladder wall changes due to subvesical stenosis. Further differentiation requires a special urological examination (**Fig. 11.12**).

Classification of Megaureter (Uretri-Vesical Function Obstruction)

- ▶ Obstructive megaureter
  - Primary, idiopathic
  - Secondary (e.g., to neurogenic bladder, subvesical obstruction)
- ▶ Refluxing megaureter
  - Primary due to reflux
  - Secondary to neurogenic bladder, subvesical obstruction
- ▶ Nonobstructive, nonrefluxive megaureter

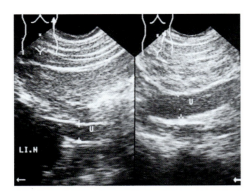 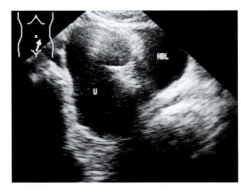

◂◂ **Fig. 11.12** Megaureter (U), probably caused by a fibrotic obstruction proximal to the bladder insertion (HBL).
  a Result: hydronephrotic sac (LI.N).
  b Iliac portion of the ureter.

◂ **c** Massive cystic dilatation at the prevesical level.

▸ Ureteropelvic Junction Obstruction

An obstruction at the ureteropelvic junction has a similar appearance to an aberrant artery. The changes range from a dilated pyelocaliceal system to hydronephrosis with loss of renal function. Ultrasound shows pyelocaliectasis or, in long-standing cases, a hydronephrotic sac whose dilatation cannot be traced into the ureter (**Figs. 11.1 and 11.13**).

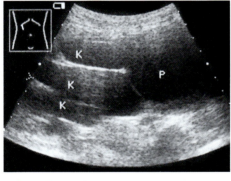 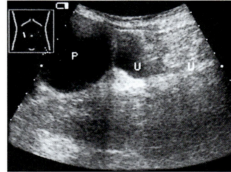 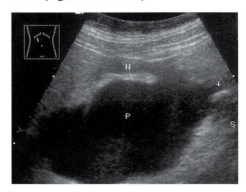

▴ **Fig. 11.13 a and b** Hydronephrotic sac. Dilated proximal ureter (U). Cause: severe ureteropelvic junction obstruction (surgery)? P, K = massive pyelocaliectasis.

▴ **c** Differential diagnosis: ureteropelvic junction stone (arrow, acoustic shadow S). Scans should always include the ureteropelvic junction to aid the differential diagnosis. N = kidney; P = pelvis.

Dilated Renal Pelvis and Ureter

Anechoic

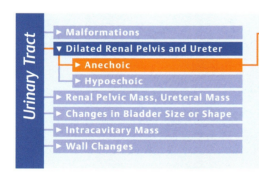

- ▸ Pyelectasis
- ▸ Subpelvic Ureteral Stenosis
- ▸ Urinary Stone Colic
- ▸ Chronic Urinary Stasis
- ▸ Retroperitoneal Fibrosis (Ormond Disease)
- ▸ Reflux

▸ Pyelectasis

Pyelectasis refers to an anechoic separation of the central renal sinus echogenicity due to dilatation of the renal pelvis with no associated expansion of the caliceal system or upper ureter. Pyelectasis may result from an ampullary renal pelvis or from fluid diuresis (**Figs. 11.14 and 11.15**).

Other frequent causes are incipient urinary stasis, like that resulting from pregnancy or stone colic with an incomplete obstruction, as well as urinary retention (**Figs. 11.16–11.19**).

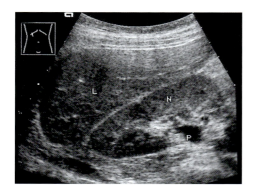
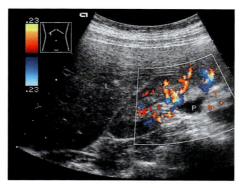

◄◄ **Fig. 11.14** Pyelectasis (P). L = liver; N = kidney.
a B-mode image: typical triangular, echo-free mass in the sinus echo complex with nonvisualization of the proximal ureter.

◄ **b** Color Doppler image: a dilated renal vein can be excluded from the differential diagnosis (see also **Fig. 11.20**).

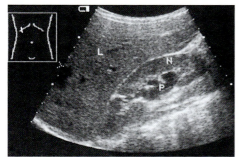
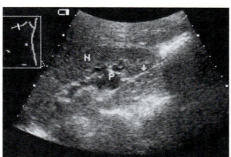
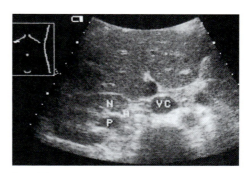

▲ **Fig. 11.15** Pyelectasis resulting from an ampullary renal pelvis. L = liver; N = kidney.
a Enlarged, anechoic pyelocaliceal system (P).

▲ **b** Scan from a more lateral angle shows a nondilated, normal-appearing ureter (arrow).

▲ **c** High transverse scan of the right kidney (N). Posterior to the artery is the ectatic renal pelvis (P) with no dilatation of the proximal ureter. VC = inferior vena cava.

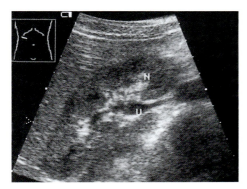
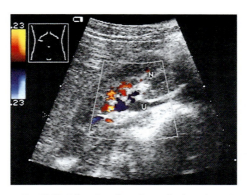
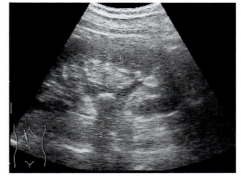

▲ **Fig. 11.16** Pyelectasis with a dilated proximal ureter (U). Obstruction? The patient presented clinically with suppurative pyelitis. IVP (i. v. urogramm) showed an ampullary renal pelvis with no outflow obstruction. N = kidney.

▲ **Fig. 11.17** Color Doppler view of the plane in **Fig. 11.16**: no vascularity, signifying fluid in the renal pelvis. N = kidney; U = ureter.

▲ **Fig. 11.18** Renal pelvic stone (arrow, acoustic shadow S) with radial anechoic streaks representing the dilated calices and infundibula. Here the renal pelvis is only minimally dilated. These stones are often missed at ultrasound, as are stones at the ureteropelvic junction (see also **Fig. 11.22**). N = kidney.

◄◄ **Fig. 11.19 a** Obstructive pyelectasis. N = kidney; P = pelvis.
b Cause: pregnancy.

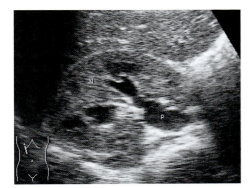
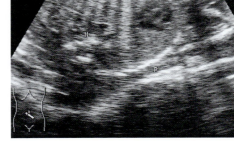

The differential diagnosis should include all conditions that cause a hypoechoic, dilated renal pelvis (see below) as well as anechoic or hypoechoic transformation of the sinus echo (**Fig. 11.20**).

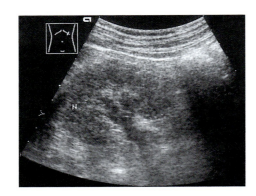
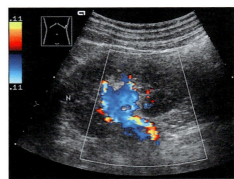

◄◄ *Fig. 11.20* Initial sonographic impression: obstructive pyelectasis of the left kidney (N).
a B-mode image shows an echo-free band in the sinus echo complex.

◄ *b* Color Doppler: a dilated renal vein!

▶ Subpelvic Ureteral Stenosis

A dilated pyelocaliceal system with no ureteral dilatation indicates a subpelvic stenosis.

Primary causes are congenital aberrant vessels and congenital ureteropelvic junction obstruction due to fibrous bands (see above). Most cases involve a partial obstruction that is not associated with progressive dilatation, and so there is no functional deterioration over time. Progressive stenoses culminate in a hydronephrotic, nonfunctioning kidney (**Fig. 11.12**).

The differential diagnosis includes secondary stenoses due to postoperative stricture, stone obstruction, or urothelial carcinoma (**Figs. 11.21–11.23**).

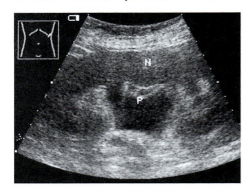
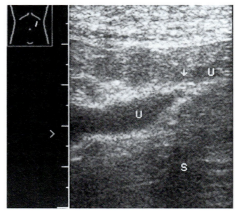

◄◄ *Fig. 11.21* Subpelvic ureteral stenosis with a clinically indeterminate cause.
a Ultrasound shows a markedly ectatic renal pelvis (P) with a broad, approximately rectangular echo-free mass. N = kidney.

◄ *b* Massive dilatation of the proximal ureter (U) with granular hyperechoic structures and an acoustic shadow (S) consistent with lithiasis. Urogram showed ureteropelvic junction stenosis of indeterminate cause with massive pyelocaliectasis. Retrograde ureterography with stenting showed ureteropelvic junction stenosis of undetermined cause.

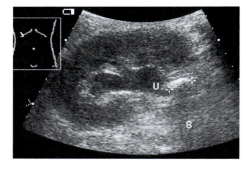
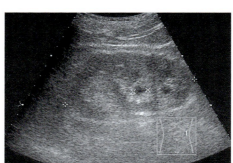

◄◄ *Fig. 11.22* Stone (cursors, acoustic shadow S) obstructing the upper ureter (U).

◄ *Fig. 11.23* Two small masses with cystlike ultrasound features in the lower moiety of a duplex kidney. Dilated pyelocaliceal system. Cause: urothelial carcinoma at the ureteropelvic junction (▣ 11.2d).

▶ Urinary Stone Colic

When the obstructing stone is not located at the ureteropelvic junction, ultrasound shows the features of pyelocaliectasis and ureteral dilatation. Stones tend to become impacted at three sites of physiological narrowing (**Figs. 11.5 and 11.3**):
▶ The ureteropelvic junction
▶ The point where the ureter crosses the iliac vessels
▶ The ureterovesical junction

Generally the ureter is not visualized by ultrasound unless it is fluid-filled owing to an obstruction. It then appears as an anechoic band that can be traced distally from the renal pelvis, in some cases as far as its insertion in the bladder floor (**Fig. 11.3**). Generally the impacted stone can be detected and localized. This is not possible with partial obstructions. In these cases it may be possible (with effort) to locate a constant, hyperechoic stony structure that casts an acoustic shadow. If the neck of the calix is enlarged to more than 4 mm and the pelvis and ureter to more than 5 mm, urinary stasis is present. This is also indicated by a unilateral decrease or absence of the ureteral jet phenomenon (3 or 4 per minute is normal) (**Figs. 11.24–11.27 and Figs. 11.49–11.52**).

Clinical Note

If a stone is detected and infection is *not* present, several days of conservative therapy may be tried under ultrasound surveillance before proceeding with invasive treatment. Intravenous urography is contraindicated, as the contrast administration could lead to rupture of the fornix or ureter (**Fig. 11.27**). If the ultrasound findings are equivocal, an abdominal plain film can be taken to check for a shadowing calculus.

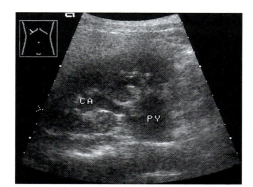
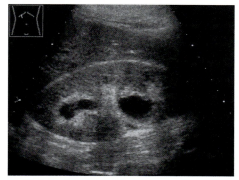

▸▸ **Fig. 11.24** Dilated pyelocaliceal system in a patient with flank pain. Suspicion of biliary colic.
a Dilated calix (CA) communicating with the dilated and obstructed renal pelvis (PY).

◂ *b* A proximal ureteral stone (arrow) causing obstructive caliceal ectasia. Scan shows two echo-free masses in the central echo complex. The upper mass represents an ectatic caliceal neck. The enlargement of a caliceal neck to more than 5 mm (here 11 mm) indicates obstruction. The lower mass is the dilated renal pelvis.

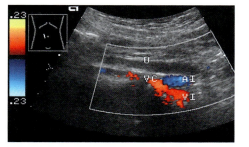

▸▸ **Fig. 11.25** Color Doppler examination.
a Course of the ureter (U) anterior to the vena cava (VC) and the iliac artery and vein (AI; VI), oblique scan through the right midabdomen.

◂ *b* Lower part of the ureter (U) in the lesser pelvis, anterior to the iliac artery (AI). The impacted stone (arrow, acoustic shadow S) is visualized.

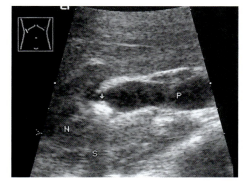
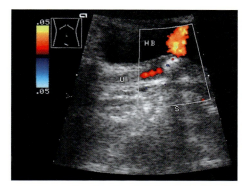
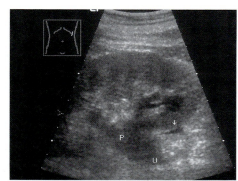

▲ **Fig. 11.26 a and b** Renal and ureteral obstruction.
a Pyelocaliceal stone (arrow, acoustic shadow S), dilated renal pelvis (P). N = kidney.

▲ *b* Cause: prevesical stone with an acoustic shadow (S); two days later, detectable urine flow (ureteral jets). HB = bladder; U = ureter.

▲ **Fig. 11.27** Fluid collection around the lower pole of the kidney: urinoma (arrows). Dilatation of the renal pelvis (P) and ureter (U).

▸ Chronic Urinary Stasis

Chronic urinary stasis is based on a disturbance of urinary transport. Urinary stasis can be classified into four grades of severity, as described by Gladish[1b], based on its sonographic appearance. This assessment includes evaluating the degree of renal pelvic distension by fluid, the integrity of the renal sinus echo complex, and the loss of renal parenchyma (▣ 11.1).

Chronic urinary stasis can have a variety of causes, most of which can be demonstrated with ultrasound. Once urinary stasis has been detected sonographically, the cause can often be discovered by starting with a posterolateral scan of the ureteropelvic junction and then moving the scan anterolaterally and inferomedially, using color Doppler as needed, until the dilated, anechoic ureter appears to terminate. This site marks the point of the obstruction.

A special form of urinary stasis due to outflow obstruction is hydronephrosis. It is identical to the grade IV hydronephrotic sac described above, but there are several special features in addition to chronic urinary stasis: the condition is usually detected incidentally and is based on an unnoticed, often congenital cause. Its significance lies in the fact that when it is bilateral (usually due to an infravesical cause), it can lead to end-stage renal failure, infection, and pyonephrosis (see below).

The various causes of chronic urinary stasis are listed in **Table 11.1** and illustrated in ▣ 11.2.

Table 11.1 Causes of chronic urinary stasis

- ▸ Ureteropelvic junction obstruction, aberrant vessel
- ▸ Impacted stone
- ▸ Clot or necrotic papilla
- ▸ Stricture
- ▸ Ectopic ureteral insertion, ureterocele
- ▸ Bladder tumor
- ▸ Prostatic hypertrophy or tumor
- ▸ Colon carcinoma
- ▸ Ovarian carcinoma
- ▸ Ureteral carcinoma
- ▸ Ormond disease

11.1 Sonographic Criteria for Grading the Severity of Urinary Stasis

▶ **Mild urinary stasis (grade I)**
- Pyelocaliectasis with anechoic separation of the renal sinus echo complex; the ureter or ureteropelvic junction may be dilated and echo-free
- Preservation of the bright sinus echoes
- Normal thickness of the renal parenchyma

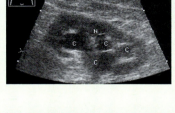

a Echo-free separation of the central renal sinus echogenicity; preservation of sinus echoes; intact parenchyma (N). This patient had metastatic colon cancer and postoperative ureteral occlusion by a suture (▣ 11.2f). PY = pelvis; U = ureter.

▶ **Moderate urinary stasis (grade II)**
- Marked caliceal dilatation to 5–10 mm, pyelectasis
- Ureteral dilatation, incipient tortuosity
- Parenchyma still normal or slightly thinned
- Diminished sinus echo complex

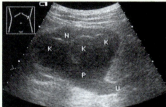

b Conspicuous, echo-free pyelocaliectasis (C) with diminished sinus echoes and incipient parenchymal thinning. Postoperative ureteral occlusion by a suture as above, six months later. N = kidney.

▶ **Severe urinary stasis (grade III)**
- Massive caliceal dilatation, pronounced anechoic pyelectasis
- Loss of the sinus echo complex
- Rarefaction of the renal parenchyma

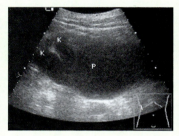

c Conspicuous, echo-free pyelocaliectasis (K, P); loss of renal sinus echogenicity; thinned parenchyma, dilated ureter (U). Patient had a metastatic ovarian tumor. N = kidney.

▶ **Hydronephrotic sac (grade IV)**
- Anechoic cystic mass in the central echo complex due to severe pyelocaliceal dilatation
- Complete loss of the renal sinus echogenicity
- Complete or almost complete loss of the renal parenchyma

d Calices (K) and renal pelvis (P) are combined to form an echo-free hydronephrotic sac with little or no evidence of any residual parenchyma.

▶ Retroperitoneal Fibrosis (Ormond Disease)

Fibrosis arising from the region of the L4 and L5 vertebrae, with the formation of collagenous connective-tissue fibers up to 2 cm thick, can lead to the extensive fibrous encasement of retroperitoneal structures including the psoas muscle, aorta, and vena cava along with the iliac vessels, mesentery, and ureters.

At ultrasound, the ureters are visibly ensheathed and obstructed, leading to chronic urinary stasis. In contrast to other occlusive diseases, a localized obstruction cannot be found. Instead there is a long, rigid, dilated ureteral segment with none of the tortuosity that is usually seen in association with chronic urinary stasis. The fibrosis itself is slightly echogenic and is poorly delineated from other retroperitoneal structures. The detection of fibrotic encasement on other retroperitoneal organs supports the ultrasound impression of fibrosis-induced urinary stasis.

Retroperitoneal fibrosis involving the ureters also occurs in inflammatory disorders such as Crohn disease, diverticulitis, sarcoidosis, and radiation-induced fibrosis. Other retroperitoneal causes of urinary stasis, such as sarcoma and malignant lymphoma, should be included in the differential diagnosis (**Fig. 11.28**).

◀◀ *Fig. 11.28* Ormond disease (retroperitoneal fibrosis).
a Grade II stasis kidney (N) with a dilated renal pelvis (P). C = calix.

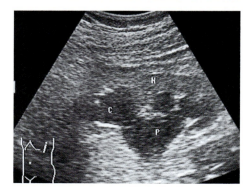

◀ *b* Broad, rigid ureter (U) encased in retroperitoneal connective tissue, recognized here only by the rigid course of the ureter. The connective tissue itself is not visualized because of its low impedance.

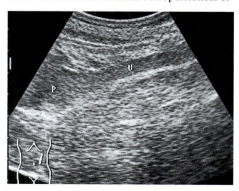

11.2 Causes of Chronic Urinary Stasis

▶ Ureteropelvic junction stone, ureteral stricture, ureterocele

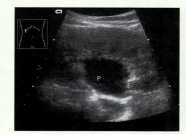
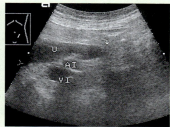
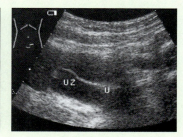

a Ureteropelvic junction obstruction? (arrow; no dilated ureter), dilated renal pelvis (P); B-mode image.

b Postoperative ureteral stricture (U, arrows): indistinct ureter in a hypoechoic scarred area. AI, VI = iliac artery and vein.

c Ureterocele (UZ) with an obstructed ureter (U).

▶ Ureteral tumor obstruction

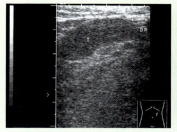
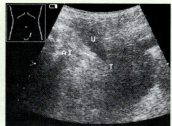
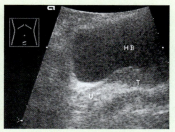

d Ureteral tumor (urothelial carcinoma, T): hypoechoic oval mass with smooth margins; indwelling drain (arrows, DR).

e Locoregional metastasis of ovarian carcinoma (T): cutoff of the obstructed ureter (U) at the level where it crosses the iliac vessels (AI).

f Metastatic prostate cancer (T) indenting the bladder (HB) and obstructing the ureter (U).

▶ Ureteral stone obstruction

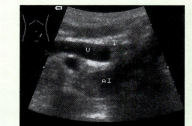
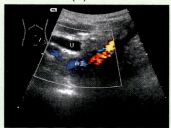
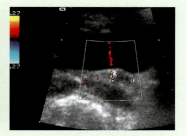

g B mode image: obstruction caused by a hypoechoic mass (arrow)

h Color doppler image: no vascularity, lack of a twinkling artifact (which mostly can be detected in renal stones. U = ureter, AI = iliac artery

i Stone obstruction of the ureteral orifice. Distinctive twinkling artifact. Ureteral jet. U = ureter.

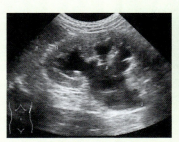
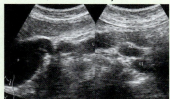
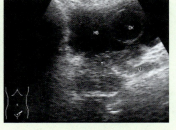

j–j Grade II urinary stasis caused by a bladder tumor.

k Ureteropelvic junction. Ureteral tortuosity over the iliac artery and vein (AI, VI). P = pelvis; U = ureter; HB = bladder.

l Invasion of the ureter (U) by a bladder tumor (T). HB = bladder; DK = catheter balloon.

▶ Reflux

Vesicoureteral and vesicorenal reflux also lead to dilatation of the ureter and renal pelvis. A distinction is drawn between primary congenital forms of reflux and secondary acquired forms.

Primary forms. Primary forms of reflux (ureterovesical junction obstruction, i.e., refluxing megaureter) are based on developmental abnormalities of the terminal ureter. These may consist of abnormal orifices, ectopic insertions, or an abnormal course of the ureter in the bladder wall. The results are partial or complete dilatation of the ureter and renal pelvis, with risk for developing progressive renal failure. Besides showing initial suggestive signs, ultrasound can furnish information on the degree of urinary obstruction. The detection of reflux is the domain of the excretory urogram and voiding cystogram. While color Doppler can demonstrate the presence of a ureteral jet, Doppler ultrasound has not yet established itself as a standard study[4].

Secondary forms. Secondary forms of vesicorenal reflux are caused by inflammatory or postoperative changes in the bladder floor or by mechanical or functional infravesical obstructions (**Fig. 11.29 and Fig. 11.53**).

The following classification system was devised by the International Reflux Study Group (1985), as quoted in Riedmiller and Köhl[9].

Classification of Reflux

- **Grade I:** Reflux causes variable dilatation of the ureter, does not reach the renal pelvis.
- **Grade II:** Reflux reaches the renal pelvis, causes no dilatation of the collecting system; the fornices remain sharp.
- **Grade III:** Mild or moderate dilatation of the ureter with or without kinking and/or mild or moderate dilatation of the collecting system; the fornices are blunted.
- **Grade IV:** Moderate dilatation of the ureter with or without kinking, moderate dilatation of the collecting system; the fornices are blunted; papillary impression is still visible.
- **Grade V:** Severe dilatation of the ureter with kinking; massive dilatation of the collecting system; papillary impression of the calices is no longer visible.

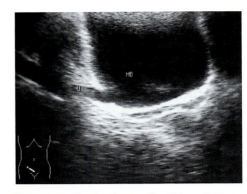

▲ **Fig. 11.29** Chronic primary reflux with grade III ureteral dilatation and chronic urinary stasis; ectopic ureteral insertion.

Hypoechoic

Urinary Tract
- Malformations
- ▼ Dilated Renal Pelvis and Ureter
  - Anechoic
  - **Hypoechoic**
- Renal Pelvic Mass, Ureteral Mass
- Changes in Bladder Size or Shape
- Intracavitary Mass
- Wall Changes

- Hemorrhage (Traumatic, Clot)
- Infected Obstruction
- Suppurative Pyelitis
- Pyonephrosis
- Hypoechoic Transformation of the Central Renal Sinus Echogenicity

▶ Hemorrhage (Traumatic, Clot)

Traumatic or postprocedure hemorrhages in the kidney appear as hypoechoic masses in the renal pelvis and ureter or may produce the features of fluid-related pyelectasis. The cause in most cases can be determined clinically (**Fig. 11.30**). Fresh hemorrhages are echogenic and show nondirectional flow with turbulent zones at color Doppler.

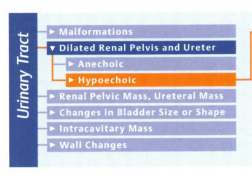

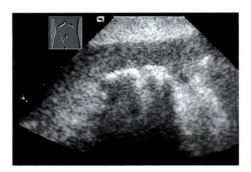

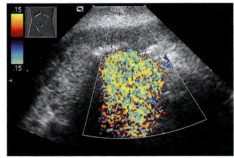

▲ **Fig. 11.30** Bleeding in the renal pelvis following the percutaneous puncture of a transplanted kidney; here, persistent echogenic bleeding.
a B-mode image shows high-level echoes with associated shadows.

▲ *b* Color duplex confirms the hemorrhage by showing the confetti-like artifact, indicating significant turbulence.

▶ Infected Obstruction

If a patient with renal stone colic becomes febrile, an infected obstruction should be suspected. Urinalysis will show signs of a urinary tract infection. Not every infected obstruction is preceded by stone colic, but an obstructive, septic urinary tract infection should be considered in patients who present with unexplained fever. This is especially likely in older patients with impaired host resistance and in poorly controlled diabetics.

Ultrasound often shows only a hypoechoic or largely anechoic dilatation of the pyelocaliceal system. A stone is frequently but not always detectable. If the obstruction can be visualized, it may appear as a hyperechoic mass in the renal pelvis (staghorn calculus), in the ureter (ureteral stone), or at the vesical or infravesical level (tumor, reflux, or prostatic hyperplasia, which is bilateral). For this reason, the sonographic investigation of fever should always include a detailed inspection of the kidneys, ureters, and bladder (**Figs. 11.31–11.33 and Fig. 11.16**).

Even if a stone is not detected and there is no ureteral dilatation, the mere suspicion of an infected obstruction warrants intervention in order to prevent urosepsis.

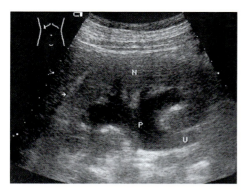

▲ **Fig. 11.31** Infected obstruction in association with a prevesical stone; septic temperatures.
a Grade I urinary stasis. The renal pelvis (P) and ureter (U) are not entirely anechoic. N = kidney.

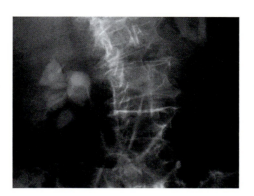

▲ **b** Prevesical obstructing stone (arrow, acoustic shadow S). HB = bladder.

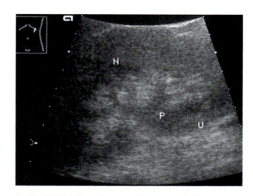

▲ **Fig. 11.32** Infected obstruction: anechoic to hypoechoic, poorly marginated dilatation of the pyelocaliceal system (P) and ureter (U). N = kidney.

◂◂ **Fig. 11.33** Infected obstruction in association with subpelvic ureteral stenosis.
a Hypoechoic, obstructed pelvis with sonographically indistinct margins.

◂ **b** Radiograph: ureteropelvic junction obstruction?, probably due to an aberrant vessel.

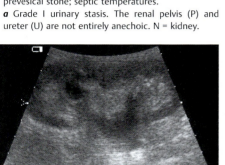

▶ Suppurative Pyelitis

Suppurative pyelitis is a pyelonephritis that has developed by the ascending route and predominantly affects the renal pelvis. Obstruction may be present or absent. Unlike pyelonephritis that arises by the hematogenous route, the findings are concentrated in the renal pelvis and consist of an anechoic mass that is clearly definable with ultrasound. Suppurative pyelitis may result from an obstruction to urine outflow such as a congenital malformation, prostatic hyperplasia, or urolithiasis, or there may be factors predisposing to infection such as diabetes mellitus, a ureteral stent, or a urinary catheter.

The sonographic signs of suppurative pyelitis range from the features of an anechoic obstruction or a dilated renal pelvis with internal echoes to circumscribed round, oval, or bandlike hypoechoic or anechoic masses. Inflammatory swelling of the renal pelvic walls over 2 mm[1a], which appear as smooth, thin, hypoechoic bands, is virtually pathognomonic of this condition (◧ **11.3, Fig. 11.1**).

▶ Pyonephrosis

An infected hydronephrosis leads to pyonephrosis. The sonographic findings are difficult to interpret because the familiar parenchymal-sinus echo pattern is absent and the normal renal shape and structure are markedly changed, which can easily lead to misinterpretation. Pyonephrosis appears as a patchy heterogeneous, tumorlike mass with a rounded or elliptical shape.

The images in ◧ **11.3** illustrate the typical sonographic features of pyelitis, pyonephrosis, and renal pelvic abscesses.

◧ 11.3 Suppurative Inflammations of the Renal Pelvis

▶ **Suppurative pyelitis**

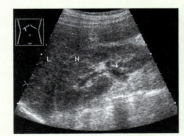 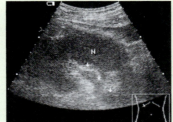 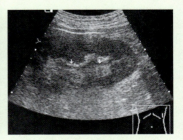

a Suppurative pyelitis. Slightly shifted scan plane shows a hypoechoic ureter with absence of central echoes (arrow). The hypoechoic "tram tracks" could represent the swollen ureteral wall. L = liver; N = kidney.

b and c Bilateral suppurative pyelitis in a young diabetic man with septic temperatures.
b Right kidney: hypoechoic bandlike mass in the renal pelvis/ureteropelvic junction (arrows). N = kidney.

c Left kidney: hypoechoic separation of the central renal sinus echogenicity due to purulent fluid in the renal pelvis and calices (arrows).

11.3 Suppurative Inflammations of the Renal Pelvis

▶ **Renal pelvic abscesses**

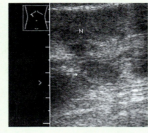 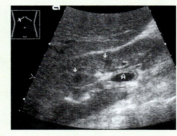 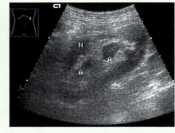

d Renal pelvic abscess (arrow) before treatment: elliptical hypoechoic mass (■ 11.3e).

e B-mode image: elliptical anechoic mass (A) with a fine, hypoechoic pelvic wall that shows inflammatory swelling.

f Pyelitis with abscessation: two hypoechoic masses in the renal pelvis (A). N = kidney.

▶ **Pyonephrosis**

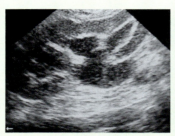 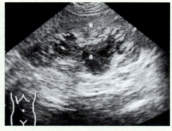 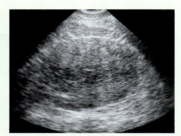

g Pyonephrosis: extensive hypoechoic, nonhomogeneous mass in the pyelocalyceal system.

h Pyonephrosis: hypoechoic abscesses with irregular margins (A) in suppurative pyelitis of the kidney (N).

i Pyonephrosis (surgery): left flank scan demonstrates an irregular mass. The kidney can no longer be identified because the entire pyelocalyceal system has acquired a solid texture due to suppuration.

Renal Pelvic Mass, Ureteral Mass

Hypoechoic

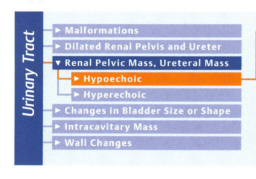

- Pyonephrosis, Renal Pelvic Abscess
- Urothelial Carcinoma
- Ureteral Clots

The differential diagnosis of hypoechoic changes in the renal sinus complex centers on the differentiation of urothelial carcinoma (see below) from other hypoechoic masses such as suppurative pyelitis, an infected obstruction, renal cell carcinoma invading the renal pelvis, atypical renal parenchymal bands, parapelvic cysts, and sinus lipomatosis. The differential diagnosis is aided by color Doppler examination, which frequently shows internal vascularity in tumors but not in abscesses, sinus lipomatosis, or cysts (see ■ **9.5, p. 305**).

▶ Urothelial Carcinoma

Classification. The majority of urinary tract tumors are urothelial carcinomas. They arise as malignant tumors from the transitional epithelium (urothelium) and therefore occur in the renal pelvis, ureter, and bladder. The following tumor types are named in the 1998 WHO classification of epithelial renal pelvic tumors[8]:

- Benign papilloma
- Malignant carcinoma
  - Transitional cell carcinoma
  - Squamous cell carcinoma
  - Adenocarcinoma
  - Medullary renal carcinoma
  - Undifferentiated carcinoma
  - Carcinosarcoma

Actual urothelial carcinomas—transitional cell carcinomas—are less common than renal cell carcinomas. They occur grossly in papillary or solid forms.

Ultrasound. The ultrasound appearance varies with tumor location. Tumors in the renal pelvis usually assume the shape of the pyelocaliceal system and may extend into the upper ureter as well as the renal parenchyma. They are somewhat more reflective than the renal parenchyma, but they may also be less echogenic. A long-standing tumor may contain foci of liquefaction, giving it a cystic or abscesslike appearance.

The differential diagnosis includes metastases, hemorrhagic cysts in the renal sinus, and extension of renal cell carcinoma into the renal pelvis (**Figs. 11.34–11.37**; ▣ **11.2d**), see also Chapter 9, p. 304).

Urothelial carcinoma in the ureter appears as a hypoechoic mass with associated obstruction to urine outflow (▣ **11.2d**).

▲ **Fig. 11.34** Urothelial carcinoma (T) (surgery): hypoechoic mass in the pyelocaliceal system with extension into the ureter, indistinguishable from suppurative pyelitis or pyonephrosis in the B-mode image. (Color Doppler can help by demonstrating intratumoral vascularity.)

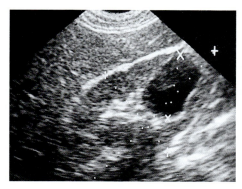

▲ **Fig. 11.35** Urothelial carcinoma (surgery): one hypoechoic and one largely anechoic mass in the renal pelvis of the right kidney (cursors). The echo-free mass (cursors) represents an area of tumor liquefaction.

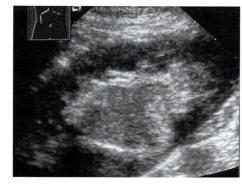

▲ **Fig. 11.36** Renal cell carcinoma located in the central echo complex: rounded, hypoechoic mass in the kidney (Dr. R.-D. Hanrath, Hagen, Germany).

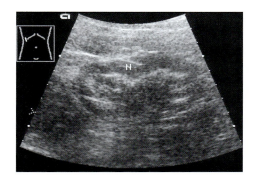

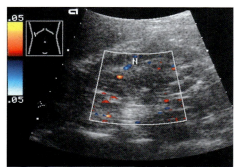

◂◂ **Fig. 11.37** Sinus lipomatosis, the main lesion requiring differentiation from urothelial carcinoma of the renal pelvis.
a B-mode image: hypoechoic streaks in the sinus echo complex of the kidney (N). Sinus lipomatosis or urothelial carcinoma?

◂ **b** Color Doppler: absence of vascularity in the hypoechoic mass is more consistent with sinus lipomatosis.

▶ **Ureteral Clots**

Ureteral clots appear as hypoechoic or heterogeneous tumorlike masses in the ureters with associated obstruction to urine outflow. They may occur in the setting of a generalized hemorrhagic diathesis, after surgical procedures, or in association with a renal tumor or urolithiasis. They are difficult or impossible to distinguish from primary tumors by ultrasound. The correct diagnosis is usually made from the history, the clinical course, or endoscopic inspection (**Fig. 11.38**).

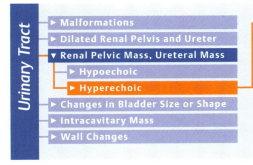

◂ **Fig. 11.38** Ureteral clot, caused by renal cell carcinoma bleeding into the ureter. Patient presented clinically with renal colic. Hypoechoic mass in the prevesical ureter (U). Arrows = echogenic ureteral ridge; HB = urinary bladder; SB = seminal vesicles.

Hyperechoic

Urinary Tract	
▶ Malformations	
▶ Dilated Renal Pelvis and Ureter	
▼ Renal Pelvic Mass, Ureteral Mass	
▶ Hypoechoic	
▶ **Hyperechoic**	▶ **Caliceal Stones** ▶ **Renal Pelvic Stone** ▶ **Staghorn Calculus** ▶ **Ureteral Stone**
▶ Changes in Bladder Size or Shape	
▶ Intracavitary Mass	
▶ Wall Changes	

Urolithiasis. Urolithiasis can have many causes: primary or secondary hyperuricemia (tumor chemotherapy!), hypercalcemia, malassimilation syndromes, inflammatory bowel diseases with increased oxalic acid absorption, and inflammatory or neoplastic renal pelvic diseases. Less frequent causes are congenital or acquired metabolic disorders such as renal acidosis or a disturbance of cystine metabolism. Often, however, lithiasis results from the crystallization of salts dissolved in the urine, with no identifiable cause. Since crystals require a relatively calm precipitation medium in order to grow, they tend to form at sites where a high salt concentration is combined with fluid stasis and a favorable pH. Stones most commonly form in the renal pelvis and bladder, therefore.

Sonographic criteria. Regardless of the stone composition—urate or cystine/xanthine stones, calcium oxalate/calcium phosphate stones, or infection stones (struvite/carbonate apatite)—ultrasound shows an intensely echogenic focus with distal acoustic shadowing. Because a stone surface echo is very difficult to discern within the high-level echoes of the renal sinus complex, the presence of an acoustic shadow is important in confirming the diagnosis of urolithiasis. Not every echo, even when associated with partial shadowing, represents a stone. It must also be consistently definable in multiple planes of section.

▶ Caliceal Stones

A renal caliceal stone is characterized by a stone echo with an acoustic shadow and by caliectasis, which occurs proximal to the site of the stone. Concomitant ectasia of the caliceal neck suggests a calculus located distal to the infundibulum, whereas a caliceal stone echo not associated with caliectasis is difficult or impossible to distinguish from papillary calcification. The history and clinical presentation in these cases will suggest the correct diagnosis (**Figs. 11.39–11.41**).

▲ *Fig. 11.39* Lower caliceal stone with caliectasis (arrow; acoustic shadow S). Scan shows a high-amplitude, hood-shaped echo below a circumscribed anechoic area.

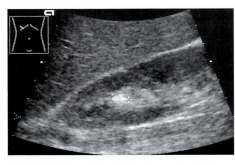

▲ *Fig. 11.40* Upper caliceal stone (cursors), similar appearance as in **Fig. 11.39**, but without caliectasis two days after renal colic. The initial obstruction has subsided due to partial outflow.

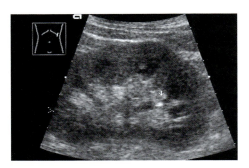

▲ *Fig. 11.41* Stone in a lower caliceal neck (arrow) with another, more distal outflow obstruction, causing very clear delineation of the caliceal stone in the fluid milieu of the pyelocaliceal system. (Without an acoustic shadow, ordinarily it would not be possible to distinguish the stone within the central echo complex.)

▶ Renal Pelvic Stone

Renal pelvic stones, like caliceal stones, may be solitary or multiple. They have the same ultrasound appearance as caliceal stones but lack the typical isolated caliectasis that occurs with the latter. They may also be obstructive for one or more caliceal groups (**Fig. 11.42**).

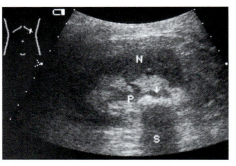

▲ *Fig. 11.42* Renal pelvic stone (arrow; acoustic shadow S).
a Here a mild obstruction of the renal pelvis (P) delineates the stone in the left kidney (N).

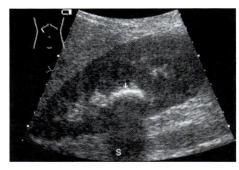

▲ *b* High-amplitude echo from a nonobstructive stone.

▶ Staghorn Calculus

Because a staghorn calculus is associated with a broad linear echo or an irregular echogenic zone, it is easily missed when nonobstructive and may be mistaken for a bright central sinus echo. Depending on the scan plane, ultrasound may show a broad echo with a single broad associated shadow, or a scan in the caliceal plane may show multiple echogenic foci that cast separate shadows (**Figs. 11.43–11.47**).

The differential diagnosis of hyperechoic masses in the renal sinus echo complex is reviewed in **Table 11.2**.

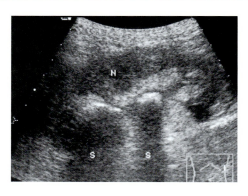

◀ *Fig. 11.43* Renal pelvic stone (partial staghorn calculus) with local obstruction of the middle and lower caliceal groups: broad hyperechoic zones with acoustic shadows (S) in the midpelvic region of the left kidney (N).

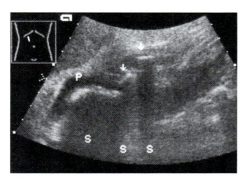 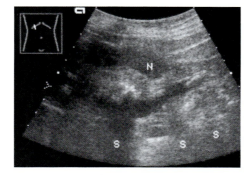 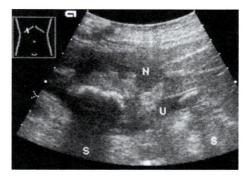

▲ **Fig. 11.44** Partial staghorn calculus, ureteropelvic junction stone. N = kidney.
a Hyperechoic calculi in the upper and middle pyelocaliceal system (P, arrows, acoustic shadows S).

▲ **b** Calcification with an acoustic shadow (S) in the mid- to lower renal pelvis.

▲ **c** Shadowing stone in the lower renal pelvis and a ureteral stone (U; acoustic shadows S).

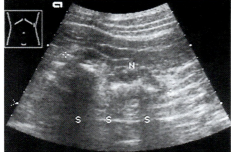 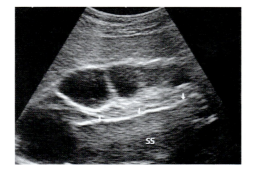

◄◄ **Fig. 11.45** Staghorn calculus: multiple high-level stone echoes with acoustic shadows (S) throughout the pyelocaliceal system. Depending on the scan plane, ultrasound may demonstrate multiple isolated stone echoes as shown here or a broad linear echo (**Fig. 11.46**). N = kidney.

◄ **Fig. 11.46** Staghorn calculus with massive caliectasis and a bright linear echo (arrows) with an acoustic shadow (SS). Massive, anechoic caliectasis with severe chronic renal congestion and parenchymal loss.

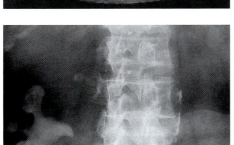

▲ **Fig. 11.47** Radiographic view of a staghorn calculus (compare with **Fig. 11.46**).

Table 11.2 Differential diagnosis of echogenic masses in the sinus echo complex

- Kidney stone (**Fig. 11.39**)
- Vascular calcification (**Fig. 9.87, p. 311**)
- Papillary calcification (**Fig. 9.86, p. 311**)
- Nephrocalcinosis (**Fig. 9.91, p. 312**)
- Tumor calcification (**Fig. 9.71, p. 304**)
- Gas-forming abscess (**Fig. 9.89, p. 312**)
- Medullary sponge kidney
- Inflammatory calcification (**Figs. 9.92, 9.93, p. 313**)
- Posttraumatic calcification

► Ureteral Stone

The most frequent cause of renal colic is a ureteral stone. Calculi tend to become impacted at sites of physiological narrowing: the ureteropelvic junction, the point where the ureter crosses the iliac vessels, and the ureterovesical junction ureter. Of these sites, the latter is the most common.

The landmark for locating the stone at ultrasound is the dilated ureter. An intravenous urogram can usually be omitted, also because of the potential for contrast-induced diuresis with risk of fornix rupture and perirenal urinoma formation (**Fig. 11.48**). **Figures 11.49–11.52** illustrate some typical locations of ureteral stones.

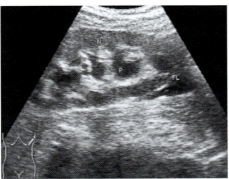

▲ **Fig. 11.48** Urinoma: perirenal echo-free fluid crescent (FL) with a dilated, congested renal pelvis (P). N = kidney.

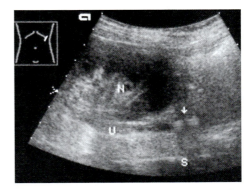

▲ **Fig. 11.49** Two high ureteral stones: hyperechoic foci in the dilated ureter (U), mild pyelectasis in the left kidney (N). S = shadowing.

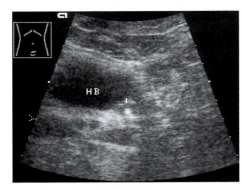
▲ **Fig. 11.50** Prevesical ureteral stone (arrow), proximal to the ureteral insertion into the bladder (HB). No ureteral obstruction.

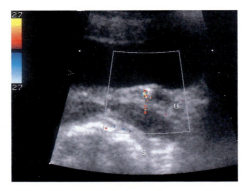
▲ **Fig. 11.51** Hyperechoic prevesical stone in the ureteral orifice (U). Color Doppler: twinkling artifact in the acoustic shadow. This artifact is over 90% sensitive in the detection of calcium stones.

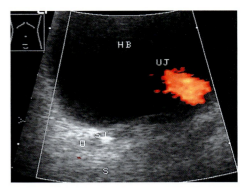
▲ **Fig. 11.52** Prevesical stone in the right ureter (ST, partial acoustic shadow S), color Doppler view: no ureteral jet on the right side with fluid diuresis, but a conspicuous color-flow jet (UJ) is visible on the left side. HB = bladder.

Changes in Bladder Size or Shape

Large Bladder

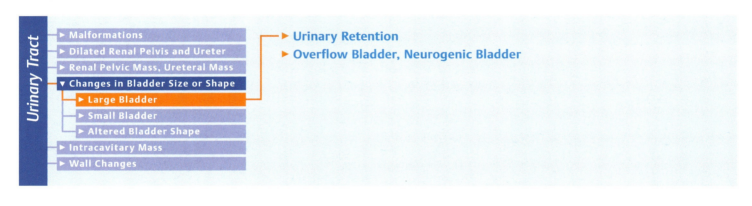

▶ Urinary Retention

Urinary retention refers to an inability to empty the bladder. All gradations can occur from mildly impaired outflow with or without residual urine to total retention. The causes are diverse and include functional and neurogenic causes (detrusor paralysis, as in Parkinson disease) as well as morphological changes (stones, tumors, foreign bodies, infravesical obstructions). Most causes can be detected and identified at ultrasound (**Table 11.3**). Idiopathic urinary retention is rare.

Volume estimation. Ultrasound in urinary retention demonstrates an overdistended bladder. The degree of enlargement can be measured by estimating the bladder volume. Normally a bladder volume of 350–450 ml triggers the urge to urinate. The maximum anatomical bladder capacity is 400–600 ml, and pathological bladder volumes may reach 2 liters or more. The sonographic estimation of bladder volume and residual urine is simple: take the product of the largest longitudinal, transverse, and anteroposterior diameters and divide by 2 (the formula for a rotational ellipsoid). The range of error is relatively large (small volumes are overestimated, large volumes are underestimated), but the formula is quite satisfactory for clinical purposes (**Figs. 11.53 and 11.54**).

Misinterpretation may be caused by paravesical anechoic masses such as ovarian cysts and loculated ascites (**Fig. 11.55**).

Table 11.3 Vesical and infravesical causes of urinary retention

Vesical causes
- ▶ Neurogenic bladder dysfunction
- ▶ Bladder neck stones
- ▶ Bladder tumors

Infravesical causes
- ▶ Prostatic hyperplasia
- ▶ Prostatic carcinoma
- ▶ Foreign bodies
- ▶ Phimosis

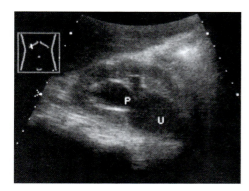
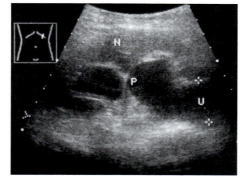
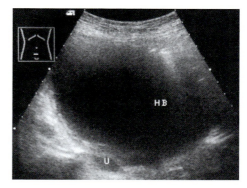

▲ **Fig. 11.53** Maximal bladder distension behind a clogged urethral catheter, with secondary reflux into the ureter (U) and renal pelvis (P). N = kidney; HB = bladder.

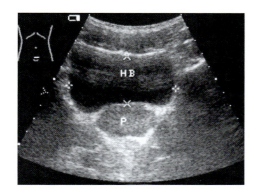
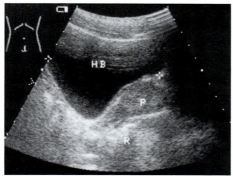
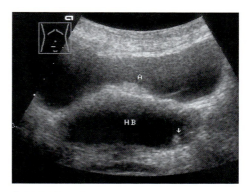

▲ **Fig. 11.54** Measurement of bladder volume in a full bladder (HB).
a Lower abdominal transverse scan: width × depth (cursors).

▲ **b** Lower abdominal longitudinal scan: greatest length (cursors). P = normal prostate; R = rectum.

▲ **Fig. 11.55** Ascites in the lower abdomen (A) assuming the shape of the bladder. The actual bladder (HB) can be positively identified as such only by scanning it after voiding and when distended (if necessary, by retrograde filling). A small papillomatous bladder tumor is noted as an incidental finding (arrow).

▶ ### Overflow Bladder, Neurogenic Bladder

Overflow bladder and neurogenic bladder are types of urine storage disorders. Their clinical hallmarks are pollakiuria, nycturia, and incontinence. Neurogenic bladder is diagnosed by exclusion and is classified on the basis of clinical findings.

The ultrasound appearance corresponds to that of urinary retention (**Fig. 11.56**).

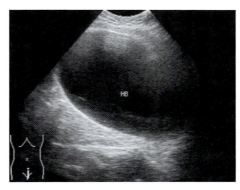

◀ **Fig. 11.56** Urinary retention with a maximally distended bladder (HB): neurogenic bladder dysfunction in a patient receiving chemotherapy for chronic lymphatic leukemia.

Small Bladder

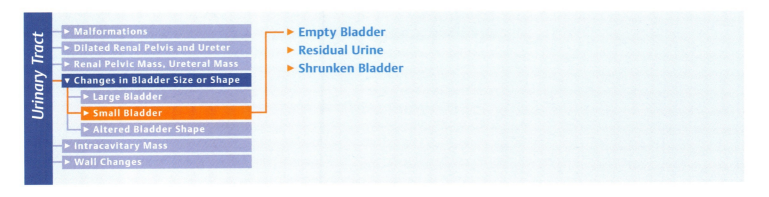

▶ Empty Bladder

When the bladder is in an empty or almost empty state, its roof sags, giving it a bowl-shaped appearance at ultrasound. Asking the patient when he or she last voided can explain a "small bladder" in doubtful cases and exclude inflammatory shrinkage (**Figs. 11.57 and 11.58**).

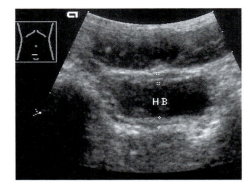

▲ **Fig. 11.57** Almost empty bladder (HB) in a lower abdominal transverse scan. Here the bladder wall appears thickened (5 mm between cursors).

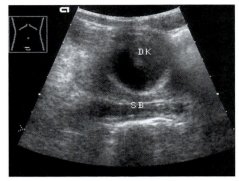

▲ **Fig. 11.58** Completely empty bladder. A lumen is no longer visualized. The bladder location is indicated by an indwelling balloon catheter (DK). SB = seminal vesicle.

▶ Residual Urine

The presence of residual urine, which can be misinterpreted as a small bladder, is demonstrated by imaging the bladder in the distended state and immediately after voiding. The volume formula is used to calculate volume (**Fig. 11.59**). Normally no residual urine is found. Small amounts less than 15 ml are not clinically significant in older adults.

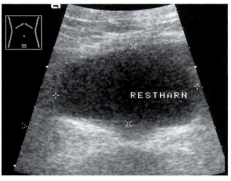

▲ **Fig. 11.59 a** Residual urine (Restharn) after complete voiding, in this case 68.6 ml. Lower abdominal transverse scan to determine the transverse and anteroposterior diameters.

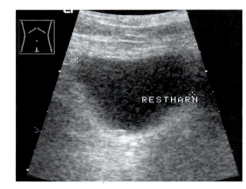

▲ **b** Lower abdominal longitudinal scan to determine the craniocaudal diameter.

▶ Shrunken Bladder

Unlike a partially emptied bladder, a shrunken bladder exhibits shape and wall changes in addition to a small size. The causes are chronic inflammatory disorders such as urinary tuberculosis and radiocystitis. The inflammatory bladder changes in urinary tuberculosis start around the ureteral orifices and then spread deep into the bladder wall, causing induration of the wall muscles and a diminished bladder capacity (**Fig. 11.60**).

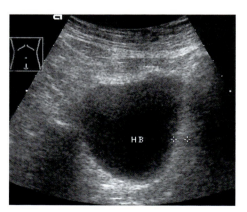

▲ **Fig. 11.60** Shrunken bladder.
a After urinary tuberculosis. HB = bladder. Maximum bladder capacity is 153 ml, residual urine volume is 43 ml. Thickened wall (cursors).

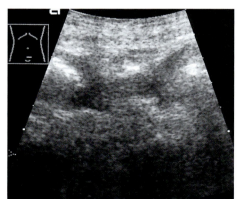

▲ **b** Neurogenic shrunken bladder with reflux. Maximum bladder capacity is 60 ml.

Altered Bladder Shape

- Malformations
- Dilated Renal Pelvis and Ureter
- Renal Pelvic Mass, Ureteral Mass
- Changes in Bladder Size or Shape
  - Large Bladder
  - Small Bladder
  - Altered Bladder Shape
- Intracavitary Mass
- Wall Changes

▶ Partially Contracted Bladder
▶ Diverticulum, Pseudodiverticulum
▶ Indented Bladder, Operated Bladder

▶ Partially Contracted Bladder

The bladder roof sags during micturition, creating a bowl-shaped lumen with tapered lateral extensions that may be mistaken for diverticula.

An almost empty bladder has a variable ultrasound appearance: crescent-shaped, rounded, or oval. The contracted muscles give the wall an irregular border and increase its thickness to as much as 6–8 mm. A wall thickness greater than 10 mm is definitely abnormal (**Fig. 11.61, Fig. 11.57**).

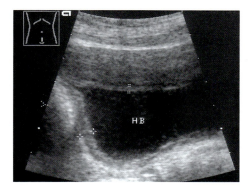

◀ **Fig. 11.61** Partially contracted bladder (HB) with apparent wall thickening due to the contracted muscles (cursors). The three-part wall structure is clearly visualized.

▶ Diverticulum, Pseudodiverticulum

Multiple pseudodiverticula resulting from a subvesical obstruction (benign prostatic hyperplasia) or large diverticula without a distinct neck can impart a bizarre shape to the bladder that is difficult to recognize sonographically as having a diverticular cause. The correct diagnosis can usually be made, however, by examining the bladder in a partially full or partially empty state or by imaging the bladder in different planes (**Figs. 11.62 and 11.63**).

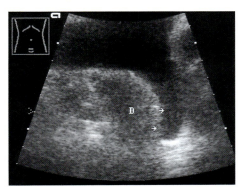

▲ **Fig. 11.62** Bladder diverticulum in a partially filled bladder. With additional distension a hypoechoic saccular mass appears, representing a large, partially filled diverticulum (D). The extension (arrows) corresponds to the elongated neck of the diverticulum.

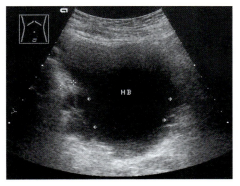

▲ **Fig. 11.63 a** Multiple pseudodiverticula (arrows) with wall hypertrophy (cursors). The protrusion of the diverticula through gaps in the bladder wall can be seen. HB = bladder.

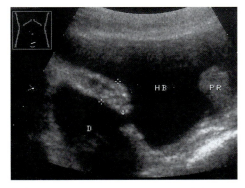

▲ **b** Large pseudodiverticulum (D), neck of diverticulum (arrow), and wall hypertrophy (12.8 mm) in benign protuberant prostatic hyperplasia (PR).

▶ Indented Bladder, Operated Bladder

Bladder shape can also be altered by extrinsic indentation from a tumor, an enlarged uterus, colonic gas, or adherent bowel loops.

A special case is a bladder substitute that has been reconstructed from bowel. The ileal neo-bladder resembles a normal full bladder but is distinguished by its asymmetry and thin wall (**Figs. 11.64 and 11.65**).

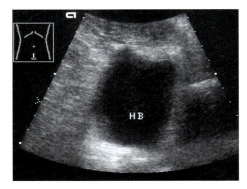

▲ *Fig. 11.64* Scarring and deformity of the bladder (HB) caused by old peritonitis following severe colitis and colostomy placement. Polygonal bladder shape with tapered extensions and ill-defined walls.

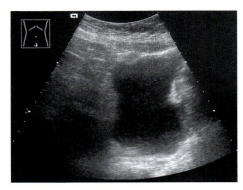

▲ *Fig. 11.65* Ileal bladder substitute following bladder tumor surgery. The substitute bladder has an irregular shape and no clearly defined wall (the ileal wall is not visualized in the standard 3.5-MHz scan).

Intracavitary Mass

Hypoechoic

- ▶ Malformations
- ▶ Dilated Renal Pelvis and Ureter
- ▶ Renal Pelvic Mass, Ureteral Mass
- ▶ Changes in Bladder Size or Shape
- ▼ Intracavitary Mass
  - ▶ Hypoechoic
  - ▶ Hyperechoic
  - ▶ Echogenic
- ▶ Wall Changes

- ▶ Blood Clots
- ▶ Bladder Sludge
- ▶ Bladder Papilloma
- ▶ Polypoid Bladder Carcinoma
- ▶ Mesenchymal Tumors

▶ Blood Clots

Blood clots in the bladder are usually iatrogenic following the construction of a suprapubic bladder fistula, but they can also result from inflammations, cytostatic therapy, coagulation disorders, and tumors. If they are mobile, the diagnosis is easily made. But clots adherent to the bladder wall require differentiation from polypoid tumors, which they resemble in their mixed hypoechoic–hyperechoic structure. This differentiation can be made by demonstrating their mobility and possible shape changes when the patient is repositioned or by instilling fluid into the bladder through an indwelling catheter (**Figs. 11.66 and 11.67**).

Bladder tamponade. Bladder tamponade is caused by extremely heavy clot formation, leading to severe compression pain and completely obstructing the outflow of urine. Generally it requires operative treatment. Sonographically, bladder tamponade appears as a tumorlike mass, usually slightly heterogeneous to hypoechoic, that completely occupies the bladder lumen. Residual anechoic urine is sometimes detectable (**Figs. 11.68 and 11.69**).

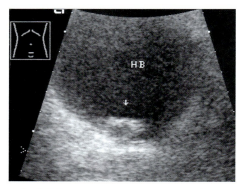

▲ *Fig. 11.66* Clotted blood in the bladder (HB), lower abdominal transverse scan.
 a Tumorlike echo texture (arrow).

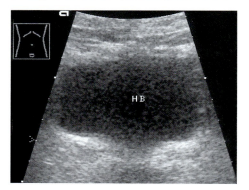

▲ *b* The mass is no longer seen after several position changes, proving that it is not a real tumor. Its position also changes on standing. Other ways to distinguish a clot from tumor are to repeat the scans with different degrees of bladder distention or rapidly fill the bladder through an indwelling catheter.

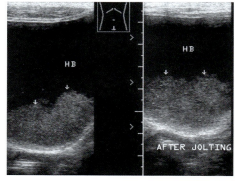

▲ *Fig. 11.67* Large polypoid blood clot (arrow), appearing as an echogenic mass on the bladder floor. The clot showed motion-dependent shape and position changes with transient swirling of clot particles. HB = bladder.

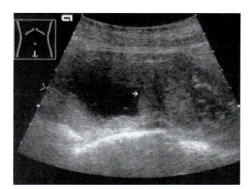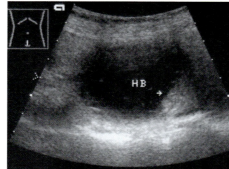

Fig. 11.68 Incomplete bladder tamponade.
a Bizarre, tumorlike hypoechoic mass (arrow) with a small amount of residual free urine.

b The clot moved after several position changes, excluding a tumor. HB = bladder.

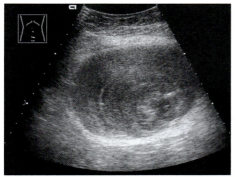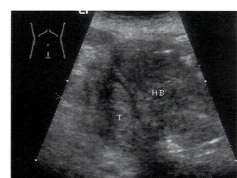

Fig. 11.69 a Bladder tamponade requiring surgery. The bladder is filled by hypoechoic clot with a nonhomogeneous structure.

b Differential diagnosis of bladder tamponade. The bladder (HB) has been invaded by sigmoid carcinoma (T), which completely fills the bladder lumen.

▶ Bladder Sludge

Sediment found in the bladder usually consists of urinary precipitates or pus. It presents a shifting or mobile sludge structure much like that seen in the gallbladder. The mobility of bladder sludge will generally distinguish it from flat, sessile bladder-wall tumors and areas of hypertrophic wall thickening (**Fig. 11.70**).

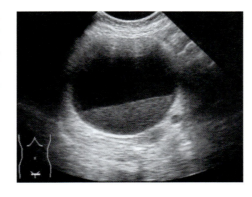

Fig. 11.70 Purulent bladder sediment in a patient with pyonephrosis.

▶ Bladder Papilloma

Most benign and malignant bladder tumors appear sonographically as exophytic intraluminal masses or as plaquelike lesions infiltrating the bladder wall. Benign bladder papilloma is an example of an exophytic tumor. Other than the loose correlation between tumor size and biological behavior, there are no sonographic criteria that can confidently distinguish a benign papilloma from papillary carcinoma. Detectable wall infiltration is suggestive of carcinoma, however. This requires differentiation from an adenoma of the prostatic median lobe protruding into the bladder (**Figs. 11.71–11.73 and Fig. 11.55**).

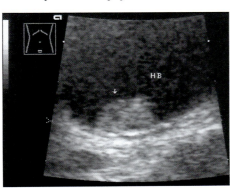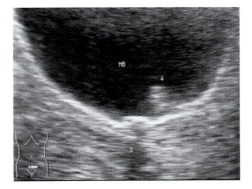

Fig. 11.71 Polypoid bladder tumor (papillary tumor by cystoscopy, urothelial carcinoma by histology): lobulated hypoechoic mass (arrow) on the bladder floor. Detected incidentally in a 46-year-old man. HB = bladder.

Fig. 11.72 Bladder papilloma (arrow): lobulated, narrow polypoid mass occupying a constant position in the bladder. Next to it is a hyperechoic mass with an acoustic shadow (S): bladder stone. HB = bladder.

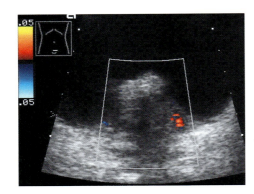
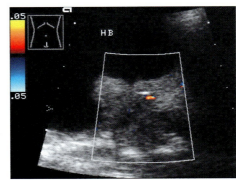

◀◀ **Fig. 11.73** Median-lobe adenoma (benign prostatic hyperplasia), color Doppler.
a Polypoid mass extending into the bladder lumen. Apparent wall infiltration, scant peripheral vascularity.

◀ **b** Longitudinal scan angled slightly downward shows that the tumor is connected to the median lobe of the prostate. HB = bladder.

▶ Polypoid Bladder Carcinoma

Most benign and malignant bladder tumors arise from the transitional epithelium (urothelium). Other tumor types include squamous cell carcinomas (often associated with schistosomiasis), adenocarcinomas, and mesenchymal tumors (rhabdomyosarcoma, seen mainly in children). The UICC staging system is shown in **Fig. 11.98**. The most common malignant bladder tumor is urothelial carcinoma. Morphologically, approximately 70% of malignant bladder tumors display a papillary, almost villous type of growth. A small percentage are solid or nodular. Bladder carcinomas metastasize chiefly to the regional lymph nodes along the iliac vessels. They can also seed hematogenously to the liver, lung, and bone marrow.

Bladder carcinomas may become ulcerated, and therefore typical complaints such as urgency are usually accompanied by hematuria.

Sonographic features. Polypoid bladder carcinoma is easily detected sonographically in a well-distended bladder when the lesion is larger than 5 mm. Exceptions are tumors located on the floor or roof of the bladder. Ultrasound demonstrates a nonhomogeneous internal echo pattern with smooth or lobulated, often hyperechoic, margins **(Figs. 11.74 and 11.75)**. Some tumors are pedunculated and exhibit a cauliflower-like structure. An intensely echogenic "hood" suggests a fibrous or partially calcified tumor surface, which reportedly is more characteristic of squamous cell carcinoma[2]. The sonographic staging[5] of a presumed or detected bladder carcinoma requires evaluating the deeper wall structures.

Sensitivity of ultrasound. Ultrasound has only about a 50% sensitivity in the diagnosis of bladder tumors[7]. This results from the low detection rate of small tumors and precancerous lesions confined to the mucosa, tumors located on the bladder roof or anterior wall, and multiple tumors. Other lesions that usually escape sonographic detection are foci of simple or atypical hyperplasia, small urothelial papillomas, carcinoma in situ, plaquelike urothelial carcinomas, and small papillary carcinomas.

Differentiation from clot. It is difficult to distinguish bladder carcinoma from intravesical clots. The following criteria are helpful in this regard:
▶ A mass on the bladder roof on sidewalls is suggestive of neoplasia.
▶ Movement of the mass when the patient is repositioned suggests a clot (no movement is more consistent with a neoplasm).
▶ Swirling echoes and a change in shape and size on rapid filling of the bladder suggest a blood clot.
▶ Color Doppler examination: vascularity suggests a tumor, while lack of vascularity (low flow velocity) is more consistent with a clot.
▶ Wall infiltration positively identifies the mass as a tumor.
▶ Repeat scans should always be obtained to check the constancy of the finding!

A bladder tumor is rarely the result of invasion by prostatic carcinoma, because that tumor arises from the outer zone of the prostate and does not extend toward the bladder floor like a median-lobe adenoma **(Fig. 11.76)**.

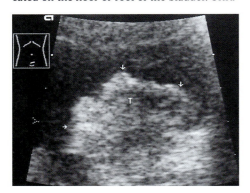
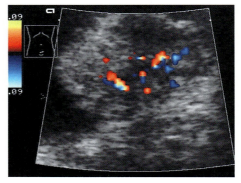
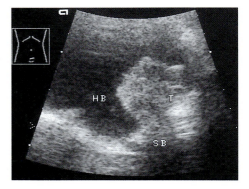

▲ **Fig. 11.74** Polypoid bladder tumor (T; papillary urothelial carcinoma).
a Intravesical mass with irregular margins (blooming effect causes the surface to appear more echogenic).

▲ **b** Irregular tumor vessels are detected, proving that the mass is not a clot.

▲ **c** Infiltration of the seminal vesicle (SB) is detected, indicating a stage T4a tumor by ultrasound **(see Fig. 11.98)**.

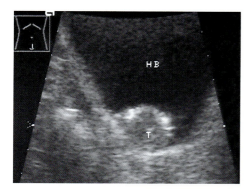

▲ **Fig. 11.75** Polypoid bladder tumor (T). Histology (after transurethral resection) indicated urothelial carcinoma without bladder wall infiltration (stage pTa).
a Hypoechoic tumor with an echogenic rim and no detectable bladder wall infiltration. HB = bladder.

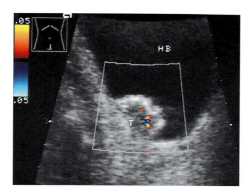

▲ **b** Color Doppler shows spotty vascularity.

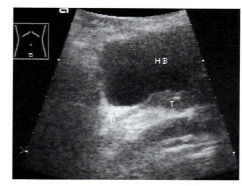

▲ **Fig. 11.76** Known local metastatic prostatic carcinoma, histologically confirmed. The tumor (T) has infiltrated the bladder floor and obstructed the ureter (U). The tumor regressed completely after combined hormonal and chemotherapy. HB = bladder.

▶ **Mesenchymal Tumors**

The rare mesenchymal tumors rhabdomyoma, rhabdomyosarcoma, and reticuloendothelial tumors are sonographically indistinguishable from urothelial carcinoma, and so the same ultrasound criteria are used for these tumors as for carcinoma.

Hyperechoic

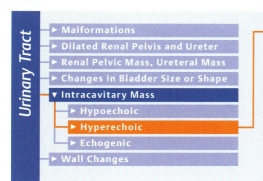

▶ **Urinary Catheter**

The most common hyperechoic mass seen in the bladder is a urinary balloon catheter. The catheter itself appears sonographically as bright parallel walls with a central anechoic fluid band. The balloon appears as a target figure with a hyperechoic wall and a bright central echo representing the catheter tip (**Figs. 11.77 and 11.78**).

Pigtail catheters and catheter fragments exhibit only a double wall with a central anechoic lumen (**Fig. 11.79**).

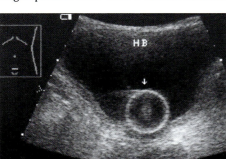

▲ **Fig. 11.77** Urinary catheter balloon (arrow): echogenic balloon wall surrounding a central high-level echo (catheter tip). HB = bladder.

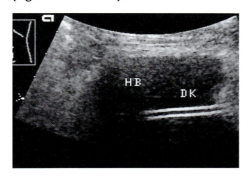

▲ **Fig. 11.78** Urinary catheter (DK) in a lower abdominal longitudinal scan: echogenic parallel walls with a central anechoic, fluid-filled lumen. HB = bladder.

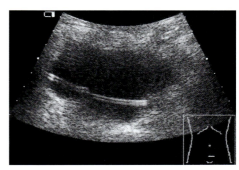

▲ **Fig. 11.79** Hyperechoic drain, placed to stent a ureter obstructed by urothelial carcinoma.

▶ Blood Clots

Clots with a hyperechoic or irregularly hyperechoic structure do occur but otherwise show the same sonographic features as the more hypoechoic-appearing forms (**Fig. 11.80**). Their diagnosis is described above.

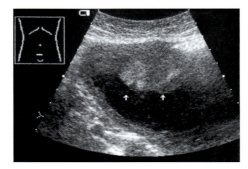
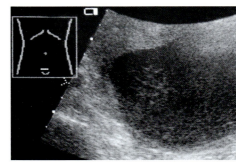

▲ **Fig. 11.80** Hyperechoic blood clots.
a Aggregate clot on the bladder roof (arrows).

▲ *b* After body movement, fragments of the clot appear as bright swirling echoes.

▶ Polypoid Bladder Tumor

Like blood clots, benign and malignant bladder tumors may appear hyperechoic owing to the blooming effect—an acoustic enhancement that occurs when sound travels through fluid spaces (**Fig. 11.81**). The true echogenicity of the mass can be appreciated by lowering the TGC (time gain compensation) setting. In other respects the tumors have the same features as the hypoechoic tumors mentioned above.

Some bladder tumors may show a high-amplitude entry echo (**Fig. 11.75**). Squamous cell carcinomas occasionally contain superficial calcifications[5].

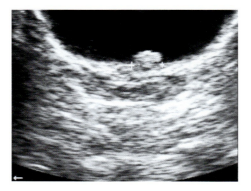

◀ **Fig. 11.81** Benign bladder papilloma (cursors), histologically confirmed. Typical location on the bladder floor near the ureteral orifices: hyperechoic lobulated mass. Here the echogenicity of the mass is enhanced due to a blooming effect.

▶ Benign Prostatic Hyperplasia

Benign prostatic hyperplasia (BPH) is a mass extrinsic to the bladder. BPH due to a median-lobe adenoma can mimic an exophytic tumor of the bladder floor. BPH may be very hypoechoic as well as hyperechoic, depending on its histology (see Chapter 12).

Unlike bladder carcinoma, BPH shows a visible connection with the prostate on dynamic ultrasound examination. It has a homogeneous echo structure, smooth margins, and a conical or globular shape (see Chapter 12) (**Fig. 11.82**).

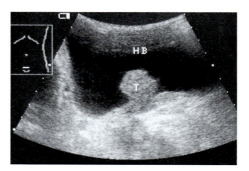
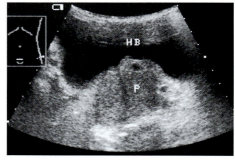

▲ **Fig. 11.82** Adenoma of the prostatic median lobe (benign hyperplasia) appears as a relatively echogenic mass protruding into the bladder (HB).
a Polypoid tumor mass (T) in the bladder.

▲ *b* Angling the scan demonstrates BPH, ruling out a primary bladder tumor. P = prostate.

▶ Lipoma, Fibroma, Myoma, Hemangioma

These somewhat rare benign tumors have smooth margins and high, homogeneous echogenicity. They cannot be reliably classified as benign or malignant by ultrasound.

▶ Ureterocele

A ureterocele, on the other hand, can be accurately diagnosed sonographically as an intraluminal mass. Its ultrasound appearance is unmistakable: a balloonlike structure with a thin echogenic wall and anechoic lumen, protruding into the bladder from the ureteral ridge. Stone formation is common in ureteroceles, however, and can produce high-level internal echoes with acoustic shadows. Only large ureteroceles are difficult to recognize as arising from the ureteral ridge, appearing as a thin, elliptical membrane within the bladder lumen (**Figs. 11.83 and 11.84**).

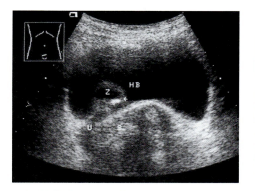

▲ **Fig. 11.83** Ureterocele (Z): anechoic urine and echogenic contents (stone, horizontal arrow, partial acoustic shadow S). The ureteral wall appears as a hyperechoic ring that has herniated into the bladder (HB). The ureter (U) is partially obstructed.

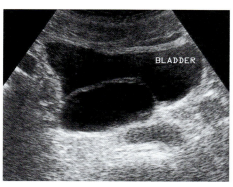

▲ **Fig. 11.84** Large right-sided ureterocele: hyperechoic elliptical membrane in the bladder lumen.
a Lower abdominal transverse scan.

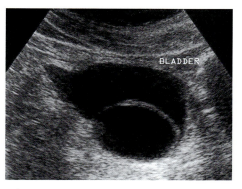

▲ *b* Lower abdominal longitudinal scan. (Dr. K. Ringewald, Hofgeismar, Germany)

▶ Artifacts

Hyperechoic bladder-wall indentations and motion-related or image artifacts can mimic true masses in the bladder.

Wall indentations. These often result from incomplete bladder distension (**Fig. 11.85a**).

Ureteral jet. A ureteral jet is a reflection caused by urine flowing into the bladder from the ureteral orifice. It appears as a hyperechoic cone that exhibits color-flow signals in color Doppler because of its motion (**Fig. 11.85b**).

Side-lobe artifact. A side-lobe artifact is caused by paravesical hyperechoic structures that are projected into the fluid medium owing to the physics of sound transmission from a convex transducer (**Fig. 11.86**).

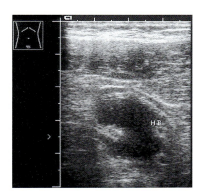

▲ **Fig. 11.85** Hyperechoic wall indentation in a partially filled bladder, with a ureteral jet.
a Slightly filled bladder (HB) with wall indentations mimicking an hourglass bladder.

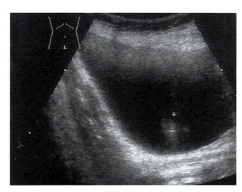

▲ *b* In color Doppler, a jet of urine entering the bladder produces a flare of color pixels, see **Fig. 11.89a**.

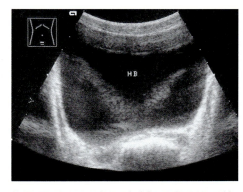

▲ **Fig. 11.86** Hyperechoic side-lobe artifacts caused by highly reflective structures located lateral to the bladder. HB = bladder.

Echogenic

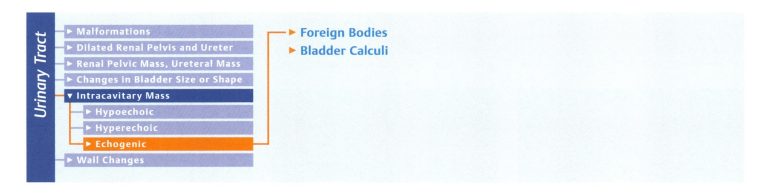

▶ Foreign Bodies

Foreign bodies such as pins, wires, or small tubes may be inserted into the urethra inadvertently during masturbation. Most foreign bodies found in the bladder are iatrogenic, however. At ultrasound they produce very high-level intraluminal echoes with acoustic shadowing (**Figs. 11.87, 11.92b**).

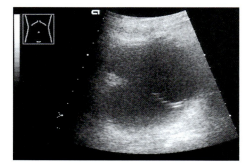

◀ **Fig. 11.87** Echogenic catheter fragment in a not entirely echo-free bladder caused by bleeding after catheter avulsion.

▶ Bladder Calculi

Stones in the bladder are common, but considerably less so than in the kidney or ureter. Uroliths that have passed through the ureter are occasionally still imaged in the bladder before entering the urethra. Otherwise, bladder calculi are found in association with incomplete bladder emptying, bladder diverticula, or a ureterocele. Their ultrasound appearance is like that of other stones: a high-level echo that casts an acoustic shadow and moves when the patient is repositioned.

Stones resting on the bladder floor may be missed if they are located in blind spots, but their mobility and acoustic shadows can confirm the diagnosis (**Figs. 11.88–11.90**).

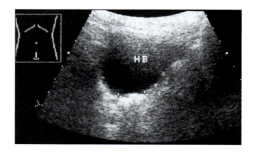

▲ **Fig. 11.88** Bladder stone: echogenic mass on the bladder floor (cursors) with partial acoustic shadowing. HB = bladder.

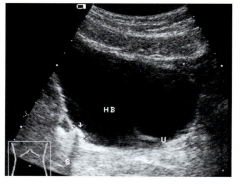

▲ **Fig. 11.89** Small bladder stone (arrow) with an acoustic shadow (S).
  a Transverse scan. HB = bladder; U = ureteral jet.

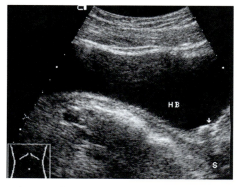

▲ **b** Longitudinal scan.

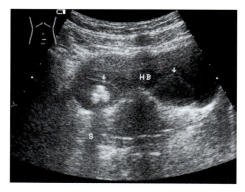

▲ **Fig. 11.90** Hyperechoic mass (left arrow, right ureteral orifice) with an acoustic shadow (S), representing a ureterocele with a stone. A second ureterocele with a thin echogenic membrane appears near the left orifice (right arrow). HB = bladder.

Wall Changes

Diffuse Wall Thickening

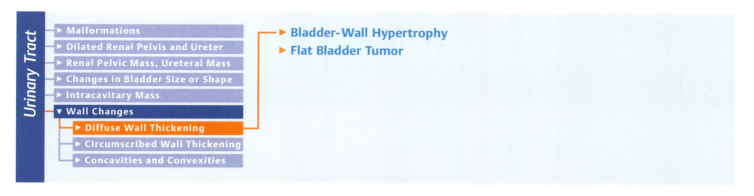

▶ Bladder-Wall Hypertrophy

The normal wall thickness of a distended bladder is 1–3 mm and does not exceed 5 mm (**Fig. 11.91**).

Diffuse bladder-wall hypertrophy greater than 5 mm may be found in association with inflammations (e.g., after prolonged catheterization) or schistosomiasis in some regions, but it most commonly results from infravesical obstruction, often combined with pseudo-diverticula (**Figs. 11.92 and 11.93**). Inadequate bladder distension may be misinterpreted as diffuse wall thickening (**Fig. 11.94**).

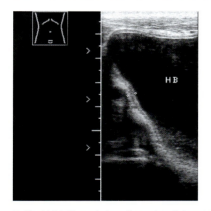

▲ **Fig. 11.91** Normal three-layered wall (cursors) of a well-distended bladder (HB).

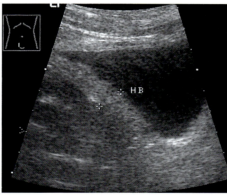

▲ **Fig. 11.92** Diffuse bladder-wall thickening secondary to an infravesical prostatic obstruction (BPH). HB = bladder.
a Bladder-wall thickening without a pseudodiverticulum (cursors).

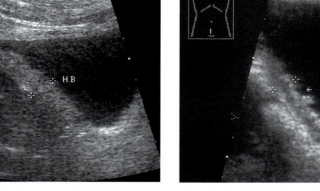

▲ *b* Diffuse wall thickening with pseudodiverticulum (arrows). IC = echogenic indwelling catheter.

◀◀ **Fig. 11.93** Massive wall thickening, measuring up to 20 mm at some sites and exceeding the wall thickness of an empty bladder (compare with **Fig. 11.94**). IC = indwelling catheter. FL = urinary fluid.

◀ **Fig. 11.94** Apparent diffuse wall thickening (cursors) in a partially distended bladder (HB).

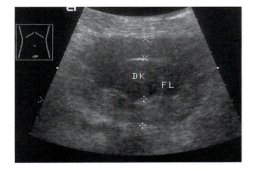

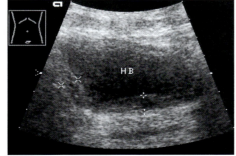

▶ Flat Bladder Tumor

It can be difficult or impossible to distinguish diffuse bladder-wall hypertrophy from a carcinoma, sarcoma, or lymphoma that has formed a plaquelike growth on the bladder wall.

If ultrasound raises suspicion of a flat carcinoma on the bladder wall, further tests such as cystoscopy, radiography, and CT should be carried out (**Fig. 11.95**).

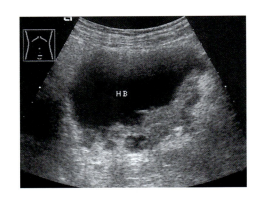
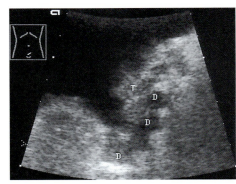

◀◀ **Fig. 11.95** Plaquelike bladder tumor (histology: papillary urothelial carcinoma, probably a diverticular tumor).
a Tumor has spread over the bladder floor and (in other planes) into both sidewalls, almost extending to the bladder roof on the left side. HB = bladder.

◀ ***b*** Tumor-encased diverticula (D). The internal echoes are caused by tumor tissue inside the diverticula. T = tumor.

Circumscribed Wall Thickening

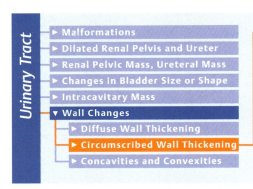

▶ Bladder-Wall Hypertrophy

Bladder-wall hypertrophy is the most frequent cause of circumscribed bladder-wall thickening demonstrated by ultrasound. The wall thickness often exceeds 7 mm in cases due to infravesical obstruction. Pseudodiverticula generally appear as anechoic, usually multiple, sharp or rounded protrusions of the bladder wall. They most commonly occur on the bladder floor and sidewalls, rarely affecting the bladder roof (**Figs. 11.96 and 11.97**).

Sites of inflammatory wall thickening due to infiltration from adjacent organs, as in Crohn disease of the terminal ileum or peridiverticulitis, are not uncommon.

The differential diagnosis should include clots or sludge adherent to the bladder wall, a flat circumscribed tumor, and especially a faulty examination technique with inadequate bladder filling.

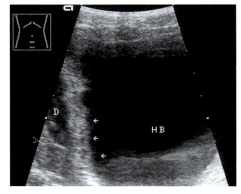

▲ **Fig. 11.96** Wall hypertrophy in a trabeculated bladder with incipient pseudodiverticula. HB = bladder.
a B-mode image, lower abdominal transverse scan: relatively long, serrated area of circumscribed wall thickening (arrows) with adherent, fluid-filled bowel segment (D). Tumor was excluded by cystoscopy. Side-lobe artifacts are also visible.

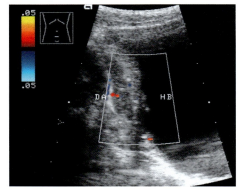

▲ ***b*** Color Doppler shows scattered vascular spots but no tumor vascularity. DA = bowel wall.

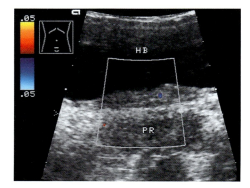
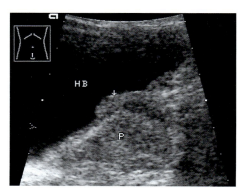

◀◀ **Fig. 11.97** Circumscribed wall thickening on the bladder floor, raising suspicion of a tumor. HB = bladder.
a Lower abdominal transverse scan. Color Doppler shows no vessels. PR = prostate.

◀ ***b*** Longitudinal scan shows a polypoid tumor mass (arrow). P = prostate. Cystoscopy showed a trabeculated bladder due to BPH.

▶ Bladder-Wall Edema

Circumscribed bladder-wall edema is usually based on mechanical irritation and inflammation from a bladder catheter, and so generally the cause is apparent.

▶ Bladder Carcinoma

The most important sonographic diagnosis is a flat, circumscribed carcinoma of the bladder wall. It is occasionally difficult to distinguish from bladder-wall hypertrophy. Tumor spread through the bladder wall to neighboring organs, especially adjacent bowel segments (e.g., the sigmoid colon), and the presence of lymph node metastases prove that the lesion is a malignant process. Conversely, it is not uncommon to find bladder invasion by tumors in adjacent organs, such as ovarian or rectosigmoid cancer.

Flat, circumscribed bladder carcinoma most commonly occurs on the bladder floor in the area of the trigone and ureteral orifices, leading to ureteral obstruction (**Figs. 11.99–11.101**).

Sonographic tumor staging is of limited accuracy in transabdominal ultrasound, but transurethral scanning is more reliable. The system for staging bladder tumors is shown in **Fig. 11.98**.

Bladder carcinoma is isoechoic to the rest of the bladder wall. Its outline is usually wavy but occasionally smooth. Sites of wall thickening near diverticula are always suspicious for carcinoma, as they are considered premalignant lesions (**see Fig. 11.105**).

TNM Involvement of urothelium, lamina propria, muscle layers, adventitia	Tis	Ta	T1	T2	T3a	T3b	T4
Involvement outside the bladder							Prostate, uterus, vagina, abdominal wall, pelvis
New TNM stage (1992)	0	I		II		III	IV

▲ **Fig. 11.98** Staging of bladder carcinoma (after reference 10).

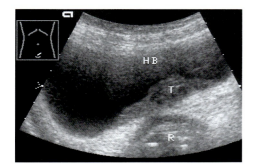

▲ **Fig. 11.99** Carcinoma involving the left side of the bladder floor. HB = bladder. R = rectum.
a Hypoechoic, slightly nonhomogeneous mass (T) spread over the bladder floor.

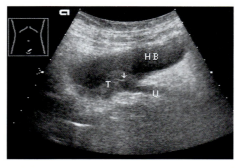

▲ *b* Shifting the probe slightly shows involvement of the left ureteral orifice (arrow) causing ureteral obstruction (U).

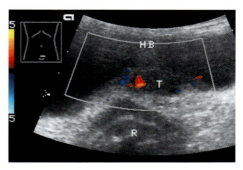

▲ *c* Color Doppler: atypical spotty vascularity.

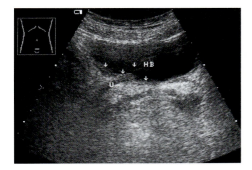

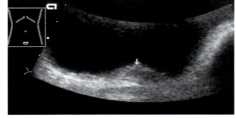

◀◀ **Fig. 11.100** Tumor spread over the bladder floor (arrows), with ureteral obstruction (U). HB = bladder.

◀ **Fig. 11.101** Recurrent urothelial carcinoma (arrow) in an 87-year-old woman two years after transurethral resection: flat, circumscribed, hypoechoic mass on the bladder floor.

▶ Blood Clots

Blood clots or viscous sludge adherent to the bladder wall may be confused with real tumors (see above).

Concavities and Convexities

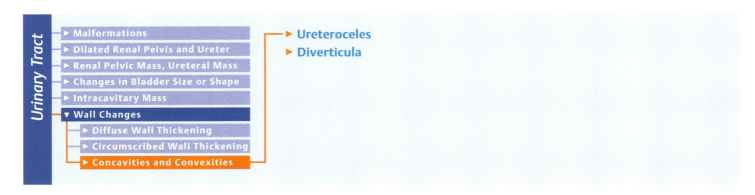

▶ Ureteroceles

Protrusions from the bladder floor near the ureteral orifices are ureteroceles. Their ultrasound appearance is described above (**Fig. 11.102**).

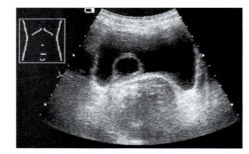

◀ **Fig. 11.102** Ureterocele: elliptical, hyperechoic ureteral wall herniating into the bladder from the area of the right ureteral orifice. The wall layers can be identified.

▶ Diverticula

Congenital bladder diverticula are based on a congenital weakness in the bladder wall, allowing a localized full-thickness herniation of the wall. They may be solitary or multiple and range in size from very small to extremely large. Diverticula predispose to stone formation and diverticular carcinoma (**Fig. 11.105**), which is why they should be surgically removed.

At ultrasound, diverticula typically appear as anechoic round or oval masses located outside the bladder wall. Most diverticula are connected to the bladder lumen by a neck or stalk. The wall of the diverticulum is thinner than the rest of the bladder wall. Diverticula may reach a size exceeding that of the bladder, often causing them to be mistaken for cysts or the bladder itself. The diagnosis of diverticula is facilitated by examining the bladder in various degrees of distension (**Figs. 11.103–11.105**).

Pseudodiverticula are secondary reactions to subvesical obstructions, and so they are usually associated with wall hypertrophy producing a trabeculated bladder (see below; **Fig. 11.106**). They represent protrusions of the bladder mucosa between bundles of hypertrophied muscle.

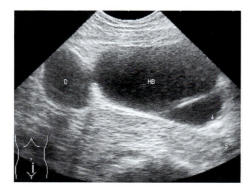

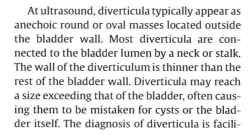

◀◀ **Fig. 11.103** Large bladder diverticula: one located cranially (D) with a well-defined diverticular neck, and one located in the bladder floor, separated from the main lumen by an echogenic wall and containing a stone (arrow; acoustic shadow S). HB = bladder.

◀ **Fig. 11.104** Diverticulum (D) in the bladder floor, with a narrow neck (arrow). The sac contains a large stone (ST) with a wide acoustic shadow (S). HB = bladder.

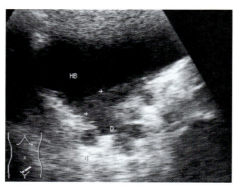

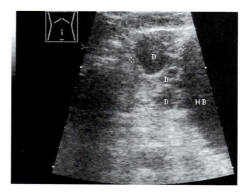

◀◀ **Fig. 11.105** Extensive diverticular tumor (arrows): hypoechoic mass spread over the bladder floor and occupying the diverticula (D). HB = bladder.

◀ **Fig. 11.106** Numerous pseudodiverticula (D), some with a diverticular neck. Bladder-wall hypertrophy. HB = bladder.

References

1a. Feuchtner G, F. Frauschner, L. Pallwein et al. Ultraschall 2000, 26. Dreiländertreffen SGUM/DEGUM/ÖGUM Basel 2002.
1b. Gladisch R. Praxis der abdominellen Ultraschalldiagnostik. 2nd ed. Stuttgart: Schattauer 1992.
2. Gottfried HW. Ultraschall in der Urologie. In: Jocham D, Miller H (eds.). Praxis der Urologie. Stuttgart: Thieme 1995; p. 55–75.
3. Hohenfellner R, Walz RH. Primärer und sekundärer Megaureter. In: Hohenfellner R, Thüroff JW, Schulte-Wissermann H. Kinderurologie in Klinik und Praxis. Stuttgart: Thieme 1986; p. 268.
4. Jequir S, Paltiel H, Lafortune M. Ureterovesical jets in infants and children: duplex and color Doppler US. Radiology 1990;175:349.
5. Jocham D. Maligne Tumoren der Harnblase. In: Jocham D, Miller H (eds.). Praxis der Urologie. Stuttgart: Thieme 1995; p. 49–115.
6. Kröpfl D. Harnleiteranomalien. In: Jocham D, Miller H (eds.). Praxis der Urologie. Stuttgart: Thieme 1995; p. 377.
7. Malone PR, Weston-Anderwood J, Aron PM. Transcutaneous ultrasound in the detection of superficial bladder cancer. Brit J Urol 1985;58:664ff.
8. Mostofi FK, Davis CJ. Histological Typing of Kidney Tumors. Berlin: Springer 1998.
9. Riedmiller H, Köhl U. Vesikoureteraler und vesikorenaler Reflux. In: Jocham D, Miller H (eds.). Praxis der Urologie. Stuttgart: Thieme 1995; p. 384–388.
10. Wilmanns W., Huhn D., Wilms K. Internistische Onkologie. Stuttgart: Thieme 2000; p. 534.

12 Prostate, Seminal Vesicles, Testis, Epididymis

Prostate 367

- ▼ The Prostate — 367
  - ▶ Anatomy and Topography
- ▼ Enlarged Prostate — 368
  - ▶ Regular — 368
    - ▶ Benign Prostatic Hyperplasia
    - ▶ Prostatic Carcinoma
    - ▶ Acute Prostatitis
  - ▶ Irregular — 370
    - ▶ Benign Prostatic Hyperplasia
    - ▶ Prostatic Carcinoma
    - ▶ Chronic Prostatitis
- ▼ Small Prostate — 371
  - ▶ Regular — 371
    - ▶ Operated Prostate
    - ▶ Radiation Therapy
  - ▶ Echogenic — 372
    - ▶ Chronic Prostatitis
- ▼ Circumscribed Lesion — 372
  - ▶ Anechoic — 372
    - ▶ Abscess, Cavity
    - ▶ Utricular Cyst, Ectopic Ureter
    - ▶ After Transurethral Resection
  - ▶ Hypoechoic — 373
    - ▶ Benign Prostatic Hyperplasia
    - ▶ Prostatic Carcinoma
  - ▶ Echogenic — 375
    - ▶ Stones, Calcifications
    - ▶ "Surgical Capsule"

Seminal Vesicles 376

- ▼ Diffuse Change — 376
  - ▶ Hypoechoic — 376
    - ▶ Vesiculitis
    - ▶ Tumor Infiltration
- ▼ Circumscribed Change — 377
  - ▶ Anechoic — 377
    - ▶ Dilatation, Cyst
    - ▶ Abscess
  - ▶ Echogenic — 378
    - ▶ Stones, Calcifications
  - ▶ Irregular — 378
    - ▶ Chronic Vesiculitis
    - ▶ Tumor Infiltration

Testis, Epididymis 379

- ▼ Testis, Epididymis — 379
  - ▶ Anatomy and Topography — 379
- ▼ Diffuse Change — 380
  - ▶ Enlargement — 380
    - ▶ Orchitis
    - ▶ Testicular Torsion
  - ▶ Decreased Size — 381
    - ▶ Anorchism, Cryptorchidism
    - ▶ Hypogonadism
    - ▶ Atrophy

- **Circumscribed Lesion** — 381
  - **Anechoic or Hypoechoic** — 381
    - Testicular Cyst
    - Hematoma
    - Abscess
    - Testicular Infarction
    - Testicular Tumor
  - **Irregular** — 383
- **Epididymal Lesion** — 383
  - **Anechoic** — 383
    - Spermatocele, Epididymal Cyst
  - **Hypoechoic** — 384
    - Epididymitis
- **Intrascrotal Mass** — 385
  - **Anechoic or Hypoechoic** — 385
    - Hydrocele
    - Varicocele
    - Hematocele
  - **Echogenic** — 386
    - Scrotal Hernia

12 Prostate, Seminal Vesicles, Testis, Epididymis

G. Schmidt

Prostatic changes. Diseases of the prostate consist of inflammatory changes (prostatitis), hyperplasias, and neoplasias. Inflammatory changes are most common in young men, while hyperplasia and carcinoma are typical diseases of aging. The incidence of prostatic carcinoma rises with aging. Its peak age incidence is the highest of all malignancies, between the seventh and eighth decades. As a result, prostate cancer has become the leading cause of death in men over age 55. Benign prostatic hyperplasia, which involves a nodular transformation of the gland, is based on a hormonal disorder.

Hyperplasia predominantly affects the upper central portion of the gland, while carcinoma tends to arise in the lower peripheral zone[2]. This is important sonographically because focal lesions located in the median lobe of the prostate generally represent hyperplasia, while cancers are typically located in the periphery of the gland. When it comes to differentiating between benign and malignant prostatic lesions, transabdominal ultrasound is less rewarding than transurethral and transrectal scanning (which are not described here but may be found in the specialized urological literature). Transabdominal scanning is of unquestioned value in assessing the size of the enlarged prostate and in the general detection of pathomorphological changes. Besides enlargement and structural abnormalities, ultrasound can demonstrate fibrotic areas, calcifications, and cysts.

Seminal vesicle changes. The seminal vesicles are paired glands that secret fluid necessary for the transport and nutrition of the sperm. Primary diseases of the seminal vesicle are extremely rare, but the gland is commonly involved by diseases spreading from adjacent organs (invasion by prostatic tumor!). Cystic dilatations and calcifications are occasionally noted at ultrasound.

Testicular changes. The location of the testes makes them easily accessible to ultrasound scanning. As a result, sonography is the modality of choice for investigating inflammatory changes and masses.

The Prostate

Anatomy and Topography

Lying against the posterior bladder floor, the prostate can be clearly visualized by placing the transducer over the distended bladder and angling the scan plane caudally (**Fig. 12.2**). The paired seminal vesicles are found posteriorly between the bladder floor and prostate (see below). The urethra runs from the funnel-shaped urethral orifice through the center of the prostate, defining a periurethral zone that can be distinguished from the inner and outer zones (**Fig. 12.1**).

This is of key importance in sonography, because it is primarily the stroma (smooth muscle) and glandular tissue in the periurethral and inner zones (transitional zone) of the posterosuperior median lobe that are susceptible to hyperplasia. The remaining portions of the gland are compressed by the hyperplastic tissue, forming an apparent capsule called the "surgical capsule." Carcinomas, on the other hand, generally arise in the predominantly glandular outer zone. These zones of predilection in the prostate aid the examiner in differentiating between carcinoma and hyperplasia. Special attention is given to the prostatic capsule surrounding the outer zone in the evaluation of transcapsular tumor spread.

Structure
- Gross anatomy: right lobe, left lobe, median lobe (posterior, superior)
- Zonal anatomy: periurethral zone, inner zone, outer zone with capsule

Relations
- Superior: bladder trigone and ureteral orifices
- Posterosuperior: seminal vesicles
- Inferior: corpora cavernosa
- Posterior: rectum

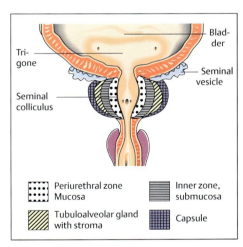

▲ **Fig. 12.1** Coronal section through the prostate, demonstrating the zones of the prostate, the bladder trigone with the ureteral orifices, and the seminal vesicles posterior to the prostate.

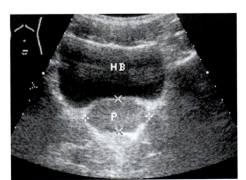 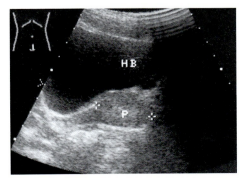

◂◂ **Fig. 12.2** Normal prostate (P, cursors).
a Lower abdominal transverse scan angled caudally demonstrates the chestnut-shaped, homogeneous prostate (P) posteroinferior to the bladder (HB).

◂ *b* Lower abdominal longitudinal scan. The rectum is visible at a more posterior level.

Enlarged Prostate

Regular

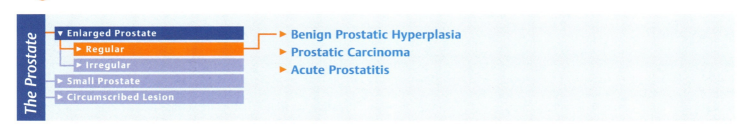

▶ Benign Prostatic Hyperplasia

Benign prostatic hyperplasia (BPH) leads to prostatic enlargement that may be either circumscribed (see below) or diffuse. The volume of the prostate is determined by multiplying length (longitudinal ultrasound section) × width × depth (in transverse section) and dividing the product by the factor 0.523 (this calculation is already built into scanners and documentation programs). This formula is fairly accurate in transabdominal ultrasound but is more accurate in transrectal scanning. Here too, however, the measured volume deviates from the actual volume or weight by up to 20%[10]. Enlargement that exceeds 80 ml is generally referred for transabdominal prostatectomy. However, estimated size alone is not a reliable indictor of clinical manifestations, which depend more on the location of the hyperplasia.

A coarser echo texture is seen with diffuse enlargement, consisting of a mixed pattern of hypoechoic and hyperechoic elements. Overall, the affected tissue appears less echogenic than the normal gland (**Figs. 12.3 and 12.4**).

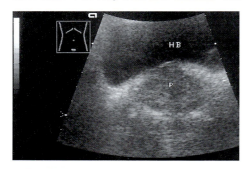

▲ **Fig. 12.3** Early benign prostatic hyperplasia (BPH) (P): homogeneous, hypoechoic enlargement of the prostate, which has a slightly irregular shape but smooth borders (cursors). Volume = 30 ml, fairly good delineation. HB = bladder.

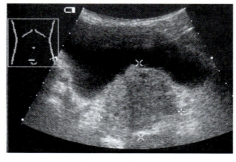

▲ **Fig. 12.4** BPH (cursors): homogeneous structure, fairly smooth borders.
a Lower abdominal transverse scan shows a large, convex indentation in the bladder floor with a small anechoic area cranially.

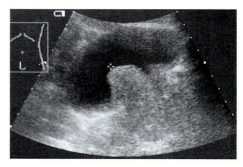

▲ **b** Lower abdominal longitudinal scan. The indentation of the bladder floor is caused by the posterosuperior median lobe. The anechoic extension from the bladder floor represents the urethral orifice. (The apparent cystic mass in **a** is cut obliquely by the scan.)

▶ Prostatic Carcinoma

Because carcinoma arises in the outer zone of the prostate in 95% of cases, considerable time passes before urinary tract obstruction occurs. As a result, early prostatic cancers are almost always an incidental finding at ultrasound, appearing as focal lesions (see below). In the advanced stage, the tumor has permeated the central portions of the prostate, penetrated the capsule, and invaded surrounding structures, particularly the seminal vesicles, bladder, and rectum. Local tumor extent is classified according to the modified TNM system[7] (**Table 12.1**).

Extent and structure. Transabdominal ultrasound is imprecise and tends to understage the extent of disease. Again, transrectal and transurethral scanning yield significantly better results.

Prostatic carcinoma usually has a predominantly hypoechoic structure with irregular outlines. Hyperechoic tumors are also seen. Differentiation from benign prostatic hyperplasia is an ever-recurring issue in routine examinations. The main criteria for malignancy are the presence of peripheral, asymmetrical tumor structures, irregular margins, and extension through the capsule; diffuse spread is not very characteristic (**Figs. 12.5 and 12.6**).

Table 12.1 Staging of prostatic carcinoma by the TNM system (after reference 7)

TX	Primary tumor cannot be assessed
T0	No evidence of primary tumor
T1	Tumor not palpable, detected incidentally at screening or TUR
T1a	Fewer than three foci, well differentiated
T1b	More than three foci, poorly differentiated
T2	Palpable tumor confined to the prostate; tumor size:
T2a	≤ 1.5 cm
T2b	> 1.5 cm or involves more than one lobe
T3	Invasion of the bladder neck or seminal vesicles
T4	Tumor fixed in the lesser pelvis, invades adjacent structures

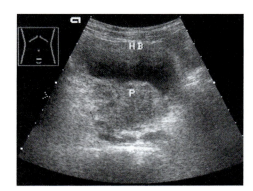

▲ **Fig. 12.5** Prostatic carcinoma: enlarged prostate (P) with an approximately normal echo structure but ill-defined margins. The malignant tumor is barely distinguishable from BPH. HB = bladder.

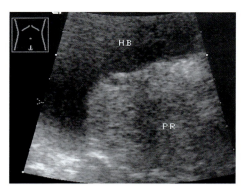

▲ **Fig. 12.6** Hypoechoic, predominantly diffuse prostatic enlargement. A circumscribed hard consistency was noted on digital rectal examination, raising strong suspicion of carcinoma. HB = bladder; PR = prostate.
a Lower abdominal longitudinal scan: enlarged prostate indenting the bladder floor, consistent with median-lobe hyperplasia. The gland appears slightly less echogenic inferiorly.

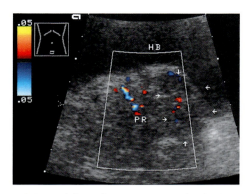

▲ *b* Lower abdominal transverse scan with color Doppler: subtle echopenic area on the left side (arrows) with atypical vascularity, creating a very high index of suspicion.

Differentiation from benign prostatic hyperplasia can be difficult or impossible by transabdominal ultrasound. Distinguishing morphological criteria are listed in **Table 12.2**.

Specificity and sensitivity. The specificity of transabdominal ultrasound is only 30%, which is slightly lower than that of transrectal scanning. Observational studies reported 33.7% attendance at digital rectal examination (DRE) plus transrectal ultrasound (TRUS) and 66.9% at prostate-specific antigen (PSA). The reported positive predictive value of digital rectal examination is 6%–33%. Both digital rectal examination and prostate-specific antigen can detect occult prostate cancer. Transrectal ultrasound is no longer considered a first-line screening test for prostate cancer, but does play a role in the investigation of patients with abnormal DRE or/and PSA.

In prostatic cancer screening, the highest detection rate (better than 98%) is achieved through the combined use of digital rectal examination, PSA testing, and transrectal or preferably transurethral ultrasound[1]. The role of transabdominal scanning is limited to detecting an abnormal echo structure and making a presumptive diagnosis or, in cases with confirmed carcinoma, assessing tumor extent and checking for locoregional metastases[4].

Clinical Diagnosis of Prostatic Carcinoma[4]

An effective early screening program for prostatic carcinoma consists of digital rectal examination with assessment of overall size, median sulcus, surface characteristics, and consistency (a circumscribed or diffuse "stony hard" consistency is suggestive of malignancy), combined with the determination of prostate-specific antigen (PSA). If induration is noted at palpation and the PSA is between 4 ng/ml (upper normal limit with men over 60 years of age; lower with younger men!) and 10 ng/ml, there is a 41% chance that carcinoma is present. With a PSA > 10 ng/ml, this rises to 72%. The incidence of carcinoma is 69% in cases where a hard, discrete nodule is found in the prostate, and 91% when the corresponding PSA is higher than 10 ng/ml. Thus, the digital findings and PSA are critical in the early detection of prostate cancer.

Transurethral sonography can support a presumptive diagnosis of carcinoma, and core biopsy can confirm the diagnosis. Even with a negative histology, however, a high PSA is still considered suspicious for carcinoma, as it is a specific tumor marker. It is extremely rare for a histological prostatic malignancy to be identified as a sarcoma or malignant lymphoma.

Table 12.2 Differentiation of prostatic carcinoma from benign prostatic hyperplasia

Prostatic carcinoma	Benign prostatic hyperplasia
▶ Predominantly hypoechoic or irregular structure ▶ Peripheral asymmetrical tumor structures ▶ Irregular outlines ▶ Capsule breached ▶ Invasion of seminal vesicles, less commonly of the bladder floor ▶ Locoregional lymphogenous spread, distant metastases	▶ Prostate shows low central echogenicity with rounded outlines ▶ Central hypoechoic tumor structure in the median lobe, indenting the bladder floor ▶ Smooth outlines ▶ Capsule intact ▶ Displacement, atrophy, and encapsulation of normal peripheral glandular tissue ▶ Possible echo-free or echogenic areas

▶ Acute Prostatitis

Five different histopathological types of prostatitis[2] can underlie the rather nonspecific symptom complex of pain, aching, burning, or pressure in the anorectal or urogenital region. Chronic complaints are often referable to a functional "prostatodynia," however.

Ultrasonography in acute prostatitis shows edematous swelling and rounding of the gland, which has a hypoechoic structure. Focal lesions (see below) may also be seen. The diagnosis is based on the clinical presentation plus corresponding sonographic findings or the detection of a causative microorganism. Swollen, hypoechoic seminal vesicles indicate concomitant inflammatory involvement of those glands (**Fig. 12.7**).

Histopathological Forms of Prostatitis

- **Purulent bacterial prostatitis**, which is often associated with abscess formation.
- **Gonorrheal prostatitis**, once the most common form, now rare.
- **Granulomatous prostatitis**, usually with an abacterial or allergic cause, marked histopathologically by destructive foci, giant cells, histiocytes, and fibroblasts.
- **Chronic nonspecific prostatitis**, in which the stasis of secretions with the formation of amyloid bodies can lead to secondary calcification and thus to prostatolithiasis and inflammation. It is diagnosed by detecting the causative organism in fluid sampled by "milking" the gland.
- **Tuberculous prostatitis**, which is associated with foci of caseous liquefaction.

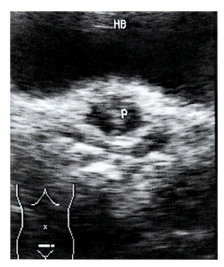
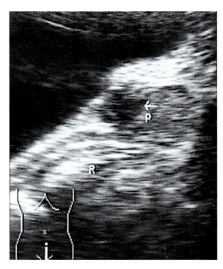

▲ **Fig. 12.7** Prostatitis (P).
a Lower abdominal transverse scan shows a largely anechoic mass. HB = bladder.

▲ *b* Lower abdominal longitudinal scan shows a small prostate with a mottled hypoechoic texture and an anechoic cystic mass (arrow). The rectum (R) appears posteriorly.

Irregular

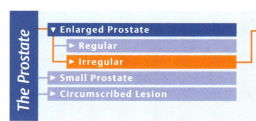

▶ Benign Prostatic Hyperplasia

Varying proportions of stromal or glandular elements affect the echo structure of benign prostatic hyperplasia: a preponderance of stroma causes the hyperplasia to appear more hypoechoic, while a preponderance of glandular elements creates a more isoechoic or hyperechoic appearance relative to the normal prostate. The result is an irregular sonographic pattern. Hyperechoic calcifications, secretory stones, and anechoic cystic areas are also seen (**Fig. 12.8**).

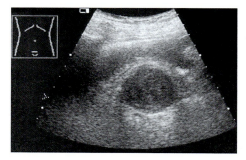
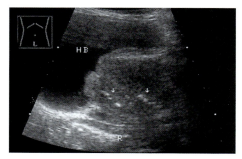

▲ **Fig. 12.8** Benign prostatic hyperplasia.
a Enlarged prostate with smooth borders, a patchy hypoechoic structure, and rounded shape.

▲ *b* Large prostate protruding into the bladder floor, nonhomogeneous texture due to numerous echogenic (arrows) microcalcifications (amyloid bodies, a common finding in chronic prostatitis). HB = bladder.

▶ Prostatic Carcinoma

Benign prostatic hyperplasia and prostatic carcinoma may present a predominantly homogeneous echo texture or a markedly irregular structure. The latter is particularly apt to occur when carcinoma is accompanied by adenomatous hyperplasia and/or fibrous, cystic, or calcifying prostatic elements. These different components cannot be distinguished by their transabdominal morphological features (**Figs. 12.9 and 12.10**).

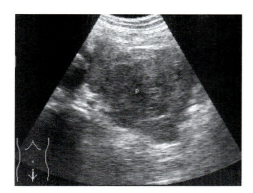 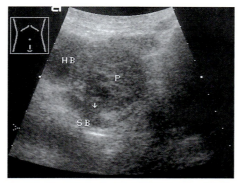 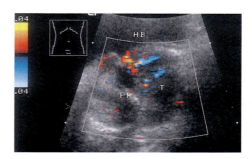

▲ **Fig. 12.9 a** Advanced prostatic carcinoma (P), which has already metastasized. Scan shows a large, tumorous prostate with irregular borders, a coarse hypoechoic texture, and tumor extension through the prostatic capsule.

▲ **b** Prostatic carcinoma (P), lower abdominal longitudinal scan: invasion of the seminal vesicle (SB), indicating a T3 tumor by ultrasound. HB = bladder.

▲ **Fig. 12.10** Prostatic carcinoma (T), color duplex: hypoechoic tumor foci in both lobes (surgery: T3 tumor). HB = bladder; PR = prostate.

▶ Chronic Prostatitis

The complaints that are associated with acute and chronic prostatitis are fairly nonspecific, and so the diagnosis can be established only by identifying the causative organism and/or detecting signs of urethral inflammation at ureterocystoscopy.

The sonographic diagnosis is also uncertain. Circumscribed hypoechoic or anechoic areas are found in acute prostatitis, while chronic prostatitis shows zones of increased density or calcification that are responsible for the irregular structural transformation (**Fig. 12.11 and 12.20**).

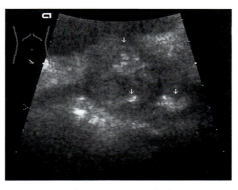 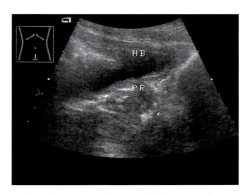

▲ **Fig. 12.11** Findings consistent with chronic prostatitis. HB = bladder; PR = prostate.
a Irregular echo structure with numerous calcifications arrows; known prostatitis.

▲ **b** Small prostate with microcalcifications and an irregular structure (45-year-old man).

Small Prostate

Regular

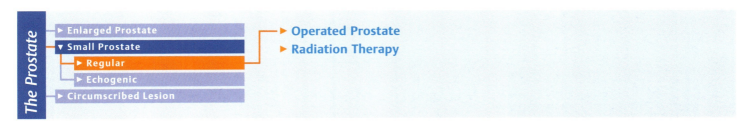

▶ Operated Prostate

A small prostate found at ultrasound is usually a result of surgery. In patients who have had a transurethral resection (TUR), the size reduction results from a complete resection of the previously enlarged median lobe. Ultrasound demonstrates a small prostatic remnant and often shows a funnel-shaped, anechoic urethral orifice formed by the resection defect at the level of the bladder neck (**Fig. 12.12**).

A transabdominal total prostatectomy involves removing the enlarged median lobe in the plane of the surgical capsule, while a transabdominal tumor resection consists of a radical prostatovesiculectomy, in which case the prostate and seminal vesicles are completely absent (**Fig. 12.13**).

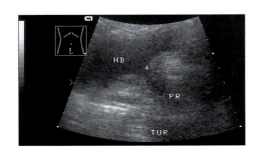 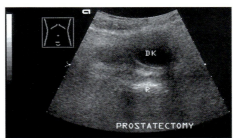

◄◄ ▶*Fig. 12.12* Small prostate (PR) following transurethral resection (TUR). The urethral orifice and prostatic urethra appear widened and anechoic after TUR. The expanded urethral orifice is funnel-shaped and fluid-filled (arrow). HB = bladder.

◄ *Fig. 12.13* Prostatectomy for carcinoma: nonvisualization of the prostate in a transabdominal low transverse scan. Urinary catheter (DK) is in place. Normally the seminal vesicle or prostate would be visualized between the bladder floor and rectum (R).

▶ Radiation Therapy

The goal of radiation therapy is complete tumor destruction. The irradiation also leads to atrophy and size reduction of the remaining gland. A tissue increase discovered at ultrasound suggests a recurrence or, more likely, the local regrowth of residual tumor.

Echogenic

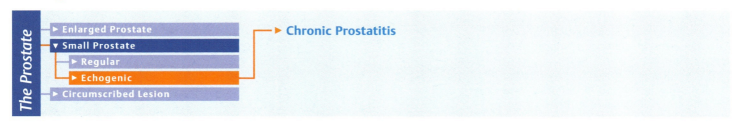

▶ Chronic Prostatitis

The prostate in the end stage of chronic prostatitis is small (**Fig. 12.11**), consisting only of glandular remnants and dense lesions such as fibrosis or calcifications. Such changes are also commonly seen in prostatic hyperplasia—at times incidentally—with no prior clinical manifestations of chronic prostatitis.

Circumscribed Lesion

Anechoic

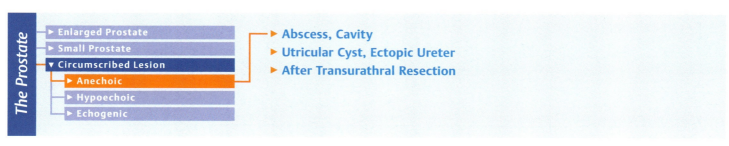

▶ Abscess, Cavity

Anechoic lesions in the prostate may be abscesses when corresponding clinical signs are present, or they may represent cavities in rare instances of urogenital tuberculosis (**Fig. 12.7**). The diagnosis is established by biopsy with culture or histological analysis.

▶ Utricular Cyst, Ectopic Ureter

Anechoic areas located in the posteromedian and cranial portion of the prostate represent harmless utricular cysts (**Fig. 12.14**). They are considered remnants of the embryonic müllerian duct. Differentiation is required from an ectopic ureter with an anomalous insertion into the wolffian duct.

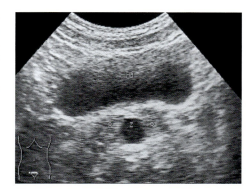
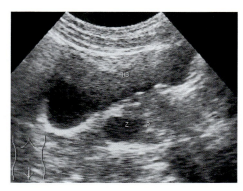

▲ **Fig. 12.14** Cystic mass (Z) in the lower midline of an otherwise normal-appearing prostate (P) in a 43-year-old man with no symptoms. Most likely a utricular cyst. HB = bladder.
a Lower abdominal transverse scan.

▲ **b** Lower abdominal longitudinal scan.

▶ After Transurethral Resection

Anechoic areas are also seen following TUR. Irregular, anechoic areas are found at the site of the resection cavity, or a funnel-shaped anechoic area may be found at the junction of the bladder neck with the proximal urethra. A prior history of TUR suggests the correct interpretation for both of these findings (**Fig. 12.12**).

Hypoechoic

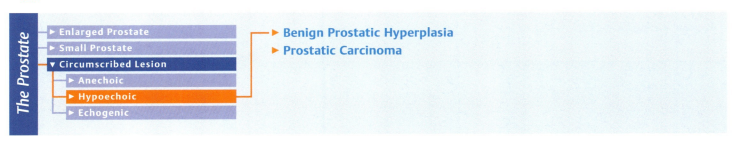

Prostatic hyperplasia and prostatic carcinoma typically appear sonographically as circumscribed hypoechoic lesions that are difficult to distinguish from each other by their ultrasound features. Every hypoechoic lesion is suspicious for carcinoma, therefore, and warrants further investigation. The location of the lesion (see above) is the only helpful sonographic sign for benign/malignant differentiation. Clinical findings (digital rectal examination, PSA) and transrectal/transurethral sonography can advance the diagnosis.

▶ Benign Prostatic Hyperplasia

A hypoechoic area in the median lobe of the prostate is suggestive of hyperplasia (**Fig. 12.15**).

Hypoechoic areas can also appear as a peripheral rim that contrasts with the more echogenic compressed tissues, forming a "surgical capsule" (**Fig. 12.16**).

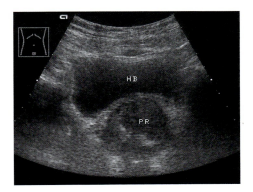
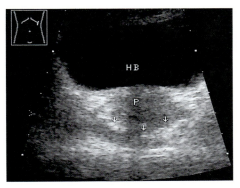

▲ **Fig. 12.15** Hypoechoic median-lobe adenoma (hyperplasia; PR), clearly demarcated from the rest of the prostate. HB = bladder.

▲ **Fig. 12.16** Hyperplastic median lobe (P), delineated by high-level echoes (arrows) from the hypoechoic displaced prostatic tissue. HB = bladder.

▶ Prostatic Carcinoma

The early stage of prostatic carcinoma usually appears sonographically as a focal hypoechoic mass[5] (**Figs. 12.17–12.19**). Irregular isoechoic structures can also occur, depending on the tumor histology and extent and any preexisting changes that are incorporated into the tumor. Tumors smaller than 5 mm are not detected by transabdominal or transrectal sonography. Differentiation from benign prostatic hyperplasia with hypoechoic fibromuscular nodules and from focal lesions in prostatitis is almost impossible, with the result that carcinoma usually cannot be detected by ultrasound screening. Generally, then, the role of ultrasonography is limited to defining tumor extent and detecting lymph node involvement in the lesser pelvis and along the iliac chain[7] (**Figs. 12.18 and 12.19**).

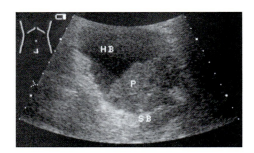
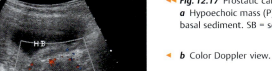

◀◀ **Fig. 12.17** Prostatic carcinoma.
   a Hypoechoic mass (P). HB = bladder with a layer of basal sediment. SB = seminal vesicle.

◀ **b** Color Doppler view.

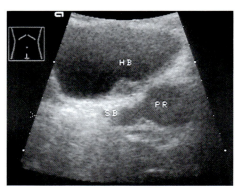

▲ **Fig. 12.18** Patchy hypoechoic prostatic carcinoma (PR), locally advanced.
a Infiltration of the bladder floor (HB, arrows) and rectum (R).

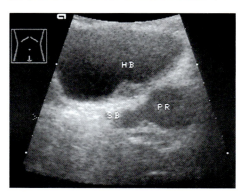

▲ **b** Infiltration of the seminal vesicles (SB).

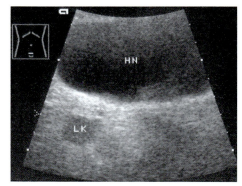

▲ **c** Locoregional lymph node (LK). All the changes regressed in response to treatment. HN = bladder.

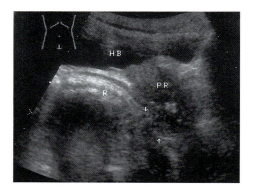

▲ **Fig. 12.19** Prostatic carcinoma infiltrating the rectum. HB = bladder; PR = prostate; R = rectum.
a Sonography: ill-defined posteroinferior margin and a thickened, infiltrated rectal wall (R; arrows).

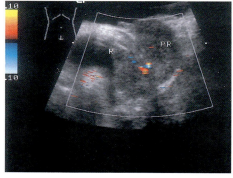

▲ **b** Color duplex image of **a**: scattered aberrant tumor vessels.

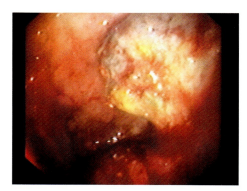

▲ **c** Endoscopy: intestinal bleeding.

Echogenic

Stones, Calcifications

Echogenic foci also occur in prostatic hyperplasia. They are consistently located in the capsulelike layer of prostatic tissue demarcated from the rest of the gland by an echogenic rim. Nonspecific inflammations, inspissated secretions, glandular hyperplasia, calculi, and calcifications are the correlates of these echogenic areas.

Stones and calcifications occur in inflammatory conditions (prostatitis in the setting of hyperplastic changes) and in carcinomas, appearing sonographically as more or less pronounced hyperechoic areas. Larger stones and calcifications cast prominent acoustic shadows, making them easy to detect with ultrasound (**Figs. 12.20 and 12.21**).

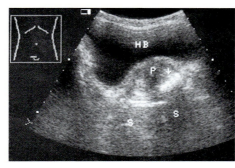

▲ **Fig. 12.20** Prostatic calculi (arrow, acoustic shadows S). Scan shows intensely echogenic, shadowing masses in the prostate (P). HB = bladder.

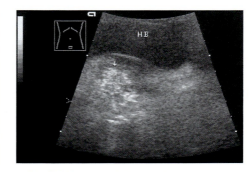

▲ **Fig. 12.21** Prostatic calcifications following hormonal ablation of prostatic carcinoma 12 years before: mottled echogenic areas with a partial acoustic shadow. HB = bladder.

▶ "Surgical Capsule"

Between a hyperplastic nodule and the displaced peripheral part of the gland is a hyperechoic fibrous layer called the "surgical capsule," so named because it defines the plane for surgical enucleation of the nodule (**Fig. 12.16**).

Seminal Vesicles

Diffuse Change

Hypoechoic

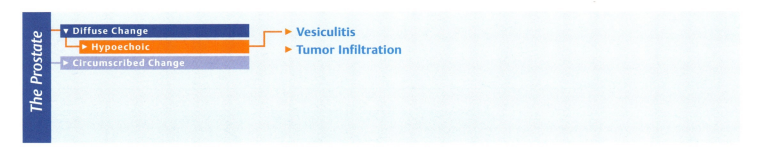

While primary tumors of the seminal vesicles are virtually unknown, vesiculitis develops occasionally, and secondary tumor infiltration (e.g., by prostatic carcinoma) is common. Transrectal sonography is used for making a detailed evaluation, but transabdominal scanning is still useful for detecting essential changes.

▶ Vesiculitis

Acute and chronic vesiculitis may be suppurative (empyema) or may consist of diffuse inflammation. Bacteriology will often identify a causative organism.

Sonographically, the seminal vesicles exhibit unilateral or bilateral hypoechoic swelling. Because of their dilatation, the vesicles may show a hypoechoic string-of-beads transformation or a plump, elliptical appearance (**Fig. 12.22**).

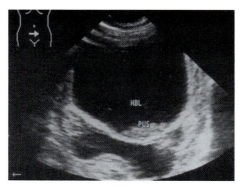

◀ **Fig. 12.22** Purulent vesiculitis: swollen, intensely echogenic seminal vesicles in a patient with suppurative pyelonephritis. Purulent bladder sediment (PUS). HBL = bladder.

▶ Tumor Infiltration

Infiltration of the seminal vesicles by prostatic carcinoma is more frequently unilateral than bilateral. The tumor structure is hypoechoic, and the vesicles show irregular expansion. The tumor extensions may arise from the surroundings, from the prostate, or even from the rectum (**Fig. 12.18**).

Circumscribed Change

Anechoic

Dilatation, Cyst

A row of elliptical, anechoic lesions found in the seminal vesicle (usually incidentally) represent foci of vesicular ectasia. They may be a manifestation of vesiculitis. Primary cysts are similar, but round and smooth (**Fig. 12.23**).

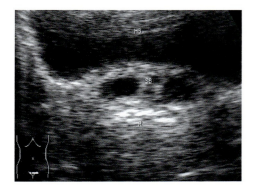
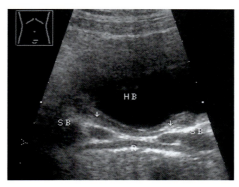
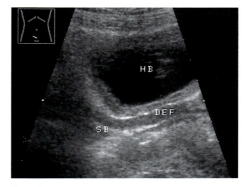

▲ **Fig. 12.23** Bilateral cystic masses in the seminal vesicles. HB = bladder; SB = seminal vesicle. R = rectum.
a Probable areas of ectasia.

▲ **b** Medially situated cystic masses (arrows).

▲ **c** When the vesicles (SB) are scanned at an oblique angle, each mass elongates into a vas deferens (DEF) (see also **Fig. 12.25**).

Abscess

Circumscribed anechoic to hypoechoic lesions in the seminal vesicles can also result from abscess formation. The diagnosis is established by the clinical features and by transabdominal or transrectal sonography, possibly combined with percutaneous drainage.

Echogenic

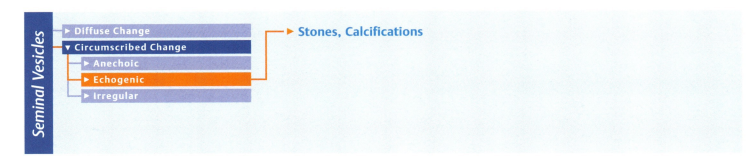

▶ Stones, Calcifications

Echogenic areas in the seminal vesicles represent stones or calcifications. Their ultrasound features are identical to those of prostatic stones and calcifications, but transabdominal ultrasound can definitely localize them to the seminal vesicle (**Fig. 12.24**).

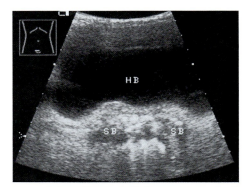

◀ **Fig. 12.24** Irregularly hyperechoic seminal vesicles with calcifications, acoustic shadows, and echogenic reverberations. HB = bladder; SB = seminal vesicle.

Irregular

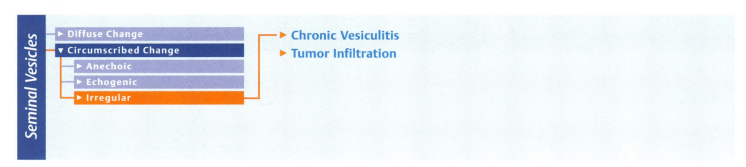

▶ Chronic Vesiculitis

Irregular structures with mixed hyperechoic/hypoechoic or cystic areas are seen in chronic vesiculitis or may be detected incidentally with no apparent cause.

▶ Tumor Infiltration

Cancer infiltrating the seminal vesicles displays structural irregularities similar to those commonly seen in prostatic carcinoma. Detection of the primary tumor confirms the diagnosis (**Fig. 12.18b**).

Testis, Epididymis

Anatomy and Topography

Structure

- Testicular lobules
- Seminiferous tubules
- Head of the epididymis
- Duct of the epididymis
- Tail of the epididymis
- Spermatic cord with the vas deferens

Testis. The testicular lobules contain spermatogonia, spermatocytes, seminal fluid, and hormones. Their secretions are carried by the seminiferous tubules to the efferent ductules of the epididymis.

Epididymis. The epididymis lies on the lateral aspect of the testis and consists of a superior head and an inferior tail, which is continuous with the vas deferens. The latter duct ascends from the scrotum in the spermatic cord, accompanied by the testicular artery and vein and the deferential artery and vein. The vas deferens crosses over the ureter and passes behind the seminal vesicles to enter the upper part of the prostate (**Figs. 12.25–12.27**).

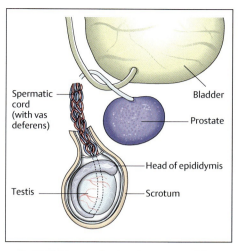

▲ **Fig. 12.25** Diagram showing the anatomy of the testis, epididymis, and vas deferens and their relation to the prostate and bladder.

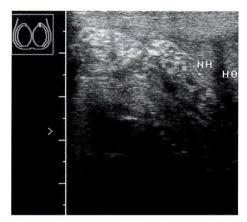

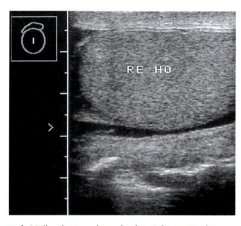

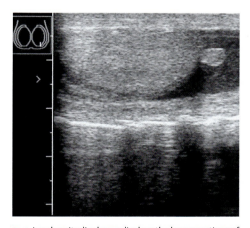

▲ **Fig. 12.26** Ultrasound scans through a normal testis and epididymis.
 a Scan through the upper part of the testis (HO) displays the head of the epididymis (NH) and the patchy hyperechoic spermatic cord with the vas deferens.

▲ **b** Midlevel scan through the right testis demonstrates a finely granular echo texture (same appearance as in uncomplicated orchitis). RE = rectum.

▲ **c** Low longitudinal scan displays the lower portions of the testis and the tail of the epididymis within the fluid medium of the scrotum.

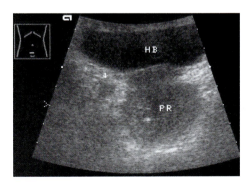

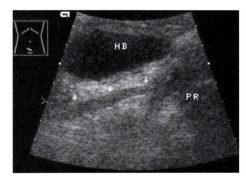

◂◂ **Fig. 12.27** Ectatic vas deferens (arrow) proximal to its entry into the prostate. HB = bladder; PR = prostate.
 a Lower abdominal transverse scan: small, anechoic, avascular mass.

◂ **b** Duct system (arrows) terminates at the prostate and has no connections with the bladder.

Diffuse Change

Enlargement

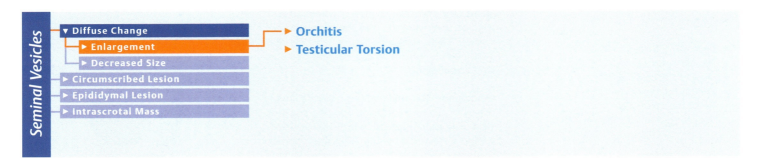

▶ Orchitis

Ultrasound contributes little to the diagnosis of orchitis, which can be inferred from the underlying disease (mumps, sarcoidosis, tuberculosis, syphilis). One or both testes are enlarged and occasionally (tuberculosis, sarcoidosis) display nonhomogeneities. Generally the epididymides are involved by the inflammation. With unilateral orchitis, the affected testis appears slightly hypoechoic relative to the opposite side (**Figs. 12.28 and 12.29**).

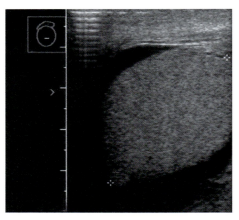

▲ **Fig. 12.28** Orchitis: enlarged, balloonlike testis (40.5 cm) with an accompanying hydrocele.

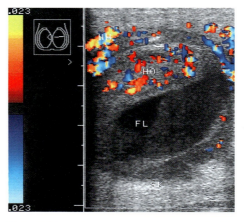

▲ **Fig. 12.29** Bacterial orchitis on the right side with abscessation (FL), confirmed at operation. HO = testis. **a** Right testis (scanned from left to right): echogenicity is slightly decreased relative to the left side, with inflammatory hypervascularity. Inflammatory edema of the scrotum (SK).

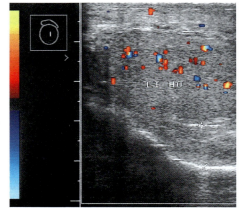

▲ **b** Compare with the normal structure and vascularity of the left testis. Patient presented clinically with poorly controlled diabetes mellitus. LI = left.

▶ Testicular Torsion

Testicular torsion occurs when the testis, epididymis, and spermatic cord are twisted on their longitudinal axis. It generally affects a testis that is abnormally mobile. The initial venous occlusion leads to unilateral enlargement with no change in echogenicity, but with passage of time the testis becomes smaller and more hypoechoic. The diagnosis is made clinically. When arterial occlusion develops, color Doppler can confirm the diagnosis based on an absence of Doppler flow signals.

Decreased Size

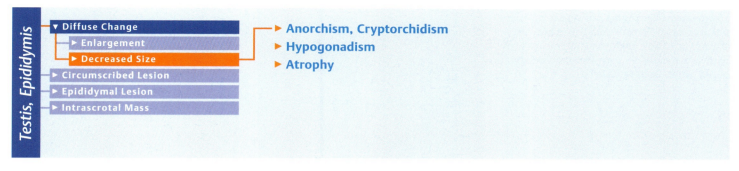

▶ Anorchism, Cryptorchidism

Unilateral or bilateral testicular aplasia is easy to diagnose with ultrasound. In cryptorchidism, ultrasound shows an ectopic, undescended testis in the groin or abdomen (e.g., iliac region). The testis is in these cases is hypoplastic.

▶ Hypogonadism

Small testes occur as an ontogenic condition in intersexuality, Klinefelter syndrome, prepubertal and postpubertal hypopituitarism (hypogonadotropic eunuchoidism, organic pituitary disease), and various other syndromes. The smallness of the testes is demonstrated by ultrasound.

▶ Atrophy

Testicular atrophy can result from insults such as testicular torsion or radiation therapy. The diagnosis is made from the underlying disorder, and ultrasound can confirm the clinical suspicion.

Circumscribed Lesion

Anechoic or Hypoechoic

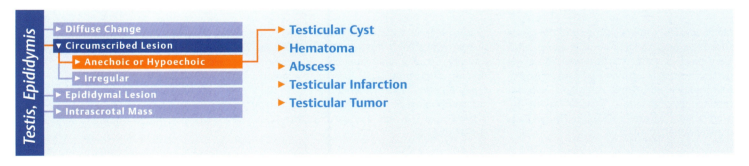

▶ Testicular Cyst

Testicular cysts occur as simple cysts without a cyst wall and in the form of very rare epidermoid cysts. Simple testicular cysts display typical cystic features at ultrasound: an anechoic interior with a rounded border and distal acoustic enhancement. Epidermoid cysts may contain distinct internal echoes.

▶ Hematoma

Posttraumatic hematoma can appear as a predominantly anechoic lesion, depending on its stage (**Fig. 12.30**). High-level internal echoes with reverberations represent bubbles produced by gas-forming bacteria.

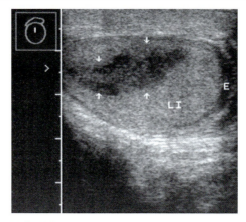
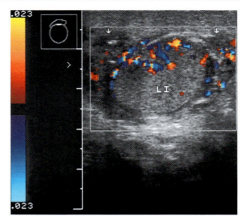

▲ **Fig. 12.30** Posttraumatic testicular hematoma. LI = left.
a B-mode demonstrates an anechoic mass.

▲ *b* Color Doppler shows an absence of vascularity in the hematoma.

▶ Abscess

Most abscesses are anechoic, but occasionally a cloudy internal structure is seen. The margins are irregular (**Fig. 12.31**). The diagnosis is established by the clinical presentation and if necessary by ultrasound-guided needle aspiration. Given the variable appearance of abscesses, there are cases in which the diagnosis can be confirmed only by demonstrating bacterial gas formation.

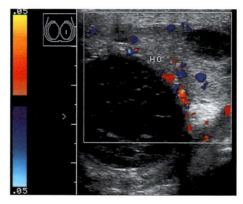

◀ **Fig. 12.31** Testicular abscess: anechoic to hypoechoic mass within the testis (HO) and scrotum. Color Doppler shows no blood flow within the mass. Patient presented clinically with septic temperatures and an infected hematoma.

▶ Testicular Infarction

On the whole, testicular infarctions are very rare. They have been characterized as hypoechoic as well as hyperechoic lesions that are virtually indistinguishable from tumors[9].

▶ Testicular Tumor

Many different tumors can occur in the testes, showing a peak incidence during adolescence. They can be classified by histological and genetic criteria into seminomas, nonseminomatous tumors (embryonic carcinoma, yolk sac tumor, choriocarcinoma), gonadal stromal tumors (Leydig cell tumor, Sertoli cell tumor), and malignant lymphomas[8].

With regard to frequency distribution, 35% of testicular tumors are seminomas, 25% are teratocarcinomas, approximately 20% are embryonic carcinomas, and 15% are combined types. All other testicular tumors are rare. The sonomorphological features described by Schwerk and Schwerk[9] are listed in **Table 12.3** (see **Fig. 12.32**).

Table 12.3 Sonomorphological features of testicular tumors (after reference 9)

- ▶ One or more foci disrupting the testicular echo texture
- ▶ Tumor outline smooth or irregular
- ▶ Great majority of tumors (approximately 90%) are hypoechoic; a few are isoechoic or hyperechoic
- ▶ Homogeneous or heterogeneous tumor structure, in some cases with focal calcifications and/or (pseudo)cystic areas

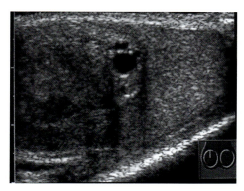
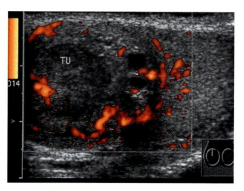
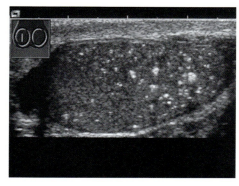

▲ **Fig. 12.32** Testicular tumor (TU).
a Testicular carcinoma: nonhomogeneous, hypoechoic mass with small anechoic cysts.

▲ **b** Color Doppler: hypervascular periphery.

▲ **c** "Starry sky" calcifications in the right testis (testicular microlithiasis) following a left orchiectomy for a germ cell tumor. Microlithiasis may have a neoplastic or inflammatory etiology or may be chemotherapy-induced.

Irregular

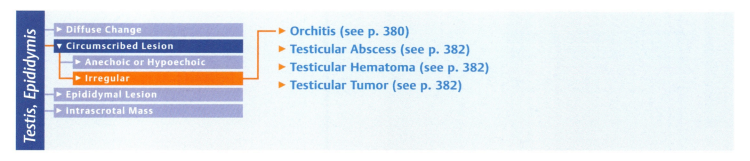

All of the focal lesions described above can also assume a heterogeneous structure. In orchitis, this is seen mainly with atypical granulomatous inflammations. Testicular microlithiasis can occur in association with inflammatory as well as neoplastic testicular lesions (**Fig. 12.32c**). Differentiation in these cases can be accomplished histologically or by reference to the history and clinical presentation (trauma, fever with inflammatory swelling, underlying disease).

Epididymal Lesion

Anechoic

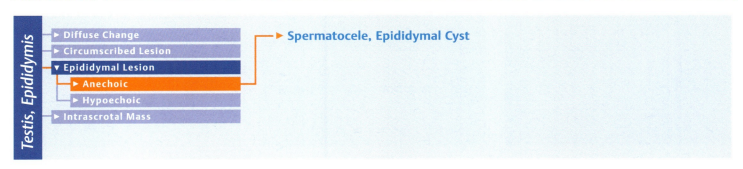

▶ Spermatocele, Epididymal Cyst

Spermatoceles and epididymal cysts are anechoic areas in the epididymis that display typical cystic features. They may be multiple and can reach considerable size (**Fig. 12.33**).

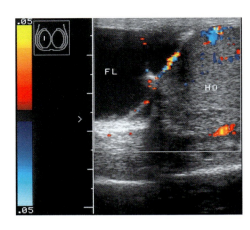 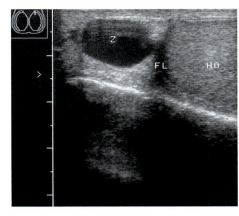

◀◀ **Fig. 12.33** Spermatocele.
 a Color Doppler of the right epididymal area: extensive, anechoic, avascular fluid collection (FL) around the testis (HO).

◀ **b** Left testis and epididymal area: fluid (FL) with a cystic area (Z) around the upper part of the testis.

Hypoechoic

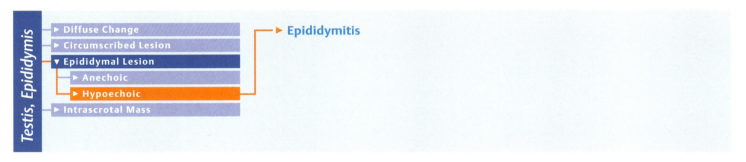

▶ Epididymitis

Inflammation of the epididymis presents clinically with gradually increasing pain and corresponding inflammatory symptoms, which distinguish this condition from testicular torsion. Epididymitis is a common entity. As in prostatitis, it may involve a nonspecific bacterial inflammation that has spread by the hematogenous route or abscessation, or it may be caused by a tuberculous, gonorrheal, or syphilitic infection.

Ultrasound reveals swelling of the head, body, or tail of the epididymis. The echogenicity is variable, and the structure is predominantly hypoechoic to heterogeneous (**Fig. 12.34**).

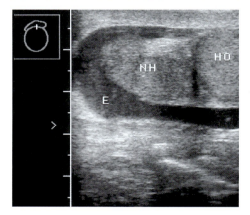 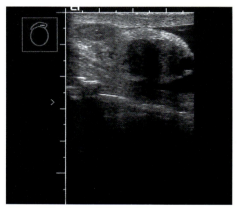 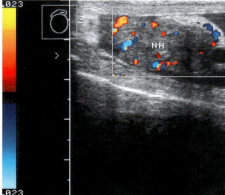

▲ **Fig. 12.34** Epididymitis.
 a Enlarged epididymis (NH) with accompanying inflammatory fluid (hydrocele; E). HO = testis.

▲ **b** Left epididymis: hypoechoic mass.

▲ **c** Color Doppler shows conspicuous vascularity.

Intrascrotal Mass

Anechoic or Hypoechoic

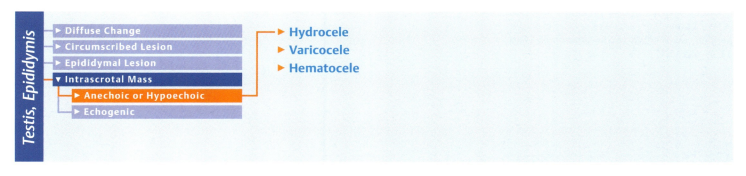

▶ Hydrocele

A hydrocele is a collection of watery fluid in the tunica vaginalis of the testis. It often communicates with ascitic fluid in the abdominal cavity, the pressure rise in the abdomen causing the previously closed processus vaginalis to become patent. Inflammatory hydroceles are also common, however (e.g., secondary to epididymitis), and cause a cystlike expansion of the tunica vaginalis. Transient hydroceles are also occasionally detected in small infants (**Fig. 12.35**).

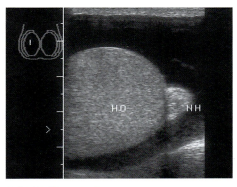

▲ **Fig. 12.35 a and b** Bilateral hydroceles.
a Right side: testis (HO) and epididymis (NH) surrounded by fluid.

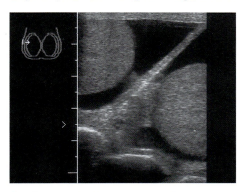

▲ **b** Sections of both testes with scrotal septum.

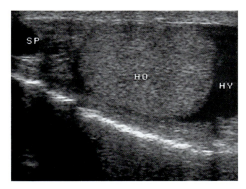

▲ **c** Hydrocele (HY) and spermatocele (SP): anechoic mass around the testis (HO). The spermatocele does not change its position, unlike the mobile fluid in the hydrocele.

▶ Varicocele

A varicocele is defined as a palpable and visible dilatation of the veins of the pampiniform plexus (WHO). It is caused by retrograde flow in the testicular vein or by an absence of venous valves. It occurs predominantly on the left side and is occasionally bilateral. Treatment is unnecessary in patients who have no complaints and a normal semen analysis or azoospermia. Otherwise, surveillance should be maintained to assess the need for operative treatment.

Ultrasound demonstrates convoluted, anechoic venous structures arranged around the testis, showing a luminal diameter greater than 2 mm. Color duplex examination reveals low-flow waveforms. If no flow is detected, the stasis may be caused by intra-abdominal or retroperitoneal tumor compression or tumor invasion of the testicular vein, which is occasionally definable with ultrasound in thin patients (**Fig. 12.36**).

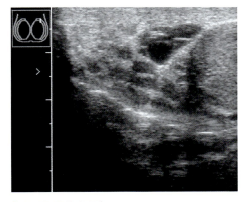

▲ **Fig. 12.36** Varicocele.
a B-mode image of the right testis: multiple anechoic foci of vascular ectasia around the epididymis.

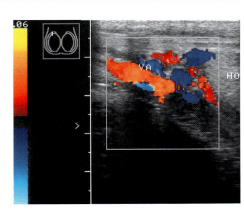

▲ **b** Color Doppler during a Valsalva maneuver shows extensive vascularity. HO = testis; VA = varicocele.

▶ Hematocele

A hematocele is a collection of free blood in the scrotal cavity. It is generally preceded by surgical or other trauma.

Ultrasound shows a predominantly anechoic, hypoechoic, or even irregular mass, depending on the age of the hematoma (**Figs. 12.30 and 12.31**).

Echogenic

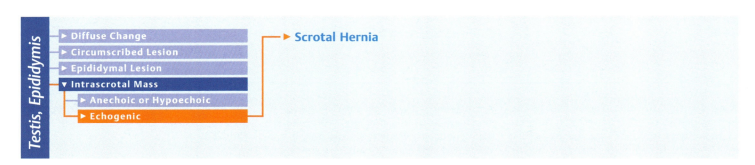

▶ Scrotal Hernia

Sonography is an excellent modality for the investigation of intrascrotal swelling. One cause of such swelling is a scrotal hernia. The hernial sac is found to contain bowel structures, which are easily identified as such with ultrasound (**Fig. 12.37**).

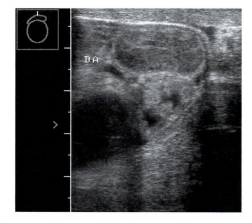

◀ **Fig. 12.37** Scrotal hernia: hyperechoic bowel structures within the scrotal cavity. DA = intestine.

References

1. Bertermann H. Transrektale Sonographie von Prostata und Samenblasen. In: Braun G, Schwerk WB (eds.). Ultraschalldiagnostik Ecomed 1996.
2. Böckung A, Riede UN. Vorsteherdrüse. In: Riede UN, Schaefer HE (eds.). Allgemeine und spezielle Pathologie. Stuttgart: Thieme 1993.
3. Giatto S, Bonardi R, Mazzotta A, et al. Comparing two modalities for screening for prostatic cancer: digital rectal exam plus transrectal ultrasound versus prostate-specific antigen. Tumor 1995;81:225–9.
4. Fabricus PG. Prostata- und Samenblasentumoren. In: Jocham D, Miller K (eds.). Praxis der Urologie. Stuttgart: Thieme 1994.
5. Frentzel-Beyme B, Schwarz I, Aurich B. Das Bild des Prostataadenoms und -karzinoms bei der transrektalen Sonographie. Fortschr Röntgenstr 1982;137:261–8.
6. Gottfried HW. Transrektale Sonographie. In: Jocham D, Miller K (eds.). Praxis der Urologie. Stuttgart: Thieme 1994.
7. Hermanek P. Neue TNM/pTNM-Klassifikation und Stadieneinteilung urologischer Tumoren ab 1987. Urologe Ausg. B 1986;26:193–7, cited after Fabricus PG. Prostata und Samenblasentumoren. In: Jocham D, Miller K (eds.). Praxis der Urologie. Stuttgart: Thieme 1993.
8. Riede UN, Wehner H. Hoden. In: Riede UN, Schaefer HE (eds.). Allgemeine und spezielle Pathologie. Stuttgart: Thieme 1993.
9. Schwerk WB, Schwerk WN. Sonographie des Skrotalinhaltes. In: Braun G, Schwerk WB (eds.). Ultraschalldiagnostik. Ecomed 1994.
10. Terris MK, Stamey TA. Determination of the prostate volume by transrectal ultrasound. J Urol 1991;145:984.

13 Female Genital Tract

Female Genital Tract 389

- **Vagina** — 390
  - Ultrasound Morphology
- **Masses** — 390
  - Imperforate Hymen with Hematocolpos
  - Vaginal Wall Cyst
  - Septate Vagina
  - Tampon
  - Vaginal Carcinoma
- **Abnormalities of Size or Shape** — 391
  - Postoperative Changes
- **Uterus** — 392
  - Anatomy
  - Ultrasound Morphology (Figs. 13.10–13.12)
- **Abnormalities of Size or Shape** — 393
  - Uterine Prolapse
  - Malformations
  - Uterine Aplasia, Atresia
  - Uterine Hypoplasia, Small Uterus
  - Hemangioma, Lymphoma, Angiomyoma, Myoma
- **Myometrial Changes** — 394
  - Uterine Myomas
  - Uterine Adenomyomatosis
  - Uterine Sarcoma
- **Intracavitary Changes** — 396
  - Foreign Body (IUD)
  - Mucocele, Serometra, Pyometra, Hematometra
  - Pregnancy
  - Ectopic Pregnancy
  - Missed Abortion, Incomplete Abortion, Cervical Pregnancy
  - Endometrial Polyps, Cervical Polyps, Placental Polyps
- **Endometrial Changes** — 398
  - Proliferative Endometrium (Midcycle)
  - Cystic Glandular Hyperplasia and Atypical Adenomatous Hyperplasia
  - Endometritis, Cervicitis
  - Corpus Carcinoma
  - Chorioepithelioma
  - Cervical Carcinoma
- **Fallopian Tubes** — 402
- **Hypoechoic Mass** — 402
  - Sactosalpinx, Hematosalpinx, Pyosalpinx
  - Tubal Carcinoma
  - Benign Tumors
  - Tubal Pregnancy
- **Ovaries** — 403
  - Anatomy and Histology
  - Topography
  - Ultrasound Morphology
- **Anechoic Cystic Mass** — 404
  - Simple Follicles
  - Functional Cysts (Follicular and Corpus Luteum Cysts)
  - Theca-Lutein Cyst
  - Paraovarian Cyst
  - Polycystic Ovaries (PCO Syndrome, Stein–Leventhal Syndrome)
  - Cystic Ovarian Tumors

Ovaries (Continue)

Solid Echogenic or Non-homogeneous Mass — 407
- Endometriotic Cysts
- Thecomatosis
- Inflammatory Adnexal Mass
- Ovarian Carcinoma
- Metastases
- Pseudomyxoma peritonei
- Ovarian Tumors (by Histological Criteria)

13 Female Genital Tract

B. Beuscher-Willems [*]

Transabdominal ultrasound. Transabdominal scanning of the lower abdomen should be done for screening purposes as part of every abdominal ultrasound examination. The use of ultrasonography in gynecology was first described by Donald in 1958[5]. Today, transvaginal sonography has become the procedure of first choice for gynecological investigations. The short penetration depth permits the use of a higher-frequency transducer, which provides higher resolution and more detailed images. Transvaginal sonography has been practiced increasingly since about 1985.

Transabdominal ultrasound is still important in gynecology, especially as an adjunct to transvaginal scanning, in defining the boundaries and extent of large masses. With its greater penetration depth, transabdominal ultrasound is also useful for evaluating positional anomalies. Other indications for transabdominal scanning exist in patients with an imperforate hymen or vaginal stenosis, or patients who refuse transvaginal ultrasound (**Table 13.1**).

Appearance of the genital tract. The physiological appearance of the female genital tract varies with hormonal changes relating to the menstrual cycle and to age. The sex hormones (estrogens, progestins, androgens) are produced in the ovaries, and ovarian function is regulated by means of a feedback control loop (hypothalamus [gonadotropin-releasing hormone = GnRH] → anterior pituitary [gonadotropins] → ovary [sex hormones]). The gonadotropins (follicle-stimulating hormone FSH, luteinizing hormone LH, and prolactin PRL) are synthesized in the anterior lobe of the pituitary gland.

The likelihood that an abnormal process exists in the female genital tract also depends on the age and hormonal status of the patient. Knowing the patient's period of life and clinical presentation is an essential part of the overall assessment and in formulating a differential diagnosis. Thus a distinction is drawn between examinations performed before menarche, during the reproductive years, during and after menopause, and in old age.

Table 13.1 **Indications for transabdominal ultrasound scanning in gynecology**

- Lower abdominal pain
- Urinary stasis
- Tumor screening
- Defining the extent of large tumors
- Follow-ups
- Positional anomalies
- Intact hymen
- Vaginal stenosis
- Refusal of transvaginal sonography

Periods of Life in the Female

- **Neonatal period,** initially still influenced by maternal hormones
- **Childhood**
- **Puberty,** including premenarche and postmenarche and marked by increasing ovarian function
- **Adolescence,** marked by feminization
- **Sexual maturity,** marked by the onset of fertility and biphasic menstrual cycles
- **Menopause,** including premenopause with relative estrogenism and luteal insufficiency
- **Postmenopause,** marked by declining estrogen production
- **Old age**

Topography (Figs. 13.1–13.3)

Relations of the genital organs
- Located in the lesser pelvis, predominantly intraperitoneal
- Anterior to the rectum
- Posterior to the bladder
- Medial to the psoas muscle
- Superior and medial to the iliac wings
- Posterior to the pubic bone and symphysis

Sonographic landmarks
- Bladder
- Rectum
- Internal and external iliac vein

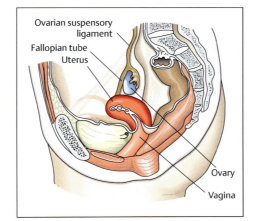

◀ **Fig. 13.1** Relations of the female internal genital organs: vagina, uterus, fallopian tubes, and ovaries.

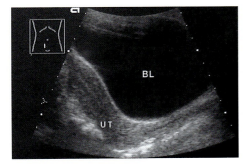
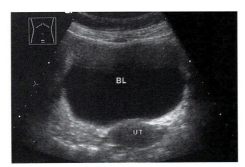

◀◀ **Fig. 13.2** Longitudinal scan of the uterus (UT) and vagina.

◀ **Fig. 13.3** Transverse scan of the uterine fundus.

---

[*] The transvaginal ultrasound images were provided by Heilbronn Womens Hospital, whose help is gratefully acknowledged.

Vagina

Ultrasound Morphology

The vagina is a flattened tube leading to the uterus. With its anterior and posterior walls composed of mucosal and muscular layers, the vagina appears as a thin, multilayered band in longitudinal and transverse ultrasound scans through the lower abdomen (**Figs. 13.4 and 13.5**). The vagina may appear echogenic to hypoechoic, depending on the angle at which it is scanned. In some cases ultrasound can distinguish a high-level entry echo followed by the hypoechoic anterior wall, a bright luminal echo at the center, the hypoechoic posterior wall, and a bright exit echo. The lumen may also be hypoechoic, depending on the fluid and mucosal content of the vagina.

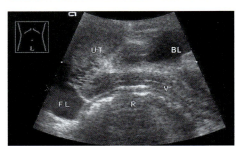
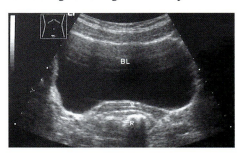

◂◂ *Fig. 13.4* Longitudinal scan of the vagina. UT = uterus; BL = bladder; V = vagina; R = rectum; FL = fluid in the cul-de-sac.

◂ *Fig. 13.5* Transverse scan of the vagina. BL = bladder; V = vagina; R = rectum.

Masses

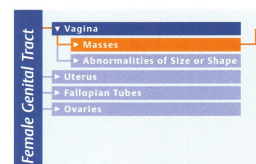

- ▶ Imperforate Hymen with Hematocolpos
- ▶ Vaginal Wall Cyst
- ▶ Double Vagina, Septate Vagina
- ▶ Tampon
- ▶ Vaginal Carcinoma

▶ Imperforate Hymen with Hematocolpos

An imperforate hymen does not become clinically apparent until puberty. With menarche, the patient experiences monthly lower abdominal pain and increasing malaise with an absence of menstrual bleeding. The blood pools in the vagina (hematocolpos) and may reflux into the uterus (hematometra) or fallopian tubes (hematosalpinx). The pseudotumor may extend to the level of the umbilicus.

Hematocolpos. Ultrasound demonstrates an almost anechoic mass of variable size and extent in the vagina, located posterior and inferior to the bladder. The uterus, which shows increased echogenicity, is displaced upward and is often barely detectable in its position above the mass (**Fig. 13.6**).

Hematometra. The blood may back up into the uterus, resulting in an enlarged anechoic mass posterior to the bladder.

Hematosalpinx. The fallopian tubes may also fill with blood, causing extension of the mass lateral to the bladder.

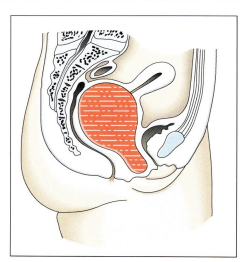

▲ *Fig. 13.6* Hematocolpos.

▶ Vaginal Wall Cyst

Vaginal wall cysts are remnants of the wolffian duct (mesonephric duct), appearing sonographically as anechoic, smooth-bordered masses located caudal to the bladder. The development of carcinoma in vaginal wall cysts is known to occur.

▶ Double Vagina, Septate Vagina

Malformations are somewhat rare and result from fusion anomalies of the müllerian ducts. In 40% of cases, malformations of the vagina are combined with anomalies of the kidneys and urinary tract.

When a double vagina is scanned with ultrasound, it initially appears thickened with a central, echogenic band. The two hypoechoic lumina can be distinguished when viewed in transverse section. Differentiation from a septate vagina is often difficult.

Only certain vaginal malformations are detectable by transabdominal scanning, and generally it is difficult to evaluate all malformations with ultrasound alone. A gynecological examination and additional tests (hysteroscopy and laparoscopy) are required.

▶ Tampon

A tampon appears caudal to the bladder as a very echogenic mass with indistinct margins and a posterior acoustic shadow (**Fig. 13.7**). The nature of the mass is easily determined by questioning the patient.

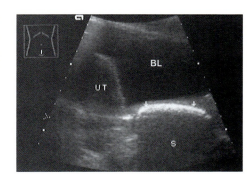

◀ **Fig. 13.7** Intravaginal tampon appears as an elongated, echogenic mass with an acoustic shadow (S). BL = bladder; UT = uterus.

▶ Vaginal Carcinoma

The most frequent site of occurrence is the posterior fornix. Squamous cell carcinomas are the most common and tend to be locally invasive (rectum, uterus, bladder) and seed locoregional metastases (**Fig. 13.8**).

Abnormalities of Size or Shape

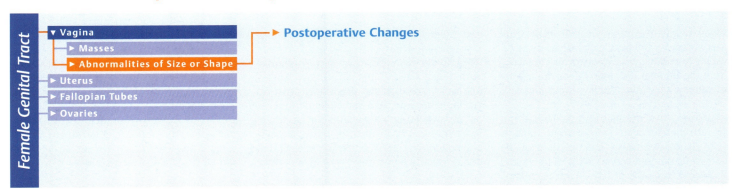

▶ Postoperative Changes

Hysterectomy and other operations can cause pronounced changes in the shape and position of the vagina (**Fig. 13.9**). A knowledge of the prior history will aid interpretation of the ultrasound findings.

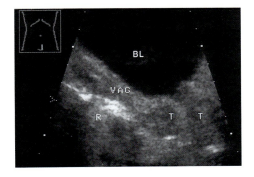

◀ **Fig. 13.8** Vaginal carcinoma (T): hypoechoic mass infiltrating the rectum (R) and bladder (BL). VAG = vagina.

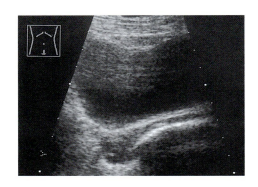
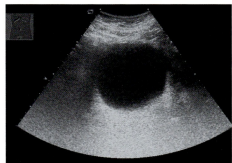

◄ **Fig. 13.9 a** Vaginal fornix after hysterectomy.

◄ **b** Bladder following resection of the uterus, vagina, and rectum: complete acoustic enhancement posteroinferior to the bladder. No organic structures are visualized.

Uterus

Anatomy

Position
- Anteversion, anteflexion (normal finding)
- Retroversion
- Straight (especially in old age, when it is more difficult to evaluate by transvaginal scanning; the fundus should be manually flexed forward)

Uterine size and shape
- Prepubertal
  - 2–3.3 cm long, 1 cm wide, 0.5–1 cm thick
  - Cervical diameter is greater than the corpus diameter. The cervix accounts for two-thirds of total uterine length
- Nullipara
  - Pear-shaped
  - 5–9 cm long, transverse diameter 1.6–4 cm, 3 cm thick
- Multipara
  - 10 × 5 × 6 cm
  - Uterine corpus comprises the upper two-thirds of the total length, the cervix the lower third
- Postmenopause
  - 4.5 cm long, 2 cm wide, 1.5 cm thick
  - Symmetrically hyperplastic

Uterine weight
- Adolescence: 44–66 g
- Childbearing age: 80–120 g
- Pregnancy: weight increases 20-fold from 50 g to 1000 g

Blood supply. The uterus (including the distal part bordering the bladder) receives its blood supply from the uterine artery, which branches from the internal iliac artery. It is drained by valveless veins of the uterine venous plexus.

Histology. The uterine wall consists of a smooth-muscle layer (myometrium) and a very glandular mucosa (endometrium of the uterine corpus and cervix). Most of the uterus is covered by a layer of serosa (perimetrium).

The endometrium of the uterine corpus consists of a single row of columnar epithelium and undergoes cyclic changes in its structure and function in response to ovarian steroids. The endocervix responds to these hormones with functional but not structural changes. The cyclic structural and size changes that occur in the myometrium and endometrium can be appreciated at ultrasound. The postmenstrual uterus is small and firm. During the second half of the cycle, the uterine wall thickens due to cellular hypertrophy. The myometrium contains abundant ovarian steroids owing to its estrogen and progesterone receptors.

Endometrium. Cyclic changes in the endometrium were first described by Hirschmann and Adler in 1908. During the proliferative phase in the first half of the cycle, estrogens stimulate an increase in endometrial thickness and vascularity that continues until the LH surge. During the second half of the cycle following ovulation, glycogen-filled vacuoles develop in response to progesterone. Mucus-filled glands develop in the later secretory phase of the cycle, and spiral arteries are formed. The regression phase begins several days before menstruation, as hormone production wanes and the thickness of the mucosa decreases by approximately 50% owing to fluid loss. The hormones decline precipitously in the desquamation phase, and the endometrial lining is sloughed. A regenerative phase follows menstruation, reinitiating the cycle.

Uterine cervix. The cervix consists mainly of connective tissue and a few smooth-muscle fibers, with the result that it undergoes minimal cyclic structural changes. The cervical canal is lined by columnar epithelium and increases its diameter at midcycle. The cervical mucus becomes more fluid in response to estrogens and then more viscous again in response to increased progesterone.

Ultrasound Morphology (Figs. 13.10–13.12)

Even the normal uterus is subject to certain variations. To interpret the findings correctly, it must be known whether the patient is prepubertal, sexually mature, premenstrual, or postmenstrual at the time of the examination. This also has an important bearing on differential diagnostic considerations. For example, lower abdominal pain in an adolescent girl is more likely due to appendicitis than to a gynecological tumor. If a tumor is present in an adolescent patient, it will tend to undergo rapid enlargement owing to the high rate of proliferation.

Echogenicity
- Outer serosa: hyperechoic
- Myometrium: uniformly hypoechoic; vessels appear as anechoic areas
- Endometrium and cervical canal: hyperechoic
- Cervix: may contain anechoic areas corresponding to nabothian follicles

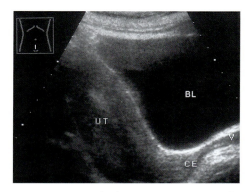
▲ **Fig. 13.10** Longitudinal uterine scan posterior to the bladder. Anteflexion is clearly defined. UT = uterine corpus; BL = bladder.

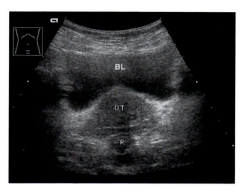
▲ **Fig. 13.11** Transverse scan through the uterus (UT) and rectum (R). BL = bladder.

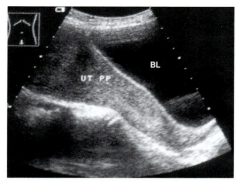
▲ **Fig. 13.12** Postpartum uterus (UT PP). Uterine length is still approximately 16 cm. BL = bladder.

Abnormalities of Size or Shape

Female Genital Tract
- Vagina
- ▼ Uterus
  - ► Abnormalities of Size or Shape
  - Myometrial Changes
  - Intracavitary Changes
  - Endometrial Changes
- Fallopian Tubes
- Ovaries

► **Uterine Prolapse**
► **Malformations**
► **Uterine Aplasia, Atresia**
► **Uterine Hypoplasia, Small Uterus**
► **Hemangioma, Lymphoma, Angiomyoma, Myoma**

► Uterine Prolapse

Atypical and abnormal positions of the uterus affect the shape of the uterus as displayed by ultrasound (**Fig. 13.13**).

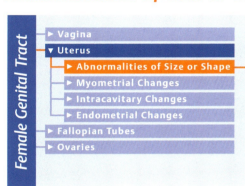
◄ **Fig. 13.13** Uterine prolapse. The uterus appears somewhat straightened, and the cervix (C) extends far caudally.

► Malformations

- Bicornuate uterus
  - Uterus bicornis unicollis
  - Uterus bicornis bicolli
- Subseptate uterus
- Uterus septus duplex (uterus bilocularis) with a septate vagina
- Arcuate uterus
- Uterus didelphys with two vaginas

Uterus bicornis unicollis is the most common malformation (**Fig. 13.14**). On the posterior aspect of the bladder, the two hypoechoic uterine horns curve around the floor and posterior wall of the bladder. This creates the appearance of a hypoechoic triangle in the lower abdominal transverse scan. Two separate endometrial echoes (thick proliferative endometrium) are seen in a transverse scan through the uterine horns at midcycle, which is the best time for detecting this anomaly when it is suspected. The malformations listed above are commonly associated with renal anomalies, and therefore the kidneys should be included in the ultrasound examination[1].

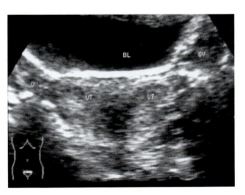
▲ **Fig. 13.14** Bicornuate uterus. UT = uterine horns; OV = ovaries; BL = bladder.

▶ Uterine Aplasia, Atresia

Uterine aplasia, characterized by a rudimentary uterus, is seen in Rokitansky–Küstner syndrome (vaginal aplasia). Despite a full bladder, the uterus either is not visualized or appears only in a rudimentary form. This aplasia is rare and congenital.

Uterine atresia, on the other hand, is an acquired condition (**Fig. 13.15**).

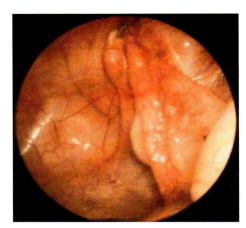

◂ *Fig. 13.15* Rudimentary uterus (snared) in uterine atresia.

▶ Uterine Hypoplasia, Small Uterus

Uterine hypoplasia occurs in patients with incomplete vaginal aplasia (affecting only the lower third). Hematometra may develop, giving the uterus an anechoic appearance.

A small uterus (4.5 cm × 1.5 cm × 2 cm) is a normal finding in postmenopausal women.

▶ Hemangioma, Lymphoma, Angiomyoma, Myoma

Benign tumors can cause significant changes in the size and shape of the uterus, depending on their size and location.

Myometrial Changes

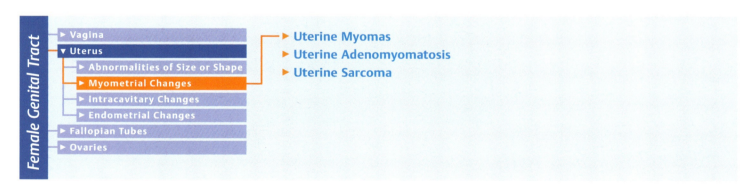

▶ Uterine Myomas

Myomas (fibroids) are muscular tumors of the uterus, generally classified histologically as fibroleiomyomas[5]. Myomas are benign tumors composed of smooth muscle and connective tissue. They are the most common type of genital tumor.

The formation and growth of uterine myomas depend on the functional status of the ovaries (relative estrogen dominance). Myomas do not occur in children or the elderly and tend to regress after menopause. Antiestrogens and progesterone inhibit their growth.

Myomas develop in the uterine corpus and cervix. They are rarely solitary and may have an intramural, subserous, submucous, or intraligamentous location. Myomas lack a true capsule. The tumor nodules are initially round but may alter their shape owing to pressure effects. Myomas undergo structural changes over time:

Malacia, characterized by the following changes:
▶ Cavernous transformation, permeation by edema
▶ Rapid myxomatous growth
▶ Tense cystic appearance, resembling an ovarian cyst
▶ Fatty degeneration (especially in the puerperium)
▶ Necrotic foci due to vascular occlusion
▶ Suppuration due to infection ascending from the uterine cavity, spreading from the bowel, or transmitted by blood vessels or lymphatics; breakdown by putrefactive bacteria, especially in submucous myomas

Induration, consisting of the following changes:
- Progressive fibrous transformation, ranging to a pure fibroma
- Irregular or eggshell calcification. Fully calcified myomas may become dislodged, resulting in the "delivery" of uterine stones.

Sonographic features. Approximately 25% of all women over age 35 have uterine myomas[10]. These tumors appear sharply circumscribed at ultrasound. Initially they are largely homogeneous and less echogenic than the rest of the myometrium owing to their copious blood supply.

Most myomas are subserous in location (■ **13.1 a**). Five percent of myomas are submucous[9]; they often cause bleeding abnormalities and are not palpable. Diffuse myomatosis is found in many multiparous women, leading to uterine enlargement with no circumscribed nodularity (■ **13.1 c**).

Degenerating myomas appear as hyperechoic masses. Calcified myomas cast an acoustic shadow that can obscure surrounding structures (■ **13.1 d, e**). Central necrosis, due, for example, to tumor growth outstripping blood supply, appears as an anechoic area (■ **13.1 f**).

Pedunculated or intraligamentous myomas can mimic an adnexal tumor. Unequivocal visualization of the stalk, as by color duplex examination, is required. Myomas cannot be distinguished sonographically from other tumors with absolute confidence. Rapid enlargement is suggestive of sarcomatous transformation.

The enlargement of a myoma is normal in early pregnancy and requires surveillance[10]. Large myomas can obstruct delivery[3].

Clinical Presentation

Myomas present clinically with bleeding abnormalities such as hypermenorrhea (usually only intramural myomas affect uterine wall contractility), menorrhagia, and metrorrhagia (caused by submucous myomas). Dysmenorrhea is caused by capsular tension or contractions and also depends on the tumor location.

Myomas can also cause bladder complaints and constipation or hydronephrosis (intraligamentous myoma) (■ **13.1 g–i**). A ruptured myoma capsule can produce the signs and symptoms of an acute abdomen. Myomas can cause infertility. A necrotic myoma can lead to an elevated ESR.

■ 13.1 Uterine Myomas

- Solitary and multiple myomas
- Diffuse myomatosis

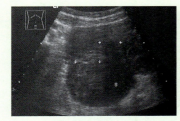 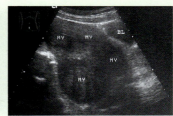 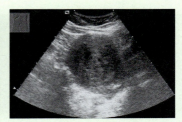

a Subserous myoma. S = shadow. *b* Multiple myomas (MY) in the uterus. BL = bladder. *c* Diffuse myomatosis with uterine enlargement.

- Calcifications and necrosis

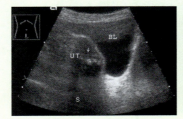 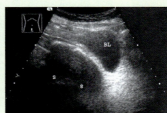 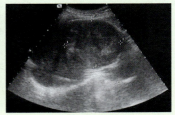

d Uterine myoma with diffuse calcification. UT = Uterine sarcoma; BL = bladder; S = shadow. *e* Uterine myoma with eggshell calcification and acoustic shadowing (S). BL = bladder. *f* Uterine myoma with central hypoechoic necrosis.

- Renal pelvic obstruction

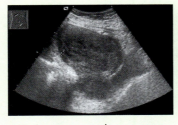 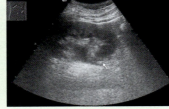 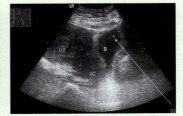

g Uterine myoma, nonhomogeneous, compressing the ureter. *h* Obstructed renal pelvis, drained with a DJ stent (arrow). *i* Uterusfornix (UF) with myoma, club-like cervix (UC), bladder (B) with indwelling DJ ureteral stent.

▶ Uterine Adenomyomatosis

The presence of endometrial cells in the myomas leads to the development of uterine endometriosis—more accurately termed adenomyosis—which may be associated with hypermenorrhea and dysmenorrhea. One-third of patients are asymptomatic.

The uterus is uniformly enlarged and shows a number of 1–5 mm sized hypoechoic zones in the myometrium, which may grow considerably larger if intramural hemorrhage occurs.

The posterior uterine wall is more commonly affected than other wall regions (**Figs. 13.16 and 13.17**).

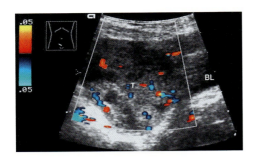
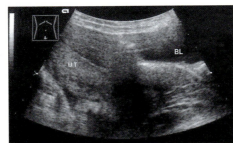

Fig. 13.16 Adenomyosis with hypoechoic foci in the myometrium. T = enlarged uterus; BL = bladder.

Fig. 13.17 Adenomyosis: hypoechoic foci in the posterior uterine wall. UT = uterus; BL = bladder.

▶ Uterine Sarcoma

Sarcomas of the uterus account for 2–4% of uterine cancers. The majority are mixed sarcomas. The most common type, leiomyosarcomas of the uterine wall (uterine wall sarcoma), can be difficult to distinguish from benign myomas. The mitotic rate is an important criterion for assessing malignancy. Sarcomas are softer than myomas, bleed easily, and show a greater degree of necrosis. There are also stromal sarcomas of the endometrium (mucosal sarcomas, see below). Carcinosarcomas are mixed mesodermal tumors that contain both sarcomatous and adenocarcinomatous elements.

Most sarcomas are detected incidentally in myomas that have been surgically removed.

Sonographic features. Sarcoma appears sonographically as a nonhomogeneous hypoechoic mass with some anechoic elements and ill-defined margins. Rapid enlargement is noted in follow-up scans (**Figs. 13.18 and 13.19**).

Treatment consists of surgical removal of the uterus and adnexa followed by irradiation. The prognosis is poorer than with uterine carcinoma.

Features Helpful in Distinguishing Uterine Carcinoma from Myoma

- ▶ Rapid uterine enlargement
- ▶ Uterine enlargement after menopause
- ▶ Change in the uterine cavity
- ▶ Secondary changes such as renal obstruction and lymph node enlargement
- ▶ Late signs such as discomfort, ascites, and cachexia

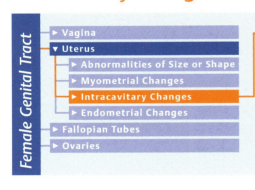
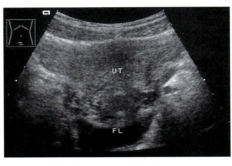

▲ *Fig. 13.18* Fast-growing uterine myoma: well-circumscribed mass showing only slight nonhomogeneity.

▲ *Fig. 13.19* Uterine sarcoma (UT): fast-growing, nonhomogeneous mass with ascites (FL).

Intracavitary Changes

- ▶ Vagina
- ▼ Uterus
  - ▶ Abnormalities of Size or Shape
  - ▶ Myometrial Changes
  - ▶ Intracavitary Changes
  - ▶ Endometrial Changes
- ▶ Fallopian Tubes
- ▶ Ovaries

- ▶ **Foreign Body (IUD)**
- ▶ **Mucocele, Serometra, Pyometra, Hematometra**
- ▶ **Pregnancy**
- ▶ **Ectopic Pregnancy**
- ▶ **Missed Abortion, Incomplete Abortion, Cervical Pregnancy**
- ▶ **Endometrial Polyps, Cervical Polyps, Placental Polyps**

▶ Foreign Body (IUD)

An intrauterine contraceptive device (IUD) appears as an intensely echogenic band with slightly indistinct margins at the center of the uterus. The shape and sharpness of the foreign body are variable, depending on the type of IUD (**Figs. 13.20 and 13.21**).

Contraceptive Protection

Today the IUD is the second most widely used contraceptive in the world. Before an IUD is inserted, transvaginal sonography should be performed to measure the size of the uterine cavity and exclude an obstructing myoma. The position of the IUD should be checked regularly to ensure contraceptive protection. The distance of the IUD from the fundus is normally 1 cm and should not exceed 2 cm. In a uterus with myomas, it is difficult to confirm correct IUD placement. The examination should be scheduled for midcycle when the uterus has a thick, proliferative endometrium.

The incidence of ectopic pregnancy is 4–5 times higher in IUD wearers.

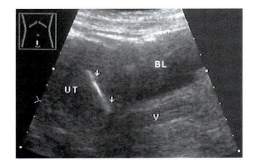
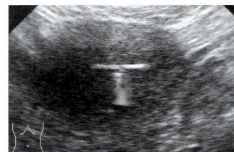

◄◄ *Fig. 13.20* IUD (arrows): very echogenic structure in the uterine cavity. Correct placement is indicated if the distance between the endometrium and IUD is less than 5 mm. UT = uterus; BL = bladder; V = vagina.

◄ *Fig. 13.21* T-shaped IUD.

► Mucocele, Serometra, Pyometra, Hematometra

Mucocele. A mucocele is a collection of secretions retained in the uterine cavity, especially around menopause. The cause of the obstructed drainage may be a carcinoma.

Serometra. This refers to an excessive accumulation of endometrial discharge due to intermittent cervical obstruction. The discharge may have a malignant or inflammatory cause (**Fig. 13.22**).

Pyometra. Pyometra occurs as a complication of endometrial carcinoma owing to stenosis of the cervical canal. Its sonographic hallmark is a dilated, hypoechoic uterine cavity. Underlying endometrial carcinoma is present in more than 50% of cases.

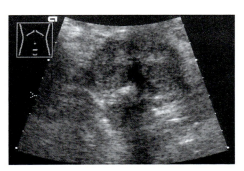
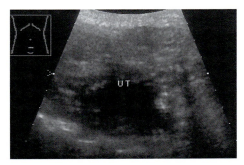

▲ *Fig. 13.22 a* Serometra: hypoechoic mass in the uterine cavity.

▲ *b* Hematometra: anechoic mass within the uterine cavity (UT), caused by anticoagulant therapy.

► Pregnancy

Pregnancy should be considered in patients undergoing ultrasound for lower abdominal pain or unexplained vomiting, and an ectopic pregnancy should be excluded.

In an intrauterine pregnancy, the normal anechoic chorionic cavity can be seen at an eccentric location in the uterus as early as 2 weeks' gestational age (**Fig. 13.23**). Its size increases by approximately 1 mm/day. By the 5th week, a ringlike structure can be seen in the chorionic cavity, representing the secondary yolk sac. This structure is of embryonic origin and affords proof of intrauterine pregnancy[1] (**Fig. 13.24**). The normal average diameter of the chorionic cavity is 5.5 cm (3–7 cm). Deviations from the norm signify a developmental anomaly, and karyotyping should be performed. The chorionic cavity is surrounded by the hyperechoic chorion, which displays a typical ringlike vascular pattern.

As gestation progresses, the product of conception becomes visible and embryofetal details can be defined and evaluated (**Figs. 13.25 and 13.26**).

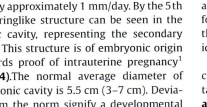
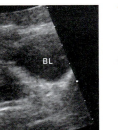
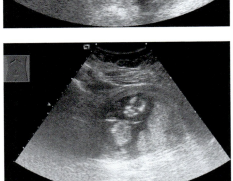
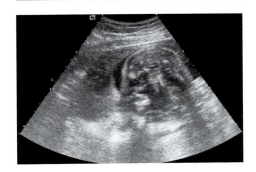

◄◄ *Fig. 13.23* Anechoic chorionic cavity in the third week of pregnancy, surrounded by the hyperechoic chorion.

◄ *Fig. 13.24* Early pregnancy with a chorionic cavity and hyperechoic conceptus. UT = uterus; BL = bladder.

◄◄ *Fig. 13.25* Embryo in the 12th week of pregnancy.

◄ *Fig. 13.26* Fetus in the 27th week of pregnancy. Male genitals are visible between the thighs.

▶ Ectopic Pregnancy

In an ectopic pregnancy (1:100 births)[10], a pseudogestational sac may appear at the center of the uterus. This fluid collection is caused by a decidual reaction within the slitlike uterine cavity. The sac rarely exceeds 2 cm in diameter, lacks an echogenic rim, and does not enlarge. A mass with a hyperechoic ring and anechoic center can be demonstrated in the adnexal region. Since this usually represents a tubal abortion, a conceptus is not present.

Ectopic pregnancy occurs more frequently when an IUD is in place (**Fig. 13.27**). It is extremely rare for an intrauterine pregnancy to coexist with an IUD: 1:35 000 pregnancies[10].

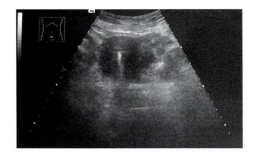

◀ *Fig. 13.27* Ectopic pregnancy: thickened, hypoechoic fallopian tube with an IUD in the uterine cavity (high-level echo).

▶ Missed Abortion, Incomplete Abortion, Cervical Pregnancy

In a missed abortion, either the chorionic cavity does not contain a conceptus or the conceptus is rudimentary and fails to develop further. The adnexa appear normal.

In an incomplete abortion, structures with irregular outlines and varying echogenicity can be demonstrated within the uterine cavity. The hyperechoic areas are retained products of conception, while hypoechoic areas represent small pockets of blood.

In some cases the remnants of an incomplete abortion may be found entirely in the cervical region. Differentiation is then required from an abnormal cervical pregnancy, which is recognized by a clublike expansion of the cervix[9].

▶ Endometrial Polyps, Cervical Polyps, Placental Polyps

Endometrial polyps. Like adenomas, polyps arise from local sites of mucosal hypertrophy and project into the uterine cavity. They are usually benign. They may be pedunculated, and the pedicle may be so long that the polyp protrudes from the cervical os. Endometrial polyps are usually solitary. Large polyps can form in response to increased estrogen production after menopause. Treatment in bleeding patients consists of dilatation and curettage. Further surveillance is indicated because of the risk of carcinoma.

Sonographically, the endometrium is hyperechoic and thickened with indistinct borders (**Fig. 13.28**). If a mucocele or serometra is present, the polyps will be clearly delineated within the anechoic or hypoechoic uterine cavity.

Cervical polyps. More common than endometrial polyps, cervical polyps are lentil-size to cherry-size growths that may be seen in the cervical os during speculum examination. Removal of these polyps should be followed by dilatation and curettage. Cervical polyps should not be removed during pregnancy.

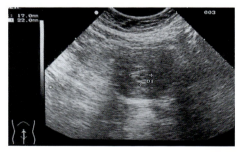

▲ *Fig. 13.28* Endometrial polyp (histological finding): thickened, hyperechoic endometrium in a menopausal patient on tamoxifen. Nonhomogeneous uterine cavity.

Endometrial Changes

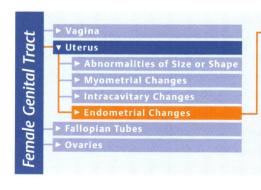

- ▶ Proliferative Endometrium (Midcycle)
- ▶ Cystic Glandular and Atypical Adenomatous Hyperplasia
- ▶ Endometritis, Cervicitis
- ▶ Corpus Carcinoma
- ▶ Chorioepithelioma
- ▶ Cervical Carcinoma

▶ Proliferative Endometrium (Midcycle)

The endometrium is more echogenic than the myometrium and appears as an oblong or elliptical structure with homogeneous echogenicity and smooth margins at the center of the uterus. Its thickness varies during the menstrual cycle.

Endometrial thickness is measured sonographically as twice the single-wall thickness, or the sum of both visible endometrial layers minus the intervening cavity.

Normal values of endometrial thickness. The normal thickness values are hormone-dependent:
- Postmenopausal (without hormone replacement) < 8 mm
- Postmenstrual 0
- Premenstrual 8–15 mm

The menstrual history is helpful in correctly interpreting the image.

Pathological findings in the endometrium. The principal findings are as follows:
- Thickness > 15 mm, or > (5–) 8 mm after menopause.
- Nonhomogeneous echo pattern with microcystic or macrocystic changes, which may be benign or malignant. Cysts smaller than 3 mm are typically benign.
- Indistinct endometrial/myometrial boundary.

A small amount of fluid in the uterine cavity does not have pathological significance.

A homogeneous endometrium more than 8 mm thick warrants ultrasound surveillance. The differential diagnosis includes hyperplasia and early endometrial carcinoma. Cytological examination is inconclusive, and the diagnosis is established by curettage.

A bright internal echo in the uterine cavity with a homogeneous endometrium, seen particularly well in the presence of serometra, may be an endometrial polyp. This is confirmed by removing the lesion for histology.

It is normal after ovulation to find a small amount of free fluid in the rectouterine pouch. Other causes of ascites should be excluded, however.

Cyclic Endometrial Changes

- *After menstruation:* no visible endometrium.
- *Proliferative phase:* central echogenic line 3 mm thick **(Fig. 13.29)**.
- *Midcycle:* hyperechoic boundary with the myometrium, bright central echo, gaping cervical canal; graafian follicle may be detectable **(Fig. 13.30)**.
- *Secretory phase:* During the secretory phase after ovulation, luteal hormones stimulate increasing transformation of the tubular glands and glandular secretions, giving the endometrium a porous, edematous appearance. The mucosa initially shows alternating hypoechoic and echogenic layers. The overall echogenicity of the endometrium increases during the luteal phase while the bright central echo disappears **(Fig. 13.31)**, culminating in a well-defined hypoechoic center caused by collected secretions **(Fig. 13.32)**.
- *Postmenopause:* The postmenopausal endometrium appears at most as an echogenic band less than 8 mm thick, usually without a detectable cavity.

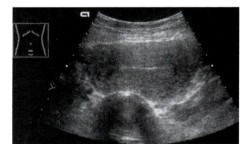

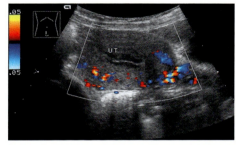

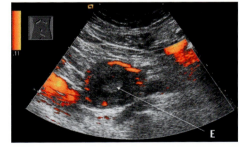

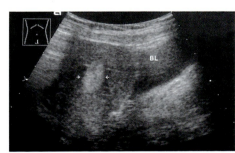

◂◂ **Fig. 13.29** Proliferative phase: endometrium with a fine central echo (first half of cycle).

◂ **Fig. 13.30** Endometrial layers at midcycle: hyperechoic – hypoechoic – hyperechoic – hypoechoic – hyperechoic.

◂◂ **Fig. 13.31** Uniformly echogenic endometrium (E) during the secretory phase after ovulation, with no central echo. Normal, circular myometrium blood flow pattern is clearly defined by power Doppler.

◂ **Fig. 13.32** Thick, proliferative endometrium (arrows), hyperechoic with a hypoechoic center. BL = bladder.

▶ Cystic Glandular Hyperplasia and Atypical Adenomatous Hyperplasia

Cystic glandular hyperplasia occurs in an anovulatory cycle with a persistent follicle[9].

Atypical adenomatous hyperplasia is diagnosed histologically by curettage. It is a precancerous lesion that progresses to corpus carcinoma in 20% of cases.

Women who take tamoxifen (antiestrogen) are at increased risk for developing endometrial carcinoma.

▶ Endometritis, Cervicitis

Inflammation of the endometrium due to tuberculosis or other diseases spreads by a descending route and may also involve the cervix (cervicitis) and vagina (colpitis) (**Fig. 13.33**). Estrogen production promotes inflammatory changes. One-third of cases of tuberculous salpingitis occur during puberty. The most common cause is an infected IUD.

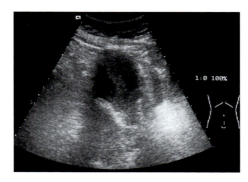

◀ *Fig. 13.33* Endometritis, myometritis.
a Hypoechoic uterus with indistinct borders, a retrouterine abscess, marked tenderness to pressure, and a foul-smelling discharge.

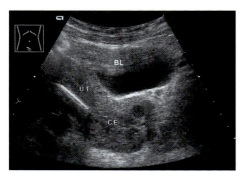

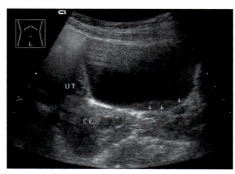

◀◀ *b* Posterior to the bladder (BL), the cervix (CE) is markedly expanded and contains hypoechoic foci signifying microabscesses. The uterus (UT) contains an IUD.

◀ *c* Cervicitis (CE) with parauterine lymph nodes (arrows).

▶ Corpus Carcinoma

Histology. Carcinoma of the uterine corpus is generally an endometrial cancer. The majority are adenocarcinomas (40%). Corpus carcinoma arises from the endometrium of the uterine fundus, usually in the cornual region. A typical lesion is adenocarcinoma of the endometrium with extensive squamous cell metaplasia, found in 28% of cases (these tumors are called adenocancroids or adenocanthomas). Squamous cell carcinoma of the uterine corpus is rare, accounting for less than 1% of lesions. Stromal cancers (mucosal sarcomas) can also arise from the endometrium.

Risk factors. Tumor growth is estrogen-dependent and is mediated by estrogen receptors on the glandular epithelial and stromal cells. This is why years of unopposed estrogen stimulation is thought to be associated with a higher risk of endometrial carcinoma (ovarian tumors, polycystic ovaries, hepatic cirrhosis, etc.).

An increased risk exists in endometrial carcinoma syndrome with overweight, hypertension, and glucose intolerance or diabetes mellitus. The principal risk factor is age, and women with a higher social standing seem to be predisposed.

Growth pattern. Corpus carcinoma grows slowly on the mucosa or may form a polypoid lesion projecting into the uterine cavity; thus it stays confined to the mucosa for some time. It eventually invades the myometrium by contiguous spread but rarely penetrates the serosa. Metastasis occurs much later than with cervical carcinoma and only after the tumor has permeated the outer third of the myometrium. Distant metastases are rare and occur at a late stage. Bleeding usually directs attention to the cancer while it is still confined to the uterine corpus.

FIGO and TNM Staging for Corpus Carcinoma

0/Tis	Carcinoma in situ
I/T1	Tumor confined to the uterine corpus
IA/T1a	Tumor confined to the endometrium
IB/T1b	Tumor invades less than half of the myometrium
IC/T1c	Tumor invades half or more of the myometrium
II/T2	Tumor invades the cervix
IIA/T2a	Spread limited to the endocervix
IIB/T2b	Tumor also invades the cervical stroma
III/T3	Spread in the lesser pelvis
IIIA/T3a	Tumor involves the serosa and/or adnexa, and/or tumor detected in ascites
IIIB/T3b	Vaginal involvement
IIIC/N1	Pelvic or para-aortic lymph node metastases
IVA/T4	Invasion of the bladder and/or rectum
IVB/M1	Distant lymph node metastases outside the lesser pelvis

Sonographic features. The sonographic hallmarks of endometrial carcinoma are as follows:
▶ Thick, hyperechoic endometrium
▶ Macrocystic changes
▶ Ill-defined margins
▶ Expansion of the uterine cavity by tumor with an exophytic growth pattern

The uterus may be larger than normal for age. Endometrial carcinoma appears more echogenic than the myometrium. The precise assessment of myometrial invasion has a crucial bearing on the prognosis. Transabdominal ultrasound is not suitable for this purpose, but transvaginal scanning can define the myometrium with great clarity (**Figs. 13.34 and 13.35**).

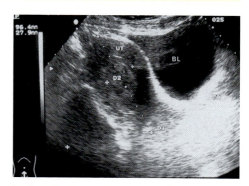

▲ *Fig. 13.34* Endometrial carcinoma (D2: 27.9 mm) in a postmenopausal patient. The uterus (UT, 96.4 mm long) is still just distinguishable from the myometrium by its greater echogenicity. BL = bladder.

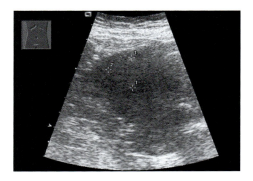
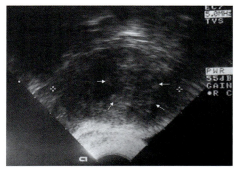

Fig. 13.35 Endometrial carcinoma.
a The tumor is just distinguishable by its higher echogenicity in the transabdominal scan.

b Transvaginal scan: 2 cm carcinoma (arrows) with ill-defined margins. Uterine width is 54 mm.

▶ Chorioepithelioma

Choriocarcinoma (malignant chorioepithelioma) arises from syncytial and Langhans cells of the placenta following a birth (20%), miscarriage (25%), or molar pregnancy (50%). It may develop after a latent period of several years. The overall incidence of chorioepithelioma is very low (1 : 100 000 births).

The tumor begins with a nodule in the endometrium, which grows rapidly into the uterine wall. Chorioepithelioma is extremely malignant and metastasizes early to lung, brain, kidney, bone, etc. Bleeding is a frequent complication. Serum levels of chorionic gonadotropins and α-hCG are elevated.

Ultrasound shows inadequate postpartum involution of the uterus in addition to an enlarging intracavitary mass. Because of the chorionic gonadotropins from chorioepithelioma, the ovaries contain corpora lutea at various developmental stages as well as granulosa and theca lutein cysts. As a result, cystic ovaries are frequently noted at ultrasonography.

▶ Cervical Carcinoma

Cervical carcinoma is usually a nonkeratinizing squamous cell carcinoma that metastasizes early to regional lymph nodes. Even with a microcarcinoma (FIGO IA2, TNM T1a2) not exceeding 5 cm in depth and 7 mm in its superficial extent, metastases are already present in 10% of cases. The tumor spreads contiguously to the vagina, uterus, and parametria. Distant metastases are rare and occur at a late stage.

Sonographic features. The carcinoma initially appears hyperechoic. Transabdominal ultrasound can detect the tumor only after it has reached an advanced stage (at least IB/T1b) (**Fig. 13.36**). With endophytic tumors, the cervix may appear greatly thickened; with exophytic tumors (less common), a cauliflower-like growth can be seen. A barrel-like distention of the cervix is most often seen with cancers of the cervical cavity. Over time the tumor may become less echogenic, particularly in response to treatment (**Fig. 13.37**). Transvaginal sonography (TVS) yields more accurate findings and permits an earlier diagnosis.

A sharply circumscribed, globular type of tumor requires differentiation from a uterine myoma. An extensive ovarian cancer can also mimic cervical carcinoma.

Complications. Ultrasound can detect the following complications due to tumor invasion:
▶ Rectal stenosis with bowel obstruction
▶ Ureteral obstruction with hydroureter and hydronephrosis

Other complications may arise:
▶ Infiltration of the sciatic nerve, causing sciatica
▶ Obstruction of the iliac vessels with inflow stasis of the vulva and lower extremities
▶ Infections, septic pyonephritis, and uremia

FIGO Staging for Cervical Carcinoma

0	Carcinoma in situ
I	Strictly confined to the cervix
II	Extends into the parametria (but not onto the pelvic sidewall) or the upper two-thirds of the vagina
III	Has spread onto the pelvic sidewall and/or involves the lower third of the vagina
IV	Has spread beyond the lesser pelvis to distant organs and/or has invaded the bladder, rectum, or both

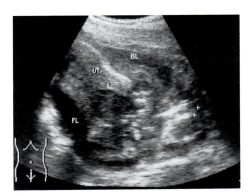
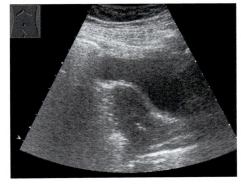

Fig. 13.36 Cervical carcinoma (arrows) spreading to the uterine corpus and vagina (arrows). Ulcerated tumor with free fluid (FL). UT = uterus; BL = bladder.

Fig. 13.37 Cervical carcinoma (stage IIIB, following irradiation and cisplatin chemotherapy): hypoechoic broadening of the cervix with tapered posterior margin due to tumor infiltration.

Fallopian Tubes

The fallopian tubes can be identified at their origin from the uterus, to the right and left of the uterine fundus. Their further course can be visualized only if pathological changes are present.

Hypoechoic Mass

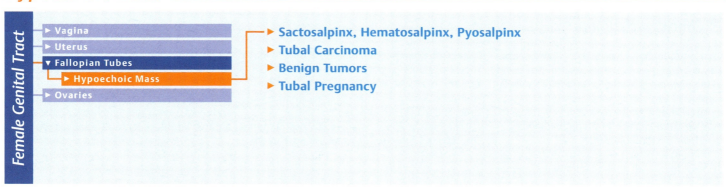

▶ Sactosalpinx, Hematosalpinx, Pyosalpinx

Definitions. Sactosalpinx is a hypoechoic mass between the uterus and ovary caused by a fluid collection in the fallopian tube due to various causes.

Hematosalpinx is a collection of blood extending into the fallopian tube, e.g., due to hymenal atresia.

Pyosalpinx is a collection of pus secondary to an inflammatory stenosis.

Sonographic features. The tubal wall appears sonographically as a pair of echogenic lines. With an abscess, the wall shows echogenic thickening (**Fig. 13.38**). The fallopian tube runs a tortuous course. When it contains a collection of clear fluid, the lumen is dilated and anechoic. With blood or pus in the tube, the lumen may appear echogenic and nonhomogeneous.

Differentiation. Color duplex examination can differentiate a fallopian tube from varicose vessels. Bowel loops generally have a hypoechoic wall that distinguishes them from the fallopian tube. Malignant masses tend to be painless, whereas inflammatory processes cause severe pain. Tubo-ovarian cysts are not true neoplasms but residua from pelvic inflammatory disease.

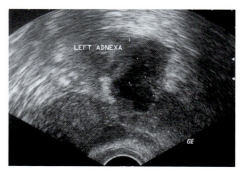

▲ **Fig. 13.38** Tubo-ovarian abscess. Transvaginal scan shows a hypoechoic mass with ill-defined margins (49.8 mm× 27 mm) in the left adnexa.

▶ Tubal Carcinoma

Only 0.3% of gynecological cancers are primary malignant tumors of the fallopian tube. The most common type is adenocarcinoma. Patients present clinically with pain on the affected side, discharge (50%), and bleeding (25%). The periodic drainage of large fluid volumes that is commonly seen with tubal carcinoma is termed hydrops tubae profluens. Thus, vaginal discharge assumes special significance in postmenopausal women and should always be investigated. Tumor cells are not found in material obtained by D&C, but the cytological examination of cervical secretions will reveal cancer cells. Given the copious lymphatic drainage of the fallopian tube region, metastases from tubal carcinoma are frequent. The prognosis is the same as for ovarian carcinoma.

Sonographic features. Tubal carcinomas are unilateral, round-to-oval lesions with a hypoechoic to hyperechoic appearance. The tube is often dilated distally and is tender to manual pressure. In its advanced stages, the tumor has the same appearance as ovarian carcinoma.

▶ Benign Tumors

Benign tumors of the fallopian tubes are very rare. The following types occur:
- Myomas
- Fibromas
- Lipomas
- Dermoids
- Lymphangiomas
- Adenomas

▶ Tubal Pregnancy

More than 90% of ectopic pregnancies are tubal pregnancies. The affected tube appears thickened and hypoechoic at transabdominal ultrasound (**Fig. 13.39**). Transvaginal sonography is definitely superior to transabdominal scanning in the diagnosis of tubal pregnancy.

With a ruptured tubal pregnancy, ultrasound will generally detect free fluid in the abdomen (**Fig. 13.40**).

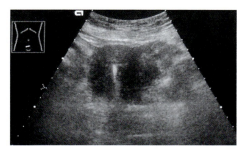

▲ *Fig. 13.39* Tubal pregnancy: thickened, hypoechoic fallopian tube with an IUD in place (high-level echo in the uterine cavity).

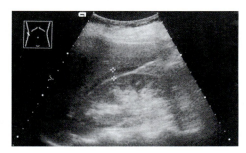

▲ *Fig. 13.40* Tubal rupture: free fluid (cursors) in the hepatorenal sinus following a tubal rupture due to ectopic pregnancy.

Ovaries

The ovaries undergo both structural and functional changes in response to gonadotropin production and aging. The sex hormones are synthesized in the ovaries.

The ovaries are highly variable in their size, shape, echogenicity, and position, making them difficult to visualize with ultrasound. Diseases of the ovaries are often detected at an extremely late stage owing to the delayed onset of symptoms.

Anatomy and Histology

The ovaries are small, firm, almond-shaped organs lying in the lesser pelvis. They are surrounded by a thin fibrous capsule (tunica albuginea). Their surface is smooth initially but becomes irregular over time owing to the pitting and scarring that result from follicular maturation and degeneration. The ovaries become scarred and atrophic after menopause.

The follicles (primordial follicles, primary and secondary follicles) are located in the very cellular cortical zone of the ovary, along with the corpora lutea and corpora albicantia. The cortical zone is continuous with the smaller medullary zone, with no distinct boundary between the two. The medullary zone is composed of connective tissue with occasional smooth-muscle cells and vessels.

Most of the ovary is intraperitoneal. Vessels enter the ovary at the hilum, which is extraperitoneal. The ovary is supplied by the ovarian arteries, which arise directly from the aorta below the renal artery, and by the ovarian branch of the uterine artery. The left ovarian artery occasionally arises from the left renal artery. The blood vessels run to the hilum in the ovarian suspensory ligament.

Arborizing valveless veins form a network, the pampiniform plexus (ovarian venous plexus), that surrounds the organs. The right ovarian vein opens directly into the vena cava, while the left ovarian vein drains into the left renal vein.

Topography

The ovaries of the nullipara lie in a small groove (ovarian fossa) in the lateral pelvic wall on both sides the uterus. They are located anterior to the ureter in the bifurcation of the common iliac artery (**Fig. 13.41**).

The ovaries are attached to the pelvic wall by the ovarian suspensory ligament and to the cornual area of the uterus by the proper ovarian ligament. They are attached posteriorly to the mesovarium by the broad ligament. During pregnancy, the enlarged uterus displaces the ovaries into the abdomen. After pregnancy, the ligaments are so stretched that the ovaries become mobile and can vary greatly in their position.

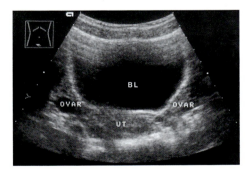

▲ *Fig. 13.41* Ovaries (Ovar) flanking the uterus (UT) posterior to the bladder (BL) in a nullipara.

Ultrasound Morphology

The ovaries can usually be visualized in women of reproductive age (**Fig. 13.41**). Both ovaries can be identified in approximately 80% of cases. The ovaries can rarely be visualized after menopause, when they are smaller and less echogenic.

The ovaries in fertile women measure approximately $2 \times 3 \times 1.5$ cm[6], which corresponds closely to the anatomical dimensions of 2.5 cm long, 2 cm wide, and 1 cm thick[2]. They may be slightly less echogenic than the uterus and display anechoic cystic changes during the ovarian cycle.

The ovarian cortex initially contains several rounded, anechoic masses up to 10 mm in diameter. Approximately seven days after menstruation, one dominant follicle appears while the others regress. The dominant follicle grows to a graafian follicle by the time of ovulation, measuring approximately 2 cm in size and projecting above the organ surface. An echogenic ringlike structure, the cumulus oophorus, appears in the follicle. After ovulation, free fluid can be demonstrated in the cul-de-sac. Now the follicle is misshapen or no longer visualized. When bleeding occurs in the corpus luteum, the follicle becomes uniformly hyperechoic.

Size and shape
- 2 × 3 × 1.5 cm
- Almond-shaped

Structure
- Medullary zone
- Cortical zone with follicles, corpora lutea, and corpora albicantia
- Capsule (tunica albuginea)

Landmarks
- Bladder
- Uterus
- Pelvic wall
- Iliac vessels

Anechoic Cystic Mass

Female Genital Tract
- Vagina
- Uterus
- Fallopian Tubes
- Ovaries
  - Anechoic Cystic Mass
  - Solid Echogenic or Nonhomogeneous Mass

- Simple Follicles
- Functional Cysts (Follicular and Corpus Luteum Cysts)
- Theca-Lutein Cyst
- Paraovarian Cyst
- Polycystic Ovaries (PCO Syndroms, Stein–Leventhal Syndrome)
- Cystic Ovarian Tumors

▶ Simple Follicles

Simple follicles appear as unilocular, anechoic masses with sharply circumscribed margins. When intraluminal hemorrhage is present, they appear hyperechoic. Simple follicles regress spontaneously.

The dominant follicle grows to a graafian follicle by the time of ovulation. It enlarges to approximately 2 cm and projects above the ovarian surface. The cumulus oophorus is visible as a ringlike structure of high echogenicity.

After ovulation, the follicle normally appears distorted in its shape or is no longer visible (**Figs. 13.42–13.44**).

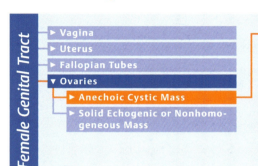

▲ **Fig. 13.42** Mature graafian follicle. BL = bladder; UT = uterus; C = follicle appearing as a cystic mass.

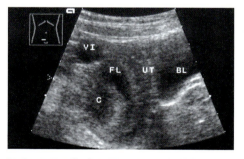

▲ **Fig. 13.43** Follicular rupture. Residual follicle (C); FL = free fluid; VI = iliac vein; UT = uterus; BL = bladder.

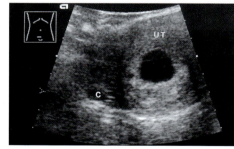

▲ **Fig. 13.44** Persistent follicle: early pregnancy with a chorionic cavity in the uterus (UT) and a follicle (C) in the ovary.

▶ Functional Cysts (Follicular and Corpus Luteum Cysts)

Most ovarian cysts are "functional cysts" such as follicular and corpus luteum cysts. Functional cysts are the response of the ovaries to elevated gonadotropin levels (FSH and LH) in the blood. A cyst no larger than 3–6 cm in a woman under age 30 may be a functional cyst. If it does not regress by the next menstruation or grows even larger, it should be surgically removed.

Follicular cyst. A follicular cyst is the most common ovarian cyst and can occur at any age. It is common after menarche and in the climacteric and is rare after menopause. A follicular cyst develops in response to estrogen stimulation when ovulation fails to occur. Generally the cyst is detected incidentally, but patients occasionally present with abdominal pain, a palpable mass, or signs of estrogen activity. The cysts may rupture when palpated, which can lead to hemorrhage, peritoneal shock, and spillage of the cyst contents into the abdominal cavity.

The sonographic criteria of a follicular cyst are as follows:
- Thin-walled
- Usually no larger than 5 cm (maximum 8 cm)
- Solitary, rarely multiple
- Unilateral, rarely bilateral
- Contains clear watery fluid, rarely hemorrhagic

Retention cysts. Retention cysts are formed by the accumulation of fluids such as blood and secretions in follicular cysts. Unlike cytomas, they grow no larger than fist-size.

Corpus luteum cyst. A corpus luteum cyst results from cystic enlargement of the corpus luteum. It develops when hemorrhage occurs within the corpus luteum and the blood is reabsorbed, leaving a cavity that contains serous fluid. Corpus luteum cysts are rarer than follicular cysts.

Most patients are clinically asymptomatic or present with irregular menstrual periods due to the overproduction of progesterone. A corpus luteum cyst is often present during pregnancy and regresses spontaneously.

The sonographic criteria of a corpus luteum cyst are as follows:
▶ Unilateral
▶ Up to 5 cm in diameter
▶ Anechoic to echogenic contents

▶ Theca-Lutein Cyst

Lutein cysts develop from atretic follicles. They represent follicular cysts that have theca-lutein cells on their inner surface. Lutein cysts result from hyperstimulation by gonadotropins and therefore occur in diseases and conditions that are associated with increased α-hCG formation, i.e., in 20% of molar pregnancies, in chorioepithelioma patients, and in multiple pregnancies. For this reason they are also commonly seen in patients with polycystic ovaries and in women treated for infertility. They may contain progesterone in high doses and regress after the cause is eliminated, although this may take several months.

Patients may become symptomatic owing to complications such as cyst torsion, intracystic hemorrhage, and rupture with hemorrhage. Ruptures and infarctions are an indication for operative treatment.

Sonographic features. Theca-lutein cysts can range from 6 to 20 cm in size[8]. A single cyst is rarely larger than a lemon; but because lutein cysts tend to be multiple and bilateral, the ovaries may be substantially enlarged. The cyst wall resembles an abscess membrane. The ovarian parenchyma is edematous. The cysts rupture easily, and pedunculated cysts often undergo torsion. Ascites may occur.

The sonographic criteria of a theca-lutein cyst are listed below:
▶ Multiple
▶ Bilateral
▶ Thin-walled
▶ Anechoic contents
▶ Echogenic with intracystic hemorrhage
▶ Moderate to massive ovarian enlargement

▶ Paraovarian Cyst

Paraovarian cysts arise from fetal tissues bordering the ovaries (epoöphoron, rests of the caudal mesonephric duct in the mesovary). They are more accurately classified as retention cysts rather than true neoplasms. They arise in the mesovary, are invariably benign, and occur at any age. Paraovarian cysts are variable in size; they may be pedunculated, and those with long pedicles tend to undergo torsion.

Their sonographic criteria are as follows:

▶ Elliptical shape
▶ Intraligamentous
▶ Well delineated from the ovary, may be pedunculated

▶ Polycystic Ovaries (PCO Syndrome, Stein–Leventhal Syndrome)

PCO syndrome develops during puberty as a result of increased androgen production by the adrenal cortex following adrenarche. It affects up to 7% of the female population. The initiating cause is poorly understood.

Stein–Leventhal syndrome develops when the hyperandrogenemia[7] gives rise to a symptom complex of polycystic ovaries, hirsuitism, menstrual abnormalities, and obesity.

The following are additional symptoms of PCO:
▶ Sterility and infertility (74%)
▶ Hirsuitism (50–70%)
▶ Amenorrhea and oligomenorrhea (approximately 50%)
▶ Dysfunctional bleeding (approximately 30%)
▶ Overweight (40%)

The estrogen stimulation of the endometrium induces hyperplasia and can also lead to well-differentiated endometrial carcinoma.

Sonographic features. The ovaries are generally larger than the uterine corpus. The smooth tunica albuginea shows echogenic thickening, and the cortex contains anechoic, usually equal-sized follicles up to 5 mm in diameter (rarely > 1 cm) arranged in a circumferential pattern. Follicular maturation does not occur. Since ovulation is absent, there is no surface pitting and no corpora albicantia.

The sonographic criteria are as follows (**Figs. 13.45 and 13.46**):
▶ Bilateral occurrence
▶ Enlarged ovaries
▶ Hyperechoic center
▶ Multiple cysts (anechoic follicles up to 5 mm in the cortex)
▶ Endometrial hyperplasia usually present

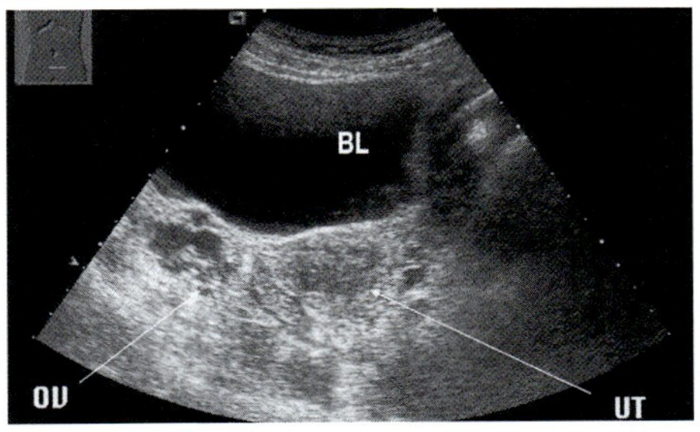

Pathogenesis of PCO Syndrome

PCO syndrome is characterized by a vicious cycle in which a stressful situation with increased ACTH secretion stimulates the formation of androstenedione in the adrenal cortex. This hormone is metabolized in the fat to estrone and sensitizes the pituitary to LHRH. The result is excessive LH secretion (FSH is unaffected), causing an unphysiological stimulation of the ovaries and increased androgen production (androstenedione) in the theca follicles and stromal cells. The androgen is again converted to estrone in the fatty tissue, and the cycle is continued.

▲ **Fig. 13.45** Polycystic ovary (OV) on the right side. Thickened endometrium in the uterus (UT). BL = bladder.

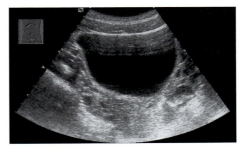

▲ **Fig. 13.46** Bilateral polycystic ovaries in menarche.

Cystic Ovarian Tumors

These lesions include benign cystadenoma, mucinous cystoma (which has a high malignant potential), and cystadenocarcinoma.

Cystadenoma. Benign cystadenoma (serous cystadenoma) is the most common benign ovarian tumor. It corresponds histologically to a cystoma serosum simplex. The wall of the cystic epithelial tumor is thin, smooth, and lined with epithelium. Cystadenoma is usually unifocal and rarely multifocal. If bilateral cystic tumors are present, they are very likely to be malignant (65–75% of carcinomas are bilateral). A cystadenoma may have serous contents (similar to the fallopian tubes) or mucinous contents (similar to the endocervix), depending on the type of epithelium and the tumor origin. The cysts are typically large and may fill the entire abdomen.

The sonographic criteria are as follows (**Figs. 13.47 and 13.48**):

- Anechoic mass
- Thin echogenic wall
- Thin septa, sometimes multilocular
- Smooth surface

Mucinous cystoma. Mucinous cystomas eventually undergo malignant transformation and therefore should be removed without delay. They account for approximately 25% of all ovarian tumors, and 10% are malignant when diagnosed. Mucinous tumors are rarely bilateral (5% of benign tumors, 10% of borderline tumors, and 20% of mucinous carcinomas are bilateral). The older the patient, the greater the likelihood that the tumor is malignant.

Mucinous cystomas are frequently septated, and their echogenicity can vary. The interior of the septated areas may show a fine to coarse echogenic pattern. Needle aspiration is not advised owing to the risk of tumor cell dissemination.

The sonographic criteria are as follows (**Fig. 13.49**):
- Cystic
- Multifocal, often septated
- Thin-walled with no deposits

Cystadenocarcinoma. Serous cystadenocarcinoma is the most common malignant ovarian tumor, accounting for approximately one-third of all ovarian cancers. The tumor is predominantly cystic, but unlike benign cystadenoma there are solid hyperechoic elements in the cyst wall, which shows circumscribed thickening (**Figs. 13.50 and 13.51**). Hyperechoic, sometimes polypoid structures may project into the cyst lumen. Nonhomogeneous, hypoechoic areas may also appear due to intratumoral hemorrhage and necrosis. Stromal infiltration can be demonstrated histologically.

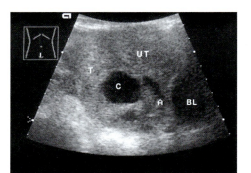
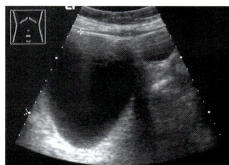

◄◄ **Fig. 13.47** Cystadenoma: anechoic mass (C) in the enlarged ovary (T). A = ascites; UT = uterus; BL = bladder.

◄ **Fig. 13.48** Serous cystadenoma: ovarian cyst (approximately anechoic mass) in menopause, 10 cm in diameter.

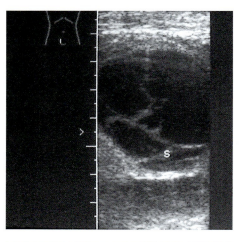
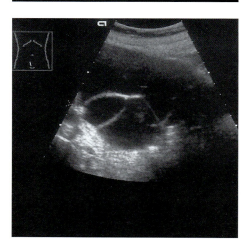

◄◄ **Fig. 13.49 a** Mucinous ovarian cystoma appears as a cystic mass with multiple septa (S).
b Cystic carcinoma: same as in **a**, but malignant. Appears as a predominantly cystic mass with internal septa.

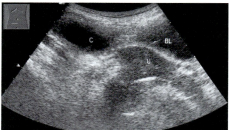
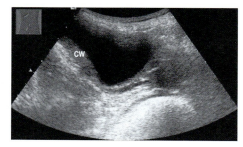

◄◄ **Fig. 13.50** Ovarian cyst (C), bladder (BL), uterus (U). The cyst wall should be scrutinized for local thickening (cystadenocarcinoma).

◄ **Fig. 13.51** Cystadenocarcinoma: circumscribed thickening of the cyst wall (CW).

Solid Echogenic or Nonhomogeneous Mass

Female Genital Tract
- Vagina
- Uterus
- Fallopian Tubes
- Ovaries
  - Anechoic Cystic Mass
  - **Solid Echogenic or Nonhomogeneous Mass**
    - **Endometriotic Cysts**
    - Thecomatosis
    - Inflammatory Adnexal Mass
    - Ovarian Carcinoma
    - Metastases
    - Pseudomyxoma Peritonei
    - Ovarian Tumors (by Histological Criteria)

▶ Endometriotic Cysts

Fifty-five percent of patients with endometriosis have ovarian involvement. The endometriotic cysts are usually located on the ovarian surface, initially have a uniformly hypoechoic cystic appearance, and later become nonhomogeneous owing to recurrent bleeding. In this case the endometriosis is no longer distinguishable from carcinoma. The full differential diagnosis is shown in **Table 13.2**.

The sonographic criteria are as follows (**Figs. 13.52 and 13.53**):
- Anechoic mass on the cortex, 1–5 mm in diameter
- With intracystic bleeding, the mass enlarges and may show homogeneous internal echoes
- Thick, echogenic wall
- Difficult to localize to a specific organ
- With recurrence, a nonhomogeneous echo pattern may be seen

Ovarian Endometriosis

Pathogenesis. The cyst wall is lined with endometrioid epithelium. This can result from the dissemination of endometrium from the uterus, but a more likely cause is the primary formation of cysts composed of coelomic epithelium. This would better explain the primary occurrence of ovarian adenocarcinoma (approximately 5% of ovarian tumors are endometrioid tumors, mostly carcinomas).

Management. Histological confirmation is always required. Ultrasound follow-ups should be scheduled at six-month intervals. Response should be monitored in cases that have been treated with GnRH analogues.

Table 13.2 Differential diagnosis of endometriotic cysts

- Hemorrhagic functional cyst
- Cystadenoma
- Ovarian carcinoma (endometrioid carcinoma)
- Intraligamentous myomas
- Inflammatory processes

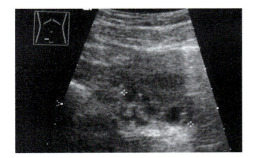

▲ **Fig. 13.52** Endometriotic cysts of the ovary.
a Multiple hypoechoic foci in the ovary.

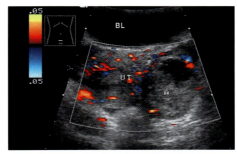

▲ **b** Large, solitary histological endometriotic cyst (surgery and histology; first sonographic diagnosis: abscess). The clinical and sonographic diagnosis was abscess. The absence of vascularity is not consistent with ovarian carcinoma. BL = bladder; UT = uterus.

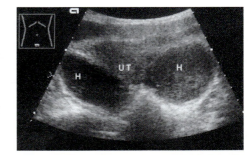

▲ **Fig. 13.53** Endometriosis with bleeding: hypoechoic mass, hematomas (H) due to bleeding in foci of endometriosis. UT = uterus.

▶ Thecomatosis

Thecomatosis is a pure stromal hyperplasia causing moderate enlargement of the ovary, which undergoes nodular changes. Histologically, the cortex is hyperplastic and shows intracellular fat deposits. Stromal hyperplasia occurs only in menopause.

▶ Inflammatory Adnexal Mass

Enlargements of the ovaries due to inflammation fall under the heading of adnexal masses. They include the following entities:
- Ovarian abscess
- Tubo-ovarian abscess originating from the fallopian tube (**Fig. 13.38**)
- Hematogenous tuberculosis. Conglomerate masses are formed, usually bilateral and densely matted (making them difficult to distinguish from carcinoma!)

▶ Ovarian Carcinoma

FIGO and TNM Staging for Ovarian Carcinoma

T1/I	Tumor confined to one ovary
T1c/Ic	Tumor on the ovarian surface, or capsule ruptured, or malignant cells in the peritoneal cavity
T2/II	Tumor extension beyond the ovary
T3/III	Peritoneal metastases outside the pelvis and/or regional lymph node metastasis
M1/IV	Distant metastases

Any kind of tissue can give rise to a malignant tumor, but only tumors derived from the germinal epithelium are classified as ovarian carcinoma. Thecalike transformation in ovarian tumors leads to small amounts of estrogen production in 15–20% of all epithelial cancers.

Tumors in postmenopausal women who are not on hormone replacement therapy are always suspicious. If findings are equivocal, diagnostic laparoscopy is always advised.

Sonographic features. Carcinoma can have almost any sonomorphological appearance: cystic, hyperechoic, hypoechoic, and nonhomogeneous. Large tumors contain nonhomogeneous solid components, may show central anechoic necrosis, and tend to invade neighboring structures, producing ill-defined margins. It is common for ovarian carcinoma to coexist with uterine or tubal cancers. Primary malignant tumors of the ovary are indistinguishable from metastases arising from other primary malignancies.

Endometrioid adenocarcinomas are more heavily permeated by cysts and papillomas. They account for approximately 5% of ovarian tumors.

Peritoneal carcinomatosis. Serous or mucinous carcinomas usually become disseminated throughout the abdominal cavity while the primary tumor itself is still relatively small. The peritoneum in these cases is studded with small tumor nodules and shows irregular hyperechoic thickening. Metastases are seeded early to the greater omentum, and a large, flat, confluent, hypoechoic tumor is formed (◻ 8.3a, d, ◻ 8.6f, Fig. 8.29). Hypoechoic masses also form on the diaphragm and along the umbilical vein. With the associated obstruction of lymphatic drainage, the serous fluid produced by the tumor cells usually leads to a copious ascites that is blood-tinged on percutaneous aspiration. Cytological analysis of the ascites has a diagnostic accuracy of 80%.

Metastasis. Lymph node metastases (para-aortic, inguinal, lesser pelvis) are of minor importance. Ovarian carcinoma spreads hematogenously to the pleura, lung, and liver and less commonly to the brain and bone.

Borderline Criteria

Borderline tumors are tumors that have a low malignant potential[2]:
- Epithelial tumors
- Confined to the organ
- No stromal invasion
- Amenable to curative surgery
- Five-year survival rate 80–90%, even with peritoneal seeding
- Occurrence in premenopausal women. Two-thirds of malignant tumors in women under age 40 are borderline tumors, as opposed to only 10% in women over age 40.

Table 13.3 Differential diagnosis of ovarian masses

- Gallbladder hydrops
- Splenic tumor
- Pelvic kidney, renal tumor, hydronephrosis
- Pancreatic cysts
- Mesenteric cysts
- Bowel tumors, diverticulosis
- Tuberculous conglomerate masses
- Nodal packages in the mesentery
- Distended bladder
- Uterine myomas
- Tumors of the pelvic connective tissue (lipoma, sarcoma, endothelioma, retroperitoneal liposarcoma, retroperitoneal pseudomyxoma, osteoma, enchondroma)
- Tumors of the bony pelvis (may invade the connective tissue)

Differential diagnosis. Differentiation from intestinal carcinoma can be difficult. Bowel cancers are frequently associated with hepatic and lymph node metastases, but they rarely show omental involvement or peritoneal carcinomatosis with ascites.

In differentiating ovarian cancer from uterine myomas, a short, firm pedicle not attached to the cornual region suggests a subserous myoma, whereas a soft, mobile pedicle connected to the cornual region suggests an ovarian tumor. The full differential diagnosis is listed in **Table 13.3**.

The sonographic criteria for carcinoma are as follows (**Figs. 13.54 and 13.55**):
- Larger than 5 cm
- Nonhomogeneous, cystic-solid
- Ill-defined margins
- Lobulated or nodulated
- Echogenic
- Broad septa
- Bilateral
- Papillary deposits
- Free fluid
- On palpation: fixed, matted, firm

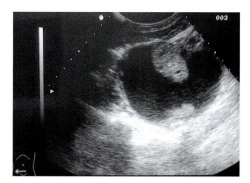
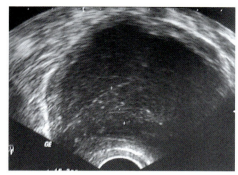

◀◀ **Fig. 13.54** Cystadenocarcinoma: hyperechoic polypoid tumors of the cystic epithelium.

◀ **Fig. 13.55** Endometrial hyperplasia (transvaginal scan) in ovarian carcinoma: uterus with endometrial hyperplasia (16.3 mm).

▶ Metastases

Ovarian metastases are very rare and originate from cancers of the bronchial system, gastrointestinal tract, breast, and gallbladder. Approximately 3% of malignant ovarian tumors are metastases.

Krukenberg tumor is the term applied to enlarged ovaries (generally both) that are diffusely permeated by epithelial signet-ring cells, usually from gastric carcinoma and occasionally from colon carcinoma. The tumor cells metastasize chiefly by the lymphogenous route and less commonly via the bloodstream.

▶ Pseudomyxoma peritonei

In pseudomyxoma peritonei, the peritoneal cavity is filled with a large quantity of mucin. Ultrasound demonstrates anechoic fluid in the peritoneal cavity.

The cause may be tumor cells seeded from a mucinous ovarian tumor or a mucinous adenocarcinoma of the appendix. Pseudomyxoma peritonei can also arise secondarily from the rupture of a mucinous cystoma (usually at operation) or possibly as a primary epithelial disease based on peritoneal metaplasia.

As there is no effective treatment, the disease runs a malignant course marked by intestinal adhesions and obstructions, with patients dying from cachexia.

▶ Ovarian Tumors (by Histological Criteria)

Because many different cell types exist in the ovaries, a large number of different neoplasms can arise. As a result, the ovaries are subject to a greater diversity of tumor types than any other organ in the human body.

Incidence data.
Epithelial tumors:
▶ 66% of all ovarian tumors are epithelial tumors.
▶ Of the malignant tumors, 85% are epithelial tumors.

Serous tumors:
▶ 50% of all ovarian tumors are serous tumors.
▶ 70% of serous tumors are benign, and 20–25% of serous tumors are true invasive carcinomas.
▶ 40% of ovarian carcinomas are serous carcinomas, making this the most common type.

Sex cord-stromal tumors:
▶ 3% of all true ovarian tumors are sex cord-stromal tumors.

Germ cell tumors:
▶ 15–20% of all ovarian tumors are germ cell tumors.
▶ 95% of germ cell tumors are benign cystic teratomas.
▶ 2–3% of germ cell tumors are malignant.
▶ Approximately 65% of malignant ovarian tumors up to age 20 are germ cell tumors.

Bilateral occurrence:
▶ 20–30% of benign tumors
▶ 30–40% of borderline tumors
▶ 65–75% of carcinomas

Classification of Ovarian Tumors[11]

▶ **Superficial epithelial-stromal tumors**
 – Serous tumors
 – Mucinous tumors
 – Endometrioid tumors
 – Clear cell tumors
 – Transitional cell tumors (Brenner tumor)
 – Squamous cell tumors
 – Epithelial mixed tumors
 – Undifferentiated car
▶ **Sex cord-stromal tumors**
 – Granulosa-stromal cell tumors
 – Sertoli-stromal cell tumors, androblastoma
 – Sex cord tumors with annular tubules
 – Gynandroblastoma
 – Unclassifiable
 – Steroid (lipid) cell tumors
▶ **Germ cell tumors**
 – Dysgerminoma
 – Yolk sac tumor
 – Embryonic carcinoma
 – Choriocarcinoma
 – Teratoma
 – Mixed types
▶ Gonadoblasotoma

▶ Germ cell-sex cord-stromal tumors
▶ Tumors of the rete ovarii
▶ Mesothelial tumors
▶ Tumors of uncertain histogenesis
▶ Gestational trophoblastic diseases
▶ Soft-tissue tumors, not ovary-specific
▶ Malignant lymphoma
▶ Unclassifiable tumors
▶ Metastases
▶ **Tumorlike lesions**
 – Solitary follicular cyst
▶ – Multiple follicular cysts
 – Luteinized cyst in pregnancy
 – Hyperreaction luteinalis (multiple lutein cysts)
 – Corpus luteum cyst
 – Gestational luteoma
 – Ectopic pregnancy
 – Stromal hyperplasia
 – Stromal hyperthecosis
 – Massive edema
 – Fibromatosis
 – Endometriosis
 – Nonclassifiable cyst
 – Inflammatory lesions

Epithelial tumors. Epithelial tumors arise from inclusion cysts in the germinal epithelium. The ovary contains numerous germinal epithelial cysts whose origin is still unexplained. Mixed epithelial tumors occur. Epithelial tumors can vary considerably in size. They may be cystic, cystic/solid, or solid. Most solid tumors are malignant.

Sex cord-stromal tumors. These tumors arise from sexually differentiated mesenchyma. They are palpable, hormone-producing ovarian tumors that are composed of one or more cell types. They produce estrogen or androgens.

Germ cell tumors. Germ cell tumors are more prevalent in Africa and Asia than in Europe (5–15% of malignant ovarian tumors), while epithelial tumors are less common. Germ cell tumors occur predominantly in childhood and from 20 to 30 years of age; they are rare after menopause. Approximately two-thirds of malignant ovarian tumors in patients under age 20 are germ cell tumors. They are derived from primordial germ cells (direct: dysgerminoma; indirect embryonic: teratoma; extraembryonic tumors: choriocarcinoma, yolk sac tumor). Germ cell tumors grow rapidly, are unilateral, and metastasize by hematogenous and lymphogenous spread. Overall, they have a favorable prognosis.

Morphological and sonomorphological criteria. Tables 13.4–13.6 summarize the principal morphological and sonomorphological criteria for the three main groups of superficial stromal tumors, sex cord-stromal tumors, and germ cell tumors. The next box then reviews the essential aspects of the clinical manifestations, diagnosis, and treatment of ovarian tumors.

Table 13.4 Features of epithelial tumors

Tumor	Tumor behavior, frequency, bilateral occurrence	Histology, morphology	Sonographic criteria	Special features
Serous tumors				
▸ Cystadenoma	– Most common benign ovarian tumor – Generally unilateral	– Thin cyst wall, lined with epithelium – Serous contents – Usually large cysts	– Anechoic mass – Smooth surface – Thin echogenic wall – Thin septa, possibly multilocular	– See Cystic Ovarian Masses
▸ Cystadenocarcinoma	– Most common malignant ovarian tumor (1/3 of all ovarian cancers)	– Predominantly cystic with solid elements – Circumscribed thickening of cyst wall – Polypoid structures, intratumoral hemorrhage, and necrosis may occur – Stromal infiltration	– Mixed anechoic (cystic elements) to hyperechoic (cyst wall) – Nonhomogeneous echogenic areas (bleeding and necrosis) – Often with ascites in metastases/peritoneal metastases	– See Cystic Ovarian Masses
Mucinous tumors				
▸ Mucinous cystoma	– 25% of all ovarian tumors – Initially benign, eventually degenerates – 5–20% bilateral (depending on malignancy)	– Multifocal – Often septated – Thin-walled	– Variable echogenicity – Fine to coarse internal echoes in the septated spaces	– See Cystic Ovarian Masses
▸ Mucinous cystadenocarcinoma	– 10% of ovarian carcinomas – 20% bilateral	– Mixed cystic and solid – Intratumoral hemorrhage and necrosis may occur	– Anechoic (cystic) to echogenic (solid) with hypoechoic areas (bleeding and necrosis)	– Often associated with pseudomyxoma peritonei
Endometrioid tumor	– 20% of ovarian carcinomas – 30–40% bilateral	– Mixed cystic and solid – Cyst contents serous or bloody – Foci of bleeding and necrosis	– Cyst contents hypoechoic to echogenic	– Coexists with endometrial carcinoma in 15–30% of cases
Clear cell tumor	– 5–10% of ovarian carcinomas – 40% bilateral	– Mixed cystic and solid	– Mixed anechoic and hyperechoic – Indistinguishable from other tumors by ultrasound	
Transitional cell tumor (Brenner tumor)	– 1–2% of all ovarian tumors – Usually benign – Unilateral	– Smooth margins – Not visible or up to 2–3 cm large – Calcifications may occur	– With calcifications: high-level internal echoes with acoustic shadows	– Patients are approximately 50 years old

Table 13.5 Features of sex cord-stromal tumors

Tumor	Tumor behavior, frequency, bilateral occurrence	Histology, morphology	Sonographic criteria	Special features
Granulosa-stromal cell tumors				
▶ Granulosa cell tumor	– Most common estrogen-producing ovarian tumor – Usually unilateral – Frequent malignant growth without correlative histology	– Solid structure – Up to 30 cm in diameter	– Hypoechoic – Possible cysts	– Estrogen production can lead to precocious pseudopuberty in adolescents, to uterine and breast enlargement in sexually mature women, to endometrial hyperplasia or carcinoma in postmenopausal women – Can recur after 10–20 years
▶ Thecoma (theca cell tumor)	– Less common than granulosa cell tumor – Unilateral – Generally benign	– 5–10 cm in diameter – Consists of fat-rich stromal cells, collagen-producing cells, and nests of granulosa cells	– Smooth margins – Hypoechoic with echogenic strands	– Estrogen production – Rare in puberty, common around menopause – Causes menstrual abnormalities and breast enlargement; endometrial hypertrophy and carcinoma may occur – Often confused with fibroma
▶ Ovarian fibroma	– Most common ovarian stromal tumor – 4% of all ovarian tumors – Usually unilateral – Usually benign	– Arises from sexually undifferentiated mesenchyma – Firm due to collagen production – "Adenofibroma": also contains glands and cysts	– Smooth margins, oval, uniformly hypoechoic – Occasional cystic degeneration – Often heavily calcified	– 40% of fibromas > 6 cm associated with ascites – Rare development of fibrosarcoma – *Meigs syndrome:* benign ovarian tumor (fibroma) with ascites and pleural effusion (usually on the right side), caused by lymphatic obstruction? – *Differentiation required from Krukenberg tumor:* metastases from bowel or breast tumors
▶ Sarcoma	– Very malignant – Pure sarcomas are rare, mostly mixed forms: fibrosarcoma, leiomyosarcoma, adenosarcoma	– Solid, less firm than fibromas – Histological structure resembles "fish meat"	– Solid, predominantly hypoechoic (less hypoechoic than fibroma)	– In young women and children
Sertoli stromal cell tumors, androblastomas	– 0.2% of all ovarian tumors – Usually benign – Unilateral	– Solid, up to 10 cm in diameter – Cells resemble Sertoli and Leydig cells	– Smooth margins, non-homogeneous hypoechoic/hyperechoic texture	– In young women (ca. 25 years) – 80% produce androgens, causing hirsuitism with beard growth, deep voice, secondary amenorrhea, clitoral hypertrophy, breast and uterine atrophy, alopecia, increased libido – *Androblastomas:* incomplete development of a testis from stroma of embryonic gonads; special form composed of ovarian hilar cells (hilar-Leydig cell tumor) may produce estrogen
Steroid (lipid) cell tumors	– Usually benign	– Resemble a hypernephroma, may arise from heterotopic adrenal tissues – Soft, slightly necrotic		– Urinary 17-ketosteroids sometimes elevated – Obesity, virilization, abdominal striae

Table 13.6 Features of germ cell tumors

Tumor	Tumor behavior, frequency, bilateral occurrence	Histology, morphology	Sonographic criteria	Special features
Dysgerminoma (gonocytoma, round cell sarcoma, seminoma)	– 5–10% of all ovarian tumors, ca. 2% of malignant ovarian tumors up to age 20 – Most common malignant germ cell tumor (50%) – Most common malignant tumor in pregnancy and intersexuality – 10% bilateral (large tumors)	– Very fast-growing, solid tumor up to about 30 cm		– Very radiosensitive – Good prognosis – Occult tumors on the opposite side
Yolk sac tumor (entodermal sinus tumor)	– 20% of immature germ cell tumors of the ovary – Malignant	– Reticular epithelial cells – Papillary structure		– Product AFP (used a tumor marker) – Better prognosis today with cytostatics
Teratomas				
▶ Dermoid (benign teratoma, dermoid cyst)	– 15% of all ovarian tumors – One-third of all benign ovarian tumors – 80% of all germ cell tumors – Benign, but the squamous portion may show malignant change (1%) – Usually unilateral	– Composed of embryonic germ cells – Grows very slowly – Rarely larger than fist-size – Surface smooth but irregular	– Ill-defined margins – Solid with high nonhomogeneous echogenicity, occasionally with calcium – Cyst with layered internal structure; pathognomonic, especially when echogenic part is anterior (floating sebum, liquid at body temperature) – May contain tooth bud and bone with acoustic shadowing	– In younger women – Strictly speaking, a retention cyst; enlarges when skin secretions expand the cyst sac – Prone to torsion, suppuration; may penetrate into the rectum
▶ Malignant solid teratomas	– Highly malignant	– Dermoid with disordered cell pattern and glial proliferation – Rapid growth		– Destructive spread – Metastases
▶ Struma ovarii		– Monodermal neoplasm, predominates in thyroid tissue	– Requires differentiation from hemorrhagic cyst, cystadenoma, fibroma	– Hormone production can cause hyperthyroidism

Clinical Aspects, Diagnosis, and Treatment of Ovarian Tumors

Symptoms
- There are no early symptoms.
- Ovarian tumors cause few if any complaints and have ample room to expand from the lesser to the greater pelvis. Often they are detected only after increasing the abdominal girth. Many of these tumors are detected incidentally.
- Uterine bleeding (7%) occurs when there is a coexisting uterine tumor or when the ovarian cancer has penetrated the vaginal wall.
- Estrogen production and its associated symptoms occur in 18% of all ovarian tumors and 25% of ovarian carcinomas.
- In 70% of cases, metastases are already present at operation.

Typical complications
- Torsion of a pedunculated uterine tumor (10–20%) may be caused by an external force acting on the tumor (sudden deceleration), especially if the mass contains fluid. A gradual occlusion of the blood supply causes a gradual increase in complaints, while sudden occlusion produces a shocklike condition with peritonitis. Torsion can lead to necrosis.
- Infections occur in 2% of ovarian tumors, usually owing to the migration of infectious microorganisms from the bowel. They can lead to suppuration (pyogenic organisms) and putrefaction (putrefactive bacteria). The results are high intermittent fever and life-threatening peritonitis.
- Incarceration occurs if the tumor cannot move upward out of the lesser pelvis.
- Rupture occurs in 3% of all ovarian cysts, usually spontaneously and often as a result of torsion. Life-threatening internal bleeding can develop. The draining cystic fluid and spillage of cells lead to chronic ascites.
- Complaints relating to the complications are low back pain, a bloated feeling, difficulties in passing urine and stool, varices, and leg edema.

Diagnosis
Gynecological examination and ultrasonography by an experienced examiner using modern equipment should ensure that no malignant tumors are discovered incidentally at operation.
Tumor locations:
- Large ovarian tumors can exert traction on the uterus, causing it to assume a transverse position in the lesser pelvis.
- Small ovarian tumors are located in the lesser pelvis adjacent to the uterus, which they may displace.
- Dermoid cysts are often located anterior to the uterus.
- Tumors of the pelvic connective tissue are difficult to define.

Rule:
- The attachment of a tumor is located opposite the site of greatest mobility. Testing this mobility sign will usually help in distinguishing between an abdominal tumor and a tumor of genital origin.

Suspicious signs during palpation:
- Tumor adherent, irregularly enlarged, or bilateral.
- Palpable nodule on the uterine attachment of the sacrouterine ligaments, in the cul-de-sac, or on the epiploic appendages of the rectum.
- Ovaries palpable after menopause.

Imaging and invasive studies
The patient may be examined by ultrasound, laparoscopy, CT (in exceptional cases), or laparotomy with extirpation and histological evaluation.

Ultrasound with a well-distended bladder:
- Criteria for malignancy: solid, irregular, mixed solid/cystic elements, ascites.
- Criteria for benignancy: smooth, unilocular or multilocular cysts.

Cysts should not be aspirated:
- Danger of rupture and possible cell spillage!
- Needle aspiration cannot exclude intracystic carcinoma.
- Cyst aspiration is never curative!

Aspiration of ascites:
- The ascites in early ovarian carcinoma is free of tumor cells.

Laparoscopy:
- Laparoscopy is unsafe owing to the risk of cell spillage and uncertain because a wedge excision may be nondiagnostic. Because every ovarian tumor ultimately should be removed, laparoscopy merely wastes time.

Computed tomography:
- Whenever possible, CT should be performed only after menopause because of radiation exposure to the ovaries.

Treatment
- Wait for menstruation to occur before performing surgery, as functional cysts will regress spontaneously.
- With malignant ovarian tumors, both ovaries and fallopian tubes should almost always be removed along with the uterus and greater omentum because of the likelihood of metastases.
- A cure is possible if the largest tumor remnant left behind is no larger than 1–2 cm.
- Ovarian tumors are responsive to chemotherapy. If tumors recur, they do so quickly after the therapy is discontinued.
- Even during pregnancy, every true ovarian tumor should be surgically removed because of the risk of torsion, rupture, and suppuration in the puerperium (10%).

Prognosis
The prognosis depends critically on the timing of the first operation and the corresponding tumor stage, the degree of tumor differentiation, and the histological type (serous tumors have a poorer prognosis than mucinous or endometrioid lesions).
- The 5-year survival rates (after surgery and chemotherapy) are as follows:

    | Stage I | 80% |
    | Stage II | 50% |
    | Stage III | 10–12% |
    | Stage IV | 1–2% |

- Today, 70% of ovarian carcinomas are diagnosed in stage III or IV; the 5-year survival rate is 30%.

References

1. Frank K, Goldhofer W. Uterus und Adnexe. In: Rettenmaier G, Seitz K (eds.). Sonographische Differentialdiagnostik. Stuttgart: Thieme 1999.
2. Innes D, Jackson J (University of Virginia School of Medicine) Basic Pathology. http://www.med.virginia.edu/med-ed/path/gyn/index.html
3. Kaiser R, Pfleiderer A. Geschwülste. In: Lehrbuch der Gynäkologie. Stuttgart: Thieme 1985.
4. Kaiser R, Pfleiderer A. Keimzelltumoren. In: Lehrbuch der Gynäkologie. Stuttgart: Thieme 1985.
5. Kozlowski P, Böhmer S. Gynäkologische Fragestellung in der Ultraschalldiagnostik. Landshut: ecomed 1991.
6. Merz E. Anatomie des weiblichen Beckens. In: Sonographische Diagnostik in Gynäkologie und Geburtshilfe. Vol 1, 2nd ed. Stuttgart: Thieme 1997.
7. Moltz L. Androgenisierungserscheinungen. In: Differentialdiagnose in Geburtshilfe und Gynäkologie. Stuttgart: Thieme 1984; p.46.
8. Schmidt-Gollwitzer K, Schmidt-Gollwitzer M. Der palpable Unterbauchtumor. In: Martius G, Schmidt-Gollwitzer M (eds.). Differentialdiagnose in Geburtshilfe und Gynäkologie. Stuttgart: Thieme 1984.
9. Schmidt-Gollwitzer M. Abnorme vaginale Blutungen. In: Martius G, Schmidt-Gollwitzer M (eds.). Differentialdiagnose in Geburtshilfe und Gynäkologie. Stuttgart: Thieme 1984; p.16.
10. Sohn C, Krapfl-Gast AS, Schiesser M. Checkliste Sonographie in Gynäkologie und Geburtshilfe. Stuttgart: Thieme 1998.
11. Soully, R. Histological typing of ovarian tumours. Deutsch: Histologische Klassifikation der Ovarialtumore. World Health Organization 1997. Berlin: Springer 1999.

14 Thyroid Gland

Thyroid Gland 417

▼ Diffuse Changes — 419

▶ Enlarged Thyroid Gland — 419
- Diffuse Parenchymatous Goiter
- Diffuse Colloid Goiter
- Hypertrophic Hashimoto Thyroiditis
- Immunogenic Basedow Hyperthyroidism
- Subacute de Quervain Thyroiditis
- Invasive Sclerosing Thyroiditis (Riedel Goiter)
- Goiter in Acromegaly
- Amyloidosis

▶ Small Thyroid Gland — 423
- Acquired Autoimmune Thyroiditis (AIT): Atrophic Lymphocytic Thyroiditis (juvenile)
- Acquired Autoimmune Thyroiditis (AIT) in Polyglandular Autoimmune Disease (PAS)
- Lithium- or Amiodarone-Induced Thyroiditis
- Neonatal Hypothyroidism
- Postoperative Thyroid/Unilateral Aplasia
- Radioiodine-Treated Thyroid
- Radiation-Induced Hypothyroidism

▶ Hypoechoic Structure — 427
- Chronic Thyroiditis with Transient Hyperthyroidism, Postpartum Thyroiditis
- Silent (Sporadic) Thyroiditis
- Lithium- or Amiodarone-Induced Thyroiditis

▶ Hyperechoic Structure — 429
- Radiation-Induced Hypothyroidism

▼ Circumscribed Changes — 429

▶ Anechoic — 429
- Cysts
- Vessels
- Abscess

▶ Hypoechoic — 431
- Microfollicular (Papillary) Adenoma
- Oncocytic Adenoma
- Lipoma
- Parathyroid Adenoma
- Abscess
- Focal de Quervain Thyroiditis
- Malignant Lymphoma
- Carcinoma
- Tumor Infiltration or Metastasis

▶ Isoechoic — 438
- Normofollicular Adenoma
- Hemorrhagic or Colloid Cyst
- Regressive Changes in an Adenoma or Adenomatous Nodule

- ▼ Circumscribed Changes (Continue)
  - ▶ Hyperechoic — 439
    - ▶ Macrofollicular Adenoma or Nodule
    - ▶ Hemorrhagic Cyst, Colloid Cyst
    - ▶ Nodule with Regressive Changes
    - ▶ Hemangioma, Myolipoma, Thyroid Regressive Changes
    - ▶ Calcifications
  - ▶ Irregular — 441
    - ▶ Nodular Goiter
    - ▶ Regressive Nodular Goiter
    - ▶ Tumor
- ▼ Differential Diagnosis of Hyperthyroidism — 443
  - ▶ Types of Autonomy — 443
    - ▶ Unifocal autonomy
    - ▶ Bifocal autonomy
    - ▶ Multifocal autonomy
    - ▶ Disseminated autonomy

14 Thyroid Gland

G. Schmidt

The thyroid gland is an endocrine gland whose function is to secrete three hormones: tetraiodothyronine (thyroxine, T_4), trace amounts of triiodothyronine (T_3; most T_3 is produced peripherally by the deiodination of T_4), and calcitonin. Thyroxine and triiodothyronine are synthesized in the thyrocytes while calcitonin is produced in the C cells of the colloid-containing follicular epithelium.

Thyroid calcitonin plays a key role in bone metabolism along with serum calcium, serum phosphate, and parathormone and is subject to a feedback control mechanism.

An intrathyroid iodine deficiency leads to a numerical increase in the thyrocyte population (follicular hyperplasia), while an increase in thyroid-stimulating hormone (TSH) leads to thyroid enlargement (follicular hypertrophy).

Both processes, then, are responsible in different ways for the development of a goiter. Ultrasonography is the method of first choice for imaging the thyroid and for evaluating the lymph nodes in the neck and thyroid region. MRI and CT are useful only in selected investigations. Radionuclide scanning (scintigraphy) is best for evaluating focal thyroid lesions and investigating hyperthyroidism.

▶ Anatomy

Shape
- Anterior aspect: butterfly-shaped
- In cross-section: horseshoe-shaped

Size
- AP diameter: 10–17 mm
- Transverse diameter: 12–20 mm
- Length of a thyroid lobe: 40–70 mm

Microanatomy
- Colloid-filled microfollicles, macrofollicles, and normal-sized follicles
- Follicular epithelium composed of thyrocytes and calcitonin cells

Blood supply
- Superior and inferior thyroid arteries (both paired)

When viewed from the front, the thyroid gland has a butterfly shape, with the head represented by the often rudimentary pyramidal lobe and the two wings by the thyroid lobes. The pyramidal lobe is a remnant of the thyroglossal duct present during embryonic development of the thyroid gland from the tongue base. Incomplete obliteration of the thyroglossal duct occasionally results in medial neck cysts.

The thyroid gland is surrounded by muscles. The sternohyoid and sternothyroid muscles are anterior to the thyroid, the sternocleidomastoid muscles are lateral, and the longus colli muscle is posterior. The blood vessels of the thyroid run through the gland in pairs: the superior thyroid artery above and the inferior thyroid artery below. Lateral to the gland are the common carotid artery and internal jugular vein (**Fig. 14.1**).

Horseshoe shape. While the thyroid gland has a butterfly shape when viewed from the front and by radionuclide scanning, it exhibits a horseshoe shape in the transverse ultrasound scan (**Fig. 14.2a**). The curved arms of the horseshoe are formed by the lobes, which are united by the thyroid isthmus. The borders of the thyroid are smooth owing to the presence of the thyroid capsule.

Size. The size of the thyroid gland is determined sonographically by measuring each lobe separately in a transverse scan on the right

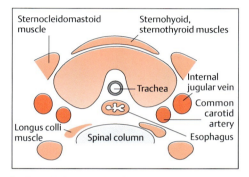

▲ **Fig. 14.1** Cross-section through the neck at the level of the thyroid gland.

and left sides (**Fig. 14.2**). This method yields the following approximate dimensions[4]: AP depth 10–17 mm, transverse diameter 12–20 mm, longitudinal dimension of each lobe 40–70 mm.

Volume. The volume of the thyroid gland is calculated using the volume formula for a rota-

Microanatomy of the Thyroid Gland

The microanatomy of the thyroid gland is determined by the follicles. The microfollicles, macrofollicles, and normal-sized follicles range from 50 to 200 αm in size and contain colloid, which consists mainly of thyroglobulin and deposits of monoiodotyrosine and diiodothyrosine. The iodination of thyroglobulin by inorganic iodide to monoiodothyrosine and diiodothyrosine, and probably their coupling to tetraiodothyronine (thyroxine) and triiodothyronine, are catalyzed by the enzyme thyroid peroxidase (TPO).

The single row of epithelial cells in the follicles consists of thyrocytes and calcitonin cells. Even the normal thyroid gland contains thyrocytes, isolated or in aggregates, that are primarily autonomous cells, i.e., not subject to the feedback control system. These cells can proliferate, especially in an iodine-deficient state, and grow into autonomous nodules (adenomas).

Table 14.1 Upper normal limits for sonographic measurements of thyroid volume

Age/sex	Volume (corresponds to weight in grams)
Newborn	1.5–2 ml
Up to 2 years	2–3 ml
3–4 years	3 ml
Up to 6 years	4 ml
Up to 10 years	6 ml
Up to 12 years	7 ml
Up to 14 years	8–10 ml
15–18 years	15 ml
Adult women	up to 18 ml
Adult men	up to 25 ml

tional ellipsoid: length of one lobe (cm) × the width of the lobe (cm) × the depth (cm) × 0.5.

Both thyroid lobes are measured separately and the results are added together to obtain the total volume (the volume of the isthmus is ignored). The normal values for age are shown in **Table 14.1**. The volume calculation is only an approximation, as it overestimates smaller volumes and underestimates larger volumes. It is difficult to make a reasonably accurate volume measurement in a nodular goiter with poorly defined margins.

Unilateral aplasia is occasionally detected incidentally in adults (previous surgery should be excluded).

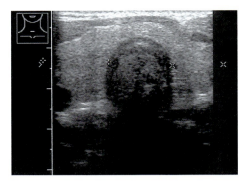

▲ **Fig. 14.2** Measuring the size of the thyroid gland (the measuring cursors are shown).
a Transverse scan through the neck.

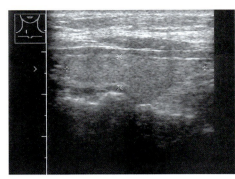

▲ *b* Longitudinal scan on the right side.

▶ Topography

Location of the thyroid gland
- Anterior to the first and fourth tracheal rings
- Isthmus and pyramidal lobe at the level of the cricoid cartilage
- Thyroid lobes anterior in the thyroid trigone
- Relates posteriorly to the pharynx and upper esophagus

Location of the parathyroid glands
- Outside the thyroid capsule
- Upper parathyroids at the level of the cricoid cartilage between the trachea and esophagus, on the posterior aspect of the upper third of the thyroid
- Lower parathyroids on the trunk and between the branches of the inferior thyroid artery; on the lateral or posterior aspect of the inferior thyroid pole or at a lower level

The thyroid gland has a horseshoe shape in anatomical cross-section. From anterior to posterior are the cervical fascia followed by the sternohyoid and sternothyroid muscles, the omohyoid muscles anterolaterally, and the powerful sternocleidomastoid muscles laterally. Posterior to these muscles are the isthmus of the thyroid gland and the left and right thyroid lobes. They are followed posteriorly by the trachea, parathyroid glands, esophagus (a little to the left), and retropharyngeal connective tissue. Behind that, placed lateral to the spinal column, are the longus colli muscles. The relations noted in this anatomical cross-section can be appreciated in the corresponding transverse ultrasound scan and longitudinal scans through each thyroid lobe (**Figs. 14.3 and 14.4**). The portion of the upper esophagus behind the thyroid gland is visible posteriorly between the left thyroid lobe and the tracheal acoustic shadow (**Fig. 14.5**).

Vessels. Ultrasound can consistently demonstrate the blood vessels that run in and around the thyroid gland. The common carotid artery and internal jugular vein run lateral to the thyroid. The superior and inferior thyroid arteries that supply the organ are consistently defined at its upper and lower poles in longitudinal scans (**Figs. 14.6–14.8**).

Parathyroid glands. The four parathyroid glands show frequent variations in their number and position; usually only two or three are present. They are located on the posterior aspect of the thyroid. Generally the upper parathyroids are extracapsular (rarely intracapsular) and are at the level of the cricoid cartilage between the trachea and esophagus. The lower parathyroids are located on the branches or trunk of the inferior thyroid artery or, in rare cases, directly on the lower poles (**see Figs. 14.35 and 14.36**).

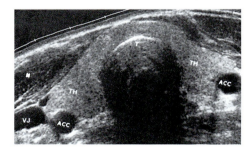

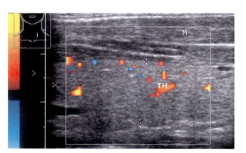

◀◀ **Fig. 14.3** Topographic relations of the thyroid gland (TH). M = sternocleidomastoid muscle; ACC = common carotid artery; JV = jugular vein; T = trachea. Posterior to the left thyroid lobe is the esophagus (appearing here as a triangular hypoechoic structure). In the right posterolateral quadrant, the inferior thyroid vein enters the jugular vein.

◀ **Fig. 14.4** Longitudinal color duplex scan of the left, structurally normal thyroid gland (TH, cursors). The less echogenic anterior neck muscles (M) are visible anteriorly. Normal, scant color spots appear at a low pulse repetition frequency (PRF) corresponding to a flow velocity of 0.06 m/s.

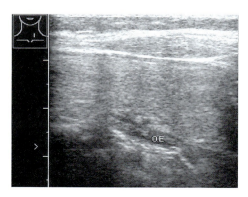

◀◀ **Fig. 14.5** Left lobe of the thyroid gland (TH), lying anterior to the cervical part of the esophagus (OE).
a Transverse scan.

◀ *b* Longitudinal scan: the anterior wall shows the typical three-part alternation between hypoechoic, hyperechoic, and hypoechoic layers. The echogenic lumen appears farther posteriorly.

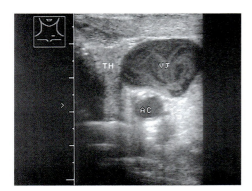
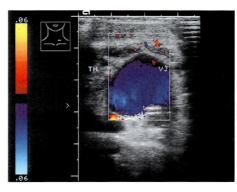

▸▸ **Fig. 14.6 a and b** Lateral to the thyroid gland (TH) are the internal jugular vein (VJ)—in this case markedly dilated with slow flow due to cardiac congestion—and, posterolaterally, the common carotid artery (AC).

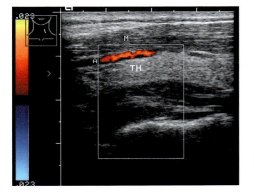
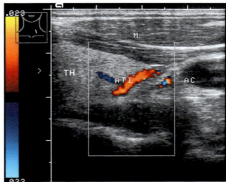

▸▸ **Fig. 14.7** Superior thyroid artery (A) in the upper part of the thyroid gland (TH). M = musculature.

▸ **Fig. 14.8** Inferior thyroid artery (ATI) at the lower pole of the thyroid gland (TH). AC = common carotid artery; M = anterolateral neck muscles.

Diffuse Changes

Diffuse thyroid changes are associated with changes in the size and/or structure of the organ. The enlarged thyroid may show a normal, hyperechoic, or hypoechoic structure, whereas the diffuse structural changes in a normal-sized thyroid are, with few exceptions (e.g., radiation-induced hypothyroidism), hypoechoic. Aside from goiters composed of multiple confluent hypoechoic nodules, these diffuse hypoechoic changes always have an inflammatory, immunogenic, or autoimmune etiology.

Micro-, macro- and normal-sized follicles as well as blood vessels determine the normal echo structure of the thyroid gland. Changes in the dominant follicle type lead to changes in this echo structure. It is best to evaluate the thyroid structure in relation to the surrounding musculature; otherwise the evaluation is subject to substantial errors. The normal thyroid tissues are more echogenic than the surrounding muscles (**Fig. 14.4**). Several factors determine the echogenicity of the thyroid: the dominant follicle type (**see Table 14.2**), vascularity, inflammation, and any regressive changes that have occurred.

Enlarged Thyroid Gland

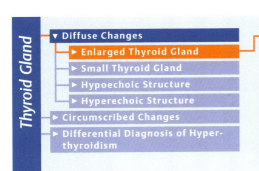

▸ Diffuse Parenchymatous Goiter

When a goiter is diagnosed clinically, adolescents and adults under age 40 are most likely to have a diffuse goiter, whereas older patients will generally have a nodular goiter or less commonly a cystic or neoplastic disease.

The underlying cause of both diffuse and nodular goiters in the United States, Germany, and several other European countries is a dietary iodine deficiency. Under the influence of various growth factors, the thyroid mounts a TSH-independent adaptive response consisting of hyperplasia with an increase in follicles, particularly microfollicles.

Sonographic features. The sonographic correlate of a diffuse goiter is an enlarged thyroid that retains a normal echo structure. Generally the structure is homogeneous, but circumscribed lesions such as adenomas, cysts, or calcifications may also be seen (**Fig. 14.9**).

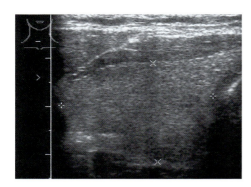
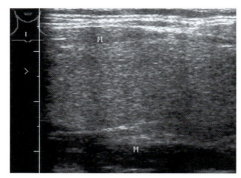

Fig. 14.9 Scans of a grade-II goiter show greatly enlarged thyroid lobes (cursors) with a normal echo structure relative to muscle tissue (M).
a Transverse scan on the right side.

b Longitudinal scan on the right side.

▶ Diffuse Colloid Goiter

Once hyperplasia of the thyroid has established a hormonal equilibrium, additional colloid storage occurs, causing an irregular increase in the size of the follicles. These macrofollicles and their colloid contents alter the structure of the gland, increasing its echogenicity (**Fig. 14.10**). Sonographically, then, the diffuse colloid goiter appears as an enlarged thyroid gland with a homogeneous hyperechoic structure. This ultrasound finding, with a normal TSH level, justifies the initiation of treatment without further diagnostic tests.

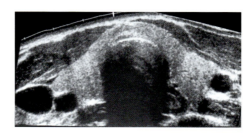

▲ **Fig. 14.10** Diffuse colloid goiter: enlarged, hyperechoic thyroid (SieScape panoramic image).

Treatment of Diffuse Goiter

Iodine therapy [17], 400 (to 500) µg/day for one year, then the following maintenance regimen:

Adults and adolescents	200 µg/day
School-age children	140–180 µg/day
Small children	100–120 µg/day
Pregnant or lactating women	230–260 µg/day

▶ Hypertrophic Hashimoto Thyroiditis

Hashimoto thyroiditis is a type of autoimmune thyroid disease and the leading cause of acquired thyroid hypofunction. A rare hypertrophic form of this disease is distinguished from an atrophic form. The Thyroid Section of the German Society for Endocrinology recognizes a chronic lymphocytic form with and without goiter, also referring to this entity as autoimmune thyroiditis, Hashimoto thyroiditis, atrophic autoimmune thyroiditis, and primary myxedema. Anglo-American authors draw a distinction between autoimmune thyroiditis and Hashimoto thyroiditis.

Sonographic features. In both the rare hypertrophic form and the atrophic form of autoimmune Hashimoto thyroiditis, ultrasound demonstrates a homogeneous, very echopenic organ that appears isoechoic to the surrounding muscles and has a bulky, often asymmetrical shape. Color duplex examination reveals an intense, speckled hypervascular pattern that is chiefly responsible for the hypoechoic structure (**Fig. 14.11; Figs. 14.19 and 14.20**).

Morphology, Clinical Aspects, and Immunology of Chronic Lymphocytic Hashimoto Thyroiditis [10, 15]

Hashimoto thyroiditis is one of a number of autoimmune thyroid diseases. Histologically, the thyroid gland shows diffuse lymphocytic and plasma cell infiltration. Consistent with the immune pathogenesis, antibodies against microsomes are found—specifically against thyroid peroxidase (anti-TPO), always present in high titers. Thyroglobulin antibodies and low titers of TSH receptor-blocking antibodies are also present.

Hyperplastic form. The hyperplastic form of the disease is associated with thyroid enlargement (usually an asymmetrical goiter) and the atrophic form with a decrease in organ size. High anti-TPO titers are always combined histologically with lymphocytic infiltrates, eliminating the need for fine-needle aspiration.

Low titers of anti-TSH receptor antibodies are responsible for a transient hyperthyroid phase. They also stimulate thyroid growth and cause thyroid enlargement, which presents clinically as an asymmetrical goiter.

Atrophic form. The atrophic form is responsible for nearly 80% of all hypothyroidism in adults. Besides lymphocytic and plasma cell infiltrates, scarring of the thyroid parenchyma is present. Hypothyroid symptoms are mild and progress slowly. Women are affected much more frequently than men.

Myxedema. Myxedema is a rare condition that represents the end stage of Hashimoto thyroiditis. Even with intensive therapy, the prognosis is poor owing to cardiovascular complications; the mortality rate is 70%.

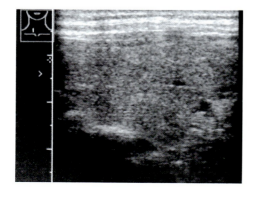
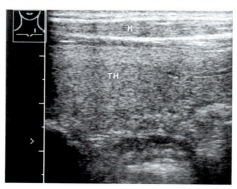

◀ **Fig. 14.11 a and b** Hashimoto goiter, hypertrophic form. TSH elevated, anti-TPO positive. The goiter is hypoechoic to the muscle tissue, and the thyroid gland (TH) is enlarged in both its longitudinal and AP dimensions. M = muscle.

▶ Immunogenic Basedow Hyperthyroidism

This condition is also commonly known as Basedow disease and Graves disease. The term "immunogenic Basedow hyperthyroidism" expresses both the autoimmune etiology of the disease and the hyperthyroid state. The hyperthyroidism is frequently associated with extrathyroid manifestations such as endocrine ophthalmopathy and pretibial myxedema. Younger women are predominantly affected. Basedow disease is the most frequent cause of hyperthyroidism in adolescents. Diagnosis is generally based on the clinical presentation and laboratory findings (autoantibody detection).

Sonographic features. Ultrasound shows a marked volume increase (up to 90 ml) and symmetrical enlargement of the thyroid. The enlargement includes the isthmus, and this is considered a significant criterion for the disease. The thyroid acquires a rounded, balloon-like appearance (**Fig. 14.12**). The volume dwindles during remissions and increases during recurrences. Because of the rich blood supply, the thyroid shows a diffuse decrease in echogenicity with densely packed hypoechoic areas, resulting in an echo-poor internal structure[14].

Color Doppler examination. Given the hypervascularity that underlies the characteristic echo structure, color Doppler reveals intense color-flow signals throughout the organ, creating a pattern described as a "thyroid inferno"[14] or "vascular inferno" (**Figs. 14.13 and 14.14**).

Diagnosis of Basedow Hyperthyroidism

Clinical features. The typical clinical symptoms present as the classic Merseburg triad of goiter, exophthalmos, and tachycardia, first described by Karl von Basedow in 1840.

Laboratory findings. The hyperthyroidism is confirmed by in-vitro suppression tests showing low TSH and elevated free T_4 and T_3. Since isolated T_3 hyperthyroidism can occur, a T_4 determination is insufficient in itself.
TRAbs. Autoantibodies against the TSH receptor (TRAbs) exert a TSH-like effect that directly stimulates the thyrocytes and produces a diffuse hyperplasia and hypertrophy of the thyroid follicular epithelium. TRAbs are positive in 90% of patients with Basedow disease. They are still positive in 46% of cases following radioiodine therapy and in 2% following strumectomy[10].
Anti-TPO. Besides TRAbs, low titers of antithyroid peroxidase antibodies (anti-TPO, formerly microsomal antibodies) are found in 76% of cases.
The diagnosis is definite when signs of endocrine ophthalmopathy are seen. Other than thyroid ultrasound, there is no need for further testing.

The internal hypervascularity does not correlate with functional status, however[1]; it is due chiefly to inflammation. But the density of the color pixels does correlate strongly with the need for thyrostatic treatment. Another indication for color duplex examination is follow-up, because thyroid blood flow is significantly higher in patients with a recurrence, and therefore vascularity becomes an important prognostic indicator. The peak flow velocity is also markedly increased to 127 cm/s[16] (**Fig. 14.15**). This is best demonstrated by Doppler sampling of the inferior thyroid artery.

Differentiation from autoimmune thyroiditis. Autoimmune thyroiditis has a similar hypoechoic structure, but Basedow goiter is distinguished by a coarser hypoechoic pattern, a more rounded shape due to concomitant isthmic enlargement, and more intense vascularity with a high arterial flow velocity. Autoimmune thyroiditis also shows marked hypoechoicity, but the vascularity on color duplex examination is less pronounced and has a finer texture.

Autonomous nodules. Autonomous nodules in a hyperthyroid Basedow goiter, or Basedow disease developing on the basis of a nodular goiter (Marine–Lenhart syndrome[11] (▯ **14.4p–r**), may occur. Autonomous nodules and adenomas do not participate in the autoimmune changes in the Basedow thyroid; this confirms their autonomous growth and identifies them as true neoplasms in Basedow goiters. At the same time, areas of regressive fibrosis may appear as focal lesions.

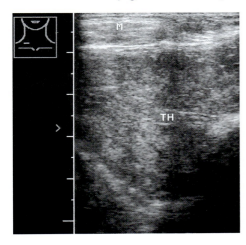

◀◀ *Fig. 14.12* Immunogenic Basedow goiter: balloonlike enlargement of the thyroid gland (TH) with a patchy echopenic structure that is isoechoic to the muscle (M). The markedly enlarged isthmus, which crosses over the trachea (TR), is a characteristic feature of Basedow goiter.
a Transverse scan through the right thyroid lobe.

◀ **b** Transverse scan through the left thyroid lobe.

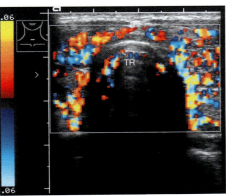
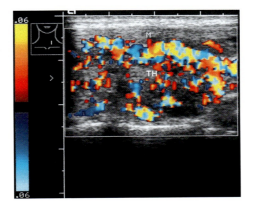

◀◀ *Fig. 14.13* Color Doppler view of a Basedow goiter, showing intense hypervascularity ("vascular inferno" pattern). In our experience, the low PRF setting (corresponding to a color Doppler velocity of 0.06 m/s) is optimal for thyroid examinations (it should be lowered to 0.025 m/s only with scant vascularity to detect very slow flows). The Doppler window should encompass the entire thyroid lobe.
a Transverse scan on the midline. TR = trachea.

◀ **b** Longitudinal scan of the right thyroid lobe (TH). M = muscle.

Diagnosis. The balloonlike shape, grainy hypoechoic texture, and intense vascularity are such typical sonographic features that, when hyperthyroidism is detected, ultrasound can establish the diagnosis of Basedow goiter even without serology.

Ultrasound[7] yields a correct diagnosis in 74% of patients with Basedow disease, radionuclide scanning in 96%. Given this high sensitivity of ultrasound and the reliability of serological testing, radionuclide scanning is indicated in Basedow disease only in cases where ultrasound has additionally detected focal changes.

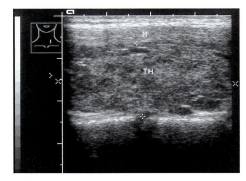

▲ **Fig. 14.14** Basedow disease: patchy hypoechoic thyroid gland (TH), isoechoic to the muscle (M) (B-mode image corresponding to **Fig. 14.13b**).

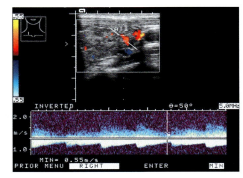

▲ **Fig. 14.15** Color Doppler with spectral analysis in Basedow disease. The peak systolic flow velocity in the inferior thyroid artery (ATI) is greatly increased, measuring 1.55 m/s.

▶ Subacute de Quervain Thyroiditis

De Quervain thyroiditis is an acute or subacute viral thyroiditis. Histologically[15], this form of thyroiditis is distinguished by giant-cell-like granulomas and by scarring in the healing stage. This can also be demonstrated by ultrasound-guided fine-needle aspiration cytology.

Sonographic features. Sonographically, the thyroid enlargement is based mainly on an increase in AP diameter. The isthmus does not appear as prominent as in Basedow disease. With regard to echo texture, this type of goiter is distinguished by its intensely hypoechoic structure with a coarse patchy, focal, or diffuse texture (**Figs. 14.16 and 14.17**)[8].

Color Doppler sonography. In color Doppler, de Quervain thyroiditis shows little or no vascularity, which positively distinguishes it from the Basedow thyroid. Unilateral focal lesions may occur (**Fig. 14.17b; Figs. 14.38 and 14.39**).

> ### Symptoms of de Quervain Thyroiditis
>
> Patients manifest the clinical signs of a viral infection (adenovirus, myxovirus, paramyxovirus) with general malaise, fever, an enlarged thyroid with local tenderness, and laboratory tests positive for inflammation. Patients often describe pain radiation to the neck region. Brief cortisone therapy can bring dramatic improvement, but most cases resolve spontaneously over a period of weeks or months.
> Hyperthyroidism (up to 50%) is often the dominant initial finding.

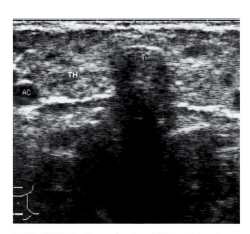

▲ **Fig. 14.16** De Quervain thyroiditis: patchy hypoechoic thyroid lobes (TH) with no isthmic enlargement. T = trachea; AC = common carotid artery.

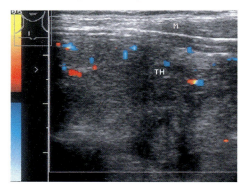
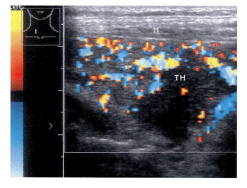

◀◀ **Fig. 14.17** De Quervain thyroiditis, color duplex. M = muscle; TH = thyroid lobe.
a Patchy low echogenicity with flow voids.

◀ **b** Four weeks later: regression of swelling, clear delineation of the hypoechoic area, marked increase in vascularity in the rest of the thyroid gland.

▶ Invasive Sclerosing Thyroiditis (Riedel Goiter)

The cause of this "stony hard" thyroid enlargement is poorly understood, but it shows similarities to other fibrosclerosis such as the retroperitoneal fibrosis in Ormond disease. In this type of goiter, inflammation spreads from an extrathyroid source to involve the thyroid gland and other tissues in the neck. It belongs in the broader category of immune thyroiditis because it is associated with lymphocytic infiltrates and leads to scarring and the formation of hyaline connective tissue.

Sonographic features. The diffuse, intense hypoechoicity reflects both the presence of hypoechoic connective tissue and the inflamed condition of the thyroid, which shows a balloonlike enlargement similar to that in Basedow disease (**Fig. 14.18**).

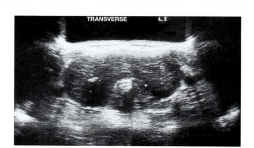

▲ **Fig. 14.18** Riedel goiter. The thyroid exhibits balloonlike swelling with an intensely hypoechoic structure.

▶ **Goiter in Acromegaly**

A goiter is almost always present in acromegaly. It may be a diffuse goiter (93%) or a nodular goiter (73%), depending on the duration of the acromegaly[8].

▶ **Amyloidosis**

Amyloid deposition in the thyroid, whether isolated or in a setting of generalized amyloidosis, is extremely rare and leads to a relatively coarse, diffuse increase in echogenicity.

Small Thyroid Gland

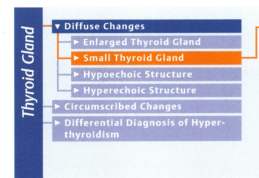

- Acquired Autoimmune Thyroiditis (AIT): Atrophic Lymphocytic Thyroiditis (primary Myxedema)
- Acquired Autoimmune Thyroiditis (AIT) in Polyglandular Autoimmune Syndrome (PAS)
- Lithium- or Amiodarone-Induced Thyroiditis
- Neonatal Hypothyroidism
- Postoperative Thyroid/Unilateral Aplasia
- Radioiodine-Treated Thyroid
- Radiation-Induced Hypothyroidism

Concept of Acquired Autoimmune Thyroiditis

Acquired autoimmune thyroiditis (AIT) is a collective term for various conditions that are probably synonymous with chronic lymphocytic Hashimoto thyroiditis:

▶ **Chronic Hashimoto-type autoimmune thyroiditis** (see above). This presents as a hypothyroidism with no other associated diseases and is characterized by the detection of anti-TPO and antithyroglobulin antibodies and a typical diffusely hypoechoic sonographic pattern. Small, hyperechoic foci of scarring appear in the late stage.

▶ **Polyglandular autoimmune syndrome (PAS).** This is an autoimmune hypothyroidism that is associated with type I diabetes and most commonly occurs in children and adolescents but is also seen in older patients with LADA diabetes (type II and III polyglandular autoimmune syndrome, PAS or PGA). Other, coexisting hormonal deficiencies occur in the following percentages of cases [10]:
- Hypoparathyroidism 80–90%
- Adrenal insufficiency (Addison disease) 60–70%
- Hypogonadism 40–50%
- IDDM 10–20%
- Autoimmune gastritis

Conversely, 70–80% of patients who have had type I diabetes for an average of 18 years also have hypothyroidism.

In the type II form of PGA, autoimmune thyroiditis and type I diabetes are accompanied by hypogonadism, myasthenia, vitiligo, and alopecia.

In type III PGA, type I diabetes is accompanied by an autoimmune thyroiditis or by adrenal insufficiency with Hashimoto autoimmune thyroiditis.

▶ **Chronic thyroiditis** (juvenile) with transient hyperthyroidism.

▶ **Postpartum thyroiditis** (see below).

▶ **Other forms of autoimmune thyroiditis** such as lithium- or amiodarone-induced thyroiditis are probably separate entities that do not fall under the heading of Hashimoto thyroiditis.

▶ **Acquired Autoimmune Thyroiditis (AIT): Atrophic Lymphocytic Thyroiditis (juvenile)**

Atrophic thyroiditis is responsible for most cases of silent hypothyroidism in adults, followed by hypothyroidism after a thyroid resection. The atrophic form is far more common than the classic Hashimoto thyroiditis associated with a goiter (see above).

Sonographic features. Ultrasound shows a markedly small thyroid, often asymmetrical, with a homogeneous grainy or patchy hypoechoic texture containing fine, hyperechoic areas of scarring. The scars may produce contour irregularities (**Figs. 14.19a and 14.20a**).

Color duplex examination shows a fine or coarse pattern of vascular signals that may still be very pronounced or already diminished owing to scarring (**Figs. 14.19b and 14.20b**).

Scans at the end stage of myxedema may still show residual areas of thyroid tissue, whose volume is less than that of a normal thyroid lobe (**Fig. 14.21**).

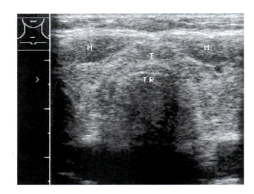
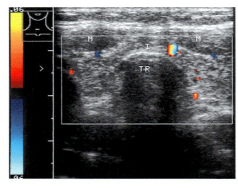

Fig. 14.19 Chronic atrophic autoimmune Hashimoto thyroiditis. M = sternocleidomastoid muscle; I = isthmus with a section of muscle; TR = trachea.
a B-mode image shows a hypoechoic background texture with small, hyperechoic inclusions, probably due to focal scarring.

b Color Doppler with a low PRF setting (corresponding to a Doppler velocity of 0.06 m/s) shows greatly decreased vascularity.

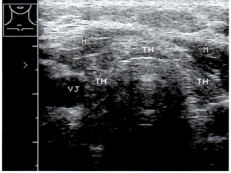
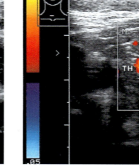
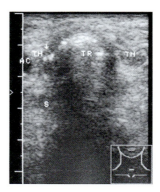

▲ **Fig. 14.20** Atrophy in autoimmune Hashimoto thyroiditis with severe hypothyroidism. M = muscle; VJ = jugular vein.
a Atrophic thyroid gland (TH) with a patchy hypoechoic texture.

▲ **b** Color duplex. The initial hypervascularity is still appreciated in the thyroid remnants.

▲ **Fig. 14.21** Myxedema due to complete thyroid atrophy (TH) with microcalcifications and acoustic shadowing (S). TR = trachea.

▶ Acquired Autoimmune Thyroiditis (AIT) in Polyglandular Autoimmune Disease (PAS)

Diabetes-associated autoimmune thyroiditis is common in long-standing cases of diabetes. For this reason, a TSH test and/or thyroid ultrasound scan should be performed in any patient who has more than a 10-year history of type I diabetes.

The echo texture and vascularity are like those seen in other types of autoimmune thyroiditis, as are the clinical manifestations and patterns of elevated anti-TPO antibodies and borderline anti-TSH receptor antibodies, although the TPO titers often do not reach the same level as in Hashimoto thyroiditis. The thyroid gland becomes small in the advanced stage, presenting a hypoechoic structure (◻ 14.1 a–c).

Largely identical patterns are also seen in nondiabetes-associated forms of autoimmune hypothyroidism (◻ 14.1 d–g).

▶ Lithium- or Amiodarone-Induced Thyroiditis

Both drugs can cause or ignite a chronic thyroiditis. Hyperthyroidism develops, and a hypothyroid atrophy of the thyroid gland can develop with long-term use (**Fig. 14.22**).

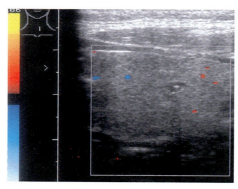
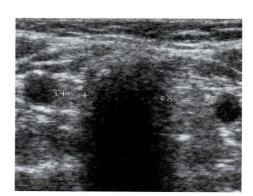

▲ **Fig. 14.22** Thyroid atrophy following 10 years of lithium therapy. Small, hypoechoic thyroid remnants.
a Lithium-induced hyperthyroidism: slightly enlarged thyroid gland with a normal echo texture and scant vascularity by color duplex.

▲ **b** Transverse scan through the neck.

14.1 Acquired Autoimmune Thyroiditis (AIT) in Polyglandular Autoimmune Disease (PAS)

▶ Autoimmune thyroiditis in type 1 diabetes mellitus

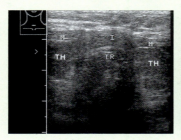
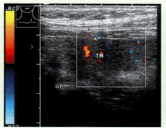
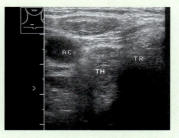

a Small thyroid lobes (TH), uniformly hypoechoic to the muscle (M). I = isthmus, TR = trachea.

b Color Doppler view of the left lobe in *a* (TH) with a very low PRF (corresponding to a V_{max} of 0.023 m/s) shows scant vascularity.

c Severely atrophic thyroid gland (TH) in long-standing diabetes mellitus. Only a greatly enlarged view can identify remnants between the common carotid artery (AC) and trachea (TR).

▶ Autoimmune thyroiditis, autoimmune gastritis, operated renal cell carcinoma

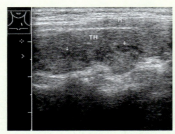
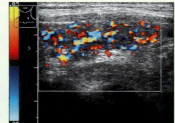

d Very high anti-TPO titers and low titers of anti-TSH receptor antibodies in a 50-year-old woman with hypothyroidism. Longitudinal scan on the left side. TH = thyroid gland; M = muscle.

e and f Color Doppler scans of the left thyroid lobe. Longitudinal scan shows intense, irregular color-flow signals with spared areas, which are also spared from hypoechoicity in the B-mode image (**d**) (may be autonomous adenomas not involved by the autoimmune thyroiditis).

▶ Neonatal Hypothyroidism

This condition is often based on ectopic thyroid tissue (lingual thyroid, aplasia), as indicated by the absence of detectable thyroglobulin.

In a study of 38 newborns with congenital primary hypothyroidism, Meller et al.[12] found 7 cases of athyrosis, 9 lingual goiters, and 15 infants with an iodine organification defect (4 with Pendred syndrome). Ectopic thyroid tissue could be detected only by radionuclide scanning. In four of the patients, the correct diagnosis could be made only by scintigraphy using the perchlorate depletion test.

Ultrasound yielded a false-negative diagnosis in two patients with hypoplasia and a false-positive diagnosis in two other patients with athyrosis. Thus, while ultrasound has limited value in terms of diagnostic accuracy, thyroid sonography is still an essential routine study for detecting an orthotopic or ectopic thyroid gland. Radionuclide scanning is still superior for locating an ectopic thyroid, however.

Immunogenic neonatal hypothyroidism often results from the transmission of maternal blocking antibodies to the fetus.

▶ Postoperative Thyroid/Unilateral Aplasia

During surgical resection of the thyroid gland, the poles are exposed and the posterior portions of the gland are dissected free in the area of the recurrent nerve. The isthmus is resected first, followed by the other parts of the gland, leaving a remnant of thyroid tissue measuring approximately 2–4 cm × 2 cm × 2 cm. Nodular areas are resected completely. Thus, a subtotal strumectomy leaves behind a greatly diminished residual gland that can be identified and measured sonographically (**Fig. 14.23**).

When a total strumectomy is performed for thyroid carcinoma, all portions of the gland are resected after the recurrent nerve has been dissected free. Ultrasound does not demonstrate a thyroid remnant in these cases.

In both operations, the parathyroid glands posterior to the upper and lower poles of the thyroid are left intact.

Unilateral aplasia is occasionally detected incidentally in adults (previous surgery should be excluded).

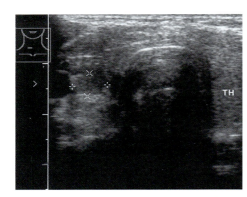 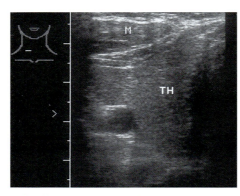 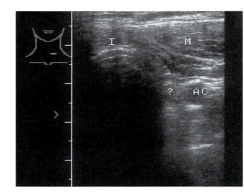

▲ **Fig. 14.23** Small residual thyroid (TH, cursors) following a subtotal strumectomy. The remnant displays a normal echo structure.
a Postoperative thyroid gland: small amount of residual thyroid tissue on the right side (cursors).

▲ **b and c** Unilateral aplasia of the thyroid gland. Normal thyroid function, no history of surgery. AC = common carotid artery; I = isthmus; M = muscle.

▶ Radioiodine-Treated Thyroid

Following radioiodine treatment with iodine-127, the thyroid volume may continue to decrease even 1–2 years after the therapy. Volume reductions of 20–40% are typically achieved, with some cases showing up to a 70% reduction. Hypothyroidism can develop in 15% of cases[17] (**Fig. 14.24**).

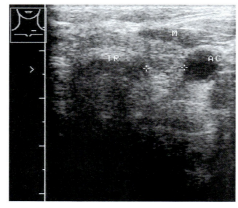 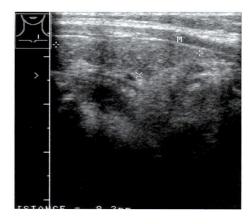

▲ **Fig. 14.24** Left thyroid lobe (cursors) following radioiodine therapy. The organ is markedly reduced in size and shows slightly irregular contours. AC = common carotid artery; M = muscle; TR = trachea.
a Transverse scan.

▲ **b** Longitudinal scan.

▶ Radiation-Induced Hypothyroidism

In these cases the cause of the hypothyroidism is determined from the history. Ultrasound generally shows a small thyroid gland with normal or slightly increased echogenicity. The contours may be irregular owing to scarring (**Fig. 14.25**).

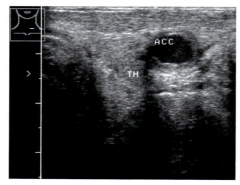 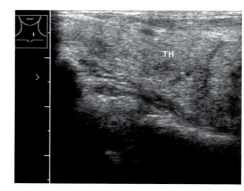

▲ **Fig. 14.25** Radiation-induced hypothyroidism. The patient underwent surgery for palatal carcinoma with radiation to the neck nodes. Hypothyroidism developed years later.
a Transverse scan on the left side shows a small thyroid lobe (TH) and irregular, indistinct vessels that are distorted due to scarring. ACC = common carotid artery.

▲ **b** Longitudinal scan on the left side. The inferior thyroid artery has a blurry, rarefied appearance.

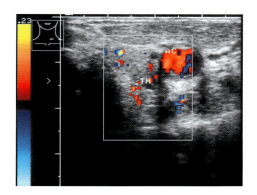 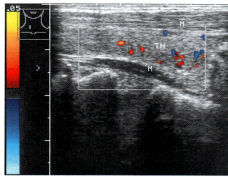

◄ *c* and *d* Scant color-flow signals at a low PRF setting (same signal pattern seen at 0.05 m/s), indicating a slight decrease in vascularity. AC = common carotid artery; M = muscle.

Hypoechoic Structure

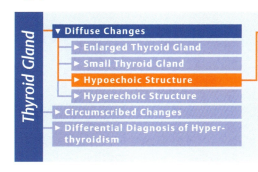

▶ Chronic Thyroiditis with Transient Hyperthyroidism, Postpartum Thyroiditis
▶ Silent (Sporadic) Thyroiditis
▶ Lithium- or Amiodarone-Induced Thyroiditis

The diffuse hypoechoic thyroid changes described below are generally associated with a normal-sized thyroid gland.

▶ Chronic Thyroiditis with Transient Hyperthyroidism, Postpartum Thyroiditis

Both chronic thyroiditis with transient hyperthyroidism (juvenile) and postpartum thyroiditis are associated with a brief period of hyperthyroidism, which should not be treated with thyrostatic agents.

Postpartum thyroiditis generally develops during a brief interval after pregnancy, showing an average incidence of 5%[8]. It is associated with transient but persistent hyperthyroidism or hypothyroidism. Postpartum thyroiditis is negative for anti-TSH receptor antibodies but positive for anti-TPO antibodies. In most cases it resolves within one year.

Ultrasound in both diseases shows diffuse or patchy hypoechoicity of the thyroid gland. Color duplex examination reveals increased vascularity as the cause of the low echogenicity (**Fig. 14.26**).

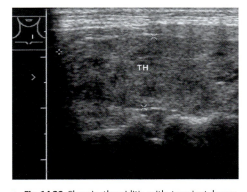

▲ **Fig. 14.26** Chronic thyroiditis with transient hyperthyroidism. Patient presented clinically with mild hyperthyroidism and no goiter. Anti-TPO and TRAbs negative, antithyroglobulin antibodies strongly positive.
Thyroid (TH) with a patchy hypoechoic structure.

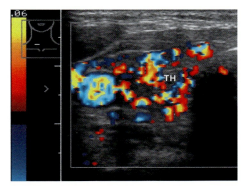

▲ **b** Color Doppler: pronounced vascularity.

▶ Silent (Sporadic) Thyroiditis

This condition runs a subacute or chronic course lasting from weeks to several months (years) with a self-limited course. It is usually associated with hyperthyroidism, rarely with hypothyroidism, but presents no other symptoms. Anti-TPO and antithyroglobulin antibodies are elevated. Silent thyroiditis is also interpreted as a painless variant of de Quervain thyroiditis, indistinguishable from postpartum thyreoiditis. It is distinguished by low radiotracer uptake in the thyroid.

The ultrasound findings are nonspecific, showing hypoechoic transformation of the gland (**Fig. 14.27**).

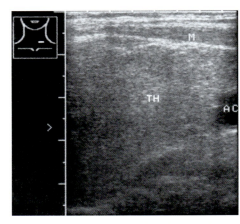

▲ **Fig. 14.27** Silent thyroiditis. Patient had mild hyperthyroidism, clinically asymptomatic and unchanged for years. TPO moderately elevated; TRAbs slightly elevated initially, now negative. Thyroid (TH) is slightly enlarged with a homogeneous, moderately hypoechoic structure.
a Transverse scan on the left side.

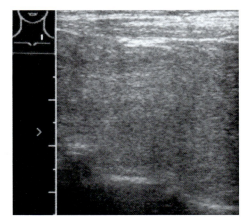

▲ *b* Longitudinal scan on the left side.

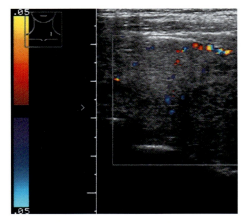

▲ *c* Color Doppler shows scant color-flow signals, contrasting with the hypervascularity in a Basedow goiter or autoimmune hyperthyroidism (**Fig. 14.13b**, ▣ **14.1e and f**, ▣ **14.4q**).

▶ Lithium- or Amiodarone-Induced Thyroiditis

Lithium. Psychiatric patients who take lithium frequently develop a thyroid disorder. This may take the form of a goiter, hypothyroidism, or both. It is assumed that lithium incites a thyroid autoimmune response. While slight enlargement is relatively common, the development of a frank autoimmune thyroiditis occurs in about 10% of cases, but this percentage rises significantly in cases with preexisting thyroid disease. Anti-TPO and antithyroglobulin antibodies are elevated.

Sonographically, the thyroid shows diffuse hypoechoicity that increases if low echogenicity was already present[9] (**Figs. 14.22, 14.28**).

Amiodarone. Treatment with amiodarone is also commonly followed by hyperthyroidism or hypothyroidism. This is based on the high iodine content of amiodarone and its structural similarity to the T_3 and T_4 hormones. Amiodarone has both agonistic and antagonistic effects on thyroid function. The fT_4 (free T4) level rises by approximately 40%, while the serum fT_3 level falls by about 50%, accompanied by a slight increase in the basal TSH.

The ultrasound findings are nonspecific and depend partly on a preexisting thyroid disorder. In Basedow disease with latent autonomy, patients frequently develop overt hyperthyroidism. Patients with Hashimoto thyroiditis tend to develop frank hypothyroidism or an exacerbation of existing hypothyroidism. If the thyroid is normal prior to amiodarone therapy, the drug may trigger an autoimmune thyroiditis, which is also associated with a hypoechoic thyroid (**Fig. 14.29**).

The changes are reversible after the drugs are discontinued.

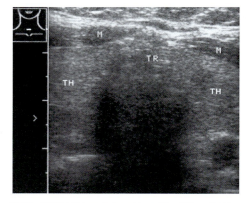

▲ **Fig. 14.28** Lithium-induced hypothyroidism. Besides minimal hypoechoicity, even color Doppler shows a normal-appearing thyroid gland (TH). TR = trachea; M = muscle.

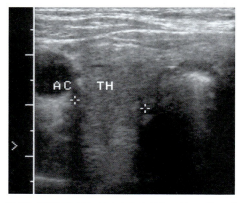
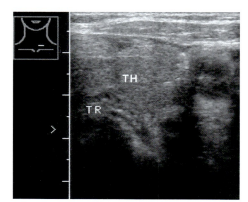

▲ **Fig. 14.29 a and b** Amiodarone-induced hypothyroidism: small, uniformly hypoechoic thyroid (TH). TR = trachea; AC = common carotid artery.

Hyperechoic Structure

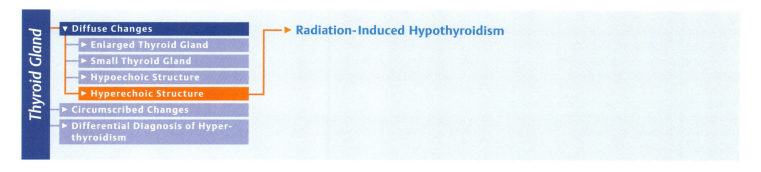

▶ Radiation-Induced Hypothyroidism

The thyroid gland is located within the radiotherapy portal when radiation is applied to the neck region, and it responds with hypothyroidism following a long latent period. The thyroid becomes smaller and undergoes a fibrous atrophy.

Accordingly, ultrasound demonstrates a small thyroid (see above) that shows a diffuse or mottled increase in echogenicity (**Fig. 14.25**).

Circumscribed Changes

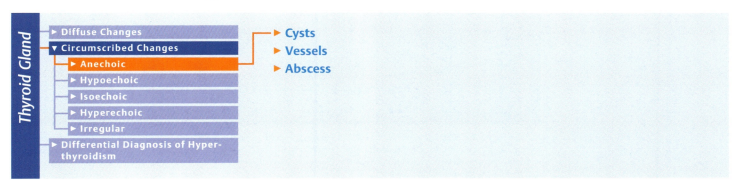

Anechoic

▶ Cysts

Cystic masses, along with thyroid nodules, are the most common focal changes that are found in the thyroid. Thyroid cysts are not true cysts and therefore do not contain cystic epithelium. Solitary cysts in an otherwise normal thyroid generally result from central hemorrhage in adenomas.

Cyst contents. Depending on their contents, cysts may appear sonographically as anechoic masses or may show a hypoechoic, hyperechoic, or irregular internal echo pattern (◧ **14.2**). Further diagnostic tests consist of color duplex sonography and fine-needle aspiration cytology. In many cases the cyst contents are unknown until fine-needle aspiration is performed. Cysts may contain various fluids:
▶ Fresh hemorrhage (◧ **14.2d and e**)
▶ Older hemorrhage (chocolate cysts, **Fig. 14.49**)
▶ Colloid (colloid cysts, ◧ **14.2f**)
▶ Lymph (lymph cysts)

Fresh hemorrhages and colloid cysts generally have a distinctive internal echo pattern and do not appear anechoic but hypoechoic or hyperechoic (◧ **14.2d and e**). With color duplex, cystic tumors show a vascularity that is never seen in cysts or hemorrhages. Other cysts extrinsic to the thyroid, such as neck cysts, should also be included in the differential diagnosis.

Solitary cysts. Uncomplicated serous cysts appear sonographically as anechoic, rounded or polygonal, sometimes lobulated, scalloped or patchy lesions with smooth margins. Like cysts in other organs, they display several typical cystic features such as absence of internal echoes, smooth borders, and distal acoustic enhancement, while a circular shape is somewhat unusual. Edge shadows are not present owing to the absence of a cyst wall. There is an additional sign, however: definite compressibility of the cysts by external transducer pressure. Solitary cysts also occur as hemorrhagic areas in diffuse goiters. Peripheral or circular remnants of the old adenomatous structure are also seen in most cases (■ 14.2a–c). Color Doppler examination shows a complete absence of vascularity in the cysts (■ 14.2e and i).

Multiple cysts. Multiple cysts are characteristic of regressive changes in the adenomatous nodules of older nodular goiters. They differ from hemorrhages in true adenomas by their multiplicity and their occurrence in the background structure of the nodular goiter.

Sonographically, they appear in various sizes ranging from microcysts to macrocysts. The latter often present clinically as circumscribed palpable nodules. Fresh bleeding in the cysts leads to the abrupt appearance or enlargement of a goiter.

Hemorrhagic cysts. Fresh bleeding in cysts produces a heterogeneous internal echo pattern that includes high-level echoes (■ 14.2d and e).

Lymph cysts. It is not uncommon for small cystic lesions to represent lymph cysts. They do not differ from other cystic lesions, except perhaps by their small size (■ 14.2g).

Colloid cysts. Because they contain colloid, these cysts display an anechoic or more or less finely granular internal echo pattern (■ 14.2f).

■ 14.2 Thyroid Cysts

▶ **Adenomas/noduls showing cystic regression**

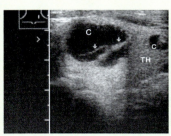
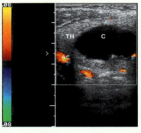
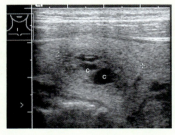

a Two cysts (C) in an otherwise unchanged left thyroid lobe (TH): anechoic masses with irregular margins. One shows septumlike partitions (arrows) and distal enhancement and creates a bulge in the thyroid contour.

b Cyst (C) in a nodular goiter (TH), the latter showing some peripheral vascularity.

c Anechoic cystic mass (C) with no internal blood flow in an isoechoic adenoma (cursors) in the left thyroid lobe (SD).

▶ **Hemorrhagic, colloid cysts**

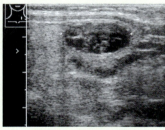
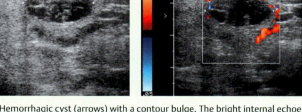
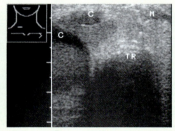

d and e Hemorrhagic cyst (arrows) with a contour bulge. The bright internal echoes are typical of fresh intracystic hemorrhage. Differentiation is required from an adenoma or tumor. Diagnosis is confirmed by the absence of internal vascularity (*e*) and by fine-needle aspiration. The peripheral vascular rim delineates the adenoma.

f Two cystic areas (C), one with internal echoes. Fine-needle aspiration yielded a creamy colloidal fluid (confirmed cytologically as colloid). M = musculature, TR = trachea.

▶ **Cysts in nodular goiters**

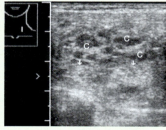
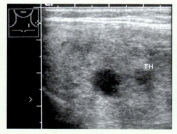
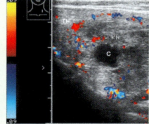

g Multiple small cysts (C) in a nodular goiter, interpreted as regressive changes. The more echogenic and more coarsely structured nodules (collagenous connective tissue) are also regressive changes. Differential diagnosis: lymph cysts.

h and i Irregular, regressive cystic mass with indistinct margins and mottled echo structure (C) in a goiter (TH). Fine peripheral vessels rim the nodular area (N).

▶ Vessels

Cysts require differentiation from anechoic lesions that can be identified as vessels only by color Doppler examination with spectral analysis **(Figs. 14.30 and 14.31; Figs. 14.6 and 14.7)**.

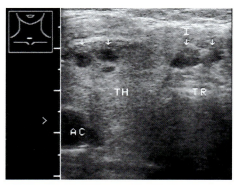
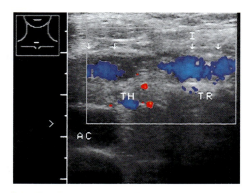

▲ **Fig. 14.30** Vessels in the thyroid. AC = common carotid artery; TR = trachea.
a Cystic areas (arrows) in gray-scale image.

▲ *b* Color Doppler identifies the areas as vessels.

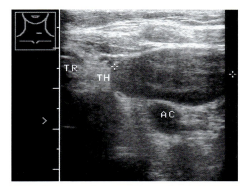
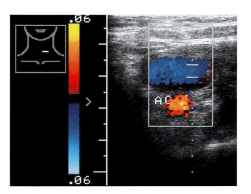

▲ **Fig. 14.31** Large, predominantly anechoic cystic mass (cursors) in the left thyroid lobe (TH). The common carotid artery (AC) is posterior. TR = trachea.
a Gray-scale image: the mass may be a large adenoma or a large cyst.

▲ *b* Color Doppler and spectral analysis identify the mass as a venous vessel (dilated internal jugular vein).

▶ Abscess

Abscesses almost always appear very hypoechoic and occasionally anechoic. The diagnosis is made clinically and/or by percutaneous aspiration **(see Fig. 14.37)**.

Hypoechoic

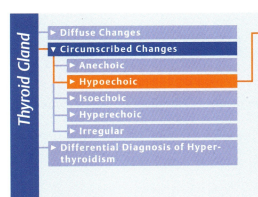

- ▶ Microfollicular (Papillary) Adenoma
- ▶ Oncocytic Adenoma
- ▶ Lipoma
- ▶ Parathyroid Adenoma
- ▶ Abscess
- ▶ Focal de Quervain Thyroiditis
- ▶ Malignant Lymphoma
- ▶ Carcinoma
- ▶ Tumor Infiltration or Metastasis

▶ Microfollicular (Papillary) Adenoma

Pathogenesis and Morphology of Thyroid Adenomas and Adenomatous Nodules

Prevalence. Thyroid nodules are found in 35–50% of people living in iodine-deficient areas. It is estimated that autonomous nodules are present in 2–6% of the general population[3] and in 10–20% of patients with a preexisting goiter.

Pathogenesis. The normal thyroid gland already contains a number of thyrocytes with an autonomous growth tendency that may give rise to adenomas, regardless of the iodine supply. A similar mechanism underlies the development of the predominantly autonomous nodules in a nodular goiter.

Morphology. True adenomas are benign neoplasms. Aside from very rare leiomyomas, they account for virtually all benign neoplasms in the thyroid. Follicular adenomas are the most common type of adenoma. Other variants are papillary adenoma and oncocytoma. Adenomas, unlike the adenomatous nodules in a nodular goiter, do not take part in autoimmune changes. Functionally, microfollicular adenomas consist mainly of autonomously functioning adenomas that appear as hot nodules at scintigraphy, whereas macrofollicular adenomas usually appear as cold nodules.

Sonographic features. Adenomas may appear as hypoechoic, isoechoic, or hyperechoic masses at ultrasound. The relationships between follicular histology and echogenicity shown in **Table 14.2** apply with fair accuracy to the echo structure of adenomas as well as to adenomatous nodules and regressive changes (◻ 14.3a–c).

Echogenicity. Hypoechoic nodules generally represent microfollicular adenomas (rarely papillary adenomas), whereas hyperechoic nodules are usually macrofollicular adenomas. Normofollicular adenomas generally appear isoechoic and are demarcated from the normal thyroid by a hypoechoic rim of displaced vessels, which can be identified with color Doppler. This vascular rim is also a feature of most other adenomas and adenomatous nodules (◻ 14.3e, f, and i). Isoechoic and hypoechoic adenomas are the most common types of adenoma, while hyperechoic adenomas are the least common.

Hypoechoic adenomas. The great majority of hypoechoic adenomas are autonomous adenomas, two-thirds of which are associated with latent hyperthyroidism (suppressed basal TSH with normal fT_3/fT_4 levels) and only one-third with overt hyperthyroidism[2]. The most common microfollicular adenomas are conspicuous by their hypoechoic structure and round shape. The anechoic rim described above is also a general characteristic of adenomas, although it is not seen with every adenoma.

Another characteristic of hypoechoic adenomas is their internal vascularity, which signifies autonomy in a high percentage of cases (73%)[5]. The absence of internal vascularity rules out autonomy with a negative predictive value of 94%[2]. Meanwhile, peripheral and internal vascularity is also found in a high percentage of malignancies, raising problems of differentiation based on ultrasound appearance.

Thyroid adenomas are also subject to regressive changes with intralesional hemorrhage and calcification, resulting in anechoic or hyperechoic internal structures (◻ 14.3f). A hypoechoic structure is insufficient in itself for evaluating functional autonomy (◻ 14.3h and I).

The above points can be summarized as follows:
- The color Doppler examination of thyroid nodules is a useful screening method for autonomous adenomas[3], especially in patients with known hyperthyroidism.

Diagnostic Evaluation of Solitary or Multiple Separate Hypoechoic Thyroid Nodules

- Sonography with color duplex scanning
- Basal TSH, also fT_3, fT_4 if necessary
- Scintigraphy of nodules > 10 mm
- Fine-needle aspiration of hypoechoic nodules that have an irregular rim and are larger than 10 mm
- With normal TSH but suspected autonomy: suppression scintigraphy
- With a sonographically hypoechoic nodule that is cold by scintigraphy: always fine-needle aspiration or surgery; also calcitonin assay (medullary C-cell carcinoma!).

- True adenomas cannot be distinguished from adenomatous nodules by their sonographic features (this cannot even be done histologically in some cases). The sonographic findings can provide clues for differentiation, however (**Table 14.3**).

Table 14.2 Histomorphology of thyroid nodules correlated with typical echogenicity at ultrasound

Histomorphological finding	Typical echogenicity
Predominance of microfollicles	Hypoechoic
Predominance of normal-sized follicles	Normal echo structure
Predominance of macrofollicles	Hyperechoic
Collagenous connective tissue	Hyperechoic
Hyaline connective tissue	Hypoechoic

Table 14.3 Sonographic clues for the differentiation of adenomas and adenomatous nodules

Adenomas	Adenomatous nodules
Usually solitary or isolated	Multiple
Usually in normal thyroid gland	Occurrence in a nodular goiter
Well-defined hypoechoic rim	Scalloped hypoechoic rim
Homogeneous internal echo pattern	Heterogeneous thyroid structure
Internal hypervascularity	Absent or scant internal vascularity

14.3 Thyroid Adenomas

- Types of adenoma
- Adenomas and nodules, color duplex

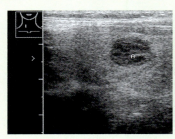 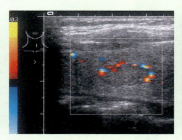 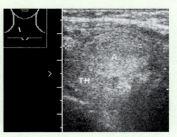

a Hypoechoic (microfollicular) adenoma (A): intensely hypoechoic mass with a subtle echo-free rim. Patient presented clinically with hyperthyroidism.

b Isoechoic adenoma, delineated only by a slightly hypoechoic peripheral vascular rim (color duplex).

c Hyperechoic.

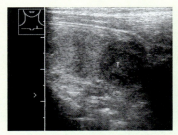 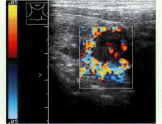 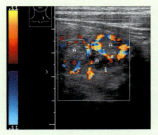

d Hypoechoic mass (T). Differential diagnosis: adenoma, malignant tumor, hemorrhagic cyst.

e Further examination with color Doppler shows intense peripheral vascularity as well as internal vessels.

f Multiple adenomas (A) of varying echogenicity in an otherwise normal thyroid, outlined by peripheral vascularity.

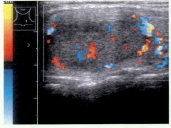 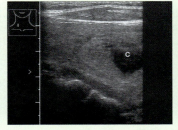 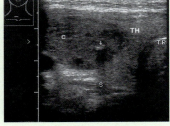

g Isoechoic adenoma with hypoechoic areas devoid of internal vascularity: adenoma with fresh intralesional hemorrhage (painful swelling; treated surgically).

h Hyperechoic adenoma with an old hemorrhagic area and cystic transformation (C).

i Thyroid adenoma with regressive changes. C = cyst, arrow = calcium with acoustic shadow. TH = thyroid; TR = trachea.

Oncocytic Adenoma

Oncocytic adenoma is another, rare type of adenoma. It is indistinguishable from a well-differentiated follicular carcinoma by ultrasonography or fine-needle aspiration cytology. Benign/malignant differentiation relies on the detection or exclusion of invasive growth in histologically examined surgical material.

Sonographically, oncocytic adenoma shows more or less pronounced internal vascularity but usually does not have a peripheral vascular rim (**Figs. 14.32 and 14.33**).

Differentiation is required from other hypoechoic tumors such as lipoma, malignant lymphoma, carcinoma, and metastases as well as rare abscesses or focal thyroiditis.

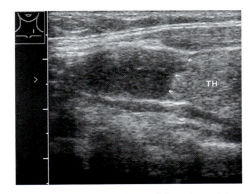 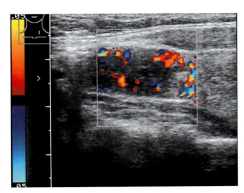

Fig. 14.32 Oncocytoma in a nodular goiter, cytological and surgical diagnosis.
a Very hypoechoic tumor with no detectable halo, relatively well demarcated (arrows) from the rest of the thyroid (TH).

b Color Doppler scan at a low PRF clearly reveals internal vascularity.

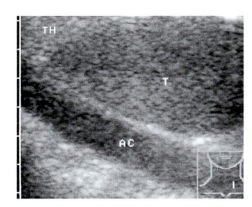 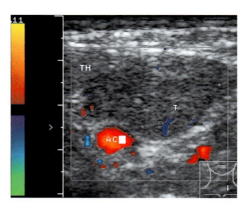

Fig. 14.33 Oncocytic adenoma, incidental finding, cytological diagnosis surgically confirmed. AC = common carotid artery.
a Homogeneous tumor (T), slightly hypoechoic to the rest of the thyroid (TH).

b Color Doppler at a relatively high PRF shows almost no vascularity.

▶ Lipoma

A lipoma is occasionally misinterpreted clinically as a nodular goiter. While its ultrasound features resemble those of adenoma or microcystic nodular transformation, it can be distinguished (when considered in the differential diagnosis) by its typical mottled or streaky hypoechoic appearance. The thyroid can usually be clearly delineated from the lipoma embedded in the anterior subcutaneous fat (**Fig. 14.34**).

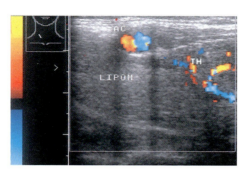

Fig. 14.34 Patient had received replacement therapy for a goiter for years. A nodule extends far toward the right side. A lipoma is delineated only by its lack of vascularity on color duplex examination of the thyroid gland (TH). AC = common carotid artery.

▶ Parathyroid Adenoma

Like lipoma, parathyroid adenoma (both primary idiopathic adenoma and secondary parathyroid hyperplasia due to renal failure and hypocalcemia) appears as a hypoechoic mass located *next to* the thyroid gland. The location of the parathyroid glands has been described above under "Topography."

Sonographic features. Parathyroid adenoma is markedly less echogenic than the thyroid, has an echo structure ranging from homogeneous to patchy-cystic with increasing size, and presents a round, oval, or polygonal shape. Internal vascularity has been variously described and may be subtle. Peripheral vascularity is believed to be uncommon, but curved vascular rims have been described around the adenomas (**Figs. 14.35 and 14.36**).

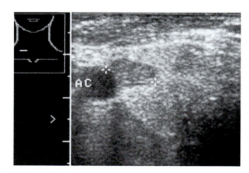 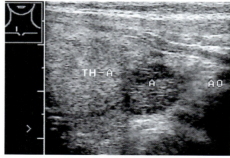 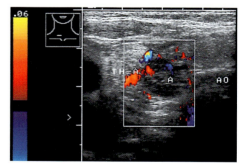

▲ **Fig. 14.35** Parathyroid adenoma (cursors) in hyperparathyroidism: rounded, hypoechoic mass bordering the common carotid artery (AC) at the inferolateral pole of the thyroid.

▲ **Fig. 14.36** Parathyroid adenoma (A).
a Located at the lower pole of the thyroid (accompanied here by an isoechoic thyroid adenoma; TH-A) and above the aortic arch (AO).

▲ *b* Color Doppler demonstrates slight internal vascularity and subtle peripheral vascularity.

▶ Abscess

Rare abscesses of the thyroid gland have a similar hypoechoic appearance to adenomas, cysts, and lymphomas. Their presence signifies an acute purulent thyroiditis.

Thyroid abscess appears sonographically as a mostly anechoic or hypoechoic mass with irregular internal echoes. Color duplex examination shows an absence of vascularity (**Fig. 14.37**).

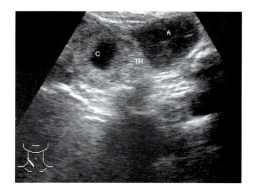

◀ **Fig. 14.37** Thyroid abscess (A) next to a thyroid adenoma with a regressive cyst (C): very hypoechoic mass opposite the cyst with faint internal echoes and blocky contours. Patient presented clinically with marked signs of inflammation and a reddish, tender neck mass.

▶ Focal de Quervain Thyroiditis

De Quervain thyroiditis is usually a diffuse thyroid disease, but infrequent unilateral cases occur. The diagnosis is established by clinical examination and fine-needle aspiration cytology.

Typical ultrasound findings consist of well-circumscribed or irregular hypoechoic areas that either are hypovascular or, in some reports, show moderate vascularity (**Figs. 14.38 and 14.39**).

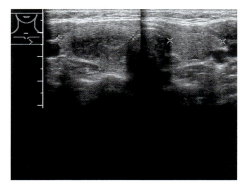

▲ **Fig. 14.38** Focal de Quervain thyroiditis of the right thyroid lobe, transverse scan through both lobes (cursors). The right lobe contains a central, ill-defined, hypoechoic mass causing an elliptical contour bulge; the left lobe appears normal. Patient had a three-month history of viral infection, high inflammatory parameters, and a circumscribed bulge with pain radiating to the right side of the neck.

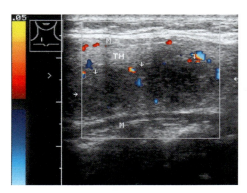

▲ **Fig. 14.39** Focal de Quervain thyroiditis. Color Doppler image shows scant peripheral vascularity and no internal vessels. Scintigraphy revealed a cold spot on the right side. Fine-needle aspiration cytology showed no evidence of an abscess or malignancy. Weeks later the left thyroid lobe was also involved. TH = thyroid; M = muscle.

▶ Malignant Lymphoma

Malignant lymphomas of the thyroid gland usually occur in the setting of generalized lymphomatous disease. Tumor clusters in the neck may be distributed about the thyroid gland. They can be difficult to delineate from the normal thyroid structure even when thyroid nodules are present.

Malignant lymphomas are characterized by a very low echogenicity. They show a variable degree of vascularity (**Fig. 14.40**).

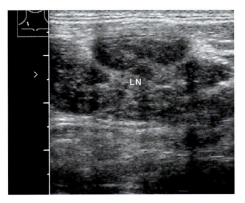

▲ **Fig. 14.40** Stage IIb Hodgkin lymphoma, nodular sclerosis.
a Markedly enlarged parathyroid lymph node (LN) with a patchy, very hypoechoic structure. Longitudinal parathyroid scan of the right neck.

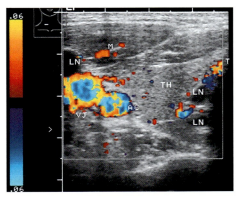

▲ **b** Lymphomas lying directly adjacent to the thyroid gland (TH) show no vascularity. T = trachea; VJ = internal jugular vein; AC = common carotid artery.

▶ Carcinoma

Thyroid carcinomas present as a clinically palpable neck mass that produces a cold nodule at scintigraphy. Ultrasound can be an effective adjunct to radionuclide scanning by showing that many cold nodules are not suspicious for cancer (cysts, calcified or hyperechoic nodules). Malignancies always have a hypoechoic or nonhomogeneous hypoechoic structure.

Histology. The following malignant thyroid tumors are listed in the WHO classification:
- ▶ Carcinoma
  - Follicular carcinoma
  - Papillary carcinoma
  - Medullary C-cell carcinoma
  - Undifferentiated (anaplastic) carcinoma
  - Special form: squamous cell carcinoma (Lindsay tumor)
- ▶ Nonepithelial tumors
- ▶ Malignant lymphoma
- ▶ Metastases from extrathyroid tumors

Papillary and follicular carcinoma are more common in the thyroid gland than medullary C-cell carcinoma, while anaplastic and squamous cell carcinoma are rare. Distant metastases are more common with follicular and medullary C-cell carcinoma, while locoregional metastases are more typical of papillary carcinoma. Medullary C-cell carcinoma grows slowly but often has already metastasized after reaching 10 mm. Undifferentiated anaplastic carcinoma is considered highly malignant owing to its propensity for rapid invasive growth and early metastasis. Only about 3% of patients survive longer than two years.

Detection. A thyroid malignancy cannot be positively detected by ultrasonography, even when color Doppler is used. Fine-needle aspiration cytology is still the most accurate method for cancer diagnosis. This pertains chiefly to papillary and medullary cancers. The diagnosis of follicular carcinoma must generally rely on surgical specimen histology. C-cell carcinoma is best diagnosed by fine-needle aspiration with a calcitonin assay or by direct histological examination.

Sonographic features. Besides their consistently hypoechoic to almost anechoic appearance, carcinomas are distinguished sonographically by a predominantly absent or incomplete (rarely closed) peripheral vascular rim. They invariably show intense central vascularity, but this is also detectable in 30% of benign nodules (**Fig. 14.41, Fig. 14.64, and Fig. 14.42**).

It can be extremely difficult to detect malignancies in nodular goiters. Most cases involve older patients with a prominent goiter. Acoustic enhancement as well as shadowing may be seen posterior to a carcinomatous lesion. Flocculent calcifications are suggestive of medullary C-cell carcinoma, while microcalcifications are often found in papillary carcinoma as well as in other forms. On the whole, the different types of carcinoma cannot be distinguished from one another by their sonographic features.

Differential diagnosis. The most difficult lesion to distinguish sonographically from carcinoma is a hypoechoic adenoma. The former belief that adenoma could be distinguished from carcinoma by its peripheral rim is no longer supported by data in the literature[2, 16]. It remains unclear whether color duplex scanning can advance the differential diagnosis. The sonographic features of adenoma are contrasted with those of carcinoma in **Table 14.4**. Ultrasound is most accurate in diagnosing carcinoma only when multiple signs (absence of a peripheral halo combined with microcalcifications and intranodal hypervascularity) are simultaneously present in a thyroid nodule with

---

Medullary Thyroid Carcinoma

MEN syndrome. Medullary thyroid carcinoma (MTC) is not a carcinoma of the actual thyroid tissue but an endocrine carcinoma located in the thyroid gland. It shows a familial occurrence and may be isolated (FMTC) or may occur in the setting of multiple endocrine neoplasia (MEN II syndrome: MTC, pheochromocytoma, parathyroid hyperplasia, cutaneous neurofibromatosis). Sporadic cases also occur.

MEN I tumors are also derived from the peripheral endocrine APUD system. The diagnosis of this syndrome relies on intestinal polypeptide screening. The age-dependent sequence of lesions occurring from early infancy to over age 50 is as follows: insulinomas, parathyroid adenomas, gastrinomas, prolactinomas (ACTH), glucagonomas, and finally VIPomas.

Laboratory values. Medullary thyroid carcinoma leads to a rise in basal or stimulated serum calcitonin levels, providing a marker for early diagnosis. Even if the tumor is not detectable, it can be inferred from elevated calcitonin levels. Carcinoembryonic antigen (CEA) is also elevated.

Growth characteristics. Medullary thyroid carcinoma grows slowly but metastasizes early to locoregional lymph nodes. Standard operative treatment should therefore include locoregional lymph node dissection in addition to total thyroidectomy. This operation is curative in 25% of cases even with positive cervical lymph nodes [6].

Table 14.4 Differentiation of microfollicular adenoma from carcinoma based on common sonographic features

	Micro- or normofollicular adenoma	Carcinoma
Structure	Hypoechoic, normal echogenicity	Hypoechoic
Regressive changes	Frequent cysts, calcification	Rarely, cystic elements
Microcalcifications	Rare	Common
Peripheral rim	Common	Variable
Internal vascularity	Common (approximately 51% of cases)	67–100%
Lymph nodes	None	Relatively common

Table 14.5 Diagnosis and treatment of a hypoechoic cold thyroid nodule

Nodule	Diagnosis	Treatment
< 10 mm	6-month ultrasound follow-ups	200 μg iodide
10–20 mm	FNAB, if benign →	200 μg iodide, follow-ups
> 30 mm	Surgery or FNAB	
De novo	Always evaluate by FNAB	Surgery if required

a high specificity of 97.2% but a low sensitivity of 16.6%. Therefore only in a small proportion of patients with thyroid carcinoma is ultrasonography and color flow Doppler information highly predictive of malignancy.

Further management. With hypoechoic thyroid nodules smaller than 10 mm, an expectant approach with 6-month follow-ups is appropriate owing to the slow growth rate of differentiated carcinomas. Any hypoechoic nodule larger than 10 mm should be investigated by thyroid scintigraphy, and a cold nodule always warrants fine-needle aspiration biopsy. **Table 14.5** shows the recommended diagnostic strategy for a scintigraphic cold nodule that is hypoechoic at ultrasound.

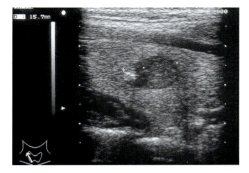
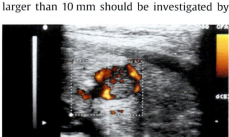

◄◄ **Fig. 14.41** Thyroid carcinoma (C-cell carcinoma).
a Hypoechoic mass (cursors) with a hypoechoic rim. It contains a small flocculent calcification with an acoustic shadow.

◄ **b** An intense vascular rim partially surrounds the mass, which shows internal vascularity.

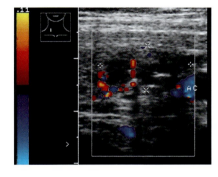

◄◄ **Fig. 14.42** Thyroid carcinoma: squamous cell carcinoma (Lindsay tumor), detected incidentally in a 45-year-old woman undergoing ultrasound for type I diabetes.
a Hypoechoic tumor (cursors, microcalcification). S = shadowing.

◄ **b** Color Doppler shows both peripheral and internal vascularity. AC = common carotid artery.

▶ Tumor Infiltration or Metastasis

Esophageal and tracheobronchial carcinomas are most likely to infiltrate the thyroid, whereas hematogenous metastasis is more common with bronchial and renal-cell carcinoma, malignant melanoma, and breast cancer.

Contiguous spread. The tumors that most commonly invade the thyroid by direct extension are esophageal carcinoma and occasionally tracheal carcinoma.

Ultrasound may show evidence of the primary tumor. Conversely, the trachea may be infiltrated by a primary thyroid carcinoma or very rarely a sarcoma. The growth of a benign nodular goiter into the trachea is extremely difficult to distinguish from the extension of carcinoma (**Figs. 14.43–14.45**).

Metastases. Metastases have the same ultrasound appearance as thyroid carcinoma. They may be microscopically small or may reach tremendous size, sometimes acquiring a scalloped shape. Their vascularity at color duplex examination ranges from hypovascular to very hypervascular (**Figs. 14.46 and 14.47**).

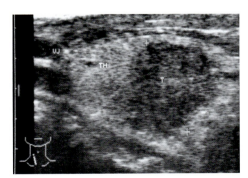

▲ **Fig. 14.43** Tracheal carcinoma invading the thyroid gland (TH). The patient presented with severe stridor. Scan shows a hypoechoic mass with ill-defined margins (T, cursors). VJ = jugular vein.

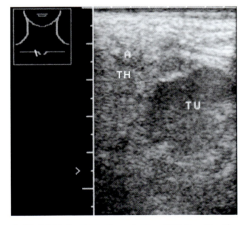

▲ **Fig. 14.44** Esophageal carcinoma (TU) invading the lower pole of the thyroid (TH). A = small thyroid adenoma.

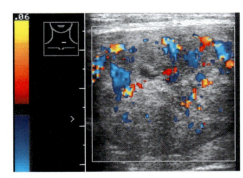

▲ **Fig. 14.45** This patient presented with a firm nodule on the left side of the neck. Color Doppler demonstrates a vascular rim encircling a large nodule that shows internal vascularity. The resistance index is increased to 0.85. The lesion shows a slightly nonhomogeneous structure with hyperechoic and hypoechoic areas. The morphological features are those of an adenomatous nodule with subtle regressive changes. A similar nodule was found on the right side. Surgery and histology: both were whitish nodules identified as metastases from a trabecular clear-cell carcinoma (renal cell carcinoma 10 years after nephrectomy! See **Fig. 1.72b, p. 30**).

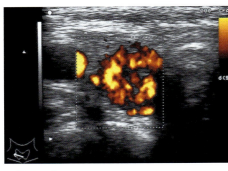

▲ **Fig. 14.46** Metastases from a malignant melanoma. Color Doppler shows marked intralesional vascularity.

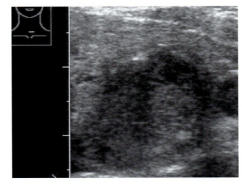

▲ **Fig. 14.47** Adenomatous nodule or metastasis?
a B-mode image shows a large, suspicious hypoechoic mass following melanoma surgery. Cytology was suspicious for metastatic melanoma, but histology confirmed an adenoma.

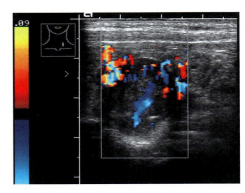

▲ **b** Color Doppler shows prominent internal vascularity.

Isoechoic

- Diffuse Changes
- ▼ Circumscribed Changes
  - Anechoic
  - Hypoechoic
  - ► **Isoechoic**
  - Hyperechoic
  - Irregular
- Differential Diagnosis of Hyperthyroidism

▶ **Normofollicular Adenoma**
▶ **Hemorrhagic or Colloid Cyst**
▶ **Regressive Changes in an Adenoma or Adenomatous Nodule**

▶ Normofollicular Adenoma

As a rule, solitary isoechoic nodules in the thyroid gland are normofollicular adenomas. They have the same echo structure as the rest of the thyroid parenchyma and can be distinguished only by their hypoechoic or anechoic rim (halo). Normofollicular thyroid nodules, like hypoechoic nodules, may show increased radiotracer uptake at scintigraphy, identifying them as autonomous adenomas. By contrast, hyperechoic adenomas almost never show uptake that indicates autonomy.

Sonographic features. Normofollicular adenomas have the same reflectivity as normal thyroid tissue, with the result that adenomas usually are not detectable with ultrasound unless they are located at the periphery of the gland and cause an appreciable contour bulge. They may be circumscribed by an echo-poor vascular rim (**Fig. 14.48, ▣ 14.3b**).

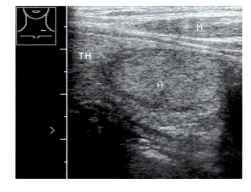
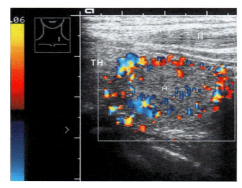

◀◀ **Fig. 14.48** Isoechoic adenoma (A) in a euthyroid patient. M = muscle.
a B-mode image shows an elliptical halo in an otherwise normal-appearing thyroid (TH).

◀ **b** Color Doppler demonstrates a vascular rim with slight internal vascularity.

▶ Hemorrhagic or Colloid Cyst

Besides adenomas, isoechoic nodules may be caused by fresh bleeding within a cyst or by large colloid-containing cysts. These cystic lesions can be identified as such by noting their compressibility at ultrasound. Subtle movements of the cyst contents may also be observed. Fine-needle aspiration can quickly resolve any doubts as to whether the mass is liquid or solid (**Fig. 14.49 and ▣ 14.2f**). Carcinomas are rarely isoechoic and are almost never hyperechoic.

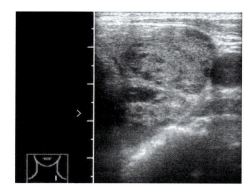

◀ *Fig. 14.49* A cyst with internal hemorrhage is predominantly isoechoic and creates a bulge in the thyroid contour. Fine-needle aspiration identified this lesion as a chocolate cyst.

▶ Regressive Changes in an Adenoma or Adenomatous Nodule

Adenomas tend to undergo regressive changes over time. As collagenous connective tissue is formed, the initially hypoechoic nodules become more echogenic. The adenomas lose their homogeneous structure, and other regressive changes such as cyst formation and calcification may supervene, giving the nodule an irregular or heterogeneous echo structure (**Fig. 14.50**).

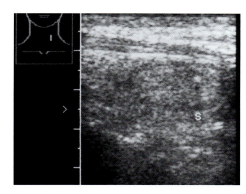

◀ *Fig. 14.50* Regressive changes in an isoechoic nodule with an echopenic halo. The lesion is isoechoic to the rest of the thyroid gland but has a somewhat coarser texture, probably due to the presence of collagenous connective tissue. It also contains a small calcification with a posterior shadow (S).

Hyperechoic

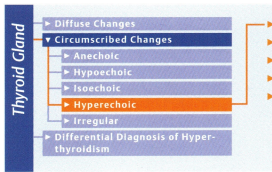

- ▶ Macrofollicular Adenoma or Nodule
- ▶ Hemorrhagic Cyst, Colloid Cyst
- ▶ Nodule with Regressive Changes
- ▶ Hemangioma, Myolipoma, Thyroid Regressive Changes
- ▶ Calcifications

Hyperechoic lesions in the thyroid gland may be macrofollicular adenomas, adenomatous nodules, nodules with regressive fibrous changes, or in rare cases benign tumors such as hemangiomas, lipomas, and myolipomas. Regressive changes may consist of cystic transformation, fibrous changes with collagenous or hyaline connective-tissue formation, and calcifications. While hyaline connective tissue has a very low reflectivity (▣ 14.1a), collagenous connective tissue is very echogenic. Thus, high echogenicity in a nodule may by caused by a histomorphological macrofollicular structure or by the presence of collagenous connective tissue in the nodule.

▶ Macrofollicular Adenoma or Nodule

Solitary hyperechoic nodules in an otherwise normal thyroid gland are generally macrofollicular adenomas. They show no tracer uptake at scintigraphy, appearing as cold nodules. Scintigraphy cannot evaluate the structural changes that underlie cold nodules, which may represent carcinoma, fibrous regressive nodules, or cysts. Sonography is an ideal complement to scintigraphy in making this kind of differentiation (**Table 14.5**).

Hyperechoic adenomas are less common than hypoechoic microfollicular adenomas. Macrofollicular nodules show little or no internal vascularity when evaluated by color Doppler.

Nodules with fibrous regressive changes, like macrofollicular adenomas, are more echogenic than normal thyroid tissue but tend to display a coarsely granular to patchy echo texture (**Fig. 14.51**).

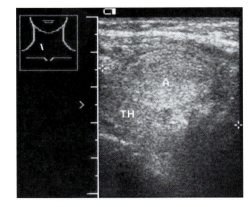

▲ **Fig. 14.51** Hyperechoic adenoma (A) in a normal thyroid gland (TH, cursors), delineated by peripheral vascularity.

▶ Hemorrhagic Cyst, Colloid Cyst

Hemorrhagic or colloid cysts may exhibit a hyperechoic or irregular echo structure. They are sharply marginated compared with other hyperechoic masses. The nature of the mass is determined by fine-needle aspiration (▣ **14.2f** and **Fig. 14.49**).

▶ Nodule with Regressive Changes

A nodular goiter of long standing will generally contain nodules with regressive changes. Cystic transformation and calcification are common along with fibrous changes (**Fig. 14.52**).

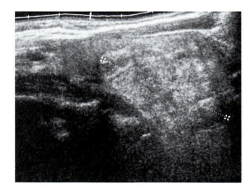

◀ **Fig. 14.52** Hyperechoic, nonhomogeneous thyroid nodule (cursors) with regressive changes.

▶ Hemangioma, Myolipoma, Thyroid Regressive Changes

These small, round, well-circumscribed lesions are quite conspicuous at ultrasound owing to their very high reflectivity. When these lesions are found, it is difficult to tell what histopathological elements are responsible for their high echogenicity. They have no real clinical significance other than the fact that they may represent a parathyroid gland that appears more echogenic due to fatty degeneration or fibrosis (**Fig. 14.53**).

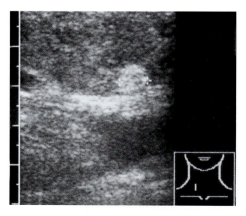

◀ **Fig. 14.53** Small, round, hyperechoic nodule (cursors) in a hypoechoic thyroid gland. The differential diagnosis consists of hemangioma, lipoma, and thyroid adenoma with regressive changes. The patient presented with renal failure and mild hyperparathyroidism.

▶ Calcifications

Calcifications occur in large, long-standing nodules that have undergone regressive change. They appear sonographically as high-amplitude echoes with acoustic shadows. They range in size from tiny specks to coarse flecks of calcification and vary markedly in their shape and conspicuity. Air echoes from the trachea may occasionally be mistaken for thyroid calcifications. Positioning the thyroid at the center of the image can help to avoid this confusion (**Figs. 14.54–14.56**).

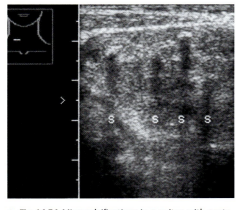

▲ **Fig. 14.54** Microcalcifications in a goiter, with posterior acoustic shadows (S).

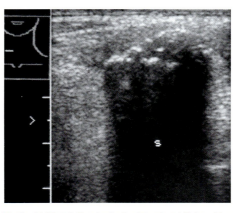

▲ **Fig. 14.55** Calcification in the right thyroid lobe with a dense acoustic shadow (S). Not to be confused with the trachea!

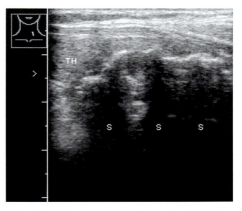

▲ **Fig. 14.56** Broad band of calcification in the left thyroid lobe with acoustic shadows (S).

Irregular

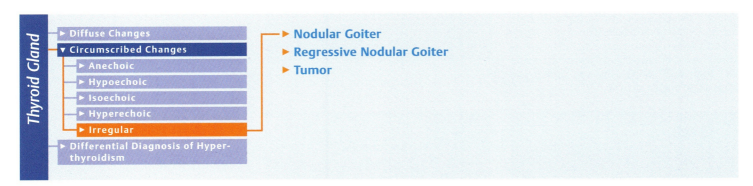

▶ Nodular Goiter

A nodular goiter generally develops in the setting of a long-standing diffuse goiter in an iodine-deficient geographic region. But nodules can form and multinodular goiters can develop even in normal thyroid glands, regardless of iodine intake, as a consequence of heterogeneous thyrocyte populations and genetic cell changes. This type of goiter is based on true adenomatous growth. For this reason alone, the goal of surgically resecting a nodular goiter is to remove all grossly visible nodules as completely as possible. Although the nodules will still be present after radioiodine treatment, their hyperthyroid activity will be eradicated.

Sonographic features. Ultrasonography is the most sensitive study for delineating nodules[18]. A nodular goiter is marked by thyroid enlargement and a disordered or heterogeneous echo structure, depending on how pronounced the regressive changes are. In the ideal case of discrete nodules in a side-by-side arrangement,

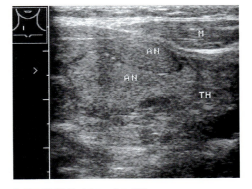

▲ **Fig. 14.57** Nodular goiter. The individual adenomatous nodules (A) are clearly delineated by their hypoechoic rims.

▲ **Fig. 14.58** Nodular goiter (TH).
a The adenomatous nodules (AN) are partially confluent.

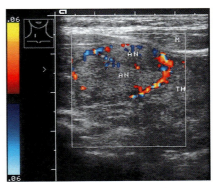

▲ **b** When viewed with color Doppler, however, the nodules are individually defined by their scalloped margins. On the whole, the thyroid appears hypoechoic to the adjacent muscle (M).

the nodular goiter is easily recognized at ultrasound by the halos that surround the nodules. Frequently, however, the nodules are confluent and of variable size, making it extremely difficult to delineate them in the B-mode image. Only color Doppler can define individual nodules in these cases (**Figs. 14.57–14.59**). It is virtually impossible, however, to distinguish autonomous nodules with ultrasound. This applies to carcinomatous nodules as well (see below).

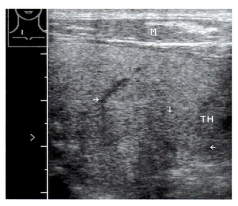

▲ *Fig. 14.59* Nodular goiter (TH). The individual nodules can no longer be identified.
a B-mode image shows only bizarre anechoic lines (arrows) that are not consistent with a diffuse goiter (which should be included in the differential diagnosis).

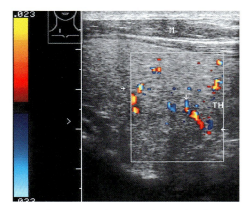

▲ *b* In the color Doppler image, the anechoic lines can be identified as remnants of peripheral vessels around the nodules.

▶ Regressive Nodular Goiter

The ultrasound appearance of a long-standing nodular goiter becomes increasingly difficult to interpret over time. The already diverse sonomorphological features of nodules are made more complex by the addition of regressive changes such as cystic transformation, hyperechoic collagenous connective tissue, hypoechoic hyaline connective tissue, and microcalcifications or macrocalcifications, which create an extremely heterogeneous appearance (**Figs. 14.60 and 14.61**).

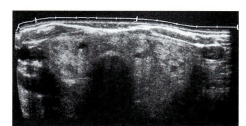

◀ *Fig. 14.60* Regressive nodular goiter. SieScape panoramic image shows an irregular thyroid structure with anechoic inclusions (cysts), hyperechoic areas (collagenous connective tissue), and hypoechoic elements (blood vessels, hyaline connective tissue?).

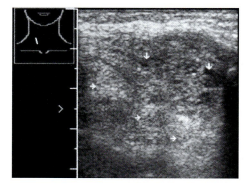
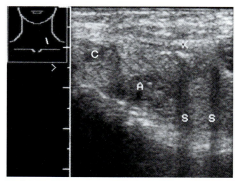

◀ *Fig. 14.61 a and b* Nodular goiter with regressive changes in a hyperthyroid patient. Scans show a patchy, hyperechoic background texture with hypoechoic adenomatous nodules (A), also calcifications with acoustic shadows (S). C = cyst.

▶ Tumor

Large tumors tend to develop areas of necrotic liquefaction. Together with calcifications, they produce a complex echo pattern with an irregular sonomorphological structure that is difficult to interpret (**Figs. 14.62–14.64**). The diagnosis relies chiefly on radionuclide findings (cold nodules), clinical manifestations (enlarging goiter), and fine-needle aspiration biopsy.

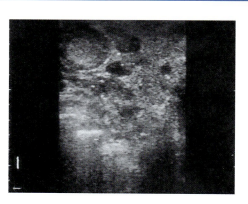

◀ *Fig. 14.62* Follicular thyroid carcinoma. Emergency surgery was performed for stridor. Ultrasound shows a large hypoechoic tumor with several hypoechoic to anechoic areas and multiple fine echogenic foci. Histology: partially necrotic follicular thyroid carcinoma.

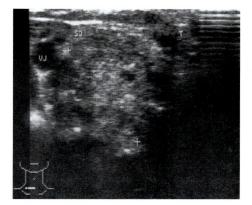
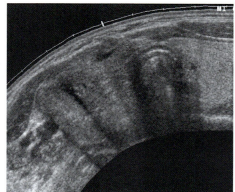

▲ **Fig. 14.63** Papillary thyroid carcinoma (histologically well-differentiated) shows a coarse heterogeneous structure with multiple confluent hypoechoic areas and small, echogenic flecks of calcification. VJ = jugular vein; T = trachea.

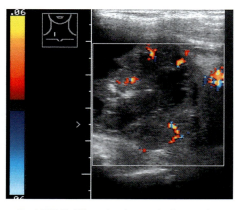

▲ **Fig. 14.64** Undifferentiated anaplastic carcinoma shows an irregular structure with a hypoechoic background, internal vascularity, central anechoic foci of liquefaction, and echogenic microcalcifications.

Differential Diagnosis of Hyperthyroidism

Types of Autonomy

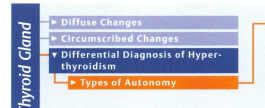

Approximately 40% of all hyperthyroidism has an immune etiology. Almost all children and adolescents with hyperthyroidism have Basedow disease as an underlying condition. In older patients with hyperthyroidism, functional autonomy (usually multifocal) is present in 70–80% of cases. In iodine-deficient areas, hyperthyroidism occurs predominantly in a latent form (low basal TSH with normal peripheral hormone levels) that is generally missed unless a routine basal TSH determination is performed (just as overt hyperthyroidism is often missed because of nonspecific clinical symptoms).

Both the sonographic and scintigraphic detection of autonomous foci in nodular goiters present major difficulties, because multiple confluent nodules give the thyroid a generally hypoechoic appearance in which these echopenic (potentially autonomous) nodules cannot be individually identified.

Special problems arise in cases where autonomously functioning nodules coexist with Basedow hyperthyroidism (Marine–Lenhard syndrome, 1% incidence) (▣ **14.4p–r**) or autonomous foci develop in a setting of autoimmune lymphocytic thyroiditis (Hashimoto) (▣ **14.4s–u**). Definitive treatment for hyperthyroidism should be withheld in these cases, and replacement therapy should be instituted despite the hyperthyroidism.

Given the important role of ultrasound in patients who present with hyperthyroid symptoms, the causes of hyperthyroidism are listed in ▣ **14.4** and illustrated with ultrasound images and correlative radionuclide scans. The examples do not include hyperthyrosis factitia (hyperthyroidism induced by the exogenous administration of thyroid hormones) or hyperthyroidism as a paraneoplastic syndrome.

Clinical Classification of Hyperthyroidism

Even isoechoic adenomas, like hypoechoic microfollicular adenomas, may be autonomous and lead to hyperthyroidism. In nodular goiters as well, the likelihood that adenomatous nodules will develop increases with the age of the goiter. The following types of autonomy can arise:
- Unifocal autonomy (one nodule)
- Bifocal autonomy (two nodules)
- Multifocal autonomy (multiple nodules)
- Disseminated autonomy involving the entire thyroid (rarer than the other types)

Autoimmune thyroid diseases that are associated with hyperthyroidism include the following:
- Immunogenic Basedow hyperthyroidism
- Hypertrophic Hashimoto thyroiditis
- de Quervain thyroiditis (including silent thyroiditis)
- Chronic thyroiditis with transient hyperthyroidism or postpartum thyroiditis
- Amiodarone-induced thyroiditis

14.4 Hyperthyroidism: Ultrasound Findings and Correlative Scintiscans

▶ Unifocal autonomy

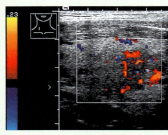 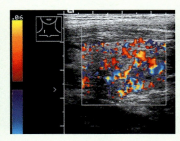 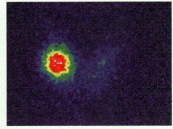

a Color Doppler scan at a relatively high PRF shows circumscribed hypervascularity only in the area of the adenoma.

b Scan at a low PRF shows diffuse vascularity that is most intense superiorly.

c Unifocal autonomy on the right side. The other portions of the thyroid are suppressed.

▶ Bifocal autonomy

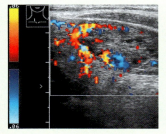 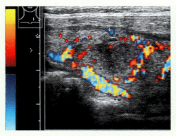 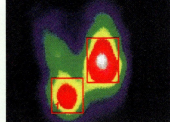

d Patchy hypoechoic adenomatous nodule in the lower part of the right lobe (A), showing marked peripheral vascularity.

e Similar adenomatous nodule in the left lobe with peripheral vascularity.

f Predominantly left-sided goiter with bifocal autonomy.

▶ Multifocal autonomy

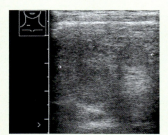 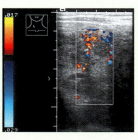 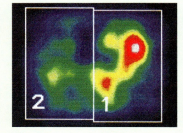

g Transverse scan on the right side shows an irregular, generally hypoechoic background pattern in the right lobe.

h Longitudinal scan on the right side shows a hypoechoic mass with scant peripheral vascularity.

i Multifocal autonomy.

▶ Disseminated autonomy

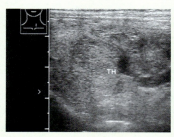 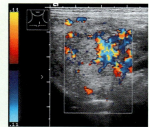 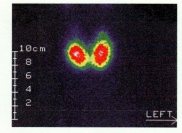

j Nodular goiter (SD).

k Coarse, patchy vascularity, subtly delineating a nodular lesion.

l Disseminated autonomy with confirmed hyperthyroidism.

▶ Disseminated autonomy in autoimmune thyroiditis (polyglandular autoimmune syndrome type II)

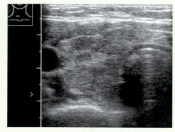 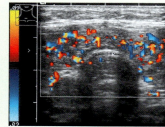 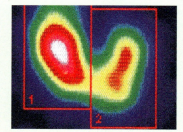

m Right thyroid lobe: coarse, patchy hypoechoic structure.

n Swelling of the isthmus. Scan at 0.09 m/s still shows definite vascularity (similar to Basedow disease). Maximally high TPO levels, no anti-TSH receptor antibodies.

o Diffuse goiter predominantly affecting the right lobe.

14.4 Hyperthyroidism: Ultrasound Findings and Correlative Scintiscans

▶ Basedow disease with focal autonomy (Marine–Lenhard syndrome)

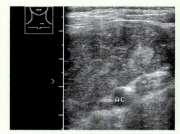
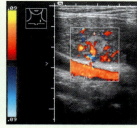
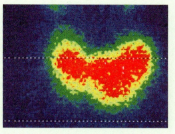

p Basedow disease: marked hypoechoicity and swelling of the left lobe, also nodules (one marked with an arrow). AC = carotid artery.

q Hypervascularity in one of the nodules, which here appears more reflective than the otherwise hypoechoic thyroid gland. AC = carotid artery.

r Basedow thyroid shows increased radiotracer uptake predominantly in the left lobe.

▶ Autoimmune thyroiditis with additional autonomous adenomas

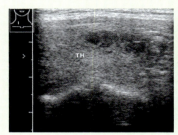
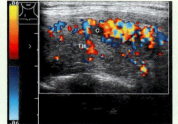
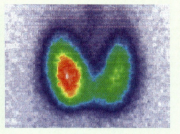

s Hypoechoic thyroid gland (TH) with a circumscribed, anechoic bandlike area on the right side; incipient thyrotoxicosis. Anti-TPO > 1000, anti-TSH receptor antibodies slightly elevated.

t Pronounced hypervascularity in the patchy echo-free lesion in *s*. The vessel-spared area is a cyst (C). The rest of the thyroid also shows increased vascularity.

u Scintiscan shows intense uptake in the right lobe and decreased uptake in the left lobe.

References

1. Baldini M, Castagnone D, Rivolta D et al. Thyroid vascularisation by color Doppler ultrasonography in Graves disease. Changes related to different phases and to the long-term outcome of the disease. Thyroid 1997;7:823–8.
2. Becker D, Bair HJ, Becker W et al. Thyroid autonomy with color-coded image-directed sonography; internal hypervascularisation for the recognition of autonomous adenomas. J clin Ultrasound 1997;25:63–9.
3. Becker D, Lohner W, Martus P, Hahn EG. Farbdopplersonographische Detektion von fokalen Schilddrüsenautonomien. Ultraschall in Med 1999;20:41–6.
4. Braun B, Günther R, Schwerk WB. Ultraschalldiagnostik. Lehrbuch und Atlas. Landshut: Ecomed 1992.
5. Clark KJ, Cronan JJ, Scola FH. Color doppler sonography: Anatomic and physiologic assessment of thyroid. J clin Ultrasound 1995;23:215–23.
6. Dralle H, Scheumann GFW, Proye C. The value of lymph node dissection in hereditary medullar thyroid carcinoma. J Intern Med 1995;238:357–61.
7. Guggenberger D. Ultraschalldiagnostik 94. Dreiländertreffen Basel 1994.
8. Junik R, Sawicka J, Kozak W, Gembicki M. Thyroid volume and function in patients with acromegaly living in iodine deficient areas. J Endocrinol Invest 1997;20(3):134–7.
9. Loviselli A, Bocchetta A, Mossa P et al. Value of thyroid echography in the long-term follow up lithium-treated patients. Neuropsychobiology 1997;31(1):37–41.
10. Mann K. Vorsymposium 33. Jahrestagung Deutsche Diabetesgesellschaft Frankfurt 1999.
11. Marine D, Lenhard CH. Pathological anatomy of exophthalmic goiter. The anatomical and physiological relations of the thyroid gland to the disease; the treatment. Arch. intern. Med. 1911;3:265–316.
12. Meller J, Zappel H, Konrad M, Roth C, Emmrich D, Becker W. 123J-Szintigraphie und Perchlorat-Depletionstest bei der Diagnostik der kongenitalen Hypothyreose. Nuklearmedizin 1998;37(1):7–11.
13. Rago T, Vitti P, Chiovato L et al. Role of conventional ultrasonography and color flow-doppler sonography in predicting malignancy in "cold" thyroid nodules. Eur J Endocrinol 1998;138:41–6.
14. Ralls PW, Mayekawa DS, Lee KP et al. Color-flow Doppler-sonography in Graves disease: "thyroidinferno". Amer J Roentgenol 1988;150:781–4.
15. Riede UN, Oberholzer M, Klöppel G. Schilddrüse. In: Allgemeine und Spezielle Pathologie. Stuttgart: Thieme 1995.
16. Saleh A, Santen R, Maims J et al. B-Mode-Sonographie und moderne dopplersonographische Methoden bei Krankheiten der Schilddrüse und der Nebenschilddrüse. Radiologe 1998;38:344–54.
17. Scherbaum WA. Kongress of Internists Wiesbaden 1999.
18. Schneider AB, Bekermann C, Cleland J et al. Thyroid nodules in the follow-up of irradiated individuals: comparison of thyroid ultrasound with scanning and palpation. J Clin Endocrinol Metab 1997;82(12):4020–7.

15 Pleura and Chest Wall

Pleura and Chest Wall 449

- **Chest Wall** — 451
  - **Masses** — 451
    - Rib and Sternal Fractures
    - Rib and Sternal Metastases
    - Cutaneous Metastases
    - Carcinoma of the Chest Wall
- **Parietal Pleura** — 456
  - **Nodular Masses** — 456
    - Metastases
    - Pleural Plaque
  - **Diffuse Pleural Thickening** — 459
    - Pleural Carcinomatosis
    - Pleural Fibrosis
    - Diffuse Malignant Mesothelioma
- **Pleural Effusion** — 462
  - **Anechoic Effusion** — 463
    - Transudative Effusion
    - Exudative Effusion
  - **Echogenic Effusion** — 464
    - Benign Effusion
    - Malignant Effusion
  - **Complex Effusion** — 466
    - Inflammatory or Malignant Effusion
    - Fibrothorax
    - Seropneumothorax, Pneumothorax

Chest Wall

Masses

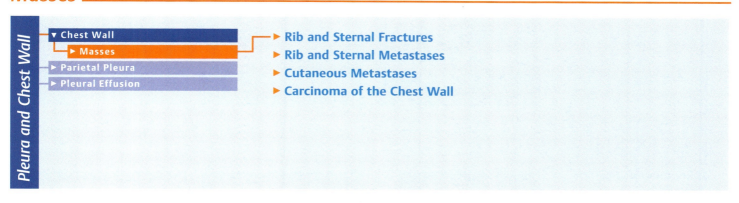

- Chest Wall
  - Masses
- Parietal Pleura
- Pleural Effusion

- Rib and Sternal Fractures
- Rib and Sternal Metastases
- Cutaneous Metastases
- Carcinoma of the Chest Wall

The ultrasound investigation of chest wall lesions is directed by the physical examination (**Fig. 15.3**). The interpretation depends on the sonographic findings, the clinical data, and also on the result of ultrasound-guided fine-needle aspiration or core-needle biopsy. Under the proper conditions, these percutaneous procedures through the chest wall can be done virtually without complications. The main value of chest-wall ultrasound lies in its ability to define the location of masses as intracutaneous, subcutaneous, intramuscular, bony, or pleural[8]. The principal masses of the chest wall are reviewed in **Table 15.1**.

Table 15.1 Differential diagnosis of masses in the chest wall

More common	Less common
Rib and sternal fractures	Abscess
Cutaneous metastases	Lipoma
Rib metastases	Benign bone tumors
Carcinoma	Sarcoma
	Malignant mesothelioma

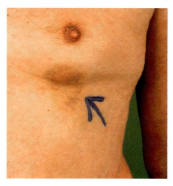

▲ *Fig. 15.3* Fractured rib.
a A man 50 years of age presented with localized left-sided chest pain (arrow) following a fall.

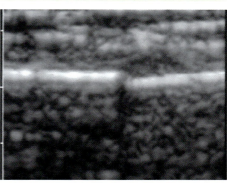

▲ *b* Minimally displaced rib fracture appears sonographically as a discontinuity in the cortical echo.

▶ Rib and Sternal Fractures

Bony thoracic lesions can be difficult to diagnose on radiographs because minimally displaced fractures are occasionally obscured by superimposed shadows.

Sonographic features. Fractures of the bony ribs and sternum can be visualized with ultrasound (◻ **15.2a–c**). A discontinuity in the linear cortical echo serves as a direct fracture sign. Indirect fracture signs are local hematoma (◻ **15.2d–f**) and a pneumothorax or hematothorax. It is not always possible to distinguish between traumatic and pathological fractures by ultrasound (◻ **15.2c**). The callus that forms during fracture healing can also be defined sonographically (◻ **15.2g–l**). The accuracy of ultrasound in the diagnosis of thoracic fractures is superior to that of conventional radiographs (**Table 15.2**).

Table 15.2 Sonographic fracture signs (after reference 1)

Direct fracture signs	Indirect fracture signs
Disruption of the cortical echo	Local hematoma
Gap between the bone ends (stepoff)	Pleural effusion
	Pneumothorax
	Hematothorax

15.2 Rib Fractures

▶ **Direct fracture sign: bony discontinuity**

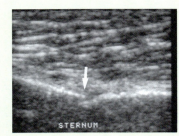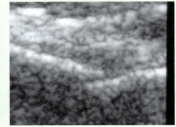

a and b Plasmacytoma, osteoporosis, and chest pain in a 78-year-old woman. Longitudinal scan shows disruption of the sternal cortical echo by a fracture.

c Bronchial carcinoma and scintigraphically confirmed rib metastasis in a 52-year-old man. Step-off with soft-tissue lesion consistent with a fracture.

▶ **Indirect fracture sign: hematoma**

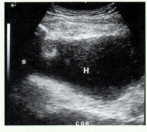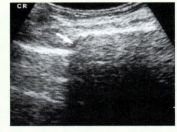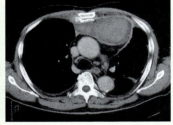

d–f Thoracic trauma in an 83-year-old man.
d and e Largely echo-free parasternal mass consistent with a hematoma (H). S = shadowing; COR = heart.

f CT demonstrates a left parasternal hematoma.

▶ **Follow-ups**

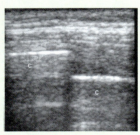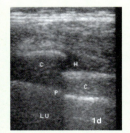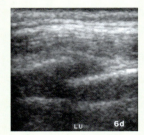

g–i A 60-year-old woman with bronchial asthma and chest pain after a fit of coughing. Ultrasound (**g**) shows a displaced rib fracture. Appearance after one day (**h**) and one week (**i**). H= hematoma; C = rib; P = Pleura-lung boundary ec; LU = lung.

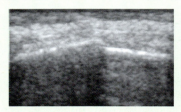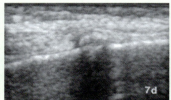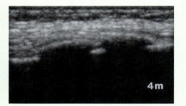

j–l Serial scans document the healing of a traumatic rib fracture with callus formation.

▶ **Rib and Sternal Metastases**

The ultrasound examination is directed by the frequent presence of localized pain. It should be noted that, in principle, a benign/malignant differentiation cannot be made based on ultrasound findings alone (■ 15.3l).

Sonographic features. With metastasis to the bony thorax, ultrasound will often show a relatively long break in the cortical echo (■ 15.3a, b). Some sites allow complete through-transmission of sound (■ 15.3i and g). Tumor extension into the soft tissue is seen with metastatic carcinoma and multiple myeloma (■ 15.3c–h). On color Doppler examination, prominent vascular signals are observed in bony metastases (■ 15.3j and k).

Ultrasound has a limited role in the diagnosis of bony metastases and should be considered only an adjunct to conventional studies[1]. Ultrasound can be helpful in monitoring response to treatment and for planning radiotherapy portals in selected cases.

15.3 Rib and Sternal Metastases

▶ **Sternal metastasis**

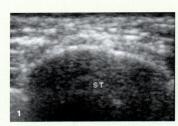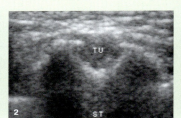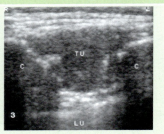

a–c Transverse scans show varying degrees of destruction including the still-intact sternum and the start of tumor involvement. ST = sternum; TU = tumor; C = rib; LU = lung.

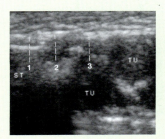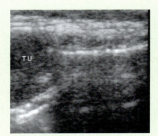

d and e Sternal metastasis from bronchial carcinoma. **d** Longitudinal scan. The sternum has been engulfed and consumed by a metastasis approximately 5 cm in size.

f CT appearance of sternal metastasis.

▶ **Bone destruction**

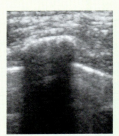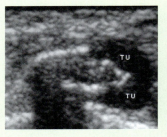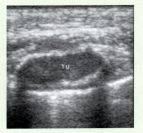

g Normal rib in transverse section.

h Rib metastasis from bronchial carcinoma. Incipient cortical destruction and tumor formation (TU) consistent with a rib metastasis.

i Plasmacytoma (TU) in a 69-year-old man. Almost complete sound transmission through a rib, consistent with tumor infiltration.

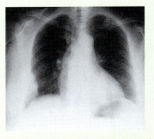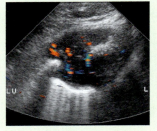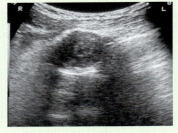

j–l Plasmacytoma in a 73-year-old woman.
j Chest radiograph shows a soft-tissue lesion in the right lateral chest wall.

k Transverse scan of a rib shows cortical destruction and a large soft-tissue mass. TU = tumor; LU = lung. Color Doppler detects flow signals in the tumor tissue.

l Benign differential diagnosis: 30-year-old man presented with a tumor in the right anterior chest wall. Ultrasound shows a complex solid lesion arising from the rib. Histology: fibrous dysplasia (Jaffe–Lichtenstein dysplasia of bone).

▶ **Cutaneous Metastases**

The ultrasound investigation of cutaneous metastases is directed by any palpable abnormalities that are noted on physical examination. The palpable mass may have a rounded or flattened shape (■ 15.4a–n).

A benign tumor (lipoma, granuloma, sebaceous cyst) in any given case can be confirmed only by histological examination (■ 15.4o).

Lipomas usually present sonographically as mobile, hyperechoic lesions with smooth margins. Granulomas are difficult to distinguish from cutaneous metastases by their ultrasound features. Granulomas frequently develop in scarred areas and usually show no vascularity on color Doppler examination.

Cutaneous metastases typically have a round to oval shape and are usually hypoechoic. Flow signals can be detected by color Doppler. Percutaneous biopsy is almost never performed, because local excision is the method of choice for establishing the diagnosis.

15.4 Cutaneous Metastases

▶ High-grade lymphoma

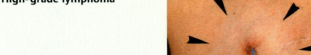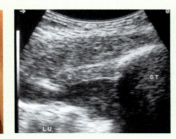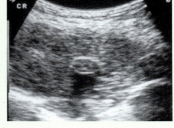

a An area of palpable induration (arrows) was noted about a Groshong catheter site in a 53-year-old woman.

b and c Longitudinal and transverse scans show a homogeneous hypoechoic lesion in the area of the cartilaginous rib (C) junction. Histology confirmed invasion by lymphoma. LU = lung; ST = sternum.

▶ Breast carcinoma

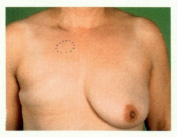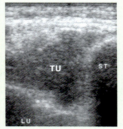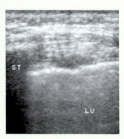

d A poorly demarcated area of palpable firmness (dotted circle) was noted in the right parasternal region of a 53-year-old woman.

e Ultrasound shows a triangular hypoechoic lesion (TU) to the right of the sternum (ST), consistent with chest-wall infiltration by known breast carcinoma. LU = lung.

f Left parasternal region appears normal. LU = lung; ST = sternum; TU = tumor.

▶ Plasmacytoma

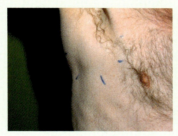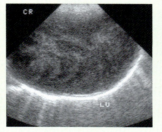

g Palm-size mass in the right lateral chest wall of a 64-year-old man.

h and i Longitudinal and transverse scans show a large, hypoechoic mass. The ribs (C) appear normal. Histology confirmed soft-tissue infiltration by plasmacytoma. LU = lung.

▶ Hodgkin disease

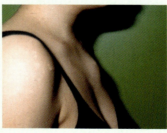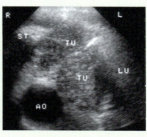

j Left parasternal swelling in a 20-year-old woman.

k and l Multiple nodular chest-wall tumors arising from the anterior mediastinum (TU). Diagnosis was confirmed by ultrasound-guided core biopsy. ST = sternum; AO = aorta; LU = lung.

▶ Bronchial carcinoma and liposarcoma

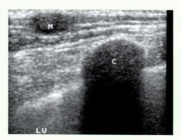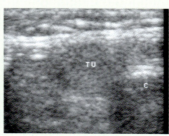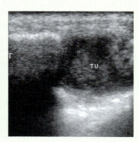

m A 53-year-old man with bronchial carcinoma and a subcutaneous nodule on the left side of the chest. Ultrasound reveals a hypoechoic cutaneous metastasis (M). C = rib; LU = lung.

n A 65-year-old man with a firm mass in the left posterior chest wall. Ultrasound shows a rounded, echogenic tumor mass (TU). Excision confirmed the diagnosis of liposarcoma. C = rib.

o Differentiation from benign lesions: tuberculous abscess in a 30-year-old HIV-positive man. Transverse and longitudinal ultrasound scans show a left parasternal mass (TU) that is fluctuant on compression.

▶ Carcinoma of the Chest Wall

Carcinomas of the chest wall are almost invariably peripheral bronchial carcinomas with the main tumor mass located in the chest wall (**Fig. 15.4**). The importance of ultrasound lies in its ability to define the extent of tumor infiltration into the various layers of the chest wall and exclude a benign lesion (hematoma, abscess, etc.).

Sonographic features. Chest-wall carcinomas are usually hypoechoic at ultrasound. Their margins are irregular. Color Doppler shows rather sparse tumor vascularity.

Pancoast tumor is a peripheral bronchial carcinoma that arises in the superior sulcus and infiltrates neighboring tissues (nerve plexus, rib, spinal column)[9] (**Fig. 15.5**).

Other malignant tumors of the chest wall, such as sarcomas and malignant lymphomas, have a similar sonographic appearance. Ultrasound-guided percutaneous biopsy is the method of choice for confirming the diagnosis.

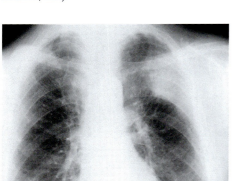
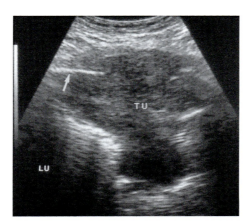

◀◀ **Fig. 15.4** Bronchial carcinoma in a 78-year-old man.
a Chest radiograph shows diffuse opacification of the left upper lung field.

◀ *b* Ultrasound shows a hypoechoic tumor mass (TU) that has penetrated the pleura (arrow) and invaded the chest wall. LU = lung.

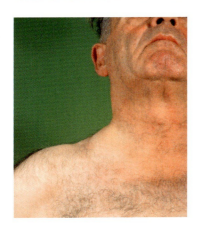
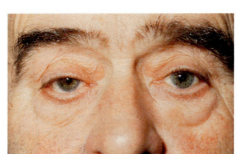

◀◀ **Fig. 15.5** A 62-year-old man with right shoulder pain.
a Palpable mass in the right supraclavicular fossa.

◀ *b* Right-sided meiosis, ptosis, and enophthalmos (Horner syndrome).

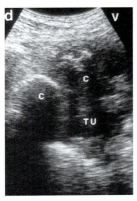
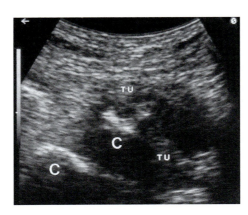

◀ *c* and *d* Posteroanterior scans of the ribs (C) show a destructive lesion (TU) infiltrating the soft tissues, consistent with a Pancoast tumor.

Parietal Pleura

Nodular Masses

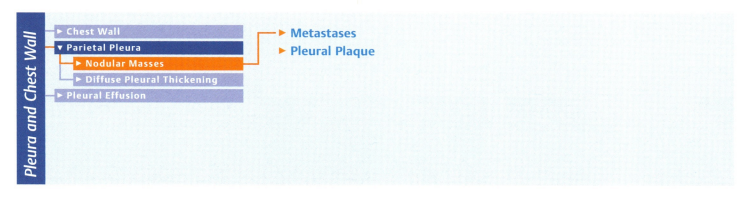

Focal nodular masses of the pleura are localized lesions that either originate from the pleura or are in intimate contact with it (**Table 15.3**). There may or may not be associated pleural effusion (**Fig. 15.6**). If effusion is absent, the lesions are usually located between the pleural layers. When pleural effusion is present, the lesion can be localized to the pleural layers[4, 5] (**Fig. 15.7**).

A confident benign/malignant discrimination is not possible based on ultrasound findings alone.

Table 15.3 Differential diagnosis of focal nodular mass lesions of the pleura

Common	Less common
Metastases	Mesothelioma
Pleural plaque	Lipoma
	Fibroma
	Fibrin bodies (in pleural effusion)
	Neurogenic tumors
	Loculated fluid
	Organized empyema

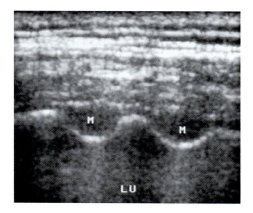

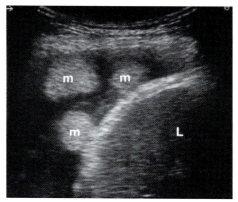

◂◂ **Fig. 15.6** Pleural metastases (M) in a 43-year-old man with hypernephroma. LU = lung.

◂ **Fig. 15.7** Hypernephroma in a 61-year-old man. Scan shows two echogenic round lesions (m) surrounded by pleural effusion on the right side of the diaphragm. L = liver.

▶ Metastases

Metastases are the most common type of focal pleural lesion. The most common primaries are bronchial carcinoma and breast cancer. The lesions may or may not be associated with pleural effusion.

Sonographic features. The lesions usually appear sonographically as round, sharply circumscribed nodules of variable echogenicity. They are frequently in contact with the parietal pleura (▣ **15.5a–c**). Infiltration of the visceral pleura should be assumed if the lesion does not move with respiratory excursions in the absence of pleural effusion[8] (**Fig. 15.8**). Even so, differentiation from peripheral lung metastases cannot always be achieved. Subcostal transhepatic scans are best for demonstrating involvement of the diaphragmatic pleura

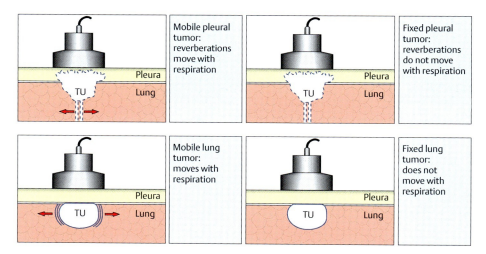

▴ **Fig. 15.8** Technique for differentiating a mobile tumor from a fixed tumor (after reference 8).

(■ **15.5d–f**). Color Doppler ultrasound can differentiate among loculated fluid (■ **15.5g–l**), hematoma, and pleural fibrin bodies (■ **15.5m, n**), which are occasionally seen in fibrin-rich exudative pleural effusions. The definitive diagnosis is established by ultrasound-guided fine-needle aspiration (■ **15.5o**).

In rare cases, malignant mesothelioma can occur as a localized tumor that is indistinguishable from pleural metastases or peripheral bronchial carcinoma by its ultrasound features.

■ 15.5 Differential Diagnosis of Pleural Metastases

▶ **Pleural metastases**

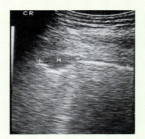 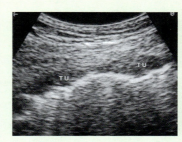 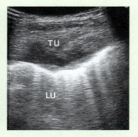

a–c Focal mass of the parietal pleura.
a Solitary nodular lesion (M), metastatic to breast carcinoma. L = lung.

b Confluent nodular metastases (TU) from breast carcinoma.

c Large focal tumor (TU) invading the chest wall. Metastasis from breast carcinoma. LU = lung.

▶ **Malignant mesothelioma**

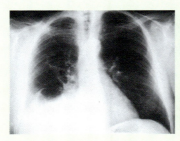 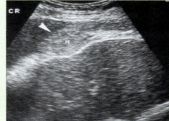

d–f Malignant mesothelioma in a 76-year-old patient.
d Chest radiograph shows moderate pleural effusion on the right side.

e and f Right lateral intercostal scan and subcostal transhepatic scan show an echogenic tumor mass in the diaphragm (arrow). PE = pleural effusion.

▶ **Local fluid: pulmonary cyst**

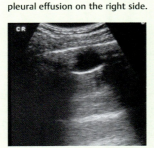 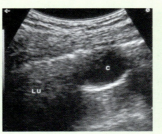

g–i Peripheral round lesion in a 64-year-old man.
g and h Rounded, sharply circumscribed, echo-free peripheral lesion (C), most likely a pulmonary cyst. LU = lung.

i CT appearance of the pulmonary cyst.

▶ **Local fluid: aortic aneurysm**

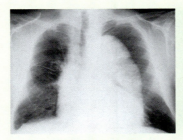 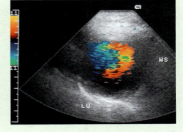

j–l A 67-year-old patient with mediastinal widening.
j Chest radiograph shows mediastinal widening.

k and l B-mode image shows an elongated, echo-free structure on the pleural wall in the left posterior paravertebral region. Color Doppler image shows zones of arterial turbulence consistent with an aortic aneurysm on the posterior chest wall. The finding was confirmed by MRI. LU = lung; WS = spinal column.

15.5 Differential Diagnosis of Pleural Metastases

▶ **Pleural effusion with a fibrin body**

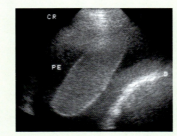 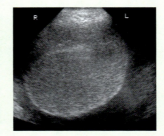

m and *n* A 76-year-old man with exudative pleural effusion (PE) on the right side. Fibrin body appears as a homogeneous mass on the pleural wall, mobile in the pleural effusion. D = diaphragm.

▶ **Parainfectious effusion**

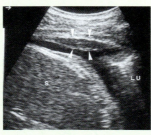

o A 20-year-old man evaluated for pleural effusion. Ultrasound two days after thoracentesis shows pleural thickening in the area of the puncture site (arrows), interpreted as a local reaction to needle insertion. The clinical course was consistent with a parainfectious effusion. LU = lung; S = spleen.

▶ **Pleural Plaque**

Pleural plaques appear as focal hypoechoic lesions that represent the end stage of pneumonia, infarction, empyema, hematoma, tumor irradiation, or chemotherapy. They are also found in the setting of asbestos exposure and other pneumoconioses (**Fig. 15.9**). Not infrequently, the pleural layers are adherent.

Sonographic features. At ultrasound the normally sharp pleural line appears irregular and fragmented. The lesions are mostly hypoechoic and oblong with ill-defined margins. The maximum thickness of the lesions is usually less than 5 mm.

Lesions of the visceral pleura cannot be distinguished from small peripheral pulmonary embolisms or pleurisy by their ultrasound features alone. The focal lesions can be localized to the visceral pleura, however, and the clinical presentation can further narrow the differential diagnosis[2]. Differentiation from pleural carcinomatosis is generally difficult.

Calcifications. Localized calcifications are occasionally found on the pleural layers. They are observed after infections (e.g., tuberculosis), after trauma (e.g., fibrothorax), in pneumoconiosis (e.g., asbestosis), and also in hypercalcemia (e.g., renal failure) (**Fig. 15.10**).

◀◀ **Fig. 15.9** A 57-year-old man with a history of asbestosis.
 a Ultrasound shows plaquelike areas of pleural thickening in addition to pleural nodules (arrow).

◀ *b* CT appearance of the pleural plaques.

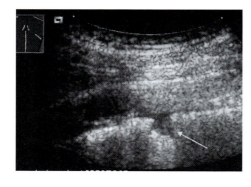 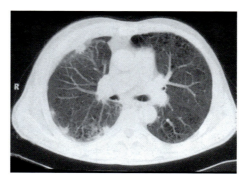

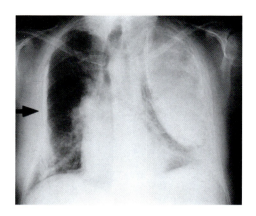
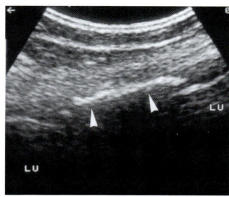

Fig. 15.10 Old pulmonary tuberculosis in a 70-year-old man.
a Chest radiograph shows a white hemithorax on the left side following surgical treatment of tuberculosis, with pleural calcifications on the right side.

b Ultrasound shows localized pleural calcifications (arrowheads). LU = lung.

Diffuse Pleural Thickening

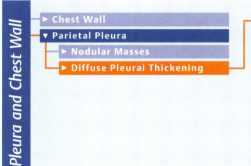

A continuum exists between nodular and more diffuse lesions of the pleura. Occasionally both infiltration patterns are encountered in the same patient.

The differentiation of malignant from benign diffuse pleural thickening has major clinical relevance. In some cases only thoracoscopy can establish the cause of the pleural thickening (**Table 15.4**). There are no definite sonographic criteria for malignant infiltration, although pleural thickening that exceeds 1 cm, additional nodular lesions, and involvement of the mediastinal pleura suggest a malignant etiology.

Table 15.4 Differential diagnosis of diffuse pleural thickening

Common	Less common
Pleural carcinomatosis	Localized pleural effusion
Chronic fibrosing pleurisy	Asbestosis
Diffuse malignant mesothelioma	Connective-tissue diseases
	Chronic empyema
	Tuberculosis
	Aspergillosis

▶ Pleural Carcinomatosis

Pleural carcinomatosis may present sonographically with pleural effusion, focal pleural metastases, or diffuse pleural thickening. The latter may occur with or without pleural effusion.

Ultrasound shows a homogeneous, hypoechoic or even hyperechoic, sheetlike tumor mass that is usually distributed along the parietal pleura (**Figs. 15.11 and 15.12**). The margins are generally well-defined, but additional nodular lesions may occasionally be seen (**Fig. 15.13**). The diagnosis is established by ultrasound-guided thoracentesis[4, 5].

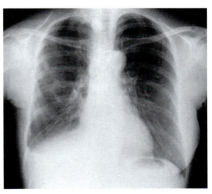

Fig. 15.11 A 38-year-old woman with breast carcinoma.
a Chest radiograph shows a small pleural effusion on the right side.

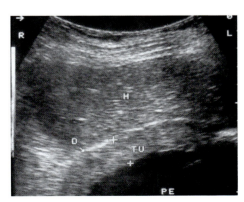

b Subcostal transhepatic scan demonstrates pleural effusion (PE) and diffuse thickening of the parietal pleura (TU) consistent with pleural carcinomatosis. D = diaphragm; L = liver.

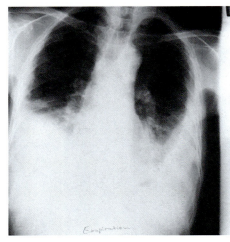

▲ **Fig. 15.12** A 69-year-old man with an ENT tumor.
a Chest radiograph shows bilateral pleural effusion.

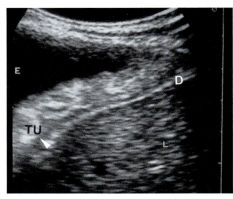 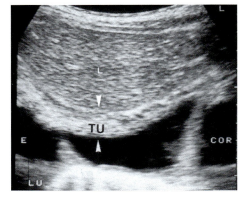

▲ *b and c* Right lateral intercostal scan (*b*) and subcostal transhepatic scan (*c*) show diffuse, hyperechoic thickening of the parietal pleura consistent with pleural carcinomatosis (TU). D = diaphragm; E = effusion; L = liver; LU = lung; COR = heart.

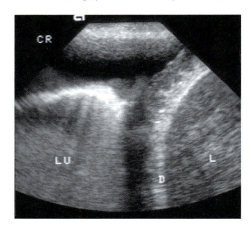 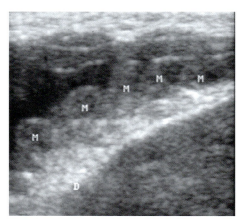

◀ **Fig. 15.13 *a* and *b*** Low-grade non-Hodgkin lymphoma in a 78-year-old man. Right lateral intercostal scan shows extensive pleural thickening in a string-of-beads pattern (M), consistent with lymphomatous infiltration. LU = lung; D = diaphragm; L = liver.

▶ Pleural Fibrosis

The pleural cavity may become diffusely permeated by fibrotic tissue during or after pneumonia and pleurisy and less commonly after a tuberculous effusion (◩ 15.6a–c), empyema (◩ 15.6d–h), pulmonary fibrosis (◩ 15.6i–n), asbestosis (◩ 15.6o, p), or hemothorax. A concomitant exudative effusion is often present.

Sonographic features. Ultrasound usually demonstrates an extended area of hypoechoic pleural thickening. Generally the thickening is less then 5 mm. Typically both the parietal pleura and visceral pleura are thickened and, in the absence of pleural effusion, cannot be defined as separate layers.

Pleural effusion. The pleural layers can be differentiated when pleural effusion is present. The effusion sometimes contains fibrin strands of varying extent ranging to a dense, honeycomb-like structure.

Scar stage. In the scar stage the visceral pleura cannot be distinguished from the parietal layer and appears as a homogeneous, hypoechoic, solid thickening of the pleural space. Calcifications due to scarring after tuberculosis or asbestosis can be visualized with ultrasound.

The pleural line is irregular and indistinct. The lung usually appears stationary on real-time ultrasound.

Lung. Additional ultrasound evaluation of the lung (e.g., pneumonia, tumor atelectasis, pulmonary metastasis, peripheral lung tumor) is helpful in determining the etiology of concomitant pleural thickening. Acute pleurisy and pleuropneumonia are discussed in Chapter 16 as diseases that arise from the pulmonary parenchyma and visceral pleura.

◩ 15.6 Various Causes of Pleural Fibrosis

▶ **Tuberculosis**

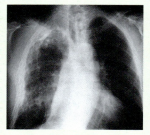 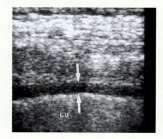 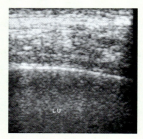

a–c Old pulmonary tuberculosis in a 75-year-old man.
a Chest radiograph shows scar changes in the right lung.

b Extensive pleural thickening (arrows). LU = lung.

c Normal pleura. LU = lung.

15.6 Various Causes of Pleural Fibrosis

▶ **Pyothorax**

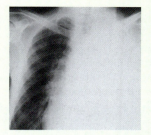 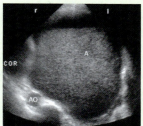 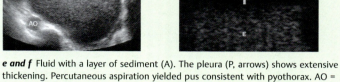

d–f Pyothorax after pneumonectomy.
d Chest radiograph shows a white left hemithorax following pneumonectomy for bronchial carcinoma.

e and f Fluid with a layer of sediment (A). The pleura (P, arrows) shows extensive thickening. Percutaneous aspiration yielded pus consistent with pyothorax. AO = aorta; E = effusion.

▶ **Old pleural empyema**

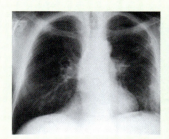 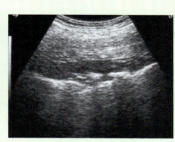

g and h Old pleural empyema in a 53-year-old man.
g Chest radiograph shows pleural thickening on the left side.

h Ultrasound shows diffuse pleural thickening with focal calcifications in the area of the former pleural empyema.

▶ **Pulmonary fibrosis**

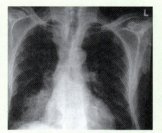 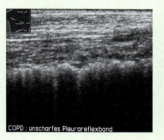 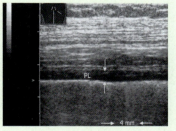

i and j A 72-year-old man with chronic obstructive lung disease.
i Chest radiograph shows signs of pulmonary emphysema with increased markings in the right lower lung field.

j The entry echo shows extended irregularity with fine fibrotic changes.

k A 74-year-old man with known pulmonary fibrosis: diffuse thickening of the pleura (PL) to 4 mm (arrows).

l–n A 32-year-old woman with left pulmonary fibrosis of undetermined cause.

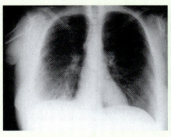 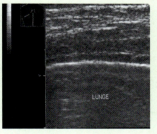

l Chest radiograph shows increased markings in the right lateral and lower lung zones.

m and n Ultrasound shows diffuse thickening of the visceral (PV) and parietal (PP) pleura. The lung is immobile. The arrows mark the entry echo at the visceral–parietal interface.

▶ **Asbestosis**

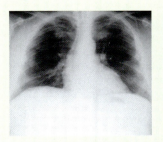 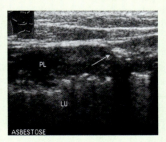

o and p Asbestosis in a 53-year-old man.
o Chest radiograph shows bilateral opacities on the pleural wall.

p Ultrasound shows diffuse thickening of the pleura (PL) to 10 mm with focal calcifications (arrow). The lung (LU) is fixed.

▶ Diffuse Malignant Mesothelioma

Almost 80% of cases occur in individuals with a history of asbestos exposure. The average latent period is 35 years. Three histological types are distinguished: epithelial, mesenchymal (sarcomatous), and mixed.

Sonographic features. Ultrasound almost always shows pleural thickening that extends into the costophrenic angle or interlobar fissures, depending on the degree of spread. Less commonly we find tumor infiltration of the chest wall or abdominal cavity. The tumor has a complex echo structure with hyperechoic elements. It cannot be distinguished from pleural carcinomatosis, metastatic adenocarcinoma, or an advanced fibrothorax by its ultrasound features alone. Pleural effusion is frequently present. In the advanced stage, the lung is encased by tumor (**Fig. 15.14**).

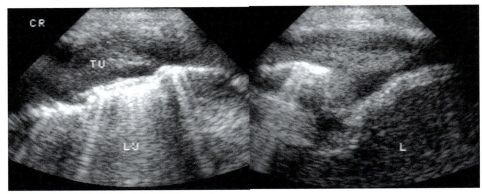

▲ **Fig. 15.14** A 40-year-old man with malignant mesothelioma.
a Chest radiograph shows encasement of the right lung.

▲ *b* and *c* Right lateral intercostal scan shows extensive hypoechoic tumor encasement (TU) of the lung (LU). L = liver.

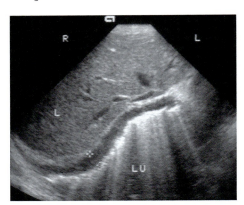
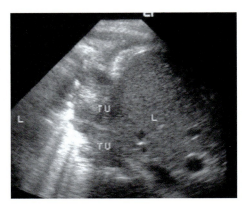
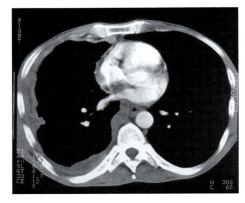

▲ *d* and *e* Subcostal transhepatic scan shows diffuse tumor spread. Scattered nodular lesions (TU) are also demonstrated in the lateral scan (*e*).

▲ *f* CT: pleural tumor.

Pleural Effusion

Pleural effusion is by far the most common space-occupying process occurring in the pleural cavity (**Table 15.5**, ▣ **15.7**). The value of ultrasound lies in its ability to distinguish an effusion from other diffuse lung opacities that are seen on radiographs. Ultrasound is superior to conventional chest films in both its sensitivity and specificity. Free effusion volumes as small as 5 ml can be identified. Sonography cannot detect a loculated interlobar effusion or localized mediastinal fluid.

A pleural effusion displays characteristic sonographic features with regard to its location (▣ **15.7a, b, d–f**) (unilateral/bilateral), extent (▣ **15.7c, g, h**), echogenicity (▣ **15.7j**), and the presence of septations (▣ **15.7i, k, l**), depending on the cause of the effusion (**Table 15.6**). Goecke et al.[3] described a volumetry technique that has proved useful for the sonographic assessment of effusion volume (**Fig. 15.15**).

The etiological classification of a pleural effusion is based on clinical presentation, sonographic findings, and the result of percutaneous aspiration. **Table 15.7** reviews the differential diagnosis of pleural effusion and the characteristic ultrasound findings.

Table 15.5 Differential diagnosis of mass lesions in the pleural cavity

Common	Less common
Anechoic effusion	Hematothorax
Echogenic effusion	Pneumothorax
Complex effusion	Fibrothorax

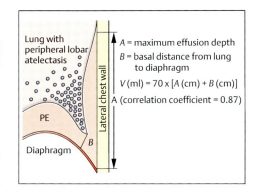

A = maximum effusion depth
B = basal distance from lung to diaphragm
$V \text{(ml)} = 70 \times [A \text{(cm)} + B \text{(cm)}]$
(correlation coefficient = 0.87)

▲ **Fig. 15.15** Diagram showing the technique of pleural effusion volumetry (after reference 3).

Table 15.6 Possible causes of pleural effusion

Metastatic/hemodynamic (usually transudate)
- Heart failure
- Hepatic cirrhosis
- Uremia
- Hypercalcemia

Inflammatory (usually exudate)
- Pleurisy
- Pneumonia
- Pulmonary infarction
- Connective tissue disease
- Pancreatitis

Neoplastic (usually exudate)
- Pleural carcinomatosis
- Malignant mesothelioma
- Malignant lymphoma
- Sarcoma

Table 15.7 Differential diagnosis of pleural effusion

	Transudate	Exudate				
		Inflammatory	Hemorrhagic	Chylous	Purulent	Malignant
Analysis of aspirate	Protein < 3 g% Hypocellular Cholesterol < 60 mg%	Protein > 3 g% Very cellular Cholesterol > 60 mg%	Protein > 3 g% Bloody	Protein > 3 g% Milky turbid Triglycerides > 100 mg%	Protein > 3 g% Debris	Protein > 3 g% Possible tumor cells
Sonographic characteristics	Anechoic Fine pleural line Frequently bilateral	Anechoic to hyperechoic Septa, fibrin strands Accentuated pleural line Parenchymal lesion	Anechoic to hyperechoic Sedimentation "Snowstorm"	Hyperechoic "Snowstorm"	Variable sedimentation Air echoes Pleural thickening	Variable septa, fibrin strands Pleural tumors Parenchymal lesion
Examples	Heart failure Hepatic cirrhosis Protein deficiency	Pneumonia Infarction Connective tissue disease	Hematothorax Tumor hemorrhage	Chest trauma	Pleural empyema Pulmonary abscess Pyothorax	Pleural carcinomatosis NHL Mesothelioma

Anechoic Effusion

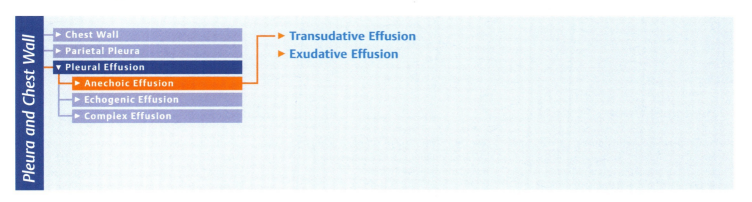

▶ Transudative Effusion

An exudative type of pleural effusion (> 2.5 g%) is distinguished from a transudative effusion (< 2.5 g%) based on the protein content of the aspirate. A transudative effusion is anechoic and is more often bilateral in varying degrees. The effusion is usually benign by aspiration cytology and occurs, for example, in heart failure due to various causes.

With extreme cardiomegaly, the heart may occasionally appear as an anechoic area on the lateral chest wall that mimics a pleural effusion (**Fig. 15.16**). An aortic aneurysm on the posterior chest wall can also appear sonographically as an anechoic liquid mass (▣ **15.5j–l**).

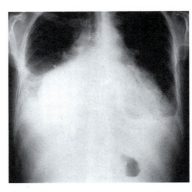

▲ **Fig. 15.16** A 54-year-old man with congestive heart failure.
a Chest radiograph shows pronounced cardiomegaly and possible pleural effusion.

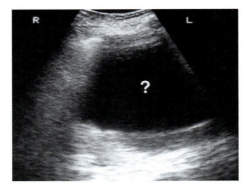

▲ **b** Right lateral intercostal scan shows an indeterminate hypoechoic mass (**?**).

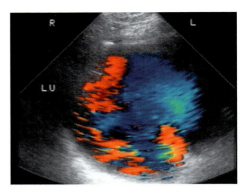

▲ **c** Conspicuous flow patterns at color Doppler confirm that the mass is an enlarged right heart. LU = lung.

▶ Exudative Effusion

In principle, even protein-rich pleural effusions may appear anechoic. They consist mainly of parainfectious effusions (e.g., due to pleurisy, pneumonia, polyserositis, or tuberculosis) and malignant effusions (e.g., due to bronchial or mammary carcinoma).

Echogenic Effusion

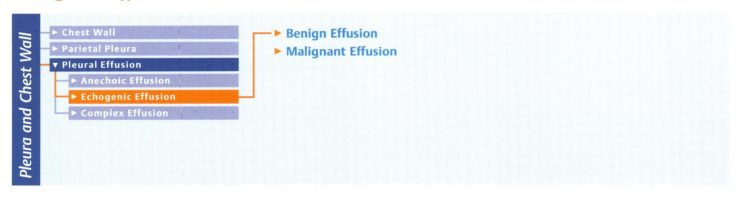

▶ Benign Effusion

An echogenic pleural effusion is caused by small corpuscular reflectors suspended in the fluid. These may consist of fibrin components, fat particles, corpuscular blood elements, air, or cellular debris. Real-time ultrasound demonstrates moving echoes within the exudative fluid.

The differential diagnosis of an echogenic pleural effusion includes the following:
▶ Inflammatory effusion
▶ Pyothorax (▣ **15.6d–f**)
▶ Hematothorax (**Fig. 15.17**)
▶ Chylothorax

Fibrin strands and septa are commonly observed in varying degrees. A benign effusion cannot be positively distinguished from a malignant effusion based on sonographic criteria alone.

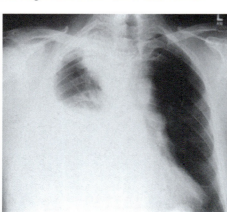
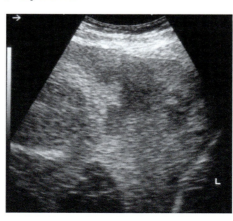

◀◀ **Fig. 15.17** Bronchial carcinoma in a 60-year-old man.
a Chest radiograph shows almost complete opacification of the right lung.

◀ **b** Right lateral intercostal scan shows a nonhomogeneous hyperechoic structure formed by echoes that move with respiration. Pleural fluid aspiration confirmed a hematothorax. L = liver.

15.7 Imaging Appearances of Pleural Effusion

▶ Basal effusion, inflammatory

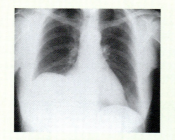 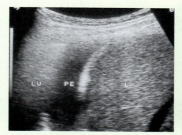 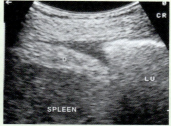

a–c Radiographic and sonographic appearances of pleural effusion.
a Chest radiograph shows elevation of the diaphragm in a 47-year-old woman.

b Right lateral intercostal scan demonstrates a subpulmonic effusion as the cause of the radiographic sign. PE = pleural effusion; L = liver; LU = lung.

c Normal chest radiograph. Ultrasound reveals a small effusion on the left side. D = diaphragm; LU = lung.

▶ Peripheral effusion, inflammatory

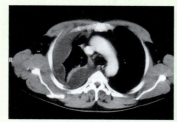 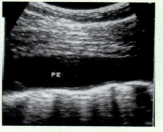

d–f A 48-year-old man with pleurisy.
d CT shows a localized fluid collection along the pleural wall.

e and f Ultrasound scans over a six-month period document resolution of the pleural effusion (PE; E) in response to antibiotic therapy. LU = lung.

▶ Malignant effusion: lymphoma

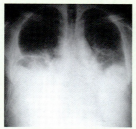 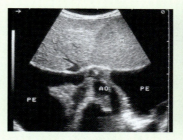 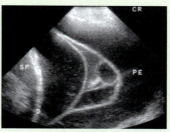

g and h A 39-year-old man with low-grade lymphoma.
g Chest radiograph shows conspicuous bilateral effusion.

h Subcostal scan angled toward the head demonstrates the bilateral effusion. PE = pleural effusion; L = liver.

i A 24-year-old man with Hodgkin disease. Ultrasound shows individual septa in an exudative pleural effusion. SP = spleen; D = diaphragm; PE = pleural effusion.

▶ Malignant effusion: bronchial carcinoma

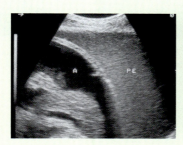 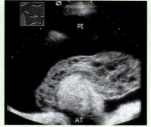 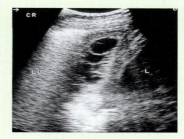

j–l Effusion in patients with bronchial carcinoma.
j Left lateral intercostal scan in a 53-year-old man. Ascites (A) appears as an echo-free area, contrasting with the more echogenic pleural effusion (PE) on the left side.

k A 74-year-old man with bronchial carcinoma and complete opacification of the hemithorax on chest radiograph. Ultrasound shows a conspicuous pleural effusion (PE) with upper lobar atelectasis (AT). The atelectasis is surrounded by a honeycomb-like fibrin mass due to exudative effusion.

l Bronchial carcinoma in a 57-year-old man. Right lateral intercostal scan shows septa in the pleural effusion with thickening of the pleura due to exudative effusion. L = liver; LU = lung.

▶ Malignant Effusion

A malignant echogenic effusion is diagnosed when tumor cells are detected by aspiration cytology. The echogenicity of the effusion (**Fig. 15.18**) and the presence of fibrin strands or septa are considered indirect but nonspecific signs. The sonographic detection of diffuse pleural thickening that exceeds 1 cm or the detection of nodular foci of pleural thickening also suggests a malignant etiology. The diagnosis should be confirmed by cytological analysis.

Frequently the effusion is unilateral, and it is not uncommon to find diffuse opacification of the hemithorax. A larger pleural effusion leads to partial atelectasis of the lung; this makes it possible to evaluate the lung parenchyma with ultrasound and detect any pulmonary nodules or a central tumor (**Fig. 15.19**).

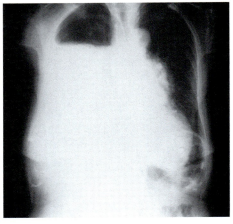
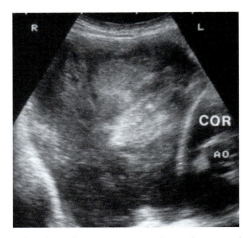
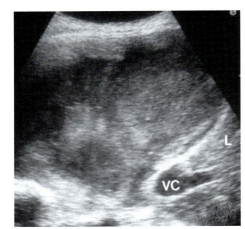

▲ **Fig. 15.18** Metastatic mucus-forming ovarian carcinoma in a 74-year-old woman.
a Chest radiograph shows almost complete opacification of the right lung.

▲ **b and c** Right anterior intercostal scan shows a nonhomogeneous echogenic mass containing faint echoes that move with respiration. Aspiration yielded mucoid material from an expansile tumor metastatic to ovarian carcinoma. COR = heart; VC = vena cava; L = liver; AO = aorta.

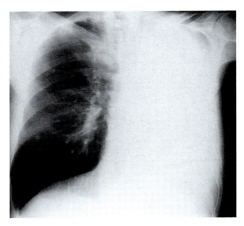
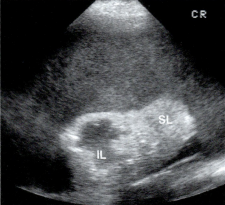
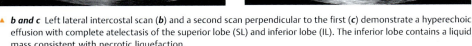

▲ **Fig. 15.19** Bronchial carcinoma in a 63-year-old man. SL = superior lobe; IL = inferior lobe.
a Chest radiograph shows complete opacification of the left lung.

▲ **b and c** Left lateral intercostal scan (**b**) and a second scan perpendicular to the first (**c**) demonstrate a hyperechoic effusion with complete atelectasis of the superior lobe (SL) and inferior lobe (IL). The inferior lobe contains a liquid mass consistent with necrotic liquefaction.

Complex Effusion

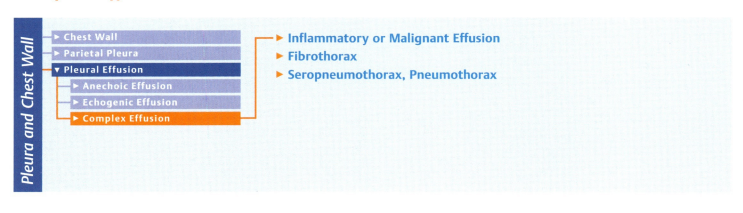

▶ Inflammatory or Malignant Effusion

Ultrasound examination of a complex pleural effusion will show varying degrees of fibrin stranding and septation, ranging to a honeycomb-like permeation of the pleural cavity in extreme cases. These structures are defined less clearly by computed tomography than by ultrasound. The ultrasound-guided aspiration of septated effusions can be rewarding in clinically symptomatic patients, consistently yielding an exudative fluid. Various degrees of pleural thickening are seen. These findings are characteristic of an inflammatory or malignant effusion.

In the latter case, it is not uncommon to find nodular tumor masses in the effusion when disease is advanced (**Fig. 15.20**). Ultrasound-guided percutaneous drainage is no longer beneficial in these cases.

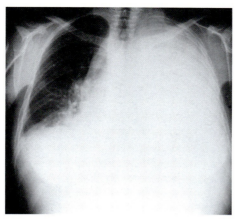

▲ **Fig. 15.20** Low-grade non-Hodgkin lymphoma in a 21-year-old woman.
a Chest radiograph shows complete opacification of the left lung.

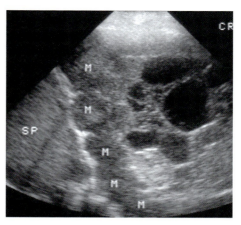

▲ *b* Left lateral intercostal scan shows an extensive, loculated pleural effusion with a string-of-beads arrangement of nodular masses (M) along the diaphragmatic pleura. Cytology confirmed lymphomatous involvement of the pleura. SP = spleen.

▶ Fibrothorax

Fibrothorax is a special type of complex effusion that develops following unilateral pneumonectomy (**Fig. 15.21**).

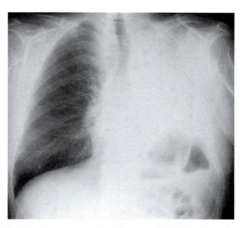

▲ **Fig. 15.21** A 65-year-old man who had previously undergone pneumonectomy for bronchial carcinoma.
a Chest radiograph shows complete opacification of the left hemithorax.

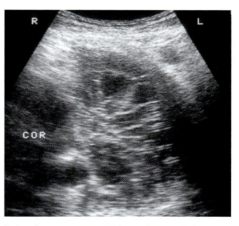

▲ *b* Left anterior intercostal scan shows a nonhomogeneous, solid/cystic-appearing mass consistent with a fibrothorax. COR = heart.

▶ Seropneumothorax, Pneumothorax

In rare cases, air or gas can be detected in the pleural cavity in addition to a serous effusion. The main causes are the iatrogenic introduction of air during the percutaneous aspiration of an effusion or an infection with air-forming or gas-forming bacteria. The air appears sonographically as a sharp, echogenic line with posterior acoustic shadowing.

A pneumothorax can also be diagnosed with ultrasound. The air in the pleural cavity appears as a sharp, highly reflective band. Unlike intrapulmonary air, the band does not move with respiration. The extent of a pneumothorax is determined by chest radiography, however.

References

1. Bitschnau R, Gehmacher O, Kopf A, Scheier M, Mathis G. Ultrasonography in the diagnosis of rib and sternal fracture. Ultraschall in Med 1997;18:158–61.
2. Gehmacher O, Kopf A, Scheier M, Bitschnau R, Wertgen T, Mathis G. Ist die Pleuritis sonographisch darstellbar? Ultraschall in Med 1997;18:214–9.
3. Goecke W, Schwerk WB. Die Real-Time Sonographie in der Diagnostik von Pleuraergüssen. In: Gebhardt J et al. (eds.). Ultraschalldiagnostik 89. Berlin: Springer 1990; p. 385–7.
4. Görg C, Görg K, Schwerk WB, Kleinsorge F. Sonographie der Pleura diaphragmatica bei Tumorpatienten. Ultraschall in Med 1988;9:274–8.
5. Görg C, Schwerk WB, Görg K, Walters E. Pleural Effusion: An "Acoustic Window" for Sonography of pleural metastases. JCU 1991;19:93–7.
6. Mathis G. Thoraxsonography-Part 1: Chest Wall and Pleura. Ultrasound in Med & Biol 1997;23:1131–9.
7. Reuß J. Sonographic imaging of the pleura: nearly 30 years experience. EJU 1996;3:125–39.
8. Wernecke K. Sonographic Features of Pleural Disease. AJR 1997;168:1061–6.
9. Yang PC, Lee LN, Luh KT et al. Ultrasonography of Pancoast Tumor. Chest 1988;94:124–8.

16 Lung

Lung 471

- **Masses** — 471
  - **Anechoic Masses** — 472
    - Loculated Pleural Effusion
    - Pulmonary Cyst, Liquefaction, Abscess
    - Aortic Aneurysm, Cardiac Cavity
  - **Hypoechoic Masses** — 474
    - Atelectasis
    - Pulmonary Embolism or Infarction
    - Pulmonary Tumors and Metastases
  - **Complex Masses** — 483
    - Pneumonia
    - Lung Abscess

16 Lung

C. Goerg

Transcutaneous ultrasound is limited in its ability to define the thoracic organs. Although sonography quickly became an established tool for pleural examination, it was not until the late 1980s that systematic studies in the lung by Mathis et al.[4] led to a greater acceptance of pulmonary ultrasound.

There are several physical and acoustic phenomena that chiefly limit the intrathoracic use of ultrasound. The ribs, sternum, spinal column, and scapula create diagnostic "dead spaces" by reflecting virtually all incident sound. Also, very large differences in acoustic impedance exist at interfaces between lung tissue and aerated alveoli, causing almost 100% sound reflection. Central lung regions cannot be scanned through normally aerated peripheral lung tissue.

As a result, thoracic ultrasound is currently used as an adjunctive, complementary procedure for investigating diffuse radiographic opacities located near the pleura[6].

Topography and Ultrasound Morphology

Relations of the lungs
- Intrathoracic
- Bounded by the ribs, sternum, and diaphragm

Sonographic landmarks
- Sharp, mobile, high-amplitude echo at the lung–pleura interface

The lungs are intrathoracic and are bounded by the thoracic skeleton. The chest cavity is bounded inferiorly by the diaphragm. The upper lobes are covered posteriorly by the scapulae. The lower lobes can be visualized by scanning through the intercostal spaces, which are directed obliquely downward. The anterior rib segments are more horizontal, and the upper lobes can be scanned at that level through the intercostal spaces on both sides. The middle lobe can be scanned from a parasternal probe position on the right side (**Fig. 16.1**). The lower lung fields can be evaluated with a subcostal scan through the liver (right lung) or through the spleen (left lung), the transhepatic scan providing the better view. The transsplenic window is frequently obscured by gas in the stomach or colon. The apical lung regions are best demonstrated by a supraclavicular scan angled toward the feet. The range of intercostal sound transmission normally extends to the visceral pleura and ends at the aerated alveoli, which reflect all incident sound. The typical echogenic pleural line is produced by total sound reflection at the pleura-lung interface (the "entry echo").

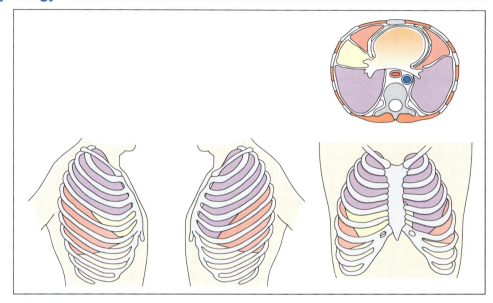

▲ **Fig. 16.1** Anatomical relations of the pulmonary lobes.

Masses

Because mass lesions of the chest wall and pleura as well as peripheral lung diseases promote sound transmission, they can be imaged with transcutaneous ultrasound. Chest-wall and pleural lesions can exert extrinsic pressure on the lung, displacing air from the tissue and enabling it to transmit sound (e.g., compression atelectasis due to pleural effusion). These lesions are distinguished from actual intrapulmonary masses that cause absent or decreased aeration of the lung parenchyma. Only the latter types of lesion will be discussed here.

Criteria for ultrasound evaluation. The sonographic evaluation of peripheral lung masses is based on their number, location, size, shape, margins, echogenicity, and homogeneity. The behavior of the focal lesion during respiratory excursions has proved to be an important criterion.

Color Doppler ultrasound can supply additional information that is useful in characterizing lesions. It can provide qualitative information on the display of color-flow signals that is useful for classifying lesions as avascular, hypovascular, or hypervascular. These signals are dependent on the quality of the equipment and the patient's ability to breath-hold for a specified period. Transmitted paracardiac pulsations also significantly limit the use of color Doppler imaging in the chest.

Qualitative Doppler flow measurements in lung tissue can help to achieve more accurate tissue discrimination in certain cases (sampling waveforms from branches of the pulmonary veins or arteries and from tumor vessels (see ■ 16.6, p. 483). The resistance index and pulsatility index have proved to be effective spectral parameters for characterizing arterial vessels[7].

The interpretation of ultrasound findings also depends on the history, the clinical presentation, and the results of follow-up scans. In some cases a definitive interpretation may require ultrasound-guided fine-needle aspiration[1].

Anechoic Masses

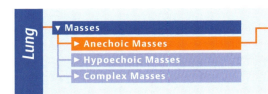

- Loculated Pleural Effusion
- Pulmonary Cyst, Liquefaction, Abscess
- Aortic Aneurysm, Cardiac Cavity

A loculated pleural effusion is the most frequent cause of an anechoic mass between the lung and chest wall. Differentiation is required from rare anechoic lung masses, which can be defined with ultrasound if they reach the parenchymal surface (**Table 16.1**, ▣ **16.1**).

Table 16.1 Differential diagnosis of echo-free masses

Common	Less common
Loculated effusion in a lobar fissure	Lung abscess
	Primary lung cyst
	Liquefying tumor
	Liquefying atelectasis
	Aortic aneurysm on the chest wall
	Cardiac cavity abutting the chest wall

▶ Loculated Pleural Effusion

Localized anechoic masses between the lung and chest wall most likely represent a loculated pleural effusion (**Fig. 16.2**). An exudative type of effusion is usually present. The underlying disease may be an infection or malignant process.

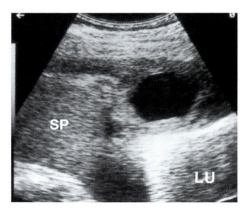

◀ **Fig. 16.2** Bronchial carcinoma in a 45-year-old man. Left lateral intercostal scan shows the bright entry echo at the interface of the pleura and lung (LU) cranial to the spleen (SP). A rounded, echo-free mass rimmed by solid echogenic material is visible in the costophrenic angle. It is consistent with a loculated effusion in pleural carcinomatosis.

▶ Pulmonary Cyst, Liquefaction, Abscess

Pulmonary cysts are rare and are subdivided into primary and secondary forms (▣ **16.1 a, d–f**).

Liquefying processes (pneumonic infiltrates, tumors, metastases) can occasionally appear anechoic (▣ **16.1 g–k**).

Lung abscesses usually have a complex echo texture but may also appear anechoic (▣ **16.1 l**). They have an echogenic wall and produce characteristic clinical symptoms. Abscessation can be confirmed by ultrasound-guided percutaneous aspiration.

▶ Aortic Aneurysm, Cardiac Cavity

An aortic aneurysm bordering the chest wall (**Fig. 16.3**) and a cardiac cavity abutting the chest wall due to cardiomegaly are rare differential diagnoses for a hypoechoic mass; they illustrate the importance of seeing the chest radiograph before making a definitive interpretation of the ultrasound findings.

16.1 Pulmonary Cysts, Liquefaction, and Abscesses

▶ Cyst, aspergilloma

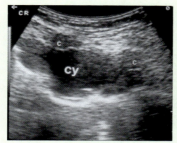
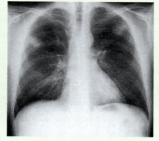
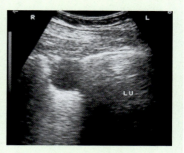

a A 67-year-old woman with a 12-year history of a constant peripheral lung mass. Parasternal scan demonstrates an echo-free mass with irregular margins in the right parasternal region, consistent with a pulmonary cyst (Cy). c = secondary cysts.

b and *c* A 49-year-old man with leukemia and fever.
b Chest radiograph shows multiple pulmonary nodules.

c Right lateral intercostal scan shows an almost echo-free mass in the lung (LU), identified histologically as an aspergilloma.

▶ Peripheral pulmonary nodule

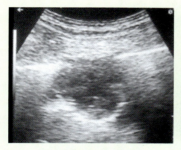
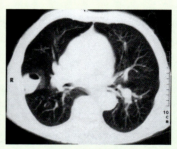

d–f Peripheral lung nodule in a 74-year-old man.
d Initially complex lung mass.

e Over the next two months the mass resolves into a cystic focus, presumably the result of pneumonia or infarction.

f CT: peripheral lung nodule.

▶ Liquefaction, cystic tumor, abscess

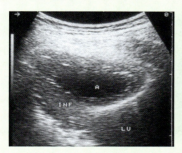
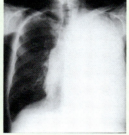
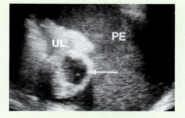

g A 38-year-old man with fever. Right anterior intercostal scan shows diffuse hypoechoic transformation of the lung with central liquefaction (A) consistent with cavitating pneumonia. INF = infarction; LU = lung.

h and *i* Bronchial carcinoma.
h Chest radiograph shows complete opacification of the left hemithorax.

i Left lateral intercostal scan shows pleural effusion (PE) with upper (UL) and lower lobar atelectasis. The lower lobe contains a central hypoechoic area (arrows) consistent with liquefaction.

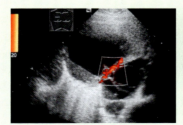
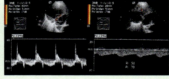
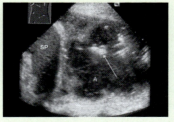

j and *k* A 33-year-old woman with known sarcoma and a large right thoracic metastasis.
j Color duplex demonstrates a cystic-solid mass with color-flow signals in the solid components.

k Sampled waveforms display a high-resistance "extremity" pattern in pulmonary arterial vessels and a low-resistance "parenchymal" pattern in tumor vessels.

l A 79-year-old man with fever and dyspnea. Left lateral intercostal scan shows a large, echo-free mass with irregular margins and central air echoes (arrow) cranial to the spleen (SP). Percutaneous aspiration of the mass yielded pus. A = abscess; SP = spleen.

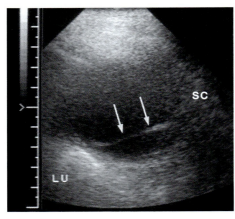
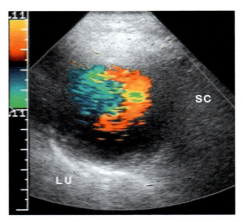
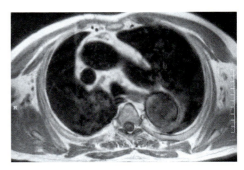

▲ **Fig. 16.3** A 67-year-old man with mediastinal widening in the chest radiograph.
a Ultrasound shows a rounded, hypoechoic mass with a septum (arrows) in the left paravertebral region. SC = spinal column; LU = lung.

▲ *b* Color Doppler shows arterial turbulence within the mass.

▲ *c* MRI confirms the diagnosis of a dissecting thoracic aortic aneurysm.

Hypoechoic Masses

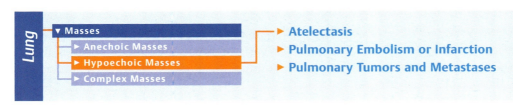

Table 16.2 reviews the differential diagnosis of hypoechoic masses in the lung.

Table 16.2 Differential diagnosis of hypoechoic masses

Common	Less common
Atelectasis	Lobar pneumonia
Pulmonary embolism or infarction	Lung abscess
Pulmonary tumor	

▶ Atelectasis

Atelectasis is characterized by an absence of aeration in pulmonary segments, lobes, or an entire lung. It is distinguished from dysatelectasis, in which aeration is decreased.

Compressive and obstructive atelectasis. Atelectasis is classified as compressive or obstructive on the basis of its pathogenesis. Compressive atelectasis is caused by a large pleural effusion in which the external fluid pressure on the lung parenchyma exceeds the internal pressure transmitted by the outside air (◧ **16.2**). Obstructive atelectasis, called also absorption atelectasis, results from bronchial obstruction and absorption of the air in the occluded area (◧ **16.3**).

Sonographic features. Compression atelectasis appears sonographically as a narrow, relatively well-defined, wedge-shaped area of peripheral lung showing homogeneous hypoechoic transformation. Real-time ultrasound may show partial reinflation of the collapsed area during inhalation. This may produce a conspicuous "air bronchogram." Partial reinflation may occur following percutaneous aspiration of the effusion (**Table 16.3**, ◧ **16.2**).

Obstructive atelectasis also shows homogeneous low echogenicity. The sectional ultrasound image of the affected lung segment resembles a scan of the liver parenchyma ("hepatization" of the lung) (◧ **16.3f**). An air bronchogram is not observed (**Table 16.3**). With longstanding atelectasis (usually caused by a central tumor mass), the retention of secretions can produce a "fluid bronchogram" (◧ **16.3a, b**). Ultrasound demonstrates hypoechoic, mucus-filled bronchial lumina surrounded by echogenic bronchial walls. Color Doppler can differentiate the fluid bronchogram from vascular structures. Increased color-flow signals are observed in the atelectatic lung tissue (◧ **16.3f, j–l**).

Central mass. Central obstructions of the bronchial tree can cause the development of atelectasis. Occasionally the obstructing central mass can be identified, the atelectatic lung serving as a kind of acoustic window for exploring mediastinal structures (◧ **16.3c, e, n**).

In principle, central masses that are sonographically defined can be aspirated through the atelectasis with a fine percutaneous needle.

Structural nonhomogeneities. The pulmonary vascular tree may account for nonhomogeneities seen with ultrasound in the postobstructive lung. Rounded, predominantly hypoechoic or anechoic areas are caused by retained secretions in the atelectatic lung. When infection is present, poststenotic foci of liquefaction may be seen due to abscess formation (obstructive pneumonitis) (◧ **16.3p–r**). The positive differentiation of hypoechoic focal masses (incipient abscess, metastasis) is occasionally difficult.

Table 16.3 Possible sonographic findings in compressive and obstructive atelectasis

	Compressive atelectasis	**Obstructive atelectasis**

B-mode ultrasound	▸ Moderate to marked pleural effusion
	▸ Triangular, peaked-cap hypoechoic transformation of the lung parenchyma
	▸ Indistinct margins with aerated lung
	▸ Partial reinflation during inhalation ("air bronchogram")
	▸ Partial reinflation after pleurocentesis
		▸ Little or no pleural effusion
		▸ Homogeneous, hypoechoic transformation of the lung parenchyma
		▸ Echogenic bands may be visible ("fluid bronchogram")
		▸ Intraparenchymal foci may appear due to:
		  – parenchymal
		  – liquefaction
		  – microabscesses or
		  – macroabscesses,
		  – metastases
		▸ A central mass may be seen
		▸ No reinflation during inhalation

Color Doppler ultrasound	▸ Increased flow signals relative to the liver	▸ Increased flow signals relative to the liver ▸ Triphasic pulmonary artery waveforms ("extremity" pattern)

16.2 Compression Atelectasis

▸ **Partial atelectasis**

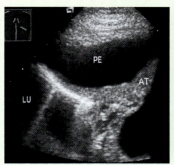 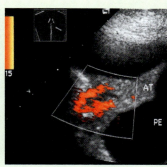 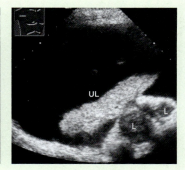

a and *b* Pleural effusion (PE) in an 87-year-old woman.
a Compression atelectasis (AT) affecting the lower lobe of the right lung (LU).

b Color Doppler shows increased flow signals in the atelectatic area (AT).

c A 73-year-old man with squamous cell carcinoma and a radiograph showing a white hemithorax on the right side. Ultrasound demonstrates effusion and upper lobe atelectasis (UL). The central hypoechoic masses are consistent with lymphnode metastasis (L).

▸ **Complete atelectasis**

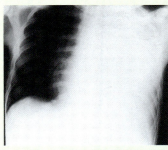 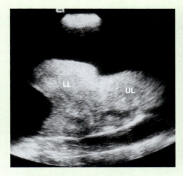 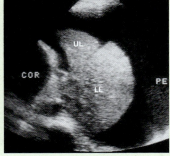

d–f A 35-year-old man with bronchial carcinoma.
d Chest radiograph shows complete opacification of the left hemithorax.

e and *f* Longitudinal and transverse scans show pronounced effusion with atelectasis of upper (UL) and lower (LL) lobes. COR = heart; PE = pleural effusion.

16.3 Obstructive Atelectasis

▶ **Middle lobe atelectasis**

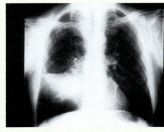 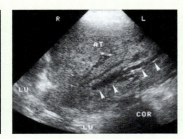 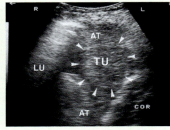

a and b Bronchial carcinoma.
a Chest radiograph shows signs of middle lobe atelectasis.

b Right anterior intercostal scan shows hypoechoic transformation of the lung with an echo-free "fluid bronchogram" caused by central obstruction. AT = atelektasis; LU = lung; COR = heart.

c Bronchial carcinoma in a 67-year-old man. Right anterior ultrasound scan shows hypoechoic transformation of the lung consistent with atelectasis (AT). A central tumor mass (TU) is identified. LU = lung; COR = heart.

▶ **Upper and lower lobe atelectasis**

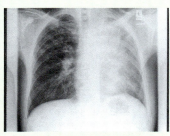 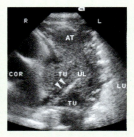 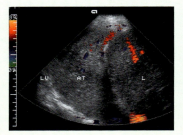

d and e Bronchial carcinoma.
d Chest radiograph shows almost complete opacification of the left hemithorax.

e Transversal scan shows upper lobe atelectasis (AT) with delineation of a central tumor (TU). The arrows point to the severely narrowed upper lobar bronchus. COR = heart; UL = upper lobe; LU = lung.

f Bronchial carcinoma. Right lateral intercostal scan shows "hepatization" of the lung characteristic of atelectasis (AT). Color Doppler shows increased flow signals in the atelectatic lung tissue. L = liver; LU = lung.

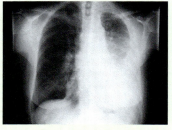 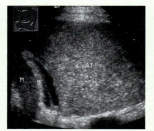 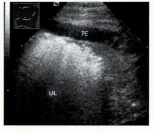

g–i Bronchial carcinoma in a 74-year-old woman.
g Chest radiograph shows opacification of the left lower lung field.

h Ultrasound shows homogeneous hypoechoic transformation of the left lower lobe consistent with atelectasis (AT). D = diagram; M = spleen.

i The central portions of the upper lobe (UL) are still aerated. Together with scant pleural effusion (PE), this suggests obstructive atelectasis of the lower lobe.

▶ **Vascular Doppler spectrum**

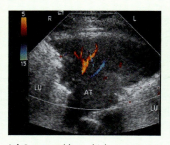 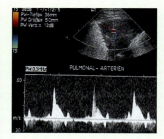 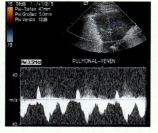

j–l Suspected bronchial carcinoma in a 74-year-old woman. In the color Doppler scanning of atelectasis, characteristic waveforms can usually be sampled from the pulmonary arteries ("extremity" pattern) and pulmonary veins. AT = atelectasis; LU = lung.

16.3 Obstructive Atelectasis

▶ Lower lobe atelectasis with tumor focus

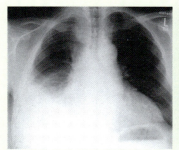 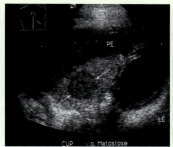 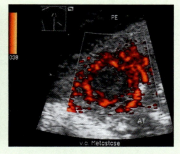

m–o A 73-year-old man with a cytologically malignant pleural effusion. **m** Chest radiograph shows a right-sided pleural effusion.

n Upper lobe atelectasis with a central hypoechoic focus. LE = liver; PE = pleural effusion.

o The absence of intralesional flow signals on color Doppler is consistent with incipient liquefaction, but a metastasis cannot be excluded. AT = atelectasis; PE = pleural effusion.

▶ Lower lobe atelectasis with obstructive pneumonitis

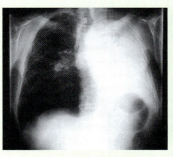 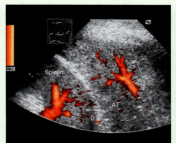 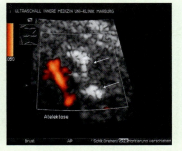

p–r Bronchial carcinoma in a 65-year-old man. **p** Chest radiograph shows a white hemithorax on the left side.

q Ultrasound scan shows homogeneous, hypoechoic transformation of the left lower lobe consistent with obstructive atelectasis. AT = atelectasis; D = diaphragm.

r Scan shows a rounded, hypoechoic, partially air-filled mass within the atelectasis in the upper lobe, consistent with obstructive pneumonitis.

▶ Pulmonary Embolism or Infarction

The results of autopsy studies prove that pulmonary embolism is among the leading causes of death (10–30%). An intravital diagnosis is made in just 20–30% of cases. An acute pulmonary embolism is accompanied by hemorrhagic lung infarction in approximately 45–60% of cases.

Diagnosis. Pulmonary embolism is diagnosed with the aid of available methods and includes an overall assessment of clinical findings, chest radiography, pulmonary scintigraphy, CT, echocardiography, and MRI.

Role of ultrasound. Although lung tissue that has undergone hemorrhagic infarction or consolidation can in principle be visualized on the basis of abnormal pulmonary sound transmission, the role of thoracic ultrasound in the diagnosis of pulmonary infarction cannot be adequately evaluated at present[3, 5]. For a pulmonary embolism to be detectable with ultrasound, there must be a significant perfusion defect causing compromise of alveolar ventilation. But in many cases a large pulmonary embolism involving pulmonary, lobar and segmental arteries will not produce an infarction owing to an adequate collateral supply, usually via branches of the bronchial rami (**Fig. 16.4**).

This type of embolism cannot be visualized with thoracic ultrasound (**16.4a–c**). Embolisms at the subsegmental level are more apt to cause hemorrhage into the alveolar airspace, making them accessible to ultrasound imaging.

Thus, thoracic ultrasound has a special role in the diagnosis of small, scintigraphically negative embolisms and infarctions that are 2 cm or less in diameter.

Whereas the hemorrhage associated with pulmonary embolism may resolve completely within a matter of days, a pulmonary infarction will show delayed regression in serial ultrasound examinations. Generally these lesions heal by scarring.

Sonographic features. Pulmonary embolism can have various ultrasound appearances (**16.5**). All possible patterns of involvement may be associated with varying degrees of pleural effusion.

Localized irregular entry echo. Irregular entry echoes are a common finding even in patients with deep lower-extremity venous thrombosis who are clinically asymptomatic for pulmonary embolism ("sentinel emboli?"). Irregular entry echo refers to a localized disruption in the sharp pleural line measuring less than 2 cm. The foci may be in the millimeter size range.

They may have a wedge or square shape with homogeneous low echogenicity. They may represent hemorrhages and may resolve within a few days. Frequently, no clinical or scintigraphic correlate is found to explain the sonographic change (**16.4d–i**).

Bandlike disruption of the entry echo. This feature is characterized by a lengthy disruption in the normal pleural entry echo. It is less common than a localized disruption and frequently has a scintigraphic correlate ("tip of the iceberg"?) (**16.4j–o**).

Wedge-shaped lesion. The classic wedge-shaped morphology of a pulmonary infarction with homogeneous low echogenicity and an absence of vascular color-flow signals in the infarcted area is rather uncommon. In serial examinations, these infarctions often show a gradual tendency to regress over a period of weeks (**16.5a–k**).

Larger areas of structural transformation. Relatively large areas of hypoechoic transformation in the lung are often associated with a pleural effusion and are considered a nonspecific feature of pulmonary embolism in thoracic ultrasound. The concomitant detection of a

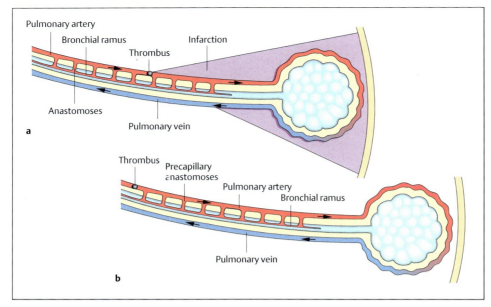

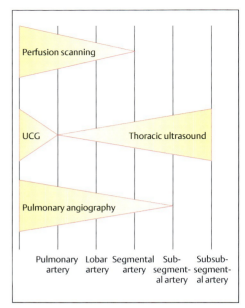

▲ **Fig. 16.4** Schematic diagram showing the occlusion of a pulmonary artery.
  a Central pulmonary artery.

▲ **b** Peripheral pulmonary artery.

deep lower-extremity venous thrombosis or of irregular entry echoes in the otherwise normal-appearing opposite lung suggests the likelihood of pulmonary embolism when corresponding clinical findings are present (▣ **16.4l–q**). Large areas of structural transformation are also seen, however, in association with pleuropneumonia and compression atelectasis due to other causes.

Color Doppler ultrasound. Color-flow signals are usually not detected in the infarcted area. In rare cases an afferent vessel may be demonstrated.

The definitive role of thoracic ultrasound in the diagnosis of pulmonary embolism remains to be determined. However, it is superior to all other modalities for selected applications, particularly the detection of smaller pulmonary embolisms (**Fig. 16.5**)[3].

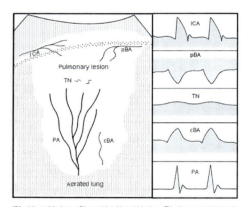

▲ **Fig. 16.5** Role of ultrasound in the diagnosis of pulmonary embolism (after reference 3) (UCG = echocardiography).

▣ 16.4 The Entry Echo in Pulmonary Embolism

▶ **Normal entry echo vs. localized irregularity**

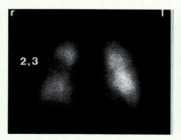

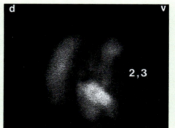

a–c Suspected pulmonary embolism in a 64-year-old man.
a and b Lung scintiscans. The findings in segments 2 and 3 of the right upper lobe are consistent with pulmonary embolism.

c Ultrasound shows a completely normal, sharp pleural entry echo along segments 2/3 of the right lung (LU).

16.4 The Entry Echo in Pulmonary Embolism

▶ Normal entry echo vs. localized irregularity

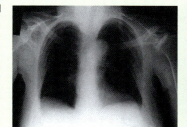 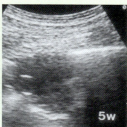 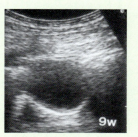

d–f A 72-year-old woman with pulmonary embolism confirmed by scintigraphy.
d Radiograph shows no lung abnormalities.

e Small foci approximately 5 mm in size are visible over both lower lung fields, consistent with pulmonary embolism.

f after 9 weeks.

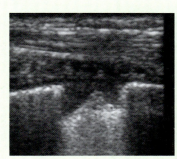 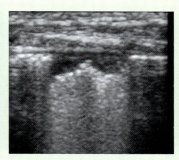 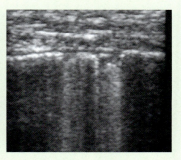

g–i A 65-year-old man with scintigraphically confirmed pulmonary embolism. Left anterior intercostal scan shows an approximately 1.5 cm pleural defect. Scans taken after one and four weeks document cicatricial healing. These findings are consistent with pulmonary infarction.

▶ Extended disruption of the entry echo

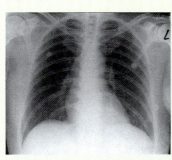 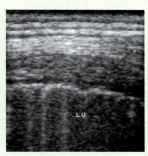 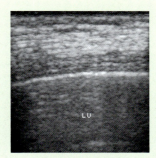

j–l Scintigraphically confirmed pulmonary embolism in a 46-year-old woman.
j Chest radiograph shows no lung abnormalities.

k Extended irregular entry echo, consistent with pulmonary embolism. LU = lung

l Normal pleural entry echo for comparison. LU = lung.

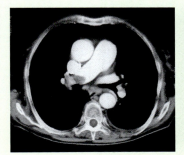 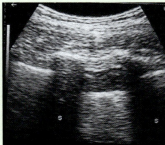

m–o Pulmonary embolism in an 80-year-old woman.
m CT shows thrombotic material in the right pulmonary artery.

n and o Ultrasound scans through different intercostal spaces show variable pleural structural defects in the posterior part of the right lower lung field. LU = lung; S = spleen.

16.5 Wedge-shaped Lesions and More Diffuse Areas of Structural Transformation due to Pulmonary Embolism

▶ **Wedge-shaped lesion**

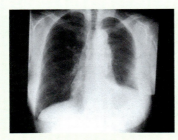 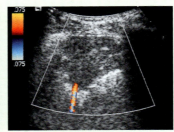

a and b Scintigraphically confirmed pulmonary embolism in a 71-year-old woman.
a Chest radiograph shows opacity in the left lower lung field.

b Left lateral intercostal scan shows a wedge-shaped hypoechoic lesion. Color Doppler shows afferent flow signals but none within the lesion. The finding is suspicious for pulmonary infarction.

▶ **Postinfarction pneumonia**

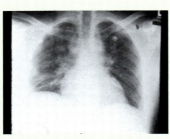 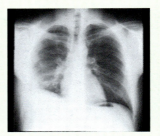 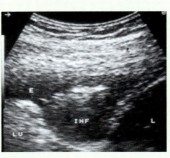

c–h Scintigraphically confirmed pulmonary embolism in a 34-year-old man.
c–e Chest radiographs show the progression of a pulmonary embolism in the right lower lobe.
c Initial radiograph shows no abnormalities.

d and e Radiographs at four and eight weeks document regression of findings in the right lower field.

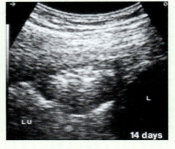 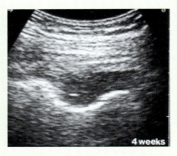 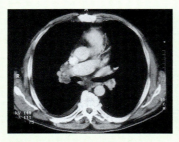

f–h Right lateral intercostal scans in postinfarction pneumonia show the progression of sonographic findings over a four-week period.

▶ **Hypoechoic transformation**

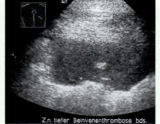 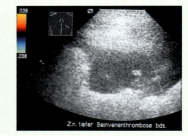

i–k Pulmonary embolism in a 56-year-old man.
i CT shows thrombotic material in the right pulmonary artery.

j Hypoechoic transformation of lung parenchyma.

k Color Doppler does not record flow signals consistent with pulmonary infarction.

16.5 Wedge-shaped Lesions and More Diffuse Areas of Structural Transformation due to Pulmonary Embolism

▶ Diffuse hypoechoic transformation

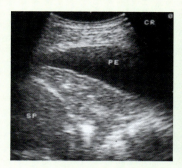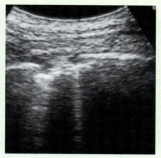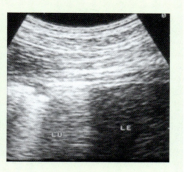

l–q Scintigraphically confirmed pulmonary embolism in a 30-year-old man.
l–n Left lateral intercostal scan shows a large area of hypoechoic transformation with moderate pleural effusion (PE). Scans through different intercostal spaces on the right side show pleural structural defects. Given the bilateral findings, the parenchymal defect on the left side is also very suspicious for postinfarction pneumonia. LE = liver; LU = lung; SP = spleen.

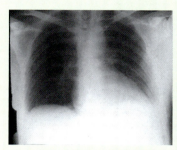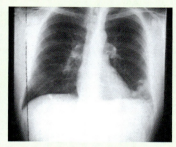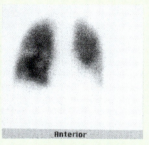

o Chest radiograph. The costophrenic angle is not defined at the edge of the lower left field.

p Follow-up radiograph shows consolidation in that region.

q Left-sided pulmonary embolism on scintigraphy.

▶ Pulmonary Tumors and Metastases

Sonography is the method of choice for accurately determining local tumor spread and should be performed before any proposed surgical treatment. The most frequent causative lesions are non-small-cell bronchial carcinomas.

Sonographic features. Peripheral lung tumors and metastases can be defined sonographically as solid hypoechoic masses when they extend to the visceral or parietal pleura (◨ **6.6a–f**). Tumor invasion of the chest wall can be diagnosed by noting fixation of the lesion to the chest wall during respiratory excursions (see **Fig. 15.8**; see also Chapter 15, p. 449) (◨ **16.6g–i**). Structural nonhomogeneities in the tumor may be due to necrosis (**Table 16.4**, ◨ **16.6j–l**). Most tumors are sharply demarcated from surrounding hyperechoic lung.

Color Doppler ultrasound. In the sonographic diagnosis of lung tumors and metastases, it should be considered that complete segmental consolidation due to pneumonia or atelectasis may also show homogeneous low echogenicity. Atelectatic areas show increased vascular flow signals in color Doppler, however. Tumors are often characterized by a scant number of vessels, which are often seen in the peripheral part of the lesion (◨ **16.6e, r–u**). An exception is alveolar cell carcinoma, which is conspicuous at color Doppler by its hypervascularity (◨ **16.6m–q**).

Table 16.4 lists the sonographic findings that are most commonly associated with peripheral lung tumors.

Ultrasound-guided percutaneous biopsy. Peripheral lung tumors and metastases can be safely punctured under ultrasound guidance. With larger lesions, tissue should be sampled from areas that exhibit color-flow vascularity. Ultrasound-guided percutaneous biopsy is particularly indicated for masses at the pleural apex (Pancoast tumors), which are difficult to biopsy by bronchoscopy.

Table 16.4 Possible sonographic findings associated with peripheral lung tumors

B-mode ultrasound
- Usually shows homogeneous, hypoechoic transformation of lung tissue
- Sharply demarcated from aerated lung
- No air bronchogram
- Occasional central necrosis

Color Doppler ultrasound
- Decreased color flow in relation to the liver
- Waveforms from tumor vessels often show high diastolic flow ("parenchymal artery" pattern)

16.6 Pulmonary Tumors and Metastases

▶ **Tumor movement with respiration**

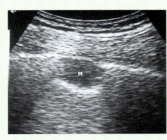 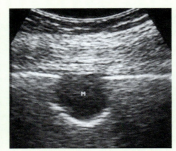 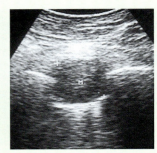

a–c The absence (*a*, *b*) or presence (*c*) of peripheral lung tumor (M) fixation to the parietal pleura can be determined by watching for tumor movement during respiration.

▶ **Adhesion to the chest wall**

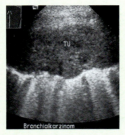 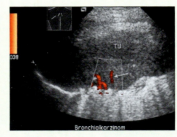 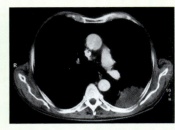

d–f Bronchial carcinoma in a 72-year-old man.
d An area of lung tissue showing homogeneous hypoechoic transformation is adherent to the chest wall. TU = tumor.

e Color flow is seen only at the periphery of the tumor (TU).

f CT: peripheral tumor mass.

▶ **Infiltration of the chest wall**

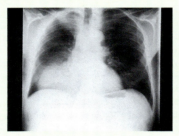 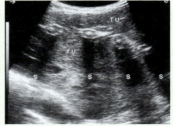 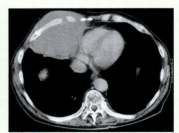

g–i Malignant lymphoma in a 70-year-old man.
g Chest radiograph shows diffuse opacity in the lower right lung.

h Right anterior scan angled caudally shows a predominantly hypoechoic lesion infiltrating the chest wall. The ribs are engulfed by tumor (TU) but are not destroyed. S = acoustic shadows.

i CT: tumor mass infiltrating the chest wall.

▶ **Necrosis**

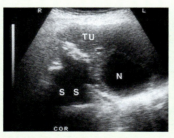 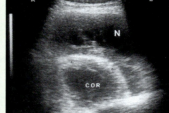 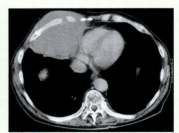

j–l Malignant histiocytoma in an 85-year-old man.
j and *k* Scans through different intercostal spaces on the left side show a complex tumor mass (TU) with signs of calcification and necrosis (N). S = acoustic shadow; COR = heart.

l CT: thoracic tumor mass.

16.6 Pulmonary Tumors and Metastases

▶ Bronchoalveolar carcinoma

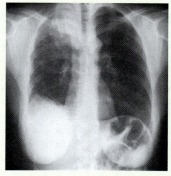 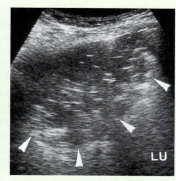 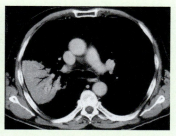

o CT: lung consolidation with a positive air bronchogram.

m–o Bronchoalveolar carcinoma in an 83-year-old man.
m Chest radiograph shows diffuse opacity in the right middle and upper zones.

n Right lateral intercostal scan shows a nonhomogeneous hypoechoic lung region with irregular margins. The tumor shows a positive air bronchogram.

▶ Color Doppler findings in bronchoalveolar carcinoma

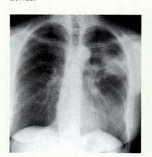 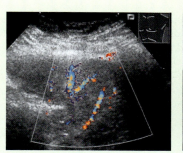 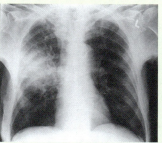

p and q Bronchoalveolar carcinoma in a 53-year-old woman.
p Chest radiograph shows diffuse shadowing in the left middle and upper zones.

q Homogeneous hypoechoic transformation of lung tissue. Color Doppler records prominent flow signals in the tumor.

r–u Bronchial carcinoma in a 77-year-old man.
r Chest radiograph shows diffuse shadowing in the right midzone.

▶ High diastolic flow in color Doppler

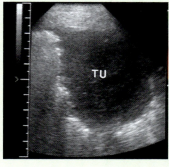 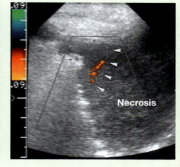 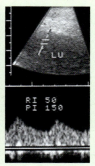

s–u Hypoechoic tumor mass (TU) in a right lateral intercostal scan. Color Doppler waveforms are recorded at the tumor periphery. The high diastolic flow ("parenchymal artery" pattern) is characteristic of tumor vessels. LU = lung.

Complex Masses

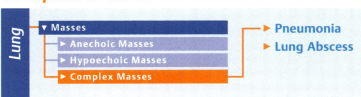

Table 16.5 Differential diagnosis of complex masses

Common	Less common
Pneumonia	Liquefying tumor
Lung abscess	Liquefying atelectasis
	Compression atelectasis

▶ Pneumonia

Ultrasound is of limited value in the diagnosis of pneumonia (◻ 16.7). It can show a more or less pronounced replacement of alveolar air, depending on the degree of pneumonic changes (◻ 16.7a–c). But the majority of inflammatory lung changes (especially central and interstitial) cannot be visualized with ultrasound (◻ 16.7d–h). **Table 16.6** reviews the sonographic findings that may be seen in pneumonia.

Lobar pneumonia. True lobar pneumonia produces a homogeneous, hypoechoic structural transformation in its early stage. The echo texture of affected lung resembles that of the liver (◻ 16.7i, j). Color Doppler shows increased vascular color-flow signals in the infiltrated lung area (◻ 16.7m–q; ◻ 16.8c). Aerated bronchi may appear as prominent echogenic bands, similar to the bronchogram seen on radiographs (◻ 16.7l). They may have a branched, string-of-beads appearance or may present as focal echogenic zones with irregular margins. The consolidated areas are usually irregular but may show segmental boundaries. The healing stage is marked by reaeration with an increase in echogenicity. Concomitant effusion is often present. The complication of cavitating pneumonia usually appears as a hypoechoic to anechoic area within the consolidated lung (◻ 16.8).

Ultrasound is not a substitute for chest radiography in pneumonia, but it is helpful as a follow-up study in detecting complications, reducing radiation exposure, and advancing the differential diagnosis (**Table 16.5**)[2].

Pleuropneumonia, pleurisy. A continuum exists between pleuropneumonia and pleurisy. The latter appears sonographically as a break in the sharp pleural line, usually combined with pleural effusion. The parenchymal defects that can be defined with ultrasound are often smaller than 1 cm and cannot be detected radiographically in the absence of pleural effusion. When combined with physical examination, ultrasonography is the method of choice in the diagnosis of pleurisy.

Table 16.6 Possible sonographic findings in pneumonia

B-mode ultrasound
- ▶ Frequent hypoechoic transformation of lung tissue
- ▶ Tends to be poorly demarcated from aerated lung
- ▶ Frequent positive air bronchogram
- ▶ Aeration often increases during inspiration
- ▶ Possible concomitant effusion

Color Doppler ultrasound
- ▶ Increased color flow in relation to the liver
- ▶ Triphasic Doppler spectrum of pulmonary artery waveforms ("extremity artery" pattern)

◻ 16.7 Interstitial and Lobar Pneumonia

▶ **Air bronchogram**

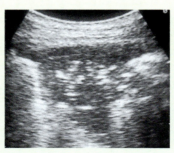
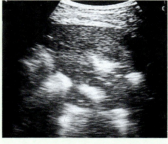
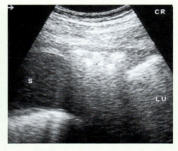

a–c Types of air bronchogram that may be seen in pneumonia. The pattern of air echoes depends partly on the course of the pneumonia.
a Branched air bronchogram.

b Patchy air bronchogram.

c Diffuse air bronchogram. LU = lung; S = spleen.

▶ **Interstitial Pneumonia**

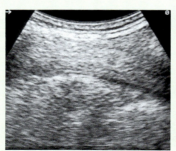
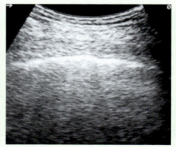
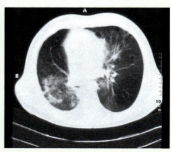

d–f Bronchial carcinoma and interstitial pneumonia in a 60-year-old man.
d The pleural line is fragmented with partial sound transmission in the lung tissue.

e Posterior scan through the lowest intercostal space on the right side (for comparison) demonstrates a normal pleural line.

f CT: interstitial pneumonia.

16.7 Interstitial and Lobar Pneumonia

▶ Interstitial Pneumonia

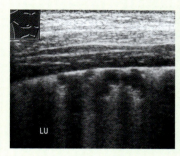 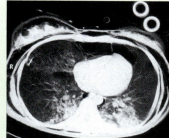

g and h Interstitial pneumonia in a 20-year-old woman.
g Ultrasound shows slight disruption of the pleural line; partial sound transmission in the lung tissue.

h CT: interstitial pneumonia.

▶ Lobar pneumonia

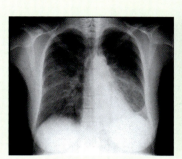 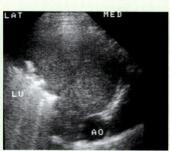 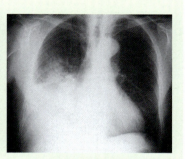

i and j Early form of lobar pneumonia.
i Chest radiograph shows opacity in the lower left lung field.

j Left posterior intercostal scan shows a largely homogeneous hypoechoic transformation of lung tissue.

k–q Pneumonia in a 73-year-old man.
k Chest radiograph shows opacity in the lower right lung field.

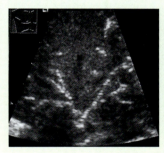 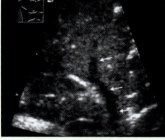 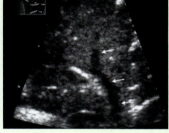

l Hypoechoic transformation of lung tissue. A branched air bronchogram is seen in the magnified view.

m and n Color Doppler image defines the course of blood vessels along the bronchial system. LA = lung artery; LV = lung vein; BR = air bronchogram.

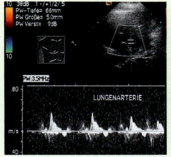 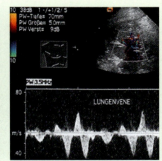

o–q The pulmonary artery (**p**) and pulmonary vein (**q**) can be identified by their color-flow image and spectral waveforms. LU = lung; LV = lung vein.

16.8 Complications of Pneumonia

▶ **Accompanying effusion**

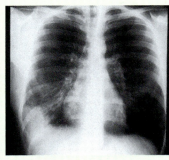 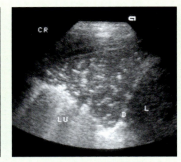 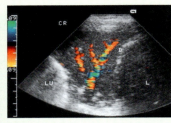

c Prominent flow signals are observed with color Doppler.

a–f Pneumonia in a 31-year-old man.
a Chest radiograph shows diffuse shadowing in the area of the right costophrenic angle.

b Right lateral intercostal scan shows a small effusion and a triangular area of hypoechoic lung tissue. A subtle, speckled air bronchogram is present.

▶ **Liquid contents**

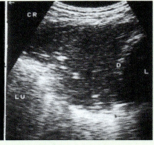 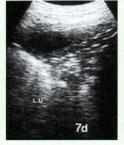 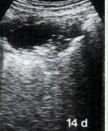 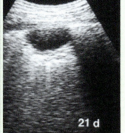

d–f Serial scans document progressive aeration over a three-week period. A small fluid collection persisted as a complication (still visible at 21 days).

▶ **Liquefaction**

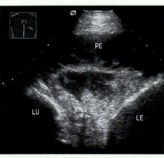 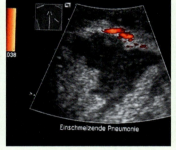 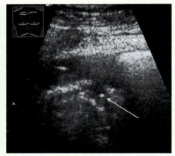

g and *h* Pneumonia in a 72-year-old man.
g Pleural effusion (PE) and a wedge-shaped area of complex lung transformation. LE = liver; LU = lung.

h Color Doppler shows peripheral flow signals. The central echo-free structure is an area of cavitating pneumonia.

i Open pulmonary tuberculosis in a 60-year-old man. Ultrasound scans show hypoechoic transformation of peripheral lung tissue. The echo-free round lesion with a central air echo in the lung parenchyma (arrow) is caused by liquefaction.

▶ Lung Abscess

Lung abscesses do not have a specific ultrasound appearance. They tend to be hypoechoic but, like abdominal abscesses, can have a variable internal echo pattern (**Table 16.7**, **16.9a–f**). Small air inclusions are evidence of gas-forming microorganisms. Larger air collections form as a result of bronchogenic fistulae.

It can be difficult to distinguish lung abscess from a pleural empyema (**16.9g–i**). The inflammatory perifocal reaction to lung abscesses bordering the pleura generally incites a local adhesion of the visceral and parietal pleura layers with corresponding fixation of the mass. This creates a more or less conspicuous hyperechoic boundary comprising the abscess membrane. Sedimentation effects may be seen if the abscess contains acoustic reflectors (sequestra, cellular debris).

Ultrasound-guided fine-needle aspiration is useful for confirming the diagnosis, sampling material, and decompressing the abscess (**16.9d–f**). Catheter drainage is recommended for abscesses that persist or cannot be decompressed with a thin needle (viscous contents).

Table 16.7 Possible sonographic findings in lung abscess/empyema

B-mode ultrasound
- Complex transformation of lung tissue
- Sharply demarcated from aerated lung
- Mass shows echogenic rim
- Possible intralesional air inclusions and moving echoes (liquefaction)

Color Doppler ultrasound
- No color-flow signals

16.9 Lung Abscess

▶ Pleural empyema

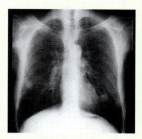
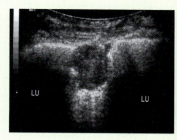
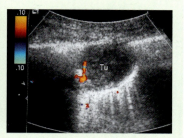

a–d Septic lung abscesses in a 54-year-old man.
a Chest radiograph shows multiple pulmonary nodules.

b Ultrasound shows a homogeneous hypoechoic peripheral lung mass (LU).

c Color Doppler shows flow signals only at the periphery of the mass (Tu). An abscess was diagnosed by ultrasound-guided core biopsy (which yielded streptococci).

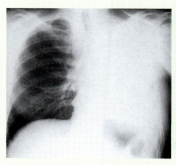
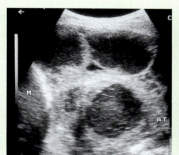
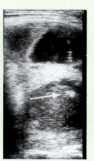

d–f Patient with bronchial carcinoma and septic temperatures.
d Chest radiograph shows diffuse opacification of the left lung.

e Loculated pleural effusion and complete lower lobe atelectasis (AT) with a central hypoechoic area of retained fluid. M = spleen.

f Diagnostic needle aspiration yielded purulent fluid consistent with a lung abscess. The arrow indicates the needle tip echo.

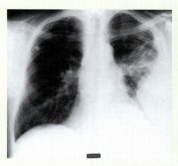
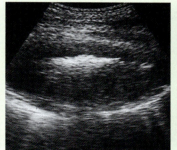
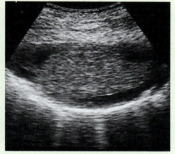

g–i Differential diagnosis: pleural empyema.
g Chest radiograph shows a large opacity bordering the chest wall on the left side.

h Scan at a higher level shows bright air echoes in the upper part of the mass.

i The lower part of the lesion contains echogenic material. The margins of the lesion are relatively smooth.

References

1. Blank W. Sonographisch gesteuerte Punktionen und Drainagen. In: Braun G, Schwerk WB (eds.). Ultraschalldiagnostik. Landsberg: ECO-Med 1994, III.II.,5–12.
2. Gehmacher O. Ultrasound pictures of pneumonia. EJR 1996;3:161–7.
3. Kroschel U, Seitz K, Reuß J, Rettenmeier. Sonographische Darstellung von Lungenembolien. Ergebnisse einer prospektiven Studie. Ultraschall in Med 1991;12:263–8.
4. Mathis G. Lungen- und Pleurasonographie. 2nd ed. Berlin: Springer 1996.
5. Mathis G, Dirschmid K. Pulmonary infarction: sonographic appearance with pathologic correlation. EJR 1993;17:170–4.
6. Schwerk WB, Görg C. Pleura und Lunge. In: Braun G, Schwerk WB (eds.). Ultraschalldiagnostik. Landsberg: ECO-Med 1993, 12.Erg.Lfg. III 2.2.,1–43.
7. Yang PC. Color Doppler ultrasound of pulmonary consolidation. EJR 1996;3:169–78.
8. Görg C, Seifart U, Görg K, Zugmaier G. Color Doppler sonographic mapping of pulmonary lesions: evidence of dual arterial supply by spectral analysis J Ultrasound Med 2003;22(10):1033–39.
9. Görg C, Seifart U, Holzinger I, Wolf M, Zugmaier G. Bronchioloalveolar carcinoma: sonographic pattern of 'pneumonia.' Eur J Ultrasound 2002;15(3):109–17.
10. Görg C, Bert T. Transcutaneous color Doppler sonography of lung consolidations: review and pictorial essay. Ultraschall Med 2004;25(3):221–6.

Index

A

abdomen
  acute 47
  wall hernia 240
  see also lymph nodes, abdominal
abdominal aorta 3–4
  aneurysms 10
  intraperitoneal branches, duplicated/variant 6–7
  retroperitoneal branches 3
    duplicated/variant 6–7
  splanchnic branches 3–4
abortion, incomplete/missed 398
abscess
  adrenal 320
  aortic 23
  diverticulitis 238–239
  epididymis 384
  gallbladder 125, 126
  gas 266
  intra-abdominal 264
  liver 77, 78, 83, 263
    amebic 78
    cholangitis 115
    gas formation 96
    hyperechoic 93
  lung 472, 473, 483, 486–487
  pancreas 154, 156
  perirenal 302
  prostate 372
  renal 299, 302, 305, 307, 309, 344
  seminal vesicles 377
  spleen 183, 188–190
  testes 382
  thyroid gland 431, 435
  tuberculous 454
abscess drain, basket 95
accessory duct of Santorini 159
acromegaly
  goiter 423
  kidneys 283
Addison disease 319
adnexal mass, inflammatory 408
adrenal glands
  abscess 320
  adenoma 321
  adjacent masses 319
  anatomy 317
  anechoic structure 318–320
  calcification 326
  carcinoma 322, 325
  complex echo structure 324–325
  cysts 319
  disease 318
  enlargement 318–327
  hematoma 319
  hemorrhage 319
  hyperechoic structure 325–327
  hyperplasia 320
  hypoechoic structure 320–324
  incidentaloma 318, 322–324
  lipoma 326
  lymphoma 322
  mass 216
  metastases 321, 324, 326
  morphology 318
  myelolipoma 326
  neuroblastoma 327
  pheochromocytoma 325, 327
  topography 317
  tumors 321–324, 326–327
    cystic 320
aerobilia 96
AIDS-induced nephropathy 286
albendazole 79
amebic liver abscess 78
amiodarone 424, 428
amyloidosis
  asplenia 180, 181
  bowel 243
  kidneys 286, 294
  liver 69
  spleen benign nonhomogeneity 176, 177
  thyroid 423
analgesic nephropathy 288, 292, 293, 295
  calcifications 312
androblastomas 411
aneurysms
  hepatic artery 214
  nonaortic 10
  renal arteries 300
  see also aorta, aneurysms
angiography, focal liver lesion differential diagnosis 99
anorchism 381
antibiotics, pseudomembranous enterocolitis 244
aorta
  abscess 23
  anatomy 3–4
  aneurysms 7–10
    chest wall 457, 472, 474
    congenital 8
    diagnosis 10
    dissecting 8, 10
    false 8, 10, 22
    intimal dissection 21
    morphology 10
    mycotic 8
    pleural effusion differential diagnosis 457, 463–464
    rupture 8
    shape 8–9
    suture-line 23
    thoracic 10
    true 7–10
    vena cava compression 32
    white thrombi 18, 21
  anomalies 5–16
  aplasia 5
  coarctation 5–6, 11
  complex arteriosclerotic lesions 17, 18
  course 3, 4
  dilatation 7–10
  duplication 5
  ectasia 7
  embolism 14–15, 20
  hematoma 23
  horseshoe kidney 24
  hypoplasia 5
  intestinal loop differential diagnosis 24
  intimal dissection 21
  kinking 6
  lumen diameter 3, 4
  lymphoma 24
  metastases 24
  microanatomy 3
  protruding arteriosclerotic plaque 20
  pseudoaneurysms 8, 10, 22
  retroperitoneal fibrosis 24
  situs inversus 5
  stenosis 11
  topography 3–4
  variant positions 5–7
  wall thickening 16–19
  see also abdominal aorta
aortic valve endocarditis 183
appendicitis 239–240
appendix 239
APUD system 436
arcuate arteries 311–312
arterial stenosis 11–14
  carcinoma 16
  lymphoma 16
  severity 13
arteries
  embolism 14–15, 20
  wall thickening 16–19
arteriosclerosis
  advanced lesions 17
  aortic stenosis 11
  complex lesions 17–18
  Mönckeberg's 19
  protruding lesions 18
  protruding plaques 20–21
  tortuous aorta 6
arteriovenous fistula 22–23
  renal 287
  spleen 187, 188
arteriovenous malformations 22–23
  intrarenal 300
  renal arteries 282
arteritis 18–19
asbestosis 457
  diffuse mesothelioma 462
  pleural fibrosis 460, 461
ascariasis 113
Aschoff–Rokitansky sinuses 130, 132
ascites 235, 254
  alcoholic cirrhosis 253
  algorithm for differentiation 256
  angle of 268
  benign 259, 268–269
  echogenic 258
  enteritis 241
  heart failure 257, 266
  hepatic cirrhosis 253, 256, 259, 266
  malignant 257, 259, 268–269
  origin 254–255
  pancreatogenous 258
  peritoneal carcinomatosis 268

ascites, peritonitis 257
   septated 263
   small bowel obstruction 271
   volume 254
aspergilloma 473
asplenia, functional 180–181
atelectasis 473, 474–477
   bronchial carcinoma 487
   complete 475
   compressive 474, 475
   lower lobe 476, 477
   middle lobe 476
   obstructive 474, 475, 476–477
   partial 475
   upper lobe 476
atheroma 17
atherosclerosis 16–19
   WHO definition 16
atherosclerotic plaque 17
axillary lymph nodes 200, 203, 210–212
   chronic lymphocytic leukemia 208

B

Baker's cyst 27
Basedow hyperthyroidism, immunogenic 421–422
   autonomously functioning nodules 443
   focal autonomy 443, 445
bezoars, small intestine 238
bile duct
   adenocarcinoma 111
   calculi 95, 109–110
   common 103
      prepancreatic 116
   congestion 116
   dilatation 107–108, 168
      cholestasis 116–117
      hilar 109–110
      intrahepatic 108–109
      intrapancreatic 111
      papillary 112
      prepancreatic 109–110
   dilated 87, 89
   disorders 166
   extrahepatic dilated 117
   foreign bodies 112–113
   gas pockets 95
   hamartoma 92
   hyperechoic 94
   intraductal pressure 107–108
   intrahepatic dilated 117
   intraluminal findings 112–114
   isoechoic 89
   malignant tumors 110
   obstruction 107, 108
      benign 109–110
      inflammatory 109
   rarefaction 106–108
   stenosis
      cicatricial 110
      intrapancreatic 157
   stents 112–113
   wall thickening 105–106, 115
      benign 105–106
      malignant 106
bile leakage 260

biliary colic 339
biliary papillomatosis, mucinous 106
biliary tree
   anatomy 103–104
   diameter 114
   extrahepatic 103, 104
   hepatocellular carcinoma 110
   intrahepatic 102, 103
   morphology 103, 104
   obstruction 114
   pressure 114
   topography 103, 104
bilioenteric anastomosis 110
bilioma 77, 264
bone marrow transplantation, asplenia 180, 181
breast cancer
   adrenal metastases 326
   chest wall cutaneous metastases 454
   metastases 60, 74, 82, 176
      lymph nodes 211
   pleural carcinomatosis 459
Brenner tumor 410
bronchial carcinoma 455
   adrenal metastases 324, 326
   atelectasis 475, 476, 477
   chest wall
      adhesion 482
      cutaneous metastases 454
   interstitial pneumonia 484
   metastases
      adrenal 324, 326
      cutaneous 454
      pleural effusion 466
      sternal 453
   opacification of hemithorax 473
   peripheral 457
   pleural effusion 465
      loculated 472
   pleural empyema 487
   pneumonectomy 467
bronchoalveolar carcinoma 483
Budd-Chiari syndrome 31–32, 42, 43
   diagnosis 62
bypass graft, infection/suture-line breakdown 23

C

calcitonin 417
calcium soap 162
Campylobacter jejuni 241
candidiasis, splenic 189, 190
carcinoid tumor, hepatic metastases 97
carcinomatosis
   peritoneal 233, 235, 257–259, 263, 267–269
      ovarian carcinoma 408
   pleural 459–460
cardiac cavity 472
cardiac cirrhosis 63
   parenchyma 73
   portal flow 37
cardiac congestion 26
cardiac insufficiency 63
cardiomegaly 464, 472
Caroli disease 57, 70, 95
carotid arteries

complex arteriosclerotic lesions 18
   stenosis 13, 16
   stents 16
carotid artery, common 418, 419
   intima-media thickness 4
celiac axis
   pancreatic carcinoma invasion 16
   stenosis 11, 12
   variants 6
celiac disease 242
cervical lymph nodes 203
   lymphoma, malignant 209
   metastases 203
cervical lymphadenopathy 207
cervicitis 400
cervix sign 231
chemotherapy, liver parenchyma 75
chest wall
   anatomy 449
   carcinoma 455
   cutaneous metastases 453–454
   lung tumor adhesion 482
   lymphoma 482
   masses 451–455
      differential diagnosis 451
   metastases 473
      cutaneous 453–454
   morphology 449–450
   necrosis 482
   topography 449
   tumor infiltration 482
chickenpox, spleen sepsis 191
cholangiectasis, prepancreatic 104, 116
cholangiocarcinoma
   bile duct dilatation 109, 110, 117
   intraductal spread 106
cholangiocellular carcinoma 105
cholangiofibroma 91
cholangiofibromatosis 57
cholangitis
   liver abscess 115
   primary sclerosing 105, 106
   pyogenic 263
   suppurative 105, 106
cholecystectomy, post-surgery status 137
cholecystic empyema 125, 126
cholecystitis 123
   acalculous 126
   acute 125–127
   calculous 127
   chronic 126, 127–128
      gallbladder carcinoma 133
   emphysematous 126
   gallbladder carcinoma differential
diagnosis 133
   phlegmonous 125, 126
   xanthogranulomatous 126
cholecystolithiasis 123, 139, 260
choleperitoneum 260
cholestasis
   differential diagnosis 114–117
   parenchymatous 115–116
   sonographic 116–117
cholesteatosis 130
cholesterol
   gallbladder deposits 130
   gallbladder pseudopolyps 131, 132
   gallbladder sludge 134, 135, 136

gallstones 134, 135
chorioepithelioma 405
chorionic cavity 397
chronic lymphocytic leukemia
   axillary lymph nodes 208
   lymph nodes 201
   spleen 194
   splenomegaly 180
chronic myelocytic leukemia, splenomegaly 177, 179–180
chyloperitoneum 261
chylothorax, pleural effusion differential diagnosis 464
cirrhosis *see* hepatic cirrhosis
clips, surgical 113
colic arteries, stenosis 11
colitis, ischemic 243–244
collagen disease, spleen benign non-homogeneity 176
colon 225–226, 227
   coprostasis 247
   Crohn's disease 242
   diverticula 238
   haustra 227
   morphology 226
   polyps 237
colon cancer 44
   carcinoma 236
   hepatic metastases 88
   peritoneal carcinomatosis 259, 269
   splenic metastases 192
comet-tail artifacts 94
computed tomography (CT), focal liver lesion differential diagnosis 99
confetti phenomenon 20, 161
congenital malformations
   arteriovenous 22–23, 282, 300
   inferior vena cava 25, 26
coprostasis 247
corpus luteum cysts 405
critical stenosis 13
Crohn's disease 105, 242–243
   complications 243
   intussusception 237
   urinary bladder wall hypertrophy 360
cryptorchidism 381
Cushing syndrome 320
cystic duct obstruction 123
cystic fibrosis 149
cytomegalovirus (CMV) hepatitis 77

D

de Quervain thyroiditis
   focal 435
   subacute 422
diabetes mellitus
   autoimmune pancreatitis 146
   autoimmune thyroiditis 424, 425
   chronic pancreatitis 168
   confetti phenomenon 20
   fatty liver 65
   large gallbladder 122
   Mönckeberg's arteriosclerosis 19
   renal abscess 299
   renal structural changes 294
diabetic foot, neuroischemic 14

diabetic glomerulosclerosis 290
diabetic nephropathy 283–284, 288–289, 290–292
   calcifications 312
   histopathology 292
   stages 292
diaphragm
   liver incisures 93
   morphology 449–450
diverticula 238
diverticulitis 238–239
diverticulosis 238–239
diverticulum, perforated 231
double-barrel shotgun sign 103, 107, 116
Douglas pouch 253, 254, 255
dromedary hump, renal 301
ductus hepatocholedochus 103
duodenal diverticulum, periampullary 112
duodenal ulcer 253
   perforated 265
duodenum
   gut signature 227
   morphology 226
   stenosis 160, 270

E

Echinococcus cysticus 184
Echinococcus granulosus 79–80, 184, 297
Echinococcus multilocularis 98, 297
endometriosis, ovarian 407
endometritis 400
endometrium 392, 393
   changes 398–401
   corpus carcinoma 400–401
   cyclic changes 399
   hyperplasia 409
      adenomatous/cystic glandular 399
   pathology 399
   polyps 398
   proliferative 399
   thickness 399
enteritis 241
   intestinal inflammation 245
enterocolitis 241
   pseudomembranous 244
epididymis
   abscess 384
   anatomy 379
   cyst 383–384
   decreased size 381
   lesions 383–384
   topography 379
epididymitis 384
erysipelas 201, 202
esophageal cancer
   lymph node invasion 203
   metastases 91
   thyroid gland metastases 437
esophageal varices 39, 40, 43
esophagus 225
   morphology 226

F

fallopian tubes
   blood in 390
   carcinoma 402
   hypoechoic mass 402–403
   pregnancy 403
   tumors 402
fat, peripancreatic 144, 145
femoral arteries
   arteriovenous fistula 22
   complex protruding lesions 20
   embolism 15
   pseudoaneurysms 10
   stenosis 13–14
femoral veins
   incompetence 28
   thrombosis 29, 30
   venous valves 31
fibrin 257, 258, 259
   fluttering strands 267
   pleural bodies 457, 458
   pleural effusion 464, 467
fibrothorax 467
fine-needle aspiration, adrenal glands 323
fistula, arteriovenous 22–23
flow velocity, diabetic foot 14
focal nodular hyperplasia, hepatic 84, 85, 87–88, 92
   diagnosis 99
follicular cysts 404
foreign bodies
   bile duct 112–113
   bowel 247
   hepatic 95
   urinary bladder 358
   uterine 396–397

G

gallbladder
   abscess 125, 126
   acute hepatitis 69
   adenoma 131, 132
   adenomyomatosis 130, 132
   agenesis 123, 137
   anatomy 119–120
   atrophic calculus 138
   atrophy 123, 124, 125
   carcinoma 110, 130, 133
      liver parenchyma 74
   cholesterol pseudopolyps 131, 132
   color-flow duplex scanning 129
   comet-tail artifacts 130
   cystic duct 119, 120
   doubling 121
   flaccid 122
   fluid level 123, 124
   hemobilia 136
   hepatic cirrhosis 73
   hepatized 89
   hydrops 122, 123
   hypoplasia 123
   intrahepatic 123
   intraluminal changes 134–136
   isoechogenicity with surrounding tissue 138–139

gallbladder, kinking 121
  large 122
  malformation 121
  malposition 139
  metastases 133
  missing 123–125, 137
  nonvisualized 137–139
  obscured 137–139
  papilloma 131, 132
  perforation 125, 126
    cholelithic 127–128
  polyps 131
  porcelain 128, 129
  pseudopolyps 131, 132
  pseudotumor 136
  septations 121
  shape variants 119, 121
  size 119
    change 122–123
  sludge 122, 134, 135, 136, 138
  small 123–125
  stomach impression 234
  strawberry 130
  topography 120
  torsion 121
  tumors 129–133
    infiltration 138
  wall
    changes 125–133
    differential diagnosis of change 127
    focal hyper-/hypo-echogenicity 128–129
    hyperechogenicity 127–128
    hypoechogenicity 125–127
    inflammation 128–129
    thickening 126, 127
    thickness 119, 124, 125
    varicosity 129
gallstones 134–136
  bile duct obstruction 109–110
  cholelithic perforation 127–128
  cholesterol 134, 135
  composition 134
  cystic duct obstruction 123
  differential diagnosis 134, 135
  gallbladder
    atrophy 124, 125
    carcinoma 133
  intrahepatic bile ducts 95, 108, 109
  microliths 134
  small intestine 238
  spherocytosis 178
gas abscess 266
gastric antrum tumors 235
see also stomach
gastric artery 6
  stenosis 11
gastric outlet obstruction 234, 270
gastric polyps 229
gastric vein, enlarged 39
gastrinoma 155, 156
gastritis 232
  autoimmune 425
gastroduodenal artery 144, 154
gastrointestinal tract
  anatomy 225–226
  extraluminal fluid 269–271
  intraluminal fluid 269–271
  morphology 226–228

  perforation 261
  topography 225–226
  tumors
    abdominal lymph nodes 206
    stromal 229
see also named regions/organs
gastrosplenic ligament 174
genital tract
  female 389
see also named organs
giant cell arteritis 18
glomerulonephritis
  acute 285, 292
  chronic 288–289, 292
glucagonoma 155, 156
goiter 419–420
  acromegaly 423
  amiodarone-induced 428
  de Quervain thyroiditis 422, 435
  diffuse colloid 420
  diffuse parenchymatous 419–420
  lithium-induced 428
  nodular 434, 441–442
    regressive 442
  Riedel 422
see also Basedow hyperthyroidism, immunogenic; Hashimoto thyroiditis
gonorrhea
  epididymitis 384
  prostatitis 370
grafts, synthetic 19
graft-*versus*-host disease, asplenia 180, 181
granulomatous disease, spleen benign nonhomogeneity 176
granulomatous prostatitis 370
Graves disease 421–422
groin lymph nodes 210–212
gut signature 227
  criteria 226, 228
  morphology 226
  ulcerative colitis 243

H

halo sign 81
Hashimoto thyroiditis 420, 443
  autoimmune 420
    atrophic 423–424
  hypertrophic 420
Hashimoto-type autoimmune thyroiditis 423
head/neck lymph nodes 200, 207–210
heart failure
  gallbladder changes 124
  inferior vena cava congestion 290
  peritoneal cavity changes 257
  pleural effusion 464
  renal congestion 285
  right-sided 266
Helicobacter pylori 232
HELPP syndrome 78
hemangiomatosis, splenic 193
hematocele 386
hematocolpos 390
hematological malignancy
  spleen 190
  splenomegaly 177, 179–180

see also chronic lymphocytic leukemia; chronic myelocytic leukemia
hematometra 390, 397
hematosalpinx 390, 402
hematothorax
  pleural effusion differential diagnosis 464
  pleural fibrosis 460
hemihepatectomy 68
hemobilia 110, 136
hemochromatosis 70, 146
  pancreas 149
hemoperitoneum 258, 260
hepatic acinus 51
see also liver
hepatic artery
  aneurysm 214
  common 6
  hepatic cirrhosis 36
  variants 104
hepatic cirrhosis 256
  alcoholic 256
  ascites 253, 256, 259, 266
  atrophic 67
  cardiac 68
  cholestasis 115–116
  diagnosis 62
  diagnostic criteria 67
  extrahepatic changes 73–74
  fatty 65, 66, 68
  flow reversal 35
  gallbladder changes 124
  hepatic artery 36
  hepatic surface 55
  hepatic vein 59
    dilatation 36
  liver size 67
  parenchymal changes 73–74
    inflammatory 56
  peritoneum 266
  portal vein flow 61
  posthepatic 68
  splenic mass 183
  splenomegaly 179
    with spontaneous bacterial peritonitis 259
  vascular changes 39
hepatic hilar lymph nodes 38
hepatic lobule 51
hepatic peliosis 79, 80
hepatic segments 52
hepatic veins 54, 58
  Budd–Chiari syndrome 31–32
  distended 63
  engorgement 26
  fatty liver hepatitis 65–66
  flow profile 37, 58–59, 63
  heart failure 257
  hepatic cirrhosis 59
  inflammatory disease 60
  liver congestion 59
  rarefied 60
  thrombosis 87
  veno-occlusive disease 60
hepatitis
  acute 69
  autoimmune 55, 73
  cholestasis 115
  chronic 72–73
  cytomegalovirus 77

fatty liver 56, 65–66
gallbladder changes 124
inflammatory lymph nodes 124, 213
toxic fatty liver 65, 66
hepatocellular adenoma 83
hepatocellular carcinoma 48, 84, 86, 91
   bile duct dilatation 109, 110
   calcification 95
   diagnosis 99
   gallbladder infiltration 138
   hepatic vein infiltration 60
   hyperechoic 92
   irregular mass 97
   isoechoic 88
   liver parenchyma 74
hepatocytes, iron deposits 70
hepatoduodenal stents 112, 113
hepatopetal flow 37
hepatosteatosis 59
hernia, abdominal wall 240
heroin-induced nephropathy 286
hilar artery 175
   hypoechoic transformation 185, 186
hilar sign 202, 203
hilar vein, hypoechoic transformation 185, 186
histiocytoma, malignant 482
Hodgkin disease 80
   bile duct dilatation 109
   chest wall cutaneous metastases 454
   lymph nodes 202, 205, 208, 211
   spleen 176, 185, 186
   splenomegaly 180
   thyroid gland 435
Horner syndrome 455
hydatid cysts 79–80
   alveolar 98
   calcification 95
   focal nodular hyperplasia differential diagnosis 85
   pancreatic 152
   renal 297
   spleen 184
hydrocele 385
hydronephrosis 300, 339
   sac 336, 340
hymen, imperforate 390
hypercalcemia, pleural calcification 458
hypertension, tortuous aorta 6
hyperthyroidism 428
   autonomy 443–445
   bifocal autonomy 443, 444
   clinical classification 443
   differential diagnosis 443–445
   disseminated autonomy 443, 444
   multifocal autonomy 443, 444
   transient 427
   unifocal autonomy 443, 444
hypoalbuminemia 124, 257
hypocortisolism 319
hypogonadism 381
hyposplenism, functional 180–181
hypothyroidism 426
   amiodarone-induced 428
   lithium-induced 428
   neonatal 425
   radiation-induced 426–427, 429
hysterectomy, vaginal changes 391–392

I

ileitis, terminal 242
ileocolic valve 227
ileum, morphology 226
ileus 245–246
   chronic 227
   mechanical 227, 246
   paralytic 246
iliac arteries
   embolism 15
   occlusion 244
   stenosis 14
iliac veins, congenital anomalies 26
infections
   bacterial
      peritonitis 257, 258, 267
      prostatitis 370
   spleen 178
      benign nonhomogeneity 176
   urinary tract obstruction 342–343
   viral in de Quervain thyroiditis 422
see also abscess
infectious mononucleosis
   hepatitis 69
   lymph node enlargement 205
   splenomegaly 178
inferior vena cava
   anatomy 4
   cardiac congestion 26
   compression 31–32
   congenital anomalies 25, 26
   congestion 59
      heart failure 290
   course 4
   dilatation 26–28
   duplication 25
   engorgement 26–27
   heart failure 257, 290
   hepatic caudate lobe enlargement 31
   infiltration 31–32
   intraluminal mass 28–30
   leiomyoma 43
   lumen diameter 4
   malignant tumors 32
   metastases 32
   microanatomy 4, 31, 32
   retroperitoneal branches 4
   splanchnic branches 4
   stenosis 27
   thrombosis 27, 29
   topography 4
inflammatory bowel disease 105, 242, 243
insulinoma 155, 156
interlobar arteries, renal 311–312
intestinal loop 24
intra-abdominal abscess 264
intra-abdominal gas 261–262
intrahepatic block, collaterals 39–42
intraperitoneal fluid
   differential diagnosis 255
see also ascites
intraperitoneal lymph nodes 200
intrauterine contraceptive device (IUD) 396–397, 398
   infected 400
iodine deficiency 417

J

Jaffe–Lichtenstein dysplasia of bone 453
jejunum 227
   morphology 226
jugular vein
   internal 418, 419
      ectasia 27
   thrombosis 30

K

Kerckring's folds 245, 246, 270–271
kidneys
   aberrant vessels 281, 335
   abscess 299, 302, 305, 307, 309, 344
   acromegaly 283
   adenoma 307
   agenesis 276–277
   AIDS-induced nephropathy 286
   amyloidosis 286, 294
   analgesic nephropathy 288, 293, 295
      calcifications 312
   anatomy 275
   anechoic structure 296–301
   angiomyolipoma 310
   anomalies 276–282
      number/position/rotation 278–280
   aplasia 276–277, 283
   arcuate arteries 311–312
   atrophic 295
   bacterial gas bubbles 312
   caliceal diverticula 281, 335
   caliceal stones 281, 300, 346
   caliectasis 335
   carbuncles 309
   cavities 299
   chronic glomerulonephritis 288–289
   circumscribed changes 296–313
   collecting system anomaly 281
   complex structure 307–308
   congestion 285
   cortex 275
   cystic malformation 277–278
   cysts 296–297, 319
      hemorrhagic 302, 309
      lymph 298
      parapelvic 305
      simple 278
      types 278
   diabetic nephropathy 283–284, 288–289, 290–292
      calcifications 312
   diffuse changes 282–296
   dromedary hump 301
   duplex 278–279, 283, 305, 334
   dysplastic cystic 278
   echogenic structure 311–313
   ectopic 279
   fetal lobulation 301
   fresh infarcts 302
   fusion anomaly 280
   heart failure 290
   hematoma 300, 303, 308
   heroin-induced nephropathy 286
   horseshoe 24, 280
   hydrocalices 300–301

kidneys, hyperechoic structure 290–295, 309–311
  hyperperfusion 291
  hypoechoic structure 289–290, 301–307
  hypoplasia 276–277, 277, 287
  hypoxemic shock 290
  infected obstruction 305
  interlobar arteries 311–312
  intracystic carcinoma 236
  intracystic hemorrhage 308
  irregular structure 295–296
  isoechoic structure 301–307
  large 282–287
  light-chain deposition disease 294
  lymphoma 306, 308
    infiltration 294
  malformations 276–282
  malrotation 280
  medulla 275
    calcification 311
  medullary pyramids 275, 284, 289, 299
  medullary sponge 278, 300
  megacalices 335–336
  megacalicosis 281, 335
  metabolic disorders 294
  metastases 306
  nephrocalcinosis 300, 312
  papillary calcification 311
  papillary necrosis 299
  paraprotein 286
  parenchymal calcification 312
  parenchymal notching 310–311
  parenchymal–pelvic ratio 283
  pelvis
    dilated 336–344
      hypoechoic mass 344–345
      mass 344–348
      obstruction by uterine myoma 395
      stone 337, 346
      suppurative inflammation 343–344
  perirenal cystic masses 297
  polycystic/polycystic disease 277–278, 284, 296–297
  putty 313
  pyelocaliceal system 339
    dilatation 343
    stones 313, 339
  pyonephrosis 286, 296, 307
  renal cell carcinoma 286, 303–304, 306, 308
    cystic 298–299, 308
    hyperechoic 309
    metastases 304, 324
    operated 425
    ureteral clots 345
  renal pelvis
    carcinoma 306
    shape 331
  renal sinus echo complex 305–306, 347
  renal stone colic 342–343
  renal tubule scarring 297
  renovascular malformations 282
  scars 310–311
  septic-toxic 284, 293
  single 283
  sinus lipomatosis 305
  size determination 282–283
  small 287–289
  staghorn calculi 313, 342, 346–347
  topography 275–276
  transplants 287
  tuberculosis 299, 313
    scars 311
  tumors 286, 310
    diffuse infiltration 295
    inflammatory 307
    parenchymal 303
  vascular anomalies 281–282
  vascular dilatations 300
  vascular ectasia 282
  vessels 275
  Waldenström disease 294
see also renal *entries*
Kimmelstiel–Wilson syndrome 290
Klatskin tumor 44, 108
  classification 111
Kupffer cells 51
kyphoscoliosis 139

L

laparoscopy
  focal liver lesion differential diagnosis 99
  hepatic metastases 100
Laplace's law 7
large intestine 235–248
  amyloidosis 243
  atrophy 248
  carcinoma 236
  diverticula 238
  foreign body 247
  hematoma 237
  hypertrophy of wall 244
  inflammation 245
  intussusception 237
  ischemia 243–244, 248
  lumen
    dilated 245–247
    narrowed 247–248
  lymphoma 236, 244
  obstruction 271
  peristalsis 228
  physiological dilatation 245
  polyps 237
  tumors 244, 247
  wall
    extended changes 241–244
    focal changes 236–240
    layers 226
leukemia *see* chronic lymphocytic leukemia; chronic myelocytic leukemia
life periods, female 389
ligamentum teres 52
  hepatis 93
  lipoma 80, 85
light-chain deposition disease 294
limb ischemia, arterial stenosis 15
lipid plaques 17
lipoma, hepatic 80, 85
liposarcoma, chest wall cutaneous metastases 454
lithium 424
liver
  abscess 77, 78, 83, 263
    amebic 78
    cholangitis 115
    gas formation 96
    hyperechoic 93
  adenoma 83–84
  amyloidosis 69
  anatomical variants 53, 54
  anatomy 52–62
  atrophy 67
  calcification 95
  cancer 82
  capsule injuries 77
  caudate lobe
    enlargement 31
    size 62
  chemotherapy 75
  cholangiofibroma 91
  comet-tail artifacts 94
  congestion 59
    acute 63, 64
    cholestasis 115
    chronic 63–64
  contour 53
  cysts 76, 78
    complicated 83
    stomach impression 234
  diaphragmatic incisures 93
  diffuse infiltration 66
  dynamic criteria 54, 57, 58
  enlarged 62–64
  extrinsic criteria 53–54
  fatty 63–66, 70
  fatty degeneration 56
  fatty focal change 87, 94
  fatty focal infiltration 65, 71–72
  fibrosis 70
  focal lesion diagnosis 98–100
  focal nodular hyperplasia 84, 85, 87–88, 92
    diagnosis 99
  foreign bodies 95
  function 51
  gas accumulation 95–96
  gas embolism 241
  hemangioma
    atypical 86, 88, 91
    differential diagnosis 91
    focal 99
    giant 90
    hyperechoic 89–91
  hematoma 83, 88
  hemorrhage/hematoma 77
  homogeneous texture
    hyperechoic 70
    hypoechoic 68–69
  hydatid cysts 79–80
    alveolar 98
  inflammatory disease 60
  inflammatory parenchymal changes 56, 59
  inhomogeneous texture
    diffuse 72–74
    regional 71–72
  intrahepatic masses 74–75
  intrinsic criteria 54–58
  lipoma 80, 85
  lymphatic infiltration 80
  lymphoma 80, 82
  metastases 74, 75, 81, 82, 91
    ascites 269
    cholestasis 115
    diagnosis 99–100

diffuse 97
hyperechoic 93
isoechoic 88
surface 55
necrosis 72, 93
parenchyma 56, 57
anechoic masses 76–87
diffuse changes 61–62
echodense masses 94–96
homogeneous texture 68–70
hyperechoic 89–94
inhomogeneous texture 71–74
irregular masses 97–98
isoechoic masses 87–89
localized changes 74–75
pathological findings 59–61
polycystic disease 76–77, 78, 263
porphyria 92
portovenous gas embolism 241
prehepatic block 38
regenerative nodules 92
resection 68
Riedel's lobe 53, 54
segments 52
shape 53
size 53, 62
small 67–68
sonographic assessment criteria 54, 57
surface 53, 55
thorotrastosis 97
topography 51
tumors
diffuse growth 74
primary 82
vascularization 82
venous flow pattern 58
see also hepatic entries
lung
abscess 472, 473, 483, 486–487
cancer and lymph node metastases 202
empyema 486–487
fluid collection 486
liquefying processes 472, 473, 486
masses 471–487
anechoic 472–474
complex 483–487
evaluation criteria 471
hypoechoic 474–483
metastases 481–483
morphology 471
percutaneous biopsy 481
topography 471
tuberculosis 486
tumors 481–483
respiration movement 482
see also atelectasis; bronchial carcinoma; pulmonary entries
lutein cyst 405
lymph nodes
abdominal 204–207
hepatic portal 212–214
iliac 220, 222
mesenteric 216–219
para-aortic 220, 222
retroperitoneal 219–222
splenic hilum 215–216
staging of involvement 206
anatomy 199

assessment 201
axillary 200, 203, 210–212
chronic lymphocytic leukemia 208
calcification 202
celiac in non-Hodgkin lymphoma 206
cervical 203
lymphoma 209
echogenicity 202, 203
enlargement 110
esophageal cancer invasion 203
extremities 210–212
groin 210–212
false aneurysm 212
head/neck 200, 207–210, 209
Hodgkin disease 202, 208, 211
inflammatory 207, 213, 215, 217
retroperitoneal 219–220
inflammatory pancreatic 156
intraperitoneal 200
invasion patterns 205, 206
location 201
lymphoma 202, 206, 209
hepatic portal 214
mesenteric 218
retroperitoneal 220, 221
splenic hilum 215–216
metastases 202, 203, 206, 207–209
axillary 211
groin 211
mesenteric 217, 218
prostate cancer 205
retroperitoneal 220, 221
splenic hilum 215
morphology 201, 202
nonperipheral 200
parapelvic cysts 297, 298
parietal 207
peripheral 199–200, 207–212
calcification 204
reactive enlargement 205
retroperitoneal 200–201
splanchnic 207
splenic hilum 215–216
supraclavicular 209
topography 199–201
vascularization 202, 204, 205
lymphadenitis, mesenteric 217
lymphadenopathy
cervical 207
differential diagnosis 199
inflammatory 207
mesenteric 241
non-Hodgkin lymphoma 206
reactive 201
lymphangioma, benign cystic 298
lymphocele, intra-/peri-renal 298
lymphoma
inferior vena cava compression 32
kidney infiltration 294
lymph node calcification 204
peripheral vein compression 32
uterus 394
lymphoma, malignant
adrenal 322
aortic 24
arterial stenosis 16
bowel wall 244
cervical lymph nodes 209

chest wall
cutaneous metastases 454
infiltration 482
hepatic involvement 80, 82
infiltrating 80
large intestine 236
lymph nodes 202, 203, 206, 209
axillary 212
groin 212
hepatic portal 214
mesenteric 218
retroperitoneal 220, 221
splenic hilum 215–216
pancreas 156, 158
pleural carcinomatosis 460
pleural effusion 465, 467
renal 306, 308
small intestine 236
spleen 176, 183, 194
invasive 184–186
splenic vein thrombosis 46
splenomegaly 177, 179–180
stomach 230, 232
thyroid gland 435
lymphoproliferative disorder, splenic infarction 186

M

magnetic resonance imaging (MRI) 99
malabsorption, gallbladder changes 124
malignancy
gallbladder infiltration 138
pancreas 145
vena cava infiltration 32
malignant melanoma
lymph nodes 203
metastases
lymph nodes 211
splenic 192
thyroid gland 438
malignant mesothelioma 457
diffuse 462
pleural fibrosis 460, 461
Marine–Lenhart syndrome 421, 443, 445
median arcuate ligament syndrome 11
megacalicosis 335
megaureter 335–336
Ménétrier disease 232
mesenteric artery, inferior 11, 12
mesenteric artery, superior 6
embolism 15
stenosis 11, 12
mesenteric lymph nodes 216–219
enlargement 217
mesenteric vein, superior 34
acute abdomen 47
lumen enlargement 36
thrombosis 46–47
mesoaortitis syphilitica 18
metabolic disorders, kidneys 294
metastases 81
adrenal 321, 324
aorta 24
breast cancer 60, 74, 82
lymph nodes 211
calcification 95

metastases, celiac lymph nodes 206
  cervical lymph nodes 203
  chest wall 453–454, 473
  cutaneous 453–454
  echogenicity 82
  focal nodular hyperplasia differential diagnosis 85
  gallbladder 133
  hepatic 74, 75, 81, 82, 91
    ascites 269
    cholestasis 115
    diagnosis 99–100
    diffuse 97
    hyperechoic 93
    isoechoic 88
    surface 55
  hepatic portal lymph nodes 213
  hepatic vein 60
  inferior vena cava 32
  lung 481–483
  lymph nodes 207–209
    axillary 211
    groin 211
    malignant melanoma 211
    mesenteric 217, 218
    prostate cancer 205
    retroperitoneal 220, 221
  malignant melanoma 211
  ovarian 409
  ovarian cancer 341
  pancreas 144, 155, 156
  peritoneal 267–268
  pleural, differential diagnosis 458
  prostate cancer 354, 355, 374
    lymph nodes 205
  rectal cancer lymph nodes 211
  renal 306
  renal cell carcinoma 304, 324
  rib 452–453
  seminal vesicles 376, 378
  spleen 176, 190, 192
    calcification 195
  sternum 452–453
  stomach 230
  thyroid gland 437–438
  ureters 341
  vena cava infiltration 32
meteorism 227
Meyenburg complexes 92
microalbuminuria 291
microliths 134
Mirizzi syndrome 109, 127
Mönckeberg's arteriosclerosis 19
Morrison's pouch 253
multiple endocrine neoplasia (MEN) 325, 436
Murphy's sign 123
myelofibrosis, splenomegaly 177, 179–180
myeloproliferative disorders
  intrasplenic varicosity 42
  spleen 194
  splenic infarction 186
  splenomegaly 177, 179–180
myometrium 392
  changes 394–396
myosarcoma, metastases 91
myxedema 420, 424

N

neck *see* head/neck lymph nodes
needle biopsy, focal liver lesion differential diagnosis 99
nephrectasia, hydronephrotic 263
nephritis, acute 289
nephrocalcinosis 300, 312
nephroma, cystic 298
nephronophthisis, familial 278
nephropathy
  adult polycystic 278
  AIDS-induced 286
  analgesic 288, 292, 293, 295
    calcifications 312
  heroin-induced 286
  infantile polycystic 278
see also diabetic nephropathy
neuroblastoma 327
non-Hodgkin lymphoma 82
  celiac lymph nodes 206
  hepatic 80
  lymphadenopathy 206
  pancreatic 156
  pleural carcinomatosis 460
  pleural effusion 467
  spleen 186

O

orchitis 380
Ormond disease 340
Osler disease 79, 80
outflow obstruction, acute 285
ovaries
  anatomy 403
  anechoic cystic mass 404–406
  cancer/carcinoma 406, 408–409, 410
    ascites 263, 269
    peritoneal carcinomatosis 259
  cystadenocarcinoma 406, 409, 410
  cystadenoma 406, 410
  cysts
    endometriotic 407
    functional 404–405
  dermoid tumors 412
  dysgerminoma 412
  endometriosis 407
  fibroma 411
  follicles 404
  follicular cysts 404
  germ cell tumors 412
  histology 403
  inflammatory adnexal mass 408
  metastases 341, 409
    pleural effusion 466
    splenic 192, 215
  morphology 403–404
  mucinous cystadenocarcinoma 410
  mucinous cystoma 406, 410
  nonhomogenous masses 407–414
  paraovarian cyst 405
  polycystic 405
  retention cysts 405
  sarcoma 411
  solid echogenic masses 407–414
  struma ovarii 412

  teratomas 412
  theca-lutein cyst 405
  thecoma 411
  thecomatosis 407
  topography 403
  tumors
    classification 409
    clear cell 410
    complications 413
    cystic 406
    diagnosis 413
    endometrioid 410
    epithelial 409–410
    germ cell 410
    granulosa cell 411
    histological criteria 409–414
    imaging 413
    prognosis 414
    sex cord-stromal 410, 411
    steroid cell 411
    symptoms 413
    transitional cell 410
    treatment 414
    yolk sac 412

P

pampiniform process 385
panarteritis nodosa 18
Pancoast tumor 455, 481
pancreas
  abscess 154, 156
  adenoma 156
  aging 146
  anatomy 143
  anechoic lesions 152–154
  annular 159–160
  atrophy 146
  blood supply 143–144
  borders 143
  calcification 161
  cancer/carcinoma 16, 41, 155–156, 158
    acinar cell 156
    cystic 263
    differential diagnosis 157
    diffuse 145
    ductal dilatation 168–169
    head 111
    hepatic metastases 88, 97
    lymph node metastases 213
    mucinous ductal 164
    papillary 112
    periampullary 107, 112, 155, 167
    splenic metastases 192
    venous infiltration 48
  congenital anomalies 159
  congenital cysts 152, 153
  cystadenocarcinoma 164, 263, 319
  cystadenoma 156, 164
  cysts 152, 153, 163
    calcified 156
    congenital 152, 153
    hemorrhagic 156
    macrocysts 148, 153
    microcysts 148, 153, 154
    neoplastic 153

retention 152, 153, 163
   stomach impression 234
diffuse change 144–151
divisum 151, 159, 166
duct system 154
endocrine 143
exocrine 143
fat necrosis 147
fibrolipomatosis 148, 150
fibromatosis 148
fibrosis 146, 148, 149, 151
focal changes 152–157
function 143
head 160
   cancer 167
   enlarged 32, 159
hemangioma 162
hemochromatosis 149
hydatid cysts 152
hyperechoic lesions 148–151, 160–162
hypoechoic lesions 147, 154–157
inflammatory lymph nodes 156
irregular lesions 163–164
isoechoic lesions 158–160
juvenile 147
large 144–145
lipoma 162
lipomatosis 148
lymphatics 144
lymphoma 16, 156, 158
macrocysts 148, 153
malignancy 145
mass 216
metastases 144, 155, 156
microcysts 148, 153, 154
microstructure 143
necrosis 153–154, 154
neoplastic cysts 153
pseudocysts 111, 153, 156, 163, 263
   malignant 164
   renal/adrenal cyst differential diagnosis 319
retention cysts 152, 153, 163
siderosis 148
small 145–146
topography 143–144
tumors
   benign 156
   cystic 164
   invasion 145
   mesenchymal 156
   neuroendocrine 155, 156
vena cava compression 32
vessels 154
pancreatectomy 146
pancreatic duct
   calculi 168
   cancer 155–156, 164
   cysts 154
   differential diagnosis of changes 165
   dilatation 148, 164–169
      causes 165
      marginal/mild 166
      marked 167–169
      prestenotic 169
   gas 162
   intraductal calculus 161
   mass 168

mucinous carcinoma 164
obstruction 112, 154
stent 162
pancreaticoduodenal artery stenosis 11
pancreatitis 267
   acute 46, 47, 144–145, 147
      calcium soap 162
      ductal dilatation 166
      focal 158
      pseudocysts 163
      splenic infarction 187
   alcohol-associated 145, 148
   autoimmune 146, 168
   biliary obstruction 111
   chronic 145, 146, 149–151, 167
      autoimmune 168
      calcifying 149, 150, 151, 161
      calculi 151
      classification 149, 150
      differential diagnosis 149, 150
      ductal dilatation 167–168
      ductal obstruction 154
      early 148
      fibrosis 151
      focal 158, 163
      irregular lesions 163
      microcalcification 162
      obstructive 151
      recurrent 148
      retention cyst 163
   classification 147, 149, 150
   edema 144, 145
   fibrin strands 267
   focal 157, 158
   groove 157
   hemorrhagic 258
   microcalcification 162
   mild 147
   necrosis 146, 151, 153–154, 265
   necrotizing 144, 258, 263, 267
   parenchymal changes 149
   recurrent 258
      ductal dilatation 166
   severe 147, 235
paracentesis, fine-needle 255, 256, 258, 259
paraovarian cyst 405
paraprotein kidney 286
parasites 113
parathyroid glands 418
parietal lymph nodes 207
peliosis, hepatic 79, 80
periampullary carcinoma 108
pericardial effusion 37
peripancreatic fat 144, 145
peripheral arteries, stenosis 13–14
peripheral lymph nodes 204
peripheral veins, duplication 26
peristalsis 228, 246
peritoneal cavity
   anatomy 251
   anechoic structure 256–258, 263–264
   collections 254
   diffuse changes 254–256
   extraperitoneal location 252, 253–254
   exudate 255
   fluid collections 252, 253, 255
   gas collections 252, 253
   hemorrhage 255

hyperechoic structure 261–263
hypoechoic structure 258–261, 264–265
intragastric processes 269–271
intraintestinal processes 270–271
intraperitoneal location 252, 253–254
irregular margin 267–269
localized perforation 265
morphology 252–254
retroperitoneal space 252, 253–254
smooth margin 266–267
topography 251–252
transudate 255
wall structures 266–269
see also carcinomatosis, peritoneal
peritoneum
   hematoma 265
   hyperechoic structure 265–266
   metastases 267–268
   reflections 251
   tumor masses 269
see also carcinomatosis, peritoneal
peritonitis 257
   bacterial 257, 258, 267
   purulent 258, 260
   viral 257
pheochromocytoma 325, 327
phleboliths 30
Phrygian cap 119, 121
   inflammation 128, 129
piano key phenomenon 245, 246, 270–271
placental polyps 398
plasmacytoma
   chest wall cutaneous metastases 454
   rib destruction 453
pleura
   anatomy 449
   calcifications 458–459
   carcinomatosis 459–460
   fibrosis 460–461
   location 449
   metastases 458
   morphology 449–450
   nodular masses 456–459
      differential diagnosis 456
   parietal 456–462
   plaque 458–459
   scar stage 460
   thickening 459–462
   thickness 449
   topography 449
pleural cavity, mass lesions 462
pleural effusion 458, 460, 462–463
   anechoic 463–464
   atelectasis 475
   basal inflammatory 465
   benign 464
   bronchial carcinoma 465
      metastases 466
   causes 463
   complex 466–467
   differential diagnosis 463
   echogenic 464–466
   exudative 464
   fibrothorax 467
   inflammatory 465, 467
   liquefaction 473
   loculated 472
   lymphoma 467

pleural effusion, malignant 465, 466, 467, 477
  ovarian cancer metastases 466
    parainfectious 458
    peripheral inflammatory 465
    pneumonia 486
    transudative 463–464
    volumetry 462
pleural empyema 486–487
  differential diagnosis 487
  pleural fibrosis 460, 461
pleurisy 484
pleuropneumonia 484
pneumobilia 96, 110, 112–113, 238
pneumoconiosis, pleural calcification 458
pneumonectomy, pyothorax 461
pneumonia 483
  air bronchogram 484
  cavitating 473
  interstitial 484, 485
  liquefying processes 486
  lobar 484, 485
  pleural effusion 486
  postinfarction 480
pneumonitis, obstructive 477
pneumoperitoneum 254, 261–262
pneumothorax 467
polycystic kidney disease 277–278, 284
polyglandular autoimmune syndrome 423
  acquired autoimmune thyroiditis 424, 425
  disseminated autonomy 444
polyneuropathy 122
popliteal artery embolism 15
popliteal vein
  duplication 26
  incompetence 28
  thrombosis 29
  venectasia 27
porphyria, hepatic 92
portal hypertension 35–43
  ascites 268
  cirrhosis 116
  collateral formation 35
  intrasplenic varicosity 42
  ligamentum teres hepatis 93
  posthepatic block 42–43
  spleen benign nonhomogeneity 176, 177
  splenomegaly 179
portal vein 33–34, 51, 54, 58, 116
  aplastic 38
  bifurcation 61
  cavernous transformation 44–45
  flow profile 37, 58, 61
  gas embolism 72
  gas pockets 95
  hepatic cirrhosis 73, 74
  hypoplasia 38
  lumen enlargement 35–43
  occlusion 44
  paraportal recanalization 44
  periportal cuffing 186
  reduced flow 36
  reflux 37
  thrombosis 43–46, 48, 87, 89, 94
    cholestasis 115
  topographic anatomy 33–34
portovenous system
  gas embolism 57, 96, 241
  tumor infiltration 48

positron emission tomography (PET) 99
posthepatic block 42–43
post-pancreatitic necrosis 146
Potter disease 278
pregnancy 397
  cervical 398
  ectopic 396, 398, 403
  multiple 405
  tubal 403
prostate
  abscess 372
  adenoma 356, 373
  anatomy 367
  anechoic 372–373
  calcifications 375
  cancer/carcinoma 368–369, 370–371, 374
    diagnosis 369
    lymph node metastases 205
    metastases 354, 355, 374
    screening 369
    staging 368
  cavity 372
  changes 367
  circumscribed lesions 372–375
  disease 367
  echogenic 372, 375
  enlarged 368–371
  hypoechoic 373–374
  operated 371–372
  radiation therapy 372
  small 371–372
  stones 375
  surgical capsule 373, 375
  topography 367
  transurethral resection 371–372, 373
prostatectomy, transabdominal total 371–372
prostatic hyperplasia, benign (BPH) 356, 368, 370, 372, 373
  prostatic carcinoma differential diagnosis 369
  urinary bladder wall hypertrophy 360
prostatitis
  acute 369–370
  chronic 371, 372
proteinuria 291
proton pump inhibitors 232
pseudoaneurysms 8, 10, 22
  femoral artery 10
  groin lymph nodes 212
  spleen 187, 188
pseudoascites 262–263
pseudomembranous enterocolitis 244
pseudomyxoma peritonei 409
pulmonary artery 485
  occlusion 478
pulmonary cyst 457, 472, 473
see also lung
pulmonary embolism 477–481
  entry echo 478–479
  hypoechoic transformation 480–481
  structural transformation 479–480
  wedge-shaped lesions 479
pulmonary fibrosis, pleural fibrosis 460, 461
pulmonary infarction 477–481, 479
  pneumonia 480
pulmonary nodule, peripheral 473
pulmonary vein 485
pulsatility index 14

lung mass evaluation 471
pulsatility index (PI) 287
pyelectasis 281, 300, 336–338
  causes 336
pyelitis, suppurative 343
pyelonephritis
  acute 285–286
  chronic 288, 292, 293
  emphysematous 312
  renal abscess 302
  scars 311
  suppurative 296
  xanthomatous 307
pyloric stenosis, hypertrophic 231
pyometra 397
pyonephrosis 286, 296, 307, 343–344
  purulent sediment 353
pyosalpinx 402
pyothorax
  pleural effusion differential diagnosis 464
  pleural fibrosis 461

R

radiotherapy
  asplenia 181
  prostate 372
  testicular atrophy 381
  thyroid gland 426–427, 429
rectal cancer metastases 211
renal agenesis 276–277
see also kidneys
renal allografts 287
renal arcuate ligament syndrome 11
renal arteries 6, 7, 275
  aneurysms 300
  arteriosclerosis/arteriolosclerosis 288
  arteriovenous malformations 282
  duplicated 6, 7
  embolism 287
  stenosis 11, 12, 13, 287
renal cell carcinoma 286, 303–304, 306, 308
  adrenal incidentaloma differential diagnosis 323
  cystic 298–299, 308
  hyperechoic 309
  metastases 304, 324
  operated 425
  ureteral clots 345
renal cysts 296–297, 319
  hemorrhagic 302, 309
  parapelvic 305
renal dysplasia, hypoplastic 277
renal failure 284
  acute 289
  diabetic nephropathy 291
  pleural calcification 458
renal infarcts, fresh 302
renal insufficiency 196
renal pelvic carcinoma 306
renal shock, hypoxemic 290
renal stone colic 342–343
renal tubules, scarring 297
renal veins 275
  congestion 300
    heart failure 290
  duplication 26

ectasia 300
 thrombosis 285, 287, 290
resistance index (RI) 287
 lung mass evaluation 471
reticuloendothelial system 51
retroperitoneal fibrosis 24, 340
 vena cava compression 32
retroperitoneal lymph nodes 200–201
retroperitoneal space 252, 253–254
ribs
 bone destruction 453
 fibrous dysplasia 453
 fractures 451–452
 metastases 452–453
 morphology 449–450
 Pancoast tumor 455
Riedel goiter 422
Riedel lobe of liver 53, 54
Rokitansky–Küstner syndrome 394

S

sactosalpinx 402
salpingitis, purulent 240
saphenofemoral junction incompetence 28
saphenopopliteal junction incompetence 27, 28
saphenous vein
 arteriovenous fistula 22
 insufficiency 27, 28
 phleboliths 30
 thrombosis 30
sarcoidosis 177
scar tissue, stellate 84, 85
scintigraphy, focal liver lesion differential diagnosis 99
scrotum
 hernia 386
 mass 385–386
scybala 227
sea anemone phenomenon 253, 254, 268, 269
seminal vesicles
 abscess 377
 anechoic 377
 calcifications 378
 changes 367
 circumscribed change 377–378
 cysts 377
 diffuse change 376
 dilatation 377
 echogenic 378
 hypoechoic 376
 prostate carcinoma infiltration 374
 stones 378
 tumor infiltration 376, 378
 vesiculitis 376, 378
sepsis, asplenia 181
seroma 300
serometra 397
seropneumothorax 467
Sertoli stromal cell tumors 411
sickle-cell anemia
 asplenia 180, 181
 splenic calcification 195
 splenic infarction 186
siderosis, pancreatic 148
sigmoid carcinoma 247–248

signet-ring carcinoma 230
sinus lipomatosis 305
small intestine 225, 235–248
 amyloidosis 243
 atrophy 248
 bezoars 238
 carcinoma 236
 diverticula 238
 foreign body 247
 gallstones 238
 hematoma 237
 hypertrophy of wall 244
 inflammation 245
 intussusception 237
 ischemia 243–244, 248
 loops 227
 lumen
  dilated 245–247
  narrowed 247–248
 lymphoma 236, 244
 obstruction 270–271
 peristalsis 228
 physiological dilatation 245
 polyps 237
 tumors 244, 247
 wall
  extended changes 241–244
  focal changes 236–240
  layers 226
spermatocele 383–384
spherocytosis, spleen 178
spiral valve of Heister 119, 120
splanchnic arteries, stenosis 11–13
splanchnic lymph nodes 207
spleen
 abscess 183, 188–190
  treatment 189
 accessory 216
  adrenal mass differential diagnosis 323
 aged 180
 anatomy 173
 anechoic mass 182–184
 arteriovenous fistula 187, 188
 benign nonhomogeneity 176–177
 calcification 195–196
 candidiasis 189, 190
 chronic lymphocytic leukemia 194
 congenital cleft 173
 cysts 182–184
  dysontogenic 182, 183
  hydatid 184
  infective 183–184
 dearterialization 186
 diffuse calcification 195
 focal calcification 195
 focal changes 182–196
 hamartoma 194
 hemangioma 193–194
 hematological malignancy 190
 Hodgkin disease 185, 186
 hyperechoic mass 193–194
 hypoechoic mass 184–192
 infarction 183, 186–188
  complications 187, 188
  healing 187
 infections 178
 intrasplenic varicosity 42
 lymphoma 176, 183, 194

 invasive 184–186
 macroabscess 188–189
 malignant invasion 176
 metastases 176, 190, 192, 215
  calcification 195
 microabscess 189–190
 myeloproliferative disorders 194
 nonfocal changes 176–181
 non-Hodgkin lymphoma 186
 parenchyma diffuse changes 176–177
 parenchymal vessels 175
 pseudoaneurysm 187, 188
 pseudocysts 183
 segmental arteries 175
 shape 173
 size 173
 small 180–182
 spherocytosis 178
 subcapsular hematoma 191, 192
 subsegmental arteries 175
 topography 173–175
 trauma 190, 191
 tumor
  benign 193–194
  solid 176
 vascular appearance 174, 175
 vascular calcification 196
 see also splenomegaly
splenic artery 6, 154, 174, 175
 calcified 161
 ectasia 319
 obstruction 176
 tortuous 319
splenic hilum
 collaterals 45
 varicosities 39, 41
splenic vein 34, 174, 175
 ectasia 319
 flow 37
 pancreatic cancer spread 169
 recanalization 46
 thrombosis 46, 179
 tortuous 319
 trunk 174
splenomegaly 36, 82, 177–180
 causes 177, 178
 hematological malignancy 177, 179–180
 hepatic cirrhosis 256
 lymphatic infiltration 80
splenorenal ligament 174
splenorenal shunt 39, 41
spontaneous bacterial peritonitis (SBP) 257, 258
sprue 227, 242
starvation gut 247, 248
steatohepatitis, non-alcoholic 65
steatosis hepatis see liver, fatty
Stein–Leventhal syndrome 405
stents 19
 bile duct 112–113
 carotid artery 16
 dilated bile duct 117
 draining varicosities 39
 endovascular 21
 hepatoduodenal 112, 113
 iatrogenic foreign body 95
 pancreatic duct 162
sternum
 fractures 451–452
 metastases 452–453

steroid cell tumors 411
stimulated acoustic emission (SAE) 89
stomach 225, 229–235
  adenocarcinoma 230
  cancer/carcinoma 230
    hepatic hilar lymph nodes 38
    hepatic vein infiltration 60
    lymph node invasion 205, 217
    malignant ascites 257
    peritoneal carcinomatosis 259, 267
    scirrhus 232, 234, 235
    splenic metastases 192
  compression 235
  congestion 233
  diverticulum 231
  edema 233
  emptying 234
  functional disorders 234
  gastritis 232
  gut signature 227
  impression 234
  inflammation 233
  lumen
    dilated 233–234
    narrowed 234–235
    postoperative status 235
  lymphoma 230, 232
  metastases 230
  morphology 226
  outlet obstruction 234, 270
  peristalsis 228
  peritoneal carcinomatosis 233
  physiological dilatation 233
  stromal tumor 229
  ulceration 231
  varices 231
  wall changes
    extended 232–233
    focal 229–231
    pancreatic cancer 41
  see also gastric entries
supraclavicular lymph nodes 209
syphilis, epididymitis 384

T

tampons 391
target sign 237
temporal arteritis 19
testes
  abscess 382
  anatomy 379
  atrophy 381
  changes 367
  circumscribed lesions 381–383
  cysts 381
  decreased size 381
  hematoma 382
  infarction 382
  microlithiasis 383
  orchitis 380
  topography 379
  torsion 380
  tumors 382–383
theca-lutein cyst 405
thecomatosis 407
thoracic ultrasound
  limitations 471
  pulmonary embolism 478
Thorotrast exposure
  liver 97
  spleen 176, 177
thorotrastosis 97
thrombi
  calcified 30
  red 21
  white 17, 18, 20, 21
thrombocytopenia, heparin-induced 263
thromboembolism, splenic infarction 186
thrombophilia, splenic infarction 186
thrombosis see venous thrombosis
thrombus, white 20–21
thymus carcinoid, lymph node calcification 204
thyroid arteries 418, 419
thyroid gland
  abscess 431, 435
  adenoma 431–432
    macrofollicular 440
    microfollicular 436
    normofollicular 438
    oncocytic 432–433
    parathyroid 434
    regressive change 439
  amyloidosis 423
  anatomy 417–418
  anechoic 429–431
  calcifications 441
  carcinoma 436–437, 442–443
    lymph node calcification 204
    strumectomy 425
  circumscribed changes 429–443
  colloid cysts 430, 439, 440
  cysts 429–431, 439, 440
  diffuse changes 419–429
  enlarged 419–423
  follicular carcinoma 436, 442
  function 417
  hemangioma 440
  hemorrhagic cysts 430, 439, 440
  hyperechoic structure 429, 439–441
  hypoechoic structure 427–428, 431–438
  irregular lesions 441–443
  isoechoic 438–439
  lipoma 434
  location 418
  lymph cysts 430
  lymphoma 435
  malignant melanoma metastases 438
  medullary C-cell carcinoma 436, 437
  metastases 437–438
  microanatomy 417
  microcalcifications 441
  multiple cysts 430
  myolipoma 440
  neonatal hypothyroidism 425
  nodules 436, 437
    adenomatous 431–432, 439
    autonomous 421
    cold 436
    isoechoic 439
    macrofollicular 440
    regressive changes 440
  papillary carcinoma 436, 443
  postoperative aplasia 425–426
  radioiodine-treated 426
  radiotherapy 426–427, 429
  regressive changes 440
  shape 417
  size 417
  small 423–427
  solitary cysts 429–430
  topography 418
  tumors 431–438, 442–443
  unilateral aplasia 425–426
  vessels 418, 431
  volume 417–418
  see also goiter; hyperthyroidism; hypothyroidism
thyroiditis
  amiodarone-induced 424, 428
  atrophic lymphocytic 423–424
  autoimmune 421
    acquired 423–425
    autonomous adenomas 445
    disseminated autonomy 444
  chronic 423
    with transient hyperthyroidism 427
  invasive sclerosing 422
  lithium-induced 424, 428
  postpartum 423, 427
  silent 427–428
  see also de Quervain thyroiditis; Hashimoto thyroiditis
thyroid-stimulating hormone (TSH) 417
thyroxine (T_4) 417
tibial veins, posterior 29
tracheobronchial carcinoma, thyroid gland metastases 437
transurethral resection of prostate 371–372, 373
transvaginal ultrasound 389
trauma
  adrenal hematoma 319
  blunt abdominal 258
  pleural calcification 458
  spleen 190, 191
  urinary tract hemorrhage 342
triiodothyronine (T_3) 417
Tripus Halleri 6
tuberculosis
  abscess 454
  ascites 260
  epididymitis 384
  lymphadenitis 217
  pleural calcifications 458–459
  pleural fibrosis 460
  prostate cavity 372
  prostatitis 370
  pulmonary 486
  renal 299, 313
    calcifications 312
    scars 311
  salpingitis 400
  splenic calcification 195
  urinary 350
tumbler phenomenon 227, 242
tympanites 138

U

ulcerative colitis 105, 243
  asplenia 181

umbilical vein
  posthepatic block 43
  recanalized 39, 40
ureteral bud 332
ureteral jet 357
ureterocele 279, 333, 341, 357, 362
ureteropelvic junction 332
  obstruction 336, 341
  tortuosity 341
ureters
  bifid 334
  clots 345
  course 332, 333
  diameter 331
  dilated 336–344
  diverticula 335
  duplex 333, 334
  ectopic 373
  hypoechoic mass 344–345
  length 331
  mass 344–348
  metastases 341
  obstruction 279, 334
  orifices 332
  stones 339, 341, 342, 347–348
  strictures 341
  subpelvic stenosis 338
  tumors 341
urethra, foreign bodies 358
urinary bladder
  artifacts 357
  blood clots 352–353, 356, 361
  calculi 358
  carcinoma 355, 361
    polypoid 354–355, 356
  diverticulum 351, 362
  empty 350
  foreign bodies 358
  ileal substitute 352
  indented 352
  mesenchymal tumors 355
  neurogenic 349
  overflow 349
  papilloma 353–354, 356
  partially contracted 351
  polypoid tumors 356
    carcinoma 354–355, 356
  pseudodiverticulum 351, 362
  purulent sediment 353
  reconstructed 352
  residual urine 350
  shape 331
    changes 347–352
  shrunken 350
  side-lobe artifact 357
  size 331
    changes 347–352
  sludge 353, 361
  small 349–350
  tamponade 352353
  topography 332–333
  tumors 341, 353–355
    flat 359–360
    polypoid 354–355, 356
    wall hypertrophy 360
  ureteral jet 357
  volume 331
    estimation 347, 348

wall
  changes 359–362
  concavities/convexities 362
  edema 361
  hypertrophy 359, 360
  indentations 357
  thickening 359–361
  see also urothelial carcinoma
urinary catheters 355
urinary retention 347–348
  acute 285
urinary stasis, chronic 339–340, 341
urinary stone colic 338–339
urinary tract
  anatomy 331–332
  anechoic 336–342
  dilatations 334–336
  duplication anomalies 333–334
  hemorrhage 342
  hyperechoic 345–348
  hypoechoic 342–344
  infected obstruction 342–343
  intracavitary mass 352–358
    echogenic 358
    hyperechoic 355–357
    hypoechoic 352–355
  malformations 333–336
  reflux 341–342
  stenoses 334–336
  topography 332–333
  tuberculosis 350
urinoma 300, 347
urolithiasis 346
urothelial carcinoma 286, 304–306, 338, 344–345, 355
  bladder wall changes 361
uterus
  adenomyomatosis 395–396
  anatomy 392
  angiomyoma 394
  aplasia 394
  atresia 394
  bicornuate 393
  blood in 390
  blood supply 392
  carcinosarcoma 396
  cervix 392
    carcinoma 401
    endometrial inflammation 400
    polyps 398
  chorioepithelioma 401
  corpus carcinoma 400–401
  diffuse myomatosis 395
  endometrial polyps 398
  foreign bodies 396–397
  hemangioma 394
  histology 392
  hypoplasia 394
  induration 395
  intracavitary changes 396–398
  lymphoma 394
  malacia 394
  malformations 393
  morphology 392–393
  mucocele 397
  myoma 394–395, 396
  prolapse 393
  pyometra 397

  sarcoma 396
  serometra 397
  size/shape abnormalities 393–394
  small 394
  tumors 394
  see also endometrium; myometrium
utricular cyst 373

V

vagina
  aplasia 394
  carcinoma 391
  double 391
  masses 390–391
  morphology 390
  postoperative changes 391–392
  septate 391
  size/shape abnormalities 391–392
  wall cyst 390
Valsalva maneuver 28
varicocele 385
vas deferens 379
vasculitis, autoimmune 205
veins
  compression 31–32
  dilatation 26–28
  filling 28
  incompressibility 29
  infiltration 31–32
  intraluminal mass 28–30, 43–48
  phleboliths 30
  tumor infiltration 48
  valves 31
venectasia 27–28
venous malformations, intramural 110
venous star 54, 58, 63
venous thrombosis 27, 28–30, 43–47
  criteria 28
  superficial 30
  see also named veins
vesicorenal reflux 279, 341–342
vesicoureteral reflux 341–342
vesiculitis 376
  chronic 378
VIPoma 155, 156
Virchow sentinel node 201
Virchow triad 27

W

Waldenström disease 294
Weigert–Meyer rule 333
Wilms tumor 303

Y

yersiniosis 241
yolk sac tumor 412

Z

Zuckerlandl organ 325